EMERGENCY MEDICINE

EMERGENCY MEDICINE

SECRETS

Fourth Edition

Vincent J. Markovchick, MD
Director, Emergency Medicine Services
Assistant Program Director, Emergency
   Medical Residency
Denver Health Medical Center
Professor of Surgery
Division of Emergency Medicine
Department of Surgery
University of Colorado Health Sciences
   Center
Denver, Colorado

Peter T. Pons, MD, FACEP
Attending Emergency Physician
Denver Health Medical Center
Professor of Surgery
Division of Emergency Medicine
Department of Surgery
University of Colorado Health Sciences
   Center
Denver, Colorado

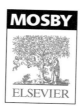

MOSBY

ELSEVIER

1600 John F. Kennedy Boulevard
Suite 1800
Philadelphia, PA 19103-2899

Emergency Medicine Secrets
Fourth Edition

ISBN-13: 978-0-323-03587-3
ISBN-10: 0-323-03587-6

NOTICE

Knowledge and best practice in this field are constantly changing. As new research and experience broaden our knowledge, changes in practice, treatment and drug therapy may become necessary or appropriate. Readers are advised to check the most current information provided (i) on procedures featured or (ii) by the manufacturer of each product to be administered, to verify the recommended dose or formula, the method and duration of administration, and contraindications. It is the responsibility of the practitioner, relying on his or her own experience and knowledge of the patient, to make diagnoses, to determine dosages and the best treatment for each individual patient, and to take all appropriate safety precautions. To the fullest extent of the law, neither the Publisher nor the Editor assumes any liability for any injury and/or damage to persons or property arising out or related to any use of the material contained in this book.

Library of Congress Cataloging-in-Publication Data

Emergency Medicine Secrets / [edited by] Vincent J. Markovchick, Peter T. Pons.–4th ed.
        p. ; cm.
    Includes bibliographical references and index.
    ISBN 0-323-03587-6
      1. Emergency medicine–Examinations, questions, etc.   I. Markovchick, Vincent J.
    II. Pons, Peter T.
      [DNLM: 1. Emergencies–Examination questions.   2. Emergency Medicine–
    Examination Questions.   WB 18.2 E53 2006]
    RC86.9.M37 2006
    616.02'5076–dc22

                                                                    2006044878

Vice President, Medical Education: Linda Belfus
Developmental Editor: Stan Ward
Project Manager: Mary Stermel
Marketing Manager: Kate Rubin

Printed in China.

Last digit is the print number: 9   8   7   6   5   4   3   2   1

Working together to grow
libraries in developing countries

www.elsevier.com | www.bookaid.org | www.sabre.org

ELSEVIER   BOOK AID International   Sabre Foundation

DEDICATION

To my wife, Leslie, and daughters, Nicole, Tasha, and Nadia—the four greatest ladies in my world. I wish to thank them for their lifelong support of all my endeavors and, in particular, for understanding the time that the editing of this manuscript has taken away from my time with them. I would also like to acknowledge all the medical students and residents with whom I have had the pleasure of working at the Denver Health Emergency Department over the past 29 years. Their enthusiasm and intellectual curiosity have stimulated many of the questions in this book.

VJM

To my wife, Kathy, whose love, support, and remarkable patience make every day worthwhile.

PTP

The editors also express their heartfelt thanks to Carol Lucas for her organizational skills, tenacity, good humor, hard work, and incredible dedication to the preparation of the fourth edition. We could not have accomplished this without her help.

CONTENTS

XIV. TOXICOLOGIC EMERGENCIES

XVII. BEHAVIORAL EMERGENCIES

XVIII. EMERGENCY MEDICINE ADMINISTRATION AND RISK MANAGEMENT

XIX. MEDICAL OVERSIGHT AND DISASTER MANAGEMENT

CONTRIBUTORS

Norberto Adame, Jr., MD, FACEP
Associate Chair, Department of Emergency Medicine, Maricopa Medical Center, Phoenix, Arizona

Stephen L. Adams, MD, FACP, FACEP
Professor of Medicine; Chief, Division of Sports Medicine; Chief Emeritus, Division of Emergency Medicine, Northwestern University Feinberg School of Medicine; Medical Director, Emergency Preparedness and Disaster Services, Northwestern Memorial Hospital, Chicago, Illinois

Ayad Al-Dharrab, MD
Division of Emergency Medicine, McMaster University, Hamilton, Ontario, Canada

Brandon H. Anderson, MD
Department of Community Health Services—Pediatrics, University of Colorado Health Sciences Center; Kids' Care Clinic, Denver Health Medical Center, Denver, Colorado

Mark E. Anderson, MD
Department of Community Health Services—Pediatrics, University of Colorado Health Sciences Center; Kids' Care Clinic, Denver, Colorado

Katherine M. Bakes, MD
Department of Emergency Medicine, Denver Health Medical Center and The Children's Hospital, Denver, Colorado

Stacey Bangh, PharmD
Clinical Instructor, College of Pharmacy, University of Minnesota; Clinical Coordinator, Hennepin Regional Poison Center, Minneapolis, Minnesota

Roger M. Barkin, MD, MPH, FAAPm, FACEP
Professor of Surgery, Division of Emergency Medicine, Department of Surgery, University of Colorado Health Sciences Center; Vice President for Pediatric and Newborn Programs, HealthONE, Denver, Colorado

Thomas B. Barry, MD
Assistant Professor of Emergency Medicine, Temple University School of Medicine, Philadelphia, Pennsylvania

Vikhyat S. Bebarta, MD
Academic Faculty, San Antonio Uniformed Services Health Education Consortium; Director of Medical Toxicology, Department of Emergency Medicine, Wilford Hall Medical Center, San Antonio, Texas

Sean P. Bender, MD
Department of Emergency Medicine, Denver Health Medical Center, Denver, Colorado

Walter L. Biffl, MD
Chief, Division of Trauma and Surgical Critical Care, Rhode Island Hospital; Associate Professor of Surgery, Brown Medical School, Providence, Rhode Island

Diane M. Birnbaumer, MD, FACEP
Professor of Medicine, David Geffen School of Medicine at the University of California, Los Angeles; Associate Program Director, Department of Emergency Medicine, Harbor-UCLA Medical Center, Los Angeles, California

Carl J. Bonnett, MD
Department of Emergency Medicine, Denver Health Medical Center, Denver, Colorado

Joan Bothner, MD
Chief, Section of Emergency Medicine; Associate Professor, Department of Pediatrics, University of Colorado School of Medicine; Emergency Services, The Children's Hospital, Denver, Colorado

Patricia A. Braun, MD
Associate Professor, Department of Pediatrics, University of Colorado Health Sciences Center; Denver Health Medical Center, Denver, Colorado

Russ Braun, MD, MPH, MBA, FACEP
Associate Clinical Professor, University of California at San Francisco School of Medicine, San Francisco, California; Vice President of Medical Affairs, Mercy San Juan Medical Center; Mercy Hospital Folsom, Carmichael, California

Gayle Braunholtz, MD
Department of Emergency Medicine, Denver Health Medical Center, Denver, Colorado

Kerry Broderick, MD
Department of Emergency Medicine, Denver Health Medical Center, Denver, Colorado

James E. Brown, MD
Department of Emergency Medicine, Cox Heart Institute, Kettering, Ohio

Michael W. Brunko, MD
Emergency Medical Services, St. Anthony Hospital, Denver, Colorado

Jennie A. Buchanan, MD
Resident in Emergency Medicine, Denver Health Medical Center, Denver, Colorado

Joanna M. Burch, MD
Assistant Professor of Dermatology and Pediatrics, University of Colorado Health Sciences Center, Aurora, Colorado

Charles B. Cairns, MD
Division of Emergency Medicine, Duke University Medical Center, Durham, North Carolina

Stephen V. Cantrill, MD
Associate Director, Department of Emergency Medicine, Denver Health Medical Center; Associate Professor, Division of Emergency Medicine, University of Colorado Health Sciences Center, Denver, Colorado

Justin C. Chang, MD
Department of Emergency Medicine, Exempla St. Joseph's Hospital, Denver, Colorado

Dane M. Chapman, MD, PhD
Clinical Professor, University of Colorado School of Medicine, Denver, Colorado

Christopher B. Colwell, MD, FACEP
Division of Emergency Medicine, Department of Surgery, University of Colorado Health Sciences Center; Denver Health Medical Center, Denver, Colorado

Elizabeth A. Criss, RN, MEd, CEN
Senior Research Associate, Department of Emergency Medicine, University of Arizona College of Medicine; Clinical Educator, Emergency Services, University Medical Center, Tucson, Arizona

Patrick G. Croskerry, MD, PhD
Department of Emergency Medicine, Dalhousie University Faculty of Medicine, Halifax, Nova Scotia; Dartmouth General Hospital, Dartmouth, Nova Scotia

Catherine B. Custalow, MD, PhD
Assistant Professor, Department of Emergency Medicine, University of Virginia Health System, Charlottesville, Virginia

Rita K. Cydulka, MD, MS
Department of Emergency Medicine, Metro Health Medical Center, Cleveland, Ohio

Daniel F. Danzl, MD
Professor and Chair, Department of Emergency Medicine, University of Louisville School of Medicine, Louisville, Kentucky

Kevin Dean, MD
Department of Emergency Medicine, University of California at Irvine, Orange, California

Wyatt W. Decker, MD
Chairman, Department of Emergency Medicine, Mayo Medical School; Mayo Clinic, Rochester, Minnesota

Jeffrey Druck, MD
Department of Emergency Medicine, Denver Health Medical Center, Denver, Colorado

James S. Eadie, MD
Academic Faculty, San Antonio Uniformed Services Health Education Consortium; Department of Emergency Medicine, Wilford Hall Medical Center, San Antonio, Texas

Bruce Evans, MD
Senior Instructor, Department of Surgery, University of Colorado Health Sciences Center; Attending Physician, Department of Emergency Medicine, University of Colorado Hospital, Denver, Colorado

Michael P. Earnest, MD
Department of Neurology, Denver Health Medical Center, Denver, Colorado

Neide Fehrenbacher, MD
Exempla Lutheran Medical Center, Wheat Ridge, Colorado; Exempla Good Samaritan, Lafayette, Colorado

Kim M. Feldhaus, MD, FACEP
Emergency Physician, Boulder Community Hospital, Boulder, Colorado

Christopher M.B. Fernandes, MD
Professor and Head of Emergency Medicine, McMaster University; Hamilton Health Sciences, Hamilton, Ontario, Canada

Sarrah Goodwin, MD
Resident in Emergency Medicine, Brown Medical School, Providence, Rhode Island

David A. Guttman, MD
Chief Resident, Department of Emergency Medicine, University of Arizona College of Medicine, Tucson, Arizona

Kent N. Hall, MD
Emergency Department Medical Director, Goodall Hospital, Sanford, Maine

Christina E. Hantsch, MD
Associate Professor, Department of Surgery, Loyola University Chicago, Chicago, Illinois; Medical Director, Illinois Poison Center, Maywood, Illinois

Luis H. Haro, MD
Department of Emergency Medicine, Mayo Medical School; Senior Associate Consultant, Department of Emergency Medicine, Mayo Clinic, Rochester, Minnesota

Corey D. Harrison, MD
Academic Faculty, San Antonio Uniformed Services Health Education Consortium; Director of Prehospital Care, Department of Emergency Medicine, Wilford Hall Medical Center, San Antonio, Texas

Jason S. Haukoos, MD, MS
Assistant Professor, Department of Emergency Medicine, Denver Health Medical Center; Assistant Professor, Department of Preventive Medicine and Biometrics, University of Colorado Health Sciences Center, Denver, Colorado

Edward P. Havranek, MD
Staff Cardiologist, Denver Health Medical Center; Professor of Medicine, University of Colorado, Denver, Colorado

Kennon Heard, MD
Division of Emergency Medicine, Department of Surgery, University of Colorado Services Center, Denver, Colorado

Philip L. Henneman, MD
Professor and Chair, Department of Emergency Medicine, Tufts University School of Medicine; Baystate Health System, Springfield, Massachusetts

Robert Hockberger, MD
Chair, Department of Emergency Medicine, Harbor-UCLA Medical Center, Torrance, California; Professor of Clinical Medicine, David Geffen School of Medicine at UCLA, Los Angeles, California

Debra Houry, MD, MPH
Assistant Professor, Department of Emergency Medicine, Emory University; Associate Director, Center for Injury Control, Atlanta, Georgia

Richard L. Hughes, MD
Chief, Department of Neurology, Denver Health Medical Center, Denver, Colorado

Katherine M. Hurlbut, MD
Department of Surgery, University of Colorado Health Sciences Center; Denver Health Medical Center, Denver, Colorado

Kenneth C. Jackimczyk, MD
Attending Physician, Department of Emergency Medicine, Maricopa Medical Center, Phoenix, Arizona

Timothy Janz, MD
Department of Emergency Medicine, Cox Heart Institute, Kettering, Ohio

Richard O. Jones, MD
Interim Chief, Obstetrics Service, Denver Health Medical Center, Denver, Colorado

Robert C. Jorden, MD
Chairman, Department of Emergency Medicine, Maricopa Medical Center, Phoenix, Arizona

Nicholas J. Jouriles, MD
Department of Emergency Medicine, Akron General Medical Center; Professor of Emergency Medicine, Northeast Ohio Universities College of Medicine, Akron, Ohio

Juliana Karp, MD
Attending Physician, Department of Emergency Medicine, Lakeland Regional Medical Center, Lakeland, Florida

John L. Kendall, MD, FACEP
Division of Emergency Medicine, Department of Surgery, University of Colorado Health Sciences Center; Denver Health Medical Center, Denver, Colorado

Eugene E. Kercher, MD
Department of Internal Medicine, University of California at Los Angeles, Los Angeles, California; David Geffen School of Medicine, Westwood, California; Chair, Department of Emergency Medicine, Kern Medical Center, Bakersfield, California

Andrew M. Kestler, MD, MBA
Assistant Professor of Surgery, Division of Emergency Medicine, University of Colorado Health Sciences Center, Denver, Colorado

Morris S. Kharasch, MD, FACEP
Assistant Professor of Medicine, Northwestern University Feinberg School of Medicine; Attending Physician, Division of Emergency Medicine, Evanston Northwestern Healthcare, Evanston, Illinois

Samuel J. Killian, MD
Department of Emergency Medicine, Swedish Medical Center, Englewood, Colorado

Daniel S. Kim, MD
Fellow in Pediatric Surgery, Brown Medical School; Hasbro Children's Hospital, Providence, Rhode Island

Michael J. Klevens, MD
Instructor of Emergency Medicine, Washington University School of Medicine in St. Louis, St. Louis, Missouri

Andrew L. Knaut, MD, PhD
Division of Emergency Medicine, Department of Surgery, University of Colorado Health Sciences Center; Department of Emergency Medicine, Denver Health Medical Center, Denver, Colorado

Carolyn S. Knaut, JD
Denver, Colorado

Michael A. Kohn, MD, MPP
Department of Epidemiology and Biostatistics, University of California at San Francisco, San Francisco, California; Mills-Peninsula Medical Center, Burlingame, California

Kenneth Kulig, MD
Associate Clinical Professor, Division of Emergency Medicine, Department of Surgery, University of Colorado Health Sciences Center; Chair, Department of Medicine, Porter Adventist Hospital, Denver, Colorado

Ryan P. Lamb, MD
Department of Emergency Medicine, Kaiser-Permanente Medical Center, Santa Clara, California

Lela A. Lee, MD
Professor of Dermatology and Medicine, University of Colorado Health Sciences Center; Director of Dermatology, Denver Health Medical Center, Denver, Colorado

Louis J. Ling, MD
Professor of Emergency Medicine and Pharmacy; Associate Dean for Graduate Medical Education, University of Minnesota, Minneapolis, Minnesota

Catherine A. Marco, MD
Department of Surgery, Medical College of Ohio; St. Vincent Mercy Medical Center, Toledo, Ohio

Vincent J. Markovchick, MD
Director, Emergency Medical Services, Denver Health Medical Center, Denver, Colorado

John P. Marshall, MD, FACEP
Department of Emergency Medicine, Maimonides Medical Center, Brooklyn, New York; Assistant Clinical Professor, Mount Sinai School of Medicine, New York, New York

John A. Marx, MD
Chair, Department of Emergency Medicine, Carolinas Medical Center, Charlotte, North Carolina; Adjunct Professor of Emergency Medicine, University of North Carolina at Chapel Hill, Chapel Hill, North Carolina

Gregory R. McGee, DMD
Denver Health Medical Center, Denver, Colorado

Robert M. McNamara, MD
Professor and Chair, Department of Emergency Medicine, Temple University School of Medicine, Philadelphia, Pennsylvania

Rick A. McPheeters, DO
Residency Director, Department of Emergency Medicine, Kern Medical Center, Bakersfield, California

Harvey W. Meislin, MD, FACEP
Professor and Head, Department of Emergency Medicine, University of Arizona Health Sciences Center; Director, Arizona Emergency Medicine Research Center, Tucson, Arizona

Gregg Miller, MD
Senior Resident, Department of Emergency Medicine, Harbor-UCLA Medical Center, Torrance, California

James C. Mitchiner, MD, MPH
Attending Physician, Emergency Department, St. Joseph Mercy Hospital; Clinical Assistant Professor, Department of Emergency Medicine, University of Michigan Medical School, Ann Arbor, Michigan

Ernest E. Moore, MD
Chief, Department of Surgery, Denver Health Medical Center, Denver, Colorado

S. Jason Moore, PA, MS
Vail Valley Medical Center, Trauma Services, Vail, Colorado

Maria E. Moreira, MD
Department of Emergency Medicine, Denver Health Medical Center, Denver, Colorado

Steven J. Morgan, MD
Residency Program Director, Denver Health Medical Center, Denver, Colorado

Larry Nathanson, MD
Director of Emergency Medicine Informatics, Beth Israel Deaconess Medical Center, Boston, Massachusetts

Christopher R.H. Newton, MD
Department of Emergency Medicine, University of Michigan Medical Center, Ann Arbor, Michigan

Edward Newton, MD, FRCPC
Professor of Emergency Medicine, University of Southern California Keck School of Medicine; Los Angeles and University of Southern California Medical Center, Los Angeles, California

Richard A. Nockowitz, MD
Neuropsychiatry Consultants, Lima, Ohio

Anna Olson, MD
Emergency Medical Services, Denver Health Medical Center, Denver Colorado

Owen P. O'Meara, MD
Department of Pediatrics, Denver Health Medical Center, Denver, Colorado

Anand A. Parekh, MRCS (Eng)
Orthopaedic Research Fellow, Denver Health Medical Center, Denver, Colorado

Peter T. Pons, MD, FACEP
Attending Emergency Physician, Denver Health Medical Center; Professor, Division of Emergency Medicine, Department of Surgery, University of Colorado Health Sciences Center, Denver, Colorado

Thomas B. Purcell, MD
Vice Chairman, Department of Emergency Medicine, Kern Medical Center, Bakersfield, California

Danielle Raeburn, MD
Denver Health Medical Center, Denver, Colorado

David B. Richards, MD
Denver Health Medical Center, Denver, Colorado

Jedd Roe, MD, MBA
Director of Emergency Medicine Residency, University of Alabama, Birmingham, Alabama

Jody J. Rogers, MD
Rocky Mountain Poison and Drug Center, Denver Health Medical Center, Denver, Colorado

Carlo L. Rosen, MD
Assistant Professor of Medicine, Harvard Medical School; Program Director, Beth Israel Deaconess Medical Center, Boston, Massachusetts

Peter Rosen, MD
St. John's Hospital, Jackson, Wyoming

Scott Rudkin, MD, MBA
Department of Emergency Medicine, University of California at Irvine, Orange, California

Douglas A. Rund, MD, FACEP
Professor and Chair, Department of Emergency Medicine; Associate Dean, Ohio State University College of Medicine and Public Health; Ohio State University Medical Center, Columbus, Ohio

Jeffrey J. Schaider, MD
Chair, Department of Emergency Medicine, Cook County Hospital; Associate Professor of Emergency Medicine, Rush Medical College, Chicago, Illinois

Nicola E.E. Schiebel, MD
Assistant Professor, Department of Emergency Medicine, Mayo Clinic; Consultant, Mayo Medical Center, Rochester, Minnesota

W. Jared Scott, MD
Swedish Medical Center, Englewood, Colorado

Donna L. Seger, MD
Associate Professor, Department of Medicine, Vanderbilt University; Medical Director, Tennessee Poison Center; Vanderbilt University Medical Center, Nashville, Tennessee

Elaine Norman Scholes, MD
Clinical Professor, Department of Pediatrics, University of Colorado Health Sciences Center; Medical Director, Denver Health Medical Plan Clinic, Denver, Colorado

Lee W. Shockley, MD
Medical Director, Emergency Department, Denver Health Medical Center, Denver, Colorado

Kaushal Shah, MD
Director of Medical Student Education, St. Luke's-Roosevelt Hospital, New York, New York

Jon Siff, MD, MBA
Department of Emergency Medicine, Metro Health Medical Center, Cleveland, Ohio

Barry Simon, MD
Chairman, Department of Emergency Medicine, Alameda County Medical Center; Associate Professor of Medicine, University of California at San Francisco, San Francisco, California

Corey M. Slovis, MD, FACP, FACEP
Professor of Emergency Medicine and Medicine; Chairman, Department of Emergency Medicine, Vanderbilt University School of Medicine; Vanderbilt University Medical Center; Medical Director, Nashville Fire and Emergency Medical Services, Nashville, Tennessee

Rodney W. Smith, MD
Department of Emergency Medicine, St. Joseph Mercy Hospital, Ann Arbor, Michigan

Daniel W. Spaite, MD, FACEP
Professor, Department of Emergency Medicine, University of Arizona College of Medicine; Director, Emergency Services, University Medical Center, Tucson, Arizona

Michelle Tartaglia, MD
Department of Emergency Medicine, Denver Health Medical Center, Denver, Colorado

Harold Thomas, MD
Professor, Department of Emergency Medicine, Oregon Health Sciences University, Portland, Oregon

Alexander T. Trott, MD
Professor, Department of Emergency Medicine, University of Cincinnati College of Medicine; Associate Chief of Staff, University of Cincinnati Hospital, Cincinnati, Ohio

David J. Vukich, MD
Department of Emergency Medicine, University of Florida at Jacksonville, Jacksonville, Florida

Joseph Wathen, MD
Emergency Department, Children's Hospital, Denver, Colorado

Robert L. Wears, MD, MS
Professor, Department of Emergency Medicine, University of Florida College of Medicine, Jacksonville, Florida

Kurt Whitaker, MD
Chief Resident, Emergency Medical Services, Denver Health Medical Center, Denver, Colorado

Stephen J. Wolf, MD
Director, Residency in Emergency Medicine, Denver Health Medical Center, Denver, Colorado

Richard E. Wolfe, MD
Chief of Emergency Medicine, Beth Israel Deaconess Medical Center, Boston, Massachusetts

Allan B. Wolfson, MD
Professor of Emergency Medicine, University of Pittsburgh; Program Director, University of Pittsburgh Affiliated Residency in Emergency Medicine, Pittsburgh, Pennsylvania

William F. Young, Jr., MD
Assistant Clinical Professor of Emergency Medicine, University of Kentucky, Lexington, Kentucky

Richard D. Zallen, DDS, MD
Director of Dentistry and Oral Maxillofacial Surgery, Denver Health Medical Center, Denver, Colorado

PREFACE TO THE FOURTH EDITION

This book is designed to be read by all of the students and practitioners of emergency medicine, both novice and experienced. As emergency medicine continues to evolve as a specialty, we have added several new chapters to our fourth edition and enhanced the format and referencing of the questions. In addition, with difficulty, we have selected the 100 top secrets from over 220 submitted by chapter authors. We hope this continues to be a valuable and enjoyable method of providing information and knowledge. Knowing some of the important questions about a particular presentation or problem is the first step to obtaining the answers needed at the patient's bedside. It is with this concept in mind that we prepared this text.

Vincent J. Markovchick, MD
Peter T. Pons, MD, FACEP

TOP 100 SECRETS

These secrets are 100 of the top board alerts. They summarize the concepts, principles, and most salient details of emergency medicine.

1. When formulating the differential diagnosis, ask "What is the most serious possible cause of this patient's presenting signs and symptoms?"

2. When uncertain of the diagnosis, communicate this truthfully to the patient and document it in the emergency department (ED) final assessment.

3. Before discharging a patient from the ED, ask, "Why did the patient come, and have I made the patient feel better?"

4. The laryngeal mask airway is the preferred backup device if a patient cannot be successfully intubated.

5. Preoxygenation is a critical component of rapid-sequence intubation preparation because it will prevent significant hypoxia despite several minutes of apnea during the intubation process.

6. When evaluating the results of a research paper, the smaller the number of patients needed to treat, the better the intervention or treatment.

7. When in doubt, remember that a p value $< .05$ is significant.

8. Neither the height of the fever nor the response (or lack thereof) to antipyretics is indicative of the seriousness of the cause of the fever.

9. In febrile patients, measuring a white blood cell count or band count is rarely useful in differentiating bacterial versus viral illness.

10. In an elderly or diabetic person, nausea and vomiting may be the only symptoms of myocardial ischemia.

11. One cannot make the diagnosis of gastroenteritis without the presence of both vomiting and diarrhea.

12. Spinal epidural abscess should be suspected as the cause of back pain in immunocompromised patients and intravenous drug users who present with localized spinal tenderness and fever.

13. An afferent pupillary defect confirms damage in the retina or optic nerve.

14. A perilimbic flush suggests iritis or glaucoma, not conjunctivitis.

15. When a mandible fracture is suspected, a panoramic radiograph is the least expensive and most accurate film to order.

16. Evaluate the mandibular condyles for fractures in patients with blunt trauma to the chin.

17. In patients with a high suspicion for meningitis, administer antibiotics promptly before the lumbar puncture is performed and after blood cultures are obtained.

18. Remember antibiotic prophylaxis for contacts of patients with meningococcal or *Haemophilus influenzae* meningitis.

19. The initial objectives of treating an asthma exacerbation are to relieve significant hypoxemia (oxygen), to reverse airflow obstruction (beta agonists + ipratropium), to reduce the likelihood of recurrence (corticosteroids), and to provide objective measure of improvement (peak expiratory flow rate [PEFR] or forced expiratory volume in 1 second [FEV_1]).

20. The initial objectives of treating a chronic obstructive pulmonary disease (COPD) exacerbation are to relieve significant hypoxemia (oxygen), to reverse airflow obstruction (beta agonists + ipratropium), to reduce of the likelihood of recurrence (corticosteroids), and to treat the underlying cause.

21. Early noninvasive ventilation combined with aggressive medical therapy may prevent the need for orotracheal intubation in patients with acute pulmonary edema and COPD.

22. The most important tool in assessing patients in whom you suspect ischemic heart disease is the history. The second most important tool is the history. The third most important tool is, well, you get the picture.

23. In a patient with an acute inferior myocardial infarction and hypotension, think about right ventricular infarction; an electrocardiogram (ECG) with right-sided precordial leads showing elevation in rV5 or rV6 or an echocardiogram may help establish the diagnosis.

24. It is not necessary to definitively identify a dysrhythmia prior to treating it.

25. An external pacemaker can be used if a permanent pacemaker malfunctions.

26. The diagnosis of atrial fibrillation (AF) can be made clinically by palpating a peripheral pulse and simultaneously auscultating the heart or visualizing the cardiac rhythm because AF is the only dysrhythmia that results in a pulse deficit (fewer beats palpated than observed or auscultated).

27. Rapidly reduce blood pressure in patients with severely elevated blood pressure and evidence of coronary ischemia, congestive heart failure (CHF), aortic dissection, acute renal failure (ARF), or preeclampsia/eclampsia.

28. Do not lower the mean arterial pressure (MAP) more than 20–25% in patients with hypertensive encephalopathy.

29. It is not necessary to gradually empty the bladder when treating an episode of acute urinary retention.

30. The indications for emergency dialysis are acute pulmonary edema, life-threatening hyperkalemia, and life-threatening intoxication or overdose by agents normally excreted by the kidneys.

31. When a patient with end-stage renal disease presents with shortness of breath, volume overload is by far the most common cause, even when physical examination and chest x-ray are not diagnostic.

32. In a young woman presenting with rash, fever, and diarrhea, consider toxic shock syndrome and inquire about last menses and tampon use.

33. Doxycycline is the drug of choice for most severe tick-borne infections; it should be used empirically and early in the febrile, severely ill patient with a possibility of tick exposure.

34. A febrile patient returning from the tropics has malaria until proved otherwise.

35. Septic arthritis can be ruled out only by a normal joint fluid analysis, not by a normal erythrocytosis sedimentation rate (ESR) or an elevated C-reactive protein (CRP).

36. Patients with myocardial infarction may get symptomatic relief from antacids, and patients with esophageal disease may get symptomatic relief from nitroglycerin. Antacids and nitroglycerin are therapeutic medications, not diagnostic tests.

37. Disproportionate tachycardia or tachypnea suggests hypothermia secondary to other diseases or injuries.

38. Elevation of liver function tests is the most consistent laboratory abnormality seen in heat stroke victims.

39. Intussusception occurs between 3 months and 3 years of age.

40. An infant with bilateral retinal hemorrhages is a victim of child abuse (shaken baby syndrome) until proved otherwise.

41. Ketamine provides sedation, analgesia, and amnesia while protecting the cardiovascular status and airway reflexes, making it an ideal agent for procedural sedation in children.

42. Because of the fast helical computerized tomography scanners of today, many infants and children can undergo this diagnostic procedure without sedation.

43. Intentional abuse of hydrocarbons (i.e., huffing, bagging, or sniffing) may lead to dysrhythmias and death.

44. Dermal exposure or ingestion of hydrofluoric acid can result in profound hypocalcemia, hypomagnesemia, and hyperkalemia.

45. The most important action to take in the event of a weapons of mass destruction (WMD) attack is simply self-protection by donning appropriate personal protective equipment.

46. Sodium bicarbonate (1–2 mEq/kg) should be considered for all poisoning patients with ventricular dysrhythmias.

47. Perform airway management early in the evaluation of patients with significant soft tissue neck injuries.

48. Delayed neurologic deficits occur more commonly than acute neurologic changes in patients with blunt carotid injury.

49. Hypotensive, tachycardic patients with penetrating chest trauma should be immediately evaluated for tension pneumothorax and pericardial tamponade because emergent decompression can be life saving.

50. A suicide attempt should be considered when the cause of a serious accident does not make logical sense.

51. Analyzing a mass gathering will allow informed decisions about the needed levels of staffing and equipment necessary to provide on-site care.

52. A computed tomography (CT) scan for appendicitis "negative" only if the entire appendix has been visualized and is normal.

53. Abdominal aortic aneurysm (AAA) can mimic renal colic.

54. Helical CT is the diagnostic modality of choice to diagnose ureteral calculus.

55. Consider testicular torsion for any male with lower abdominal pain.

56. Early goal-directed therapy in patients with severe sepsis reduces short-term mortality by 10–20% compared with an unstructured traditional treatment regimen.

57. Culture and antibiotics are not indicated in nonimmunocompromised patients with a cutaneous abscess and normal host defenses.

58. Necrotizing fasciitis should be considered in any patient with a soft tissue infection who has pain and tenderness out of proportion to the visible degree of cellulitis.

59. If antibiotics are used in the outpatient treatment of abscesses, assume methicillin-resistant *Staphylococcus aureus* (MRSA) is the causative agent.

60. Amphetamine and cocaine toxicity should be treated with intravenous (IV) benzodiazepine in incremental doses titrated to adequate control of heart rate, blood pressure, and temperature.

61. Beta blockers are contraindicated in the treatment of stimulant toxicity because they may potentiate alpha effects and cause coronary artery vasoconstriction.

62. No diagnostic studies are indicated in an asymptomatic patient exposed to smoke in a nonenclosed space.

63. In the presence of CO, pulse oximetry will yield a falsely elevated reading.

64. A blood pressure (BP) greater than 140/90 mmHg in a pregnant woman is suspicious for preeclampsia.

65. A pregnant woman with hypertension and seizures should be treated with IV magnesium sulfate and emergent delivery of the fetus.

66. The most deceptive of serious hand injuries is the high-pressure injection injury from a hydraulic paint or oil gun because, despite a seemingly innocuous appearance on initial presentation, these injuries require aggressive, surgical management.

67. In children with tenderness over an open epiphysis, assume a fracture of the physis and immobilize.

68. An elevated osmolal gap (calculated serum osmolarity subtracted from measured serum osmolality; greater than 10 is considered elevated) suggests the possibility of toxic alcohol

poisoning (methanol, ethylene glycol), but a normal osmolal gap *cannot* be used to rule out methanol or ethylene glycol poisoning.

69. With very few exceptions, procedures performed in the ED can be done with fewer complications and greater success using ultrasound as a guide.

70. Any elderly patient with flank, back, abdominal pain, hypotension, syncope, or pulseless electrical activity (PEA) should have an emergency ultrasound exam to evaluate for an AAA.

71. IV bolus administration of epinephrine to a patient with an obtainable BP and pulse can result in ischemic cardiac pain, hypertension, supraventricular tachycardia, and ventricular tachycardia.

72. Examine every patient with urticaria for mucosal edema, stridor, wheezing, and hypotension to rule out life threats associated with anaphylaxis.

73. A contaminated wound is one with a high degree of bacterial inoculum at the time of wounding and is not synonymous with a dirty wound.

74. Determination of a pretest probability for venous thromboembolism (VTE) is critical in knowing when to initiate a diagnostic work-up and how to interpret your diagnostic test.

75. Only in low to low-moderate pretest probability patients can a negative D-dimer rule out the diagnosis of VTE.

76. The problem of "error" in medicine and the adverse events that sometimes follow are problems of psychology and engineering, not of medicine.

77. Emergency medicine, because of its nature, has more failure-producing conditions than any other specialty in medicine.

78. CT of the head will identify 95% of patients with subarachnoid hemorrhage (SAH). Lumbar puncture (LP) is recommended for patients with a strong suspicion of SAH and negative CT of the head.

79. The patient with a posterior nasal packing in place must be monitored in the hospital for recognition of hypoxia and/or apnea secondary to stimulation of the nasopulmonary reflex.

80. In the treatment of hyperkalemia, calcium chloride should only be used for a wide QRS; it narrows the QRS but does not lower the serum potassium.

81. When hypoxatremia is treated, serum sodium should never be raised by more than 10–12 mEq/day to prevent the development of central pontine myolysis.

82. Consider a retropharyngeal space infection in a young child who presents with a history of fever, refusal to drink or decreased oral intake, a suspicion of a sore throat, significant cervical adenopathy, and reluctance to move the neck.

83. The concomitant ingestion of ethanol (ETOH) with methanol or ethylene glycol protects against their toxic metabolites.

84. In addition to a threatened or spontaneous abortion, first-trimester vaginal bleeding requires the exclusion of an ectopic pregnancy.

85. Suspect ectopic pregnancy if there is no evidence of intrauterine pregnancy (IUP) by transvaginal ultrasound and the quantitative human chorionic gonadotropin (HCG) concentration is greater than 2000 IU/L.

86. In head injured patients, hyperventilation to a pCO_2 of 30–35 mmHg is used only if the patient has elevated intracranial pressure (ICP) and is clinically deteriorating.

87. In a lucid patient with blunt abdominal trauma, the clinical examination is the best guide to selection of diagnostic tests.

88. A negative abdominal ultrasound does not reliably exclude significant intraperitoneal injury.

89. Children manifest shock later than adults with the same percentage of blood volume loss.

90. In the case of vascular and/or skin compromise of a deformed limb, urgent realignment and splinting of the involved extremity should precede radiography.

91. Always exclude associated fractures of the spine and lower extremities in patients presenting with calcaneal fractures.

92. Never restrain a patient in the prone position; restrain on the side to minimize risks of aspiration and sudden death.

93. Consider domestic violence in women with depression or suicidal ideations, chronic pain, or psychosomatic complaints.

94. Only 2 weeks of chronic steroid use (prednisone > 20 mg/day) will cause adrenal suppression, making a patient more prone to adrenal crisis.

95. Lightning strike is the one exception to the usual multiple casualty incident (MCI) triage rules: the first priority should go to those who are not breathing and not moving because only those who present in cardiac arrest are at high risk of dying.

96. Arborescent superficial erythema (known as Lichtenberg's flowers, ferning, arboration, or fractals) is pathognomonic for lightning injury. It is seen in only 20% of confirmed cases and fades away over hours. It is not a true burn but the effect of a strong electromagnetic field on wet skin.

97. Follow potassium closely when treating patients with insulin.

98. Glucose should not be withheld due the unfounded fear of precipitating Wernicke-Korsakoff syndrome.

99. Zoos usually keep antivenin on hand for the exotic venomous animals in their collections.

100. In pregnant patients, all clinically necessary radiologic investigations should be performed regardless of radiation concerns.

DECISION-MAKING IN EMERGENCY MEDICINE

Vincent J. Markovchick, MD

1. **Is there anything unique about emergency medicine?**

   Although there is significant crossover between emergency medicine and all other clinical specialties, emergency medicine has unique aspects, such as the approach to patient care and the decision-making process.

2. **Describe the conventional method of evaluating a patient.**

   A comprehensive history, physical examination, "routine" laboratory diagnostic studies, special diagnostic procedures, and the formulation of a problem-oriented medical record and rational course of therapy constitute the "ideal" approach to patient care because it is so comprehensive.

3. **Why is the conventional methodology not ideal for use in the emergency department (ED)?**

   Even though in retrospect only 10–20% of patients presenting to an ED truly have emergent problems, it must be presumed that every patient who comes to an ED has an emergent condition. Therefore, the first and most important question that must be answered is *What is the life threat?* The conventional approach does not ensure an expeditious answer to this question. Time constraints also impede the use of conventional methodology in the ED.

4. **How do I identify the life-threatened patient?**

   Three components are necessary to quickly identify the life-threatened patient:
   - A chief complaint and a brief, focused history relevant to the chief complaint
   - A complete and accurate set of vital signs in the field and in the ED that are accurately taken and critically interpreted
   - An opportunity to visualize, auscultate, and touch the patient

5. **What is so important about the chief complaint?**

   The chief complaint, which sometimes cannot be obtained directly from the patient but must be obtained from family members, observers, emergency medical technicians (EMTs), or others at the scene, will immediately help categorize the general type of problem (e.g., cardiac, traumatic, respiratory).

6. **Why are vital signs important?**

   Vital signs are the most reliable, objective data that are immediately available to ED personnel. Vital signs and the chief complaint, when used as triage tools, will identify the majority of life-threatened patients. Familiarity with normal vital signs for all age groups is essential.

7. **What are the determinants of (normal) vital signs?**

   Age, underlying physical condition, medical problems (e.g., hypertension), and current medications (e.g., β blockers) are important considerations in determining normal vital signs for a given patient. For example, a well-conditioned, young athlete who has just sustained major trauma and arrives with a resting, supine pulse of 80 bpm must be presumed to have significant blood loss because the normal pulse is probably in the 40–50 bpm range.

8. **What is the most inaccurate vital sign taken in the field and ED?**
   In the field, the most common inaccurate vital sign is the respiratory rate, because it is sometimes estimated rather than counted. In the ED, the temperature may be inaccurate if a tympanic membrane thermometer was used or if the patient was hyperventilating or mouth breathing when the oral temperature was taken.

9. **Why do I need to compare field vital signs with ED vital signs?**
   Most prehospital care systems with a level of care beyond basic transport also provide therapy to patients. Because this therapy usually makes positive changes in the patient's condition, the patient may look deceptively well on arrival in the ED. For example, a 20-year-old woman with acute onset of left lower quadrant abdominal pain, who is found to be cool, clammy, and diaphoretic, with a pulse of 116 bpm and a blood pressure of 78 palpable, and who receives 1500 ml of intravenous (IV) fluid en route to the ED, may arrive with normal vital signs and no skin changes. If one does not read and pay attention to the EMT's description of the patient and the initial vital signs, the presumption may be made that this is a stable patient.

10. **When are "normal" vital signs abnormal?**
    This is where the chief complaint comes in. For example, a 20-year-old man who states he has asthma and has been wheezing for hours arrives in the ED with a respiratory rate of 14 breaths/minute. An asthmatic who is dyspneic and wheezing should have a respiratory rate of at least 20–30 breaths/minute. Thus, a "normal" respiratory rate of 14 breaths/minute in this setting indicates the patient is fatiguing and is in respiratory failure. This is a classic example of when "normal" is extremely abnormal.

11. **Why do I need to visualize, auscultate, and touch the patient?**
    In many instances, these measures help to identify the life threat (e.g., is it the upper airway, lower airway, or circulation). Touching the skin is important to determine whether shock is associated with vasoconstriction (hypovolemic or cardiogenic) or with vasodilatation (septic, neurogenic, or anaphylactic). Auscultation will identify life threats associated with the lower airway (e.g., bronchoconstriction, tension pneumothorax).

12. **Once I have identified the life threat, what do I do?**
    Do not go on. Stop immediately and intervene to reverse the life threat. For example, if the initial encounter with the patient identifies upper airway obstruction, take whatever measures are necessary to alleviate upper airway obstruction such as suctioning, positioning, or intubating the patient. If the problem is hemorrhage, volume restoration and hemorrhage control (when possible) are indicated.

13. **I have identified and stabilized or ruled out an immediate life threat in the patient. What else is unique about the approach?**
    The differential diagnosis formulated in the ED must begin with the most serious condition possible to explain the patient's presentation and proceed from there. An example is a 60-year-old man who presents with nausea, vomiting, and epigastric pain. Instead of assuming the condition is caused by a gastrointestinal disorder, one must consider that the presentation could represent an acute myocardial infarction (MI) and take the appropriate steps to stabilize the patient (i.e., start an IV and place the patient on O_2 and a cardiac monitor) and rule out an MI (an adequate history, physical exam, and electrocardiogram [ECG]).

14. **Why does formulating a differential diagnosis sometimes lead to problems?**
    The natural tendency in formulating a differential diagnosis is to think of the most common or statistically most probable condition to explain the patient's initial presentation to the ED. If one does this, one will be right most of the time but may overlook the most serious, albeit sometimes a very uncommon, problem. Therefore, the practice of emergency medicine involves

some degree of healthy paranoia in that one must consider the most serious condition possible and, through a logical process of elimination, rule it out and thereby arrive at the correct and generally more common diagnosis.

15. **Is a diagnosis always possible or necessary with information I can obtain in the ED?**

Of course not. Sometimes it takes days, weeks, or months for the final diagnosis to be made. It is unreasonable to expect that every patient evaluated in the ED should or must have a diagnosis made in the ED. If you have an obsessive-compulsive personality with a need to be absolutely certain before you can act to stabilize or treat a patient, then the ED is an unhealthy work environment for you.

16. **Suppose I cannot make the diagnosis, What do I do?**

It is advisable to be intellectually honest and admit to the patient and document in the medical record the inability to make a diagnosis. As stated earlier, it is the role of the ED physician to rule out serious or life-threatening causes of a patient's presentation, not to arrive at the definitive diagnosis. For example, a patient who presents with acute abdominal pain, who has had an appropriate history taken, who has had a physical exam and diagnostic studies performed, and who in your best judgment does not have a life-threatening or acute surgical problem should be so informed. The discharge diagnosis would be abdominal pain of unknown etiology. This avoids the trap so often encountered of labeling the patient with a benign diagnosis such as gastroenteritis or gastritis that is not supported by the medical record. More importantly, it avoids giving the patient the impression that there is a totally benign process occurring and will help to avoid the medical (and legal) problem of the patient presenting 2 days later with a ruptured appendix (see Chapter 103).

17. **What is the most important question to ask a patient who presents with a chronic, persistent, or recurrent condition?**

What's different now? This question should be asked of all patients who have a chronic condition that has resulted in their visit to the ED. The classic example is migraine headache. The patient with a chronic, recurrent migraine headache who is not asked this question may, on this presentation, have had an acute subarachnoid bleed. Such a patient may not volunteer that this headache is different from the pattern of chronic migraines unless asked.

18. **How do I decide if the patient needs hospitalization?**

Obviously, the medical condition is the first factor to consider. The question that must be answered is "Is there a medical need that can be fulfilled only by hospitalization?" For example, does the patient need oxygen therapy or cardiac monitoring? Another factor to weigh in the decision regarding hospitalization is whether the patient can be safely observed in the outpatient setting. For example, a patient who has sustained head trauma and needs to follow head trauma precautions at home, and who is either homeless or lives alone, cannot be safely discharged. Unfortunately, the patient's ability to pay for services is also sometimes inappropriately used in ED disposition decisions.

19. **If the patient does not need admission, how do I arrange a satisfactory disposition?**

Every patient seen in the ED must be referred to a physician or referred back to the ED for follow-up care. Failure to do so constitutes patient abandonment. Appropriate and specific follow-up instructions should be given to all patients.

20. **What is meant by specific follow-up instructions?**

All follow-up instructions must include specific mention of the most serious potential complication of the patient's condition. For example, a patient who is being discharged home with the diagnosis of a probable herniated L4-5 intervertebral disk should be instructed to return immediately if any bowel or bladder dysfunction develops. This takes into account the most serious complication of a herniated lumbar disk, which is a central midline disk herniation (cauda equina syndrome) with bowel or bladder dysfunction, and constitutes an acute neurosurgical emergency.

21. **What two questions should always be asked (and answered) before a patient is discharged from the ED?**
    - Why did the patient come to the ED?
    - Have I made the patient feel better?

    Generally, most patients present to the ED because of pain, somatic or psychological, and a reasonable expectation is that this pain will be acknowledged and appropriately treated. If such pain cannot be alleviated, a thorough explanation should be given to the patient regarding the reasons why. An example of this is a patient with abdominal pain of unknown etiology, which may evolve into appendicitis since narcotics may delay the recognition of worsening symptoms and localized abdominal pain. Reassurance is sometimes all that is needed to relieve anxiety about serious medical conditions such as cancer or heart attack. Other agents such as antiemetics or antianxiety medications should be administered in the ED to alleviate presenting symptoms.

KEY POINTS: DECISION-MAKING IN EMERGENCY MEDICINE

1. Stabilize the patient before performing diagnostic procedures.

2. Always inquire about a patient's social situation prior to ED discharge.

3. Remember to focus on alleviating the patient's somatic or psychological pain.

22. **Why is the previous question and answer one of the most important in this chapter?**
    Attention to treating and alleviating a patient's pain will dramatically reduce subsequent complaints concerning care in the ED and remove one of the significant risk factors for initiation of a malpractice suit. It is also how you would want to be treated.

23. **What about the chart?**
    The chart must reflect the answers to the preceding questions in this chapter. It need not list the entire differential diagnosis, but one should be able to ascertain from reading the chart that the more serious diagnoses were indeed considered. It also must contain appropriate follow-up instructions.

CHAPTER 2

MANAGEMENT OF CARDIAC ARREST AND PRINCIPLES OF RESUSCITATION

Jason S. Haukoos, MD, MS, and Charles B. Cairns, MD

1. **What are the ABCs of resuscitation?**
   Airway, breathing, and circulation. The ABCs should be used to guide the resuscitation of all critically ill patients, including all patients who experience cardiac arrest.

2. **How should cardiopulmonary resuscitation (CPR) be performed?**
   If the arrest is in the out-of-hospital setting, activate emergency medical services (EMS) by calling 911; if it occurs in the hospital, activate the hospital's cardiac arrest team.
   1. Open the airway by performing a head tilt-chin lift or a head tilt-jaw thrust maneuver. These maneuvers cause anterior displacement of the mandible and lift the tongue and epiglottis away from the glottic opening. To improve airway patency, suction the mouth and oropharynx, and insert an oropharyngeal or nasopharyngeal airway.
   2. Assist breathing by performing mouth-to-mouth, mouth-to-mask, or bag-value-mask breathing. The recommended technique depends on the clinical setting, the equipment available, and the rescuer's skill and training. Although these techniques can sustain oxygenation and ventilation indefinitely in ideal situations, they can be suboptimal in the emergency setting. Air leaks around the facemask may result in inadequate ventilation, insufflation of the stomach, and emesis and aspiration. To reduce the probability of such problems, deliver slow, even breaths, pausing for full deflation between breaths to avoid excessive peak inspiratory pressures. Use the Sellick maneuver (using your fingers to apply continuous posterior pressure to the cricoid cartilage) to compress the esophagus to reduce the risk of vomiting and aspiration.
   3. After opening the airway and initiating rescue breathing, check for spontaneous circulation by palpating for a carotid or femoral pulse. If the patient is pulseless, begin chest compressions. Compress the chest smoothly and forcefully 100 times per minute, providing a compression-ventilation ratio of 30:2. Allow for complete chest recoil during CPR and avoid interruptions in chest compressions.

   2005 American Heart Association Guidelines for Cardiopulmonary Resuscitation and Emergency Cardiovascular Care. Circulation 112:1–211, 2005.

3. **What is the "squeeze, release, release" method of providing mechanical ventilation?**
   "Squeeze, release, release" was first described in 1997 as a bag-valve-mask technique to provide an appropriate level of ventilation to pediatric patients. Subsequently, this technique has been extended to adult patients and consists of performing ventilation at a rate consistent with someone saying "squeeze, release, release" to maintain an appropriate ventilation rate.

   Gausche M, Lewis RJ, Stratton SJ, et al: Effect of out-of-hospital pediatric endotracheal intubation on survival and neurologic outcome: a controlled clinical trial. JAMA 283:783–790, 2000.

4. **What are the exceptions to the rule of the ABCs?**
   - **Monitored cardiac arrest.** When a patient in a monitored setting experiences sudden pulseless ventricular tachycardia (VT) or ventricular fibrillation (VF), immediate electrical defibrillation is the priority.

- **Traumatic arrest.** In traumatic cardiac arrest, closed-chest CPR is usually ineffective. In trauma, the cause of the arrest may be a tension pneumothorax, cardiac tamponade, or exsanguinating hemorrhage from the thorax or abdomen. An immediate thoracotomy, not CPR, is indicated. When neck injury is possible, a jaw thrust (never a head tilt) should be used to open the airway.

5. **Explain the mechanism of blood flow during CPR.**

   Two basic models explain the mechanism of blood flow during CPR. In the "cardiac pump model," the heart is squeezed between the sternum and the spine. Chest compressions result in systole, and the atrioventricular valves close normally, ensuring unidirectional, antegrade blood flow. During the relaxation phase (diastole), intracardiac pressures fall, the valves open, and blood is drawn into the heart from the lungs and vena cavae. In the "thoracic pump model," the heart is considered a passive conduit. Chest compressions result in uniformly increased pressures throughout the thorax. Forward blood flow is achieved selectively in the arterial system because the stiff-walled arteries resist collapse and because retrograde flow is prevented in the great veins by one-way valves. In addition, chest recoil results in increased negative intrathoracic pressures, which improve ventricular filling and coronary blood flow. These mechanisms have all been substantiated in animal models, and all probably contribute to blood flow during CPR.

6. **Is blood flow to the brain and heart adequate during CPR?**

   Even when performed by experts, CPR provides only approximately 30% of normal blood flow to the brain and 10–20% of normal blood flow to the heart. Blood flow to the heart occurs during the relaxation phase of CPR, whereas blood flow to the brain occurs during the compression phase of CPR. This is the foundation for the American Heart Association's recommended CPR duty cycle of 50% (the ratio of time spent in compression to the time spent in relaxation).

7. **What is coronary perfusion pressure (CPP)?**

   CPP is defined as the aortic pressure minus the right atrial pressure during diastole.

8. **What is the association between CPR, CPP, and return of spontaneous circulation (ROSC)?**

   Better CPR produces better CPPs. Higher CPPs translate into higher rates of ROSC. This emphasizes the importance of performing good CPR and explains how vasopressors (e.g., epinephrine) impact rates of ROSC by increasing CPPs.

   Paradis NA, Martin GB, Rivers EP, et al: Coronary perfusion pressure and the return of spontaneous circulation in human cardiopulmonary resuscitation. JAMA 263:1106–1113, 1990.

9. **Describe "hands off" CPR?**

   "Hands off" CPR refers to lifting the hands off the chest wall during decompression to maximize chest recoil. Incomplete chest wall recoil during CPR has been shown to result in hemodynamic deterioration of forward blood flow in animal models. In addition, in an observational human study, incomplete chest recoil was common during CPR.

   Aufderheide TP, Pirallo RG, Yannopoulos D, et al: Incomplete chest wall decompression: A clinical evaluation of CPR performance by EMS personnel and assessment of alternative manual chest compression-decompression techniques. Resuscitation 64:353–362, 2005.

10. **Discuss the role of pharmacologic therapy during CPR.**

    The immediate goal of pharmacologic therapy is to improve CPPs, and thus, myocardial blood flow, which correlates with ROSC. Adrenergic agonists (e.g., epinephrine) augment the aortic-to-right-atrial diastolic gradient by increasing systemic vascular resistance. Reports suggest that nonadrenergic agonists (e.g., vasopressin) may be more effective than adrenergic agonists in improving myocardial blood flow. Additional clinical studies suggest that amiodarone improves rates of successful defibrillation and prevents recurrent postarrest dysrhythmias. These antifibrillatory effects may be independent of myocardial blood flow.

KEY POINTS: STANDARD DOSES OF CARDIAC ARREST MEDICATIONS

1. Epinephrine: 1 mg IV push
2. Vasopressin: 40 units IV push
3. Atropine: 1 mg IV push
4. Amiodarone: 300 mg IV push
5. Lidocaine: 1.0–1.5 mg/kg IV push

11. Under what circumstances should "CPR before defibrillation" be used?

A growing body of research suggests that patients with untreated prolonged VF may benefit from CPR for 2 to 3 minutes prior to defibrillation, and several prehospital care systems have incorporated this into their protocols.

Wik L, Hansen TB, Fylling F, et al: Delaying defibrillation to give basic cardiopulmonary resuscitation to patients with out-of-hospital ventricular fibrillation: A randomized trial. JAMA 289:1389–1395, 2003.

12. What are the indications for open chest cardiac massage?

The primary indication for open chest cardiac massage is traumatic arrest. However, several other non-trauma-related indications include hypothermia, pulmonary embolism, cardiac tamponade, abdominal hemorrhage, third-trimester pregnancy, and chest wall deformities that prevent adequate chest compressions.

13. What are the most common causes of cardiopulmonary arrest?

Although the incidence of **ventricular fibrillation** (VF) appears to be declining, it still remains the most common initial rhythm encountered in patients suffering from cardiac arrest. Underlying coronary artery disease accounts for the majority of VF arrests. Other etiologies of VF include drug toxicity, electrolyte disturbances (e.g., hyperkalemia), and prolonged hypoxemia.

The second most common initial rhythm encountered is **asystole.** This commonly results from prolonged untreated VF and is due to severe hypoxia and acidemia. Other causes of asystole include drug toxicity, electrolyte disturbances, and hypothermia.

Pulseless electrical activity (PEA) is the third most commonly encountered initial arrest rhythm. As with asystole, PEA commonly results from prolonged untreated VF or defibrillation of VF after a prolonged untreated period (usually > 5 minutes). Other causes of PEA include hypovolemia, hypoxia, cardiac tamponade, tension pneumothorax, hypothermia, massive pulmonary embolism, drug toxicity, electrolyte disturbances, acidemia, or myocardial infarction.

14. What are other reversible causes and immediate treatments of cardiopulmonary arrest?

- Always begin with the ABCs.
- **Hyperkalemia:** Treatment includes calcium chloride, sodium bicarbonate, insulin-glucose, and nebulized albuterol.
- **Anaphylaxis:** Volume expansion (using crystalloid) and epinephrine are used.
- **Cardiac tamponade:** Pericardiocentesis is performed.
- **Tension pneumothorax:** Immediate chest decompression is used.
- **Hypovolemia:** Treatment includes immediate intravenous (IV) access and administration of crystalloid solutions. In the setting of trauma, blood products should be given judiciously and

concomitantly with crystalloid. Always consider using a level I infuser when large volumes are required over a short period of time.

- **Torsades de pointes:** Treatment includes defibrillation, magnesium, isoproterenol, or overdrive pacing.
- **Toxic cardiopulmonary arrest:** *Carbon monoxide* poisoning occurs after prolonged exposure to smoke and inhalation of exhaust from incomplete combustion. High-flow and hyperbaric oxygen and management of acidosis are the cornerstones of treatment. *Cyanide* poisoning occurs after intentional ingestion or after exposure to fire involving synthetic materials. The antidote for this includes IV sodium nitrite and sodium thiosulfate. *Tricyclic antidepressants* act as type Ia antidysrhythmic agents and cause cardiac conduction slowing, ventricular dysrhythmias, hypotension, and seizures.
- **Primary asphyxia:** In addition to anaphylaxis, obstructive asphyxia may occur after foreign body aspiration, inflammatory conditions of the hypopharynx (e.g., epiglottitis or retropharyngeal abscess), or neck trauma. The latter results in edema or hematoma formation, subcutaneous emphysema, or laryngeal or tracheal disruption. Treatment includes establishment of a patent airway via endotracheal intubation or by cricothyrotomy and assisted ventilation with 100% oxygen.

15. **How should VF be treated?**
Rapid treatment is essential, as the prognosis worsens with each untreated minute. Standard treatment consists of immediate defibrillation. Recommended energy levels are 200 J (biphasic) or 360 J (monophasic). Escalation of energy levels is no longer recommended. The antidysrhythmic agent of choice is amiodarone, which enhances the rate of successful defibrillation and reduces the rate of recurrent VF after successful conversion. Administration of epinephrine or vasopressin before defibrillation may improve defibrillation success; in addition, CPR before defibrillation (*see* question 11) may also improve defibrillation success in the setting of prolonged VF.

16. **What is the difference between monophasic and biphasic defibrillation?**
The terms "monophasic" and "biphasic" refer to the energy waveforms produced by the defibrillation device. Monophasic waveforms vary in speed in which the waveform returns to the zero voltage point, whereas biphasic waveforms deliver current that first flows in a positive direction for a specific duration then reverses direction for a specific duration. Biphasic defibrillation achieves the same defibrillation success rates as monophasic defibrillation, but at significantly lower energy levels, resulting in less postresuscitation cardiac dysfunction.

17. **What about persistent VF?**
   1. Perform endotracheal intubation and ensure adequate oxygenation and ventilation.
   2. Continue CPR.
   3. Administer epinephrine (1 mg IV push) or vasopressin (40 units IV push) to augment aortic diastolic blood pressure and to improve myocardial perfusion.
   4. Administer amiodarone (300 mg IV push). Amiodarone can be repeated at 150 mg IV push after 3 to 5 minutes.
   5. Consider the administration of lidocaine (1.0–1.5 mg/kg IV push) or procainamide (17 mg/kg at a rate of 30 mg/minute IV). However, neither lidocaine nor procainamide has been shown to improve defibrillation success rates or restore perfusing rhythms in patients with VF, however.

18. **Describe the three-phase model of cardiac arrest.**
The first phase, called the "electrical phase," suggests that immediate defibrillation is the most efficacious treatment within the first 4 minutes of VF. The second phase, called the "circulatory phase," follows the first phase and suggests that successful ROSC and overall survival are maximized with a period of CPR before defibrillation. The third phase, called the

"metabolic phase," is reached after about 10 minutes and is associated with a profound systemic inflammatory response syndrome; no current directed therapies offer survival benefit in this setting.

19. Is PEA treatable after defibrillation from VF?
Delayed defibrillation frequently results in asystole or PEA, both of which are commonly untreatable and result in death. In animal experiments, high-dose epinephrine (0.1 mg/kg) has helped to restore cardiac contractility and pacemaker activity. In humans, high-dose epinephrine has been shown to improve ROSC rates but without significant long-term survival.

20. How should asystole be treated?
1. Confirm the absence of cardiac activity in more than one electrocardiogram (ECG) lead. Check for loose or disconnected cables and monitor leads. Finally, increase the amplitude to detect occult, fine VF.
2. Administer epinephrine (1 mg IV push) or vasopressin (40 units IV push).
3. Administer atropine (1 mg IV push) to counteract high vagal tone.

KEY POINTS: MANAGEMENT OF CARDIAC ARREST

1. CPR and defibrillation are the most important components to the initial management of the cardiac arrest patient.

2. Treat VF with immediate defibrillation, CPR then defibrillation, and/or amiodarone.

3. If the arrest is due to PEA, remember its common causes (hypovolemia, hypoxia, cardiac tamponade, tension pneumothorax, hypothermia, massive pulmonary embolism, drug toxicity, electrolyte disturbances, acidemia, or myocardial infarction) and treat them appropriately.

4. If the arrest is due to asystole, remember to exclude fine VF.

21. Is defibrillation or electrical pacing useful for asystole?
Defibrillation is reserved for cases in which differentiation between asystole and fine VF is difficult. In these ambiguous situations, defibrillation should be used after administration of epinephrine. Electrical pacing is occasionally attempted for asystole but is rarely effective in restoring pulses.

22. What are the appropriate routes of drug administration?
IV administration is the preferred route of drug therapy during CPR. If a central venous catheter is in place, the most distal port should be used. Otherwise, use of a peripheral venous catheter results in a slightly delayed onset of action, although the peak drug effect is similar to that for the central route. Intracardiac administration should be reserved for cases of open cardiac massage. Many drugs (e.g., lidocaine, epinephrine, atropine, naloxone) are absorbed systemically after administration through the endotracheal tube, yet the effectiveness of this route during CPR is questionable. Pulmonary blood flow and systemic absorption are minimal during CPR. Studies in animals suggest comparable hemodynamic responses when 10 times the IV dose is given endotracheally. All drugs used for resuscitation can be given in conventional

doses by the intraosseous route; this method is useful in pediatric or adult patients when an IV line cannot be established.

23. **When may prehospital resuscitation efforts be terminated?**

According to the most recent American Heart Association advanced cardiac life support (ACLS) guidelines, prehospital resuscitation may be discontinued by EMS authorities when a valid no-CPR order is presented to the rescuers or when a patient is deemed nonresuscitable after an adequate trial of ACLS, including successful endotracheal intubation, achievement of IV access, and administration of appropriate medications. Additional criteria for stopping resuscitation include a persistent asystolic or agonal rhythm is determined; and no reversible cause for the arrest is identified.

CONTROVERSY

24. **Which vasopressor should I administer in the setting of cardiac arrest, epinephrine or vasopressin?**

This remains controversial. Epinephrine has been evaluated in human trials in approximately 9000 patients. The recommended 1 mg dose was extrapolated from animal research, and trials comparing this dose with high-dose regimens (i.e., 0.1 to 0.2 mg/kg) demonstrated increased rates of ROSC in patients who received high-dose epinephrine; however, these studies have not shown improvements in survival or survival with good neurologic outcomes. Vasopressin acts directly on V_1-receptors and, unlike epinephrine, is more effective in an acidemic environment. Vasopressin has been compared with epinephrine in three human trials, totaling approximately 1500 patients without a significant difference in survival.

Wenzel V, Krismer AC, Arntz HR, et al: A comparison of vasopressin and epinephrine for out-of-hospital cardiopulmonary resuscitation. N Engl J Med 350:105–113, 2004.

25. **Should I use amiodarone in the setting of cardiac arrest?**

Amiodarone is a class III antidysrhythmic agent used, in part, to treat VT or VF. Two randomized clinical trials have demonstrated a survival to hospital admission benefit for amiodarone over placebo and lidocaine, respectively. Neither study demonstrated survival benefit to hospital discharge, however. In most settings amiodarone has become the first-line agent for treating VT or VF.

Dorian P, Cass D, Schwartz B, et al: Amiodarone as compared with lidocaine for shock-resistant ventricular fibrillation. N Engl J Med 346:884–890, 2002.

26. **Should I routinely administer sodium bicarbonate during resuscitation?**

Sodium bicarbonate is not recommended as routine therapy in the setting of cardiac arrest. A no- or low-flow state causes progressive respiratory and metabolic acidosis as a result of accumulation of PCO_2 and lactate. Neither state can be corrected without adequate oxygenation, ventilation, and tissue perfusion. At present, no clinical data support its routine use except in cases of hyperkalemia, tricyclic antidepressant overdose, cocaine-induced arrest, or preexisting metabolic acidosis.

27. **Should I routinely administer calcium during resuscitation?**

Calcium is not recommended as routine therapy in the setting of cardiac arrest. No data exist to support its routine use in this setting. Calcium administration, however, may be beneficial in the setting of hyperkalemia, hypocalcemia, or calcium channel blocker toxicity.

28. What should I do after ROSC?

Once ROSC is achieved, the vulnerable postresuscitation period begins. This period is marked by a profound systemic inflammatory response syndrome resulting from whole-body ischemia and reperfusion. Patients commonly develop hemodynamic instability, resulting in multiple organ dysfunction and subsequent death (hours to days later). Prompt recognition and treatment of the inciting event and meticulous intensive care unit support are required to provide patients with the best probability for survival. Use of hemodynamic and inotropic agents is important for supporting patients during this period. Also, mild therapeutic hypothermia should be considered to improve neurologic recovery.

Hypothermia after Cardiac Arrest Study Group: Mild therapeutic hypothermia to improve the neurologic outcome after cardiac arrest. N Engl J Med 346:549–556, 2002.

29. What percentage of all cardiac arrest patients survive to hospital discharge?

5%.

30. Where can I find more information about the management of cardiac arrest?

http://www.americanheart.org/

FURTHER READING

1. Aufderheide TP, Pirallo RG, Yannopoulos D, et al: Incomplete chest wall decompression: A clinical evaluation of CPR performance by EMS personnel and assessment of alternative manual chest compression-decompression techniques. Resuscitation 64:353–362, 2005.

2. Dorian P, Cass D, Schwartz B, et al: Amiodarone as compared with lidocaine for shock-resistant ventricular fibrillation. N Engl J Med 346:884–890, 2002.

3. Gausche M, Lewis RJ, Stratton SJ, et al: Effect of out-of-hospital pediatric endotracheal intubation on survival and neurologic outcome: a controlled clinical trial. JAMA 283:783–790, 2000.

4. Hypothermia after Cardiac Arrest Study Group: Mild therapeutic hypothermia to improve the neurologic outcome after cardiac arrest. N Engl J Med 346:549–556, 2002.

5. Paradis NA, Martin GB, Rivers EP, et al: Coronary perfusion pressure and the return of spontaneous circulation in human cardiopulmonary resuscitation. JAMA 263:1106–1113, 1990.

6. Wik L, Hansen TB, Fylling F, et al: Delaying defibrillation to give basic cardiopulmonary resuscitation to patients with out-of-hospital ventricular fibrillation: A randomized trial. JAMA 289:1389–1395, 2003.

7. Wenzel V, Krismer AC, Arntz HR, et al: A comparison of vasopressin and epinephrine for out-of-hospital cardiopulmonary resuscitation. N Engl J Med 350:105–113, 2004.

CHAPTER 3

AIRWAY MANAGEMENT

Barry Simon, MD

1. **Do I really need to know about airway management?**
   Yes. Expeditious airway management saves lives.

2. **How is the adequacy of ventilation assessed?**
   First, look at the patient. Cyanosis suggests profound hypoxia. Diaphoresis and somnolence
   indicate hypercapnia and respiratory acidosis. Measure the respiratory rate and assess the tidal
   volume by placing your hand over the endotracheal tube or the patient's mouth and nose. If you
   are still concerned, use a pulse oximeter. Mild-to-moderate hypoxia can be monitored with pulse
   oximetry, which measures arterial oxygen saturation. If there is a question of inadequate
   ventilation, an arterial blood gas or measurement of end-tidal CO_2 should be considered.

3. **Why do patients need airway management?**
   Assisted ventilation can help to decrease intracranial pressure or correct hypercarbia and
   acidosis. **Oxygenation** may be needed in patients with severe lung disease or injury who are
   unable to maintain an acceptable PaO_2. **Overcoming or preventing airway obstruction** is
   imperative in patients with neck trauma, epiglottitis, or airway burns from smoke inhalation or
   ingestion of caustic substances. **Prevention of aspiration** in patients with altered mentation is
   best accomplished with endotracheal intubation. **Administration of intratracheal drugs
   (epinephrine, atropine, lidocaine)** through the endotracheal tube is indicated in resuscitation
   until an intravenous (IV) line can be established.

4. **What is the most common cause of airway obstruction?**
   The tongue obstructs the airway far more commonly than do foreign bodies or edema.
   With decreasing levels of consciousness, the supporting muscles in the floor of the mouth
   lose tone, and the tongue falls posteriorly, obstructing the oropharynx. The fastest, least
   invasive treatment modality is repositioning via the head tilt-chin lift maneuver. A
   nasopharyngeal or oral airway should be inserted in a patient with ongoing upper airway
   obstruction unrelieved by repositioning. Care must be taken in patients with potential or
   suspected cervical spine injury.

5. **What is a Combitube?**
   The Combitube is a dual-lumen, dual-cuffed airway. The two lumens allow ventilation whether
   the tube is placed into the esophagus or in the trachea. The tube differs from the esophageal
   obturator airway because it does not require an adequate mask seal to affect adequate
   ventilation. This device is placed blindly and is usually placed in the esophagus. Dual balloons
   are inflated to seal the device. Tube/lumen 1 is ventilated if the device ended up in the esophagus
   and lumen 2 is inflated if it was placed in the trachea. End-tidal CO_2 detectors are used to
   confirm placement and ventilation.

Vrocher D, Hopson L: Basic airway management and decision making. In Roberts JR, Hedges JR (eds):
Clinical Procedures in Emergency Medicine, 4th ed. Elsevier, 2004, pp 53–68.

6. **What are the indications for the Combitube?**
   The Combitube is most useful in the prehospital setting when assisted ventilation is needed and the providers are not trained or authorized to perform endotracheal intubation.

7. **Is the Combitube safe?**
   The Combitube is safer than its predecessor, the esophageal obturator airway. However, if the tube ends up in the esophagus, then the patient is still at risk for aspiration of secretions, bleeding, and emesis. Esophageal rupture has been reported when the distal balloon is overinflated.

8. **What are the relative contraindications to blind nasotracheal intubation (BNTI)?**
   Apnea is the most important contraindication because the chance of esophageal intubation is unacceptably high. Because epistaxis complicates BNTI in one third of cases, the procedure is contraindicated in patients with coagulopathies. Other routes of intubation are advisable in patients with maxillary facial or severe nasal fractures because a false passage, severe epistaxis, or, rarely, cranial placement may occur. Hematomas, epiglottitis, and infections of the upper neck are relative contraindications because of the risk of sudden airway obstruction or laryngospasm.

9. **Name some complications of BNTI.**
   Hypoxia may occur during the intubation process. In addition to epistaxis and esophageal intubation, there are acute complications, such as avulsion of the turbinates, avulsion of the vocal cords, and pharyngeal perforations with retropharyngeal dissection. Significant elevation in intracranial pressure with coughing may precipitate uncal herniation in head-injured patients. Sinusitis may occur several days later from obstruction of the paranasal ostia.

10. **What is the laryngeal mask airway (LMA)?**
    The LMA (Fig. 3-1) is an irregular ovoid-shaped silicone mask with an inflatable rim connected to a tube that allows ventilation. The device can be passed blindly with a high degree of success. The nose of the mask is seated in the esophagus. When the rim is inflated, it prevents air from going into the esophagus and forces air into the trachea. This is a good temporizing device until a definitive airway can be established. All practicing emergency physicians should be familiar with the use of the LMA.

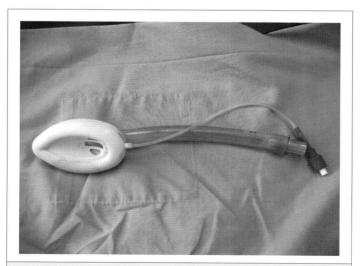

Figure 3-1. Laryngeal mask airway.

11. What are the benefits of the LMA?
The LMA is relatively simple to place with a high degree of success even for those who are inexperienced. The LMA should be considered the alternative airway device of choice in cases in which traditional endotracheal intubation is not successful. The LMA has the added benefit of allowing practitioners to pass an endotracheal tube through the device into the trachea for definitive airway management.

12. What is rapid-sequence intubation (RSI)?
A method of paralyzing and intubating a patient with a full stomach. Because all emergency patients are at risk for aspiration, the airway must be secured as quickly as possible. Paralysis with succinylcholine facilitates visualization and tube placement and reduces complications that occur with attempts to intubate an awake, struggling patient.

Vrocher D, Hopson L: Basic airway management and decision making. In Roberts JR, Hedges JR (eds): Clinical Procedures in Emrergency Medicine, 4th ed. Elsevier, 2004, pp 53–68.

13. What are the predictors of a difficult intubation?
- Morbid obesity
- Abnormal facial shape
- Buck teeth
- Protruding/prominent tongue
- Prominent mandible
- Short neck/limited motion

The Mallampati score helps to predict the level of difficulty with intubation. A higher class score predicts a greater degree of difficulty (Fig. 3-2).

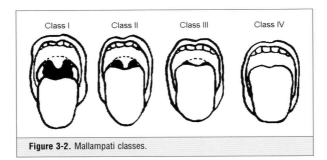

Figure 3-2. Mallampati classes.

14. Don't you need to be an anesthesiologist to perform RSI? How is it done?
No. The basics can be remembered as the **five Ps**: preparation, preoxygenation, priming, pressure, and paralysis (Table 3-1).
1. **Prepare** equipment (e.g., suction, endotracheal tube, bag, mask, laryngoscope).
2. **Preoxygenate** with 100% oxygen (no positive-pressure) ideally for 5 minutes.
3. Pretreat with a defasciculating dose of vecuronium or pancuronium (0.01 mg/kg).
4. **Prime** with thiopental, 3 to 4 mg/kg, or etomidate, 0.3 mg/kg rapid IV push.
5. Apply **pressure** with Sellick's maneuver (cricoid pressure) as consciousness is lost to prevent regurgitation and aspiration.
6. Follow thiopental or etomidate immediately with 1.5 mg/kg of succinylcholine to **paralyze.**
7. Intubate the trachea and verify accurate placement with an end-tidal CO_2 detector.
8. Release cricoid pressure.

TABLE 3-1.   PARALYTIC DRUGS

	Succinylcholine (Anectine)	Rocuronium (Zemuron)	Pancuronium (Pavulon)	Vecuronium (Norcuron)
Uses	Skeletal muscle relaxation	Skeletal muscle relaxation	Skeletal muscle relaxation	Skeletal muscle relaxation
Supplied	200-mg vial, 20 mg/mL	100-mg vial, 10 mg/mL	10-mg vial, 1 mg/mL	10-mg powder, 1 mg/mL
Cost	*	***	*	**
Pregnancy class	C	B	C	C
Adult dose	1–1.5 mg/kg	0.9–1.2 mg/kg RSI	0.1 mg/kg	0.25 mg/kg RSI
	3–4 mg/kg IM (max. 150 mg)		0.01 mg/kg priming dose	0.1 mg/kg standard dose
	0.15 mg/kg priming dose			0.01 mg/kg priming dose
Pediatric dose	1–2 mg/kg + atropine 0.01 mg/kg	0.6–1.2 mg/kg	0.04–0.1 mg/kg	0.1 mg/kg
Onset	30–60 sec	45–90 sec	1–3 min	60-sec RSI
Duration	5–10 min	20–40 min	40–60 min	0.3–5 min standard
				60–120 min RSI
				20–40 min standard
Class	Ultrashort-acting depolarizing muscle relaxant	Rapid-acting nondepolarizing neuromuscular blocker	Long-acting nondepolarizing neuromuscular blocker	Intermediate-acting nondepolarizing neuromuscular blocker
Effects	Fasciculations, increased IOP, ICP, and IGP	Prolonged recovery with liver failure, vagolytic activity may increase HR, BP, and CO	Prolonged recovery with liver and renal failure	Prolonged recovery with liver and renal failure

Continued

TABLE 3-1. PARALYTIC DRUGS—CONT'D

	Succinylcholine (Anectine)	Rocuronium (Zemuron)	Pancuronium (Pavulon)	Vecuronium (Norcuron)
	Caution: exaggerated hyperkalemic response with burns, spinal injury, stroke, paraplegia, neuromuscular disease (maximum at 7–10 days after injury) and acidosis, sepsis, crush muscle injury	Onset and duration are dose-dependent.	Vagolytic activity may increase HR, BP, and CO.	Onset and duration are dose-dependent.
				Minimal histamine or CV effects
	Histamine release, cardiac arrhythmias, especially bradycardia, consider atropine 0.01 mg/kg			
Comments	Refrigerate or use in 14 days	Refrigerate or use in 30 days	Refrigerate or use in 6 months	Mix with 10 cc sterile H_2O

IM = intramuscular, RSI = rapid-sequence induction, IOP = intraocular pressure, ICP = intracranial pressure, IGP = intragastric pressure, HR = heart rate, BP = blood pressure, CO = cardiac output, CV = cardiovascular.

Alternative RSI
1. Prepare equipment (e.g., suction, endotracheal tube, bag, mask, laryngoscope).
2. Preoxygenate with 100% oxygen (no positive-pressure ventilation), ideally for 5 minutes.
3. Prime with thiopental, 3 to 4 mg/kg, or etomidate, 0.3 mg/kg IV push.
4. Paralyze with rocuronium, 1.0 mg/kg IV push.
5. Apply Sellick's maneuver (cricoid pressure) as consciousness is lost.
6. Intubate the trachea and verify accurate placement with an end-tidal CO_2 detector.
7. Release cricoid pressure.

15. **How do I preoxygenate a patient before intubation?**
Bag-valve-mask ventilation is the only option in the apneic patient, even though this increases the risk of aspiration by raising gastric pressure. If a patient is making effective respiratory efforts, he or she should receive passive oxygenation via a nonrebreather mask on 100% oxygen for a full 5 minutes. In the apneic patient, eight vital capacity breaths using high-flow oxygen should be administered. Adequate preoxygenation will protect the patient against hypoxia for several minutes despite becoming apneic after induction and paralysis.

Walls R: Airway. In Marx JA, Hockverger RS, Walls RM (eds): Emergency Medicine Concepts and Clinical Practice, 5th ed. St. Louis, Mosby, 2002, pp 2–21.

16. **Which patients are likely to be difficult to ventilate with a bag-valve-mask?**
- Excess facial hair
- Severe facial burns
- Morbid obesity
- Angioedema/facial fractures
- Unstable facial fractures

17. **What is Sellick's maneuver?**
Sellick described a method of applying pressure over the cricoid cartilage to help prevent aspiration. Pressure should equal the amount of force it takes to cause discomfort when pressing over the bridge of one's nose. Pressure is applied after loss of consciousness and is maintained until the endotracheal tube balloon is inflated and tube placement is confirmed.

18. **How do I remember the size of the endotracheal tube for children?**
The easiest way is to carry a card in your wallet. The following formula works for persons 2 to 20 years old:

$$\text{Tube size} = (\text{age in years} + 16)/4$$

19. **Describe some of the induction drugs available for RSI.**
- **Thiopental** is a short-acting barbiturate that has been used by anesthesiologists for decades. It is safe and effective with few serious complications but is a little longer acting than many of the newer agents (10–15 minutes).
- **Methohexital** is an ultra-short-acting barbiturate with a similar safety profile. The benzodiazepine **midazolam** has the added benefit of being reversible.
- **Propofol** is a diisopropylphenol induction agent that has become popular among anesthesiologists for outpatient procedures. Its major disadvantage is a significant decrease in blood pressure.
- **Etomidate** has become the most popular induction drug in emergency settings for its rapid action, short duration, and absence of any effects on the cardiovascular system.
  Table 3-2 summarizes sedation and induction drugs.

Blanda M, Gallo EU: Emergency airway management. Emerg Med Clin North Am 21:11–26, 2003.

TABLE 3-2. SEDATION AND INDUCTION DRUGS

	Methohexital (Brevital)	Thiopental (Pentothal)	Propofol (Diprivan)	Etomidate (Amidate)	Ketamine (Ketalar)
Uses	Sedation, induction, anesthesia	Sedation, induction, anesthesia	Sedation, induction, anesthesia	Sedation, induction, anesthesia	Sedation, induction, analgesia, dissociative anesthesia
Supplied	500 mg powder	500 mg powder	200 mg ampule	20 mg ampule	500 mg vial
	10 mg/mL	25 mg/mL	10 mg/mL	2 mg/mL	100 mg/mL
Cost	*	*	***	*	*
Pregnancy	B	D	B	C	?
Adult dose	1–1.5mg/kg induction dose	3–5 mg/kg induction dose	1.5–3.0 mg/kg induction dose	0.2–6 mg/kg induction dose	1.0–2.5 mg/kg induction dose
	0.25–1.0 mg/kg sedation	0.5–1.0 mg/kg sedation	5.1 mg/kg sedatopm	1.3 mg/kg sedation	0.5–1.0 mg/kg IV sedation
					5–10 mg/kg IM sedation
Pediatric dose	1–2 mg/kg	4–6 mg/kg	1.3–3.0 mg/kg	0.3–4 mg/kg	1–2 mg/kg IV, 4 mg/kg IM
	5–10 mg/kg IM				6–10 mg/kg PO 30 min prior
Onset	30–60 sec	30 sec	30 sec	30 sec	30 sec
Duration	5–10 min	3–5 min	3–5 min	3–10 min	5–15 min IV, 10–25 min IM

TABLE 3-2. SEDATION AND INDUCTION DRUGS—CONT'D

	Methohexital (Brevital)	Thiopental (Pentothal)	Propofol (Diprivan)	Etomidate (Amidate)	Ketamine (Ketalar)
Class	Ultra-short acting oxybarbiturate	Ultra-short thiobarbiturate	Diisoproplylphenol hypnotic	Imidazole derivitive nonbarbiturate hypnotic	Rapid-acting dissociative anesthetic
Effects	Rapid hypnosis: hypotension, apnea, no analgesia, excitatory phenomena (>children and elderly), seizure potential, bronchospasm, pain on injection, less fat uptake and faster onset/recovery than thiopental	Rapid hypnosis: hypotension, apnea, no analgesia, decreased ICP and CBF, maintains CPP, bronchospasm, decreased IOP, pain on injection, retrograde amnesia	Rapid hypnosis: hypotension, apnea, antiemetic and 10x more rapid recovery than thiopental, decreased IOP, ICP, MAP, and CPP, pain on injection, myoclonus, anaphylaxis with soy and egg allergy	Rapid hypnosis, relative CV and respiratory stability, no analgesia, decreased IOP, ICP, and CBF, maintain CPP, pain on injection, myoclonus (decreased with benzo/opioids), potential adrenal suppression	Rapid dissociative state, increased HR, BP, and maintenance of airway reflexes although apnea and hypotension possible in catechol-depleted patients, bronchodilation, analgesia, increased IOP and ICP, nystagmus, mydriasis, peds: 01 mg/kg atropine + versed 0.05 mg/kg
Comments	Mix with 50 mL NS	Mix with 20 mL NS	Slow IV increments, 20–40 mg q 10 sec		Push slowly over 1–2 min

IV = intravenous, IM = intramuscular, ICP = intracranial pressure, CBF = cerebral blood flow, CPP = coronary perfusion pressure, IOP = intraocular pressure, MAP = mean arterial pressure, HR = heart rate, BP = blood pressure, NS = normal saline.

20. Why is succinylcholine the most common paralyzing agent in RSI?
No other neuromuscular blocking agent has as rapid an onset of action (45–60 seconds) or as brief a duration of activity (4–7 minutes). This provides added safety, with the return of spontaneous respiration within 7 minutes.

21. What are the theoretical risks of succinylcholine?
Despite its significant benefits, succinylcholine has many undesirable characteristics, some of which may be dangerous. It increases intragastric, intraocular, and intracranial pressure. Life-threatening hyperkalemia may occur in patients with neuromuscular disease or 3 to 4 days after major burns and trauma. Severe muscle contractions cause delayed pain and occasionally rhabdomyolysis. Rarely, it can precipitate malignant hyperthermia.

22. Are there any alternative paralytics?
- **Rocuronium** is gaining popularity, and many providers prefer rocuronium over succinylcholine. It has few complications and has an onset of action nearly as fast as succinylcholine. Its only significant drawback is a duration of action of 20 to 40 minutes.
- **Vecuronium** is another alternative, but its duration is even longer at 60 to 90 minutes. Pancuronium is a poor choice for RSI because of its slow onset of action. Newer nondepolarizing drugs with properties similar to succinylcholine are on the horizon.

23. Are there any contraindications to RSI?
Yes. Paralyze a patient only when you are sure he or she can be bag-mask ventilated if intubation is unsuccessful. Anticipation of a difficult airway based on anatomic features or traumatic anatomic distortion (e.g., patients with massive facial trauma or severe facial burns) is a relative contraindication. Inability to preoxygenate patients (e.g., patients with severe chronic obstructive pulmonary disease or asthma) is a relative contraindication to RSI. Patients with airway obstruction (foreign body, allergic reaction, airway infections, malignancies) who continue to make some respiratory effort should not be paralyzed.

24. How do I manage patients who have contraindications to RSI?
Nasotracheal intubation is a good alternative in patients with pulmonary disease. If unsuccessful, or if there is a contraindication to nasotracheal intubation, awake oral intubation with an induction agent, such as ketamine, allows the patient to maintain a certain degree of ventilation and airway protection during the procedure. Ketamine should not be used in head-injured patients because it dramatically increases intracranial pressure. Benzodiazepines, such as midazolam, may be useful for induction because they can be reversed easily with flumazenil if the need arises.

KEY POINTS: AIRWAY MANAGEMENT

1. Never paralyze a patient unless you are certain that he or she can be ventilated using a bag-valve-mask device.

2. Assume that all ED patients that require active airway management have a full stomach and require rapid-sequence intubation.

3. Objective measures like end-tidal CO_2 must be used to confirm endotracheal intubation in every patient.

4. The laryngeal mask airway device is an invaluable rescue tool that every practicing emergency physician should be familiar with.

5. Preoxygenation with 100% O_2 for 5 minutes is a critical component of rapid-sequence intubation preparation.

25. **Summarize the alternatives (rescue devices) available if these standard techniques fail.**
   1. **Cricothyrotomy,** a surgical airway through the cricothyroid membrane, can be done rapidly, although it often is complicated by hemorrhage and is contraindicated in children younger than 8 years.
   2. **Tracheotomy** is more time-consuming but is the surgical airway of choice in children and patients with tracheal injury.
   3. **Fiberoptic intubation** allows visualization of the cords and trachea but is technically difficult and time consuming.
   4. In **tactile intubation,** the practitioner uses his or her index and middle fingers to palpate the epiglottis and guide the tube through the cords. The patient needs to be comatose or heavily sedated, and the success rate is lower than that of RSI.
   5. **Retrograde intubation** involves placing a wire through the cricoid membrane and securing it through the mouth. The wire is used as a guide to pass the endotracheal tube.
   6. **Percutaneous transtracheal ventilation** involves inserting a catheter into the trachea and ventilating the patient with high-pressure oxygen.
   The two last techniques are used rarely and require prior training or special equipment.

26. **When the patient is intubated, how do I determine if the endotracheal tube is placed correctly?**
   The best method of confirming placement is to see the tube pass through the cords. Monitoring of oxygen saturation and the use of capnography or colorimetric end-tidal CO_2 devices are standard-of-care adjuncts. Other findings are helpful but are not definitive: The tube fogs and clears with ventilation, breath sounds are heard in both axillae but not over the stomach, and chest expansion is noted and symmetric.

   Walls R: Airway. In Marx JA, Hockverger RS, Walls RM (eds): Emergency Medicine Concepts and Clinical Practice, 5th ed. St. Louis, Mosby, 2002, pp 2–21.

27. **Doesn't the chest radiograph confirm placement in the trachea?**
   No. Although the chest radiograph is helpful in ruling out bronchial intubation, the tube easily can be placed in the esophagus and appear to be in the trachea proximal to the carina.

CHAPTER 4

SHOCK

Jason S. Haukoos, MD, MS

1. **Define shock.**

   Shock is a clinical syndrome characterized by widespread *inadequate* oxygenation and supply of nutrients to tissues and organs, resulting in cellular dysfunction.

2. **How common is shock?**

   Shock constitutes approximately 1% of all emergency department visits.

   > Kline JA: Shock. In Marx J (ed): Rosen's Emergency Medicine: Concepts and Clinical Practice, 5(th) ed. St. Louis, Mosby, 2002, pp 33–47.

3. **What is the overall mortality rate of patients who develop shock?**

   The mortality rate exceeds 20% for patients across all categories of shock.

4. **Name the five categories of shock and give examples of each.**

   - **Hypovolemic:** Trauma, gastrointestinal bleeding, ruptured ectopic pregnancy, ruptured abdominal aortic aneurysm, diabetic ketoacidosis
   - **Cardiogenic:** Acute myocardial infarction, cardiomyopathy, valvular dysfunction
   - **Distributive:** Sepsis, anaphylaxis, spinal cord injury
   - **Obstructive:** Pulmonary embolism, cardiac tamponade
   - **Toxic/metabolic:** Carbon monoxide, cyanide, beta blocker, calcium-channel blocker

5. **How do you identify a patient in shock?**

   A patient in shock will generally appear ill. Shock is a clinical syndrome that reflects hypoperfusion. A brief focused history and targeted physical examination will help determine if shock is present and identify its underlying etiology. Examples of system-based symptoms and signs include the following:

   - Central nervous system: Altered mental status
   - Cardiovascular: Decreased cardiac output, tachycardia, hypotension, weak rapid pulses
   - Pulmonary: Tachypnea, hyperpnea, pulmonary edema
   - Renal: Insufficiency, decreased urine output
   - Skin: Delayed capillary refill, cool in the setting of hypovolemic or cardiogenic shock and warm in the setting of distributive shock

6. **What other marker is used to identify someone in shock?**

   Serum lactate is a commonly used marker to assess the extent of systemic hypoperfusion and the degree to which a patient may be responding to resuscitation. Serum lactate concentrations > 4 mEq/L are associated with the highest mortality rates.

   > Shapiro NI, Howell MD, Talmor D, et al: Serum lactate as a predictor of mortality in emergency department patients with infection. Ann Emerg Med 45:524–528, 2005.

7. **What is the lactate clearance index? How can it be used during resuscitation of a patient in shock?**

   The lactate clearance index refers to measuring serum lactate concentrations at two or more times during the course of the resuscitation. If the serum lactate concentration has not decreased by 50% one hour after resuscitation has begun, additional steps should be undertaken to improve systemic perfusion.

Abramson D, Scalea TM, Hitchcock R, et al: Lactate clearance and survival following injury. J Trauma 35:584–588, 1993.

8. **Describe compensated and decompensated shock.**
Shock initiates a sequence of stress responses intended to preserve perfusion to vital organs. Compensated shock occurs soon after the onset of shock and is marked by the maintenance of tissue perfusion pressures. Such patients typically have evidence of a stress response (e.g., tachycardia and tachypnea) but also have a normal or high blood pressure and normal or mildly elevated serum lactate concentrations. If left untreated, compensated shock will progress to decompensated shock, which is characterized by profound global tissue hypoperfusion, elevated serum lactate concentrations, and hypotension.

9. **What is the initial management of a patient who presents in shock?**
Management of patients in shock begins with the ABCs (airway, breathing, and circulation). Due to poor delivery and uptake of oxygen, all patients should be placed on either 15 L of oxygen by nonrebreather or intubated. Simultaneously, all patients should have large-bore intravenous access and be placed on a cardiac monitor.

10. **Define oxygen delivery.**
Oxygen delivery is the product of the cardiac output and arterial oxygen concentration. Arterial oxygen concentration is defined by the hemoglobin level, the arterial oxygen saturation, and the arterial oxygen partial pressure. Maximizing cardiac output, hemoglobin, arterial oxygen saturation, and the arterial partial pressure of oxygen will maximize oxygen delivery.

$$DO_2 = CaO_2 \times CO$$

where DO_2 = oxygen delivery, CaO_2 = arterial oxygen concentration, and CO = cardiac output.

$$CaO_2 = (1.34 \times Hgb \times SaO_2) + (0.003 \times PaO_2)$$

where Hgb = hemoglobin, SaO_2 = arterial oxygen saturation, and PaO_2 = arterial oxygen partial pressure.

Marino PL: The ICU Book, 2nd ed. Baltimore, Williams & Wilkins, 1998.

11. **How useful are vital signs in assessing and treating someone in shock?**
Although cliché, vital signs are vital. Heart rate, respiratory rate, blood pressure, and pulse oximetry should be monitored closely in patients in shock. Physiologic compensation and decompensation (see question 7) are commonly reflected in a patient's vital signs. Additionally, normalization of abnormal vital signs is one indicator of a patient's response to resuscitation.

12. **If a patient has normal vital signs, should I be reassured?**
Not always. A patient's heart rate and blood pressure may be normal in the setting of severe illness. In the setting of shock, heart rate and blood pressure correlate poorly with cardiac output and often underestimate the severity of systemic hypoperfusion.

13. **What is the shock index (SI)?**
SI was first described in 1967 and is defined as the heart rate divided by the systolic blood pressure. Normal SI ranges from 0.5 to 0.7, and a SI > 0.9 is highly specific for global oxygen deficiency and ischemia and is associated with significant cardiac dysfunction, global hypoxia, and mortality.

14. **Are orthostatic vital signs a sensitive indicator of hypovolemia? What determines a positive orthostatic test?**
To know what is abnormal, you first must know what is normal. Studies on healthy euvolemic people showed an average increase in pulse of 13 to 18 beats/minute with a large standard

deviation. A pulse increase of 20 beats/minute as a determinant for hypovolemia is nonspecific because many normal individuals fall within this range. However, a 30 beats/minute increase in heart rate is more specific. A 20% volume loss is required to produce this change in heart rate, making this an insensitive test at best. The development of symptoms (e.g., lightheadedness on standing) does not occur in healthy euvolemic individuals on standing and should be considered abnormal. Patients in shock should not be allowed to stand to assess changes in vital signs.

15. **What is a normal central venous pressure (CVP)? How is it measured?**
A normal CVP ranges from 5 to 10 cm H_2O. CVP is measured by attaching an electronic pressure transducer or a water manometer to the end of a central line placed into the central venous system. The zero reference point for measuring a CVP is at the point that bisects the fourth intercostals space and the midaxillary line in a supine patient. This point corresponds to the position of the right atrium.

16. **How is CVP used during resuscitation of a patient in shock?**
The guiding principle for the CVP centers on normalizing or supranormalizing its value. The target CVP should range from 10 to 15 cm H_2O to maximize cardiac preload. In many shock states, the heart becomes stiff and its function depressed. A supranormal CVP thus allows for improved cardiac filling.

17. **How should urine output be used during resuscitation of a patient in shock?**
Patients in shock should have a Foley catheter placed to accurately measure urine output. Urine output is an excellent indicator of organ perfusion, assuming the patient has normal renal function. A normal urine output is > 1.0 mL/kg/hour, a *reduced* urine output ranges from 0.5 to 1.0 mL/kg/hour, and a *severely reduced* urine output is < 0.5 mL/kg/hour. During resuscitation, targeted therapy should additionally focus on improving or normalizing urine output.

18. **What is early goal-directed therapy?**
Goal-directed therapy refers to the practice of resuscitating patients to defined physiologic endpoints (e.g., mean arterial pressure, CVP, urine output, serum lactate concentration, cardiac output, hemoglobin level, venous oxygen saturation), indicating that systemic tissue perfusion and vital organ function have been restored. This has only been systematically studied in patients with sepsis; however, it is likely that early goal-directed therapies will be evaluated in other forms of shock, including those suffering from trauma and during the postresuscitation period following cardiac arrest.

Rivers EP, Nguyen B, Havstad S, et al: Early goal-directed therapy in the treatment of severe sepsis and septic shock. N Engl J Med 8:1368–1377, 2001.

19. **List the primary resuscitation goals in patients suffering from shock.**
   - Maximize oxygenation to improve delivery to tissues.
   - Establish adequate ventilation.
   - Improve hemodynamic dysfunction.
   - Treat the underlying etiology.

20. **What is the Trendelenburg position? What purpose(s) does it serve?**
Trendelenburg refers to the patient placed in a supine, approximately 45-degrees head-down position. The purposes of this position have been reported to include improving blood pressure, redistributing circulating blood volume, placing central lines, and improving the sensitivity of abdominal ultrasound for intra-abdominal fluid. Although commonly used for the purpose of improving hemodynamic parameters, several studies have not demonstrated its utility in significantly improving blood pressure or redistribution of blood volume.

KEY POINTS: SHOCK

1. The five categories of shock are hypovolemic, cardiogenic, distributive, obstructive, and toxic/metabolic.

2. Serum lactate is a commonly used marker to assess the extent of systemic hypoperfusion and the response to resuscitation.

3. Shock index (SI) is defined as the heart rate divided by the systolic blood pressure. Normal SI ranges from 0.5 to 0.7.

4. The primary resuscitation goals in patients suffering from shock are to maximize oxygenation, establish adequate ventilation, improve hemodynamic distribution, and treat the underlying cause.

21. **Define systemic inflammatory response syndrome (SIRS).**
SIRS is defined by two or more of the following:
- Temperature $> 38°C$ or $< 36°C$
- Heart rate > 90 beats/minute
- Respiratory rate > 20 breaths/minute or $PaCO_2 < 32$ mmHg
- Serum white blood cell count $> 12,000$ mm^3 or < 4000 mm^3 or 10% band forms

It is important to note that this definition, although standardized, is highly nonspecific for defining serious illness. Although most commonly related to sepsis, SIRS can result from a variety of noninfectious insults, including trauma, burns, pancreatitis, and overdose.

> Bone R: American College of Chest Physicians/Society of Critical Care Medicine Consensus Conference: Definitions for sepsis and organ failure and guidelines for the use of innovative therapies in sepsis. Crit Care Med 20:864–874, 1992.

22. **Define sepsis, severe sepsis, and septic shock, and discuss their specific therapies.**
See Chapter 46.

23. **How do I treat cardiogenic shock?**
The treatment of cardiogenic shock should focus on improving myocardial contractility and overall pump function. Provide oxygen and ventilatory support, including the judicious use of noninvasive positive-pressure ventilation when pulmonary edema is present. Initiate inotropic support using dobutamine (5 μg/kg/min), and identify the etiology and administer specific treatment (e.g., thrombolysis or percutaneous coronary intervention in the setting of acute coronary syndrome). Consider intra-aortic balloon counterpulsation or cardiopulmonary bypass for patients with refractory shock.

24. **Explain the mechanism of dobutamine.**
Dobutamine is a synthetic catecholamine with primarily β$_1$-receptor (cardiac stimulation) and mild β$_2$-receptor (vasodilation) agonism.

> Rivers EP, Amponsah D: Shock. In: Wolfson AB (ed): Harwood-Nuss' Clinical Practice of Emergency Medicine, 4th ed. Philadelphia, Lippincott Williams & Wilkins, 2005, pp 36–43.

25. **Explain the mechanism of dopamine.**
Dopamine is an endogenous catecholamine that when administered intravenously produces a dose-dependent activation of adrenergic and dopaminergic receptors. When given in low doses (e.g., 5 μg/kg/min), dopamine preferentially activates dopaminergic receptors, producing vasodilatation in renal, mesenteric, and cerebral circulations. When given in intermediate doses

(e.g., 5–10 µg/kg/min), dopamine stimulates ß-receptors, thus increasing cardiac output. When given in high doses (e.g., > 10 µg/kg/min), dopamine activates α-receptors, producing a dose-dependent increase in systemic vascular resistance. It is important to note that dopamine has modest inotropic characteristics when compared with dobutamine and that tachyphylaxis may result from its use if used for a prolonged period of time.

26. **How do I treat shock due to anaphylaxis?**
Anaphylaxis results in a distributive form of shock. As always, control the airway and provide appropriate levels of oxygenation and ventilation. Administer crystalloid in doses of 20 mL/kg to maximize intravascular volume and cardiac filling pressures. If the patient remains hypotensive or if airway compromise is present, administer either intramuscular (1:1000 at 0.3 mL or 0.01 mL/kg in children) or intravenous epinephrine (beginning at 0.02 µg/kg/minute and titrating to effect). Finally, administer intravenous diphenhydramine (25–50 mg in adults and 1.25 mg/kg in children) and methylprednisolone (1–2 mg/kg).

27. **Explain the mechanism of epinephrine.**
Similar to dopamine, epinephrine is a primary ß-receptor agonist at low doses and an α-receptor agonist at high doses. However, epinephrine is significantly more potent than dopamine.

28. **How do I treat shock due to pulmonary embolism (PE)?**
Massive PE causes shock by reducing the cross-sectional area of the pulmonary outflow tract, thus increasing right-sided heart pressures, reducing blood flow to the left side of the heart, all of which results in hemodynamic instability. Treatment centers on provision of oxygenation and ventilation, hemodynamic support using crystalloids and vasopressors, as necessary, and use of thrombolytics and/or surgical embolectomy in the setting of refractory shock.

29. **How do I treat shock due to cardiac tamponade?**
As always, ensure adequate oxygenation and ventilation. Administration of intravenous fluids may help overcome increased cardiac filling pressures. However, the principal therapies for cardiac tamponade are pericardiocentesis or pericardiotomy.

30. **What is neurogenic shock? How is it treated?**
Neurogenic shock is a form of distributive shock resulting from spinal cord injury in which central or peripheral sympathetic tone is lost. Such patients are commonly hypotensive with either a normal or low heart rate. Administer intravenous fluids to normalize intravascular volume. If hypotension persists, several vasopressor options exist, although intravenous phenylephrine (0.15–0.75 µg/kg/min) is considered the classical first-line agent.

Bell RM, Krantz BE: Initial assessment. In: Mattox KL, Feliciano DV, Moore EE (eds): Trauma, 4th ed. New York, McGraw-Hill, 2000, pp 153–170.

31. **Explain the mechanism of phenylephrine.**
Phenylephrine is a pure and potent α-agonist. Administration of this agent can induce a reflex bradycardia, resulting in decreased cardiac output.

CHAPTER 5

EMERGENCY ULTRASOUND

John L. Kendall, MD, and Katherine M. Bakes, MD

1. **What is emergency department (ED) ultrasound all about?**

   An ultrasound probe in the hands of the clinician is the stethoscope of the 21st century. It is noninvasive; it is safe; and when used appropriately, it can be another tool with which to perform certain focused aspects of the physical examination.

2. **Why should ultrasound be performed in the ED?**

   Limited ultrasound examinations performed by ED physicians allow for more timely, less invasive, and safer evaluations of patients. Ectopic pregnancy and biliary colic may be evaluated rapidly, intra-abdominal traumatic hemorrhage may be diagnosed without the invasiveness of diagnostic peritoneal lavage or the delay of a computed tomography (CT) scan, and patients with major trauma or suspected abdominal aortic aneurysm (AAA) may be evaluated quickly in the safety of the ED.

3. **How does emergency ultrasound differ from ultrasound performed by the radiology department?**

   Emergency ultrasound is meant to be a limited, goal-directed examination. Specific findings, such as the presence of intraperitoneal fluid in blunt abdominal trauma; intrauterine pregnancy (IUP) in suspected ectopic pregnancy; gallstones, wall thickness, or sonographic Murphy's sign in right upper quadrant pain; aortic dilation in suspected AAA; and pericardial fluid in patients with possible pericardial tamponade, are used to guide patient care. In contrast, a radiologist-performed ultrasound is more comprehensive. All of the structures in the requested type of ultrasound are evaluated and commented on.

4. **How about some basic ultrasonography physics?**

   Ultrasound images are generated as sound waves at various frequencies (MHz) that reflect off tissue interfaces. The higher the ultrasound frequency, the greater the resolution but at the cost of reduced tissue penetration. Dense tissues, such as bone or gallstones, appear bright because most of the ultrasound energy is absorbed or reflected. Solid organs, such as the liver or spleen, show a gray scale of tissue architecture. All of the ultrasound energy passes through fluid or blood, leaving a black, or anechoic, area on the screen. Ultrasound energy does not propagate through air well, so lung and hollow viscous structures are difficult to visualize. In general, abdominal and cardiac examinations are done using 3.5- to 5-MHz probes; transvaginal ultrasound examinations use 7.5- to 10-MHz probes, and vascular studies use 10- to 12-MHz specialized probes.

5. **Describe the basics of the trauma ultrasound examination.**

   The trauma ultrasound examination is done rapidly at the patient's bedside during the secondary survey. The primary goal is to detect free intraperitoneal fluid, which appears as anechoic areas within the peritoneal cavity. Sites in the abdomen that are evaluated are the potential spaces that occur at dependent sites within the peritoneal cavity. These include the hepatorenal recess or Morison's pouch (Fig. 5-1), splenorenal recess, retrovesicular recess (pouch of Douglas), and both pericolic gutters. Oblique views of the right and left chest are obtained to search for hemothorax, and a subxiphoid or left parasternal cardiac image is obtained to locate pericardial effusion (Fig. 5-2).

KEY POINTS: PRIMARY CHARACTERISTICS OF THE EMERGENCY ULTRASOUND EXAM

1. Performed for a defined indication

2. Focused, not complete

3. Easily learned and quickly performed

4. Directed toward one or two easily recognizable findings

5. Directly impacts clinical decision making

6. Performed at the bedside

6. **Where is the best place to look for intraperitoneal fluid?**
The sonographic examination should include all of the sites mentioned previously. The sensitivity increases from approximately 60% if one site is viewed to almost 90% if all sites are used. At least one study has shown the most sensitive site to be the pouch of Douglas (58% sensitive).

Ma OJ, Kefer MP, Mateer JR, Thoma B: Evaluation of hemoperitoneum using a single- vs multiple-view ultrasonographic examination. Acad Emerg Med 2:581–586, 1995.

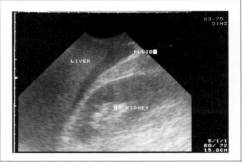

Figure 5-1. View of Morison's pouch shows intraperitoneal fluid.

7. **How does ultrasound compare with traditional means of evaluating the traumatic abdomen?**
Physical examination is only 50–60% sensitive for detecting abdominal injuries after blunt trauma. Diagnostic peritoneal lavage is 95% sensitive but is not specific, resulting in unnecessary laparotomies. CT is sensitive for detecting abdominal injuries ($> 95\%$) but is costly, is time consuming, and requires the patient to leave the ED. Prospective studies of ultrasound showed an 85–90% sensitivity for

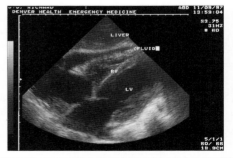

Figure 5-2. Subxiphoid cardiac view shows a pericardial effusion.

the detection of hemoperitoneum, with sensitivity approaching 100% in patients who were hypotensive from an abdominal source. The accuracy of ultrasound to detect the underlying parenchymal lesion varies widely.

8. **How should I use ultrasound in my evaluation of blunt trauma patients?**
A good start would be to consider it for patient scenarios based on vital signs and ultrasound findings: (1) stable vital signs, negative ultrasound; (2) stable vital signs, positive ultrasound; (3) unstable vital signs, negative ultrasound; and (4) unstable vital signs, positive ultrasound. Patients with stable vital signs and a negative ultrasound who have no other significant injuries, have normal mental status, and are not intoxicated can be managed with observation, serial physical examinations, and serial ultrasound studies. Patients with stable vital signs and a positive ultrasound warrant an abdominal CT scan. If the vital signs are unstable and ultrasound is negative or indeterminate, a bedside diagnostic peritoneal lavage should be done. If the vital signs are unstable and the ultrasound is positive for free fluid, the patient should go directly to laparotomy.

Branney SW, Moore EE, Cantrill SV, et al: Ultrasound based key clinical pathway reduces the use of hospital resources for the evaluation of blunt abdominal trauma. J Trauma 42:1086–1090, 1997.

9. **Can I tell how much intraperitoneal fluid is present based on the ultrasound image?**
No. Conflicting data exist, but no study has yet shown any accurate means of quantifying the amount of intraperitoneal fluid that is present based on its sonographic appearance.

10. **What are some of the pitfalls I may encounter during a trauma ultrasound examination of the abdomen?**
Although relatively rare, one of the more concerning aspects of emergency ultrasound is the false-negative study. In terms of abdominal trauma, clotted blood is the finding that mimics a negative study the closest. An example of clotted blood found in Morison's pouch is shown in Fig. 5-3. It initially was interpreted to be liver parenchyma because of a similar echogenic pattern. False-positive findings simulate hemoperitoneum. Examples are ascites, urine from a ruptured bladder, bowel contents from bowel perforation, perinephric fat, and fluid-filled bowel.

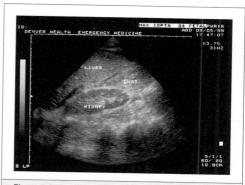

Figure 5-3. Clotted blood in Morison's pouch.

11. **What is the sonographic appearance of the gallbladder and related structures?**
The gallbladder is cystic, so the sonographic appearance is a pearlike structure that is anechoic. Surrounding this anechoic area is a ring of midechogenicity that corresponds to the gallbladder wall. Normally, it is less than 4 mm wide, but can be thicker immediately after eating or if in edematous states, such as liver disease, ascites, congestive heart failure, renal disease, or acquired immunodeficiency syndrome (AIDS). Stones are typically circular in nature, can be of any size, and are bright, or hyperechoic, on their proximal side. Ultrasound does not penetrate stones well, so distal to the stone there is a shadow (Fig. 5-4). This also is called the *headlight*

sign, signifying the presence of a calcified gallstone. Sludge is a collection of the precipitants of bile that layers within the gallbladder and appears sonographically as mildly echogenic material without any shadowing.

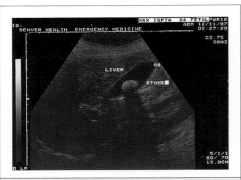

Figure 5-4. Long-axis view of the gallbladder shows a gallstone. The gallstone is represented by an echogenic proximal surface and distal attenuation shadow.

12. **What findings are suggestive of acute cholecystitis?**
    The primary findings of the emergency gallbladder ultrasound are the presence of stones, sonographic Murphy's sign (defined as maximal tenderness over an ultrasound-detected gallbladder), and wall thickening (> 4 mm). The presence of all three primary findings has a 99% positive predictive value for the presence of gallbladder disease. Other findings, such as ductal dilation, pericholecystic fluid, sludge, and an emphysematous gallbladder, are considered to be secondary findings and are less reliably seen by emergency sonographers. Ultrasound is insensitive at detecting choledocholithiasis.

    Kendall JL, Shimp RJ: Performance and interpretation of focused right upper quadrant ultrasound by emergency physicians. J Emerg Med 21:7–13, 2001.

    Ralls PW, Colletti PM, Chandrasoma P, et al: Real-time sonography in suspected acute cholecystitis. Radiology 155:767–771, 1985.

13. **What are the indications for pelvic ultrasonography in the ED?**
    Ultrasonography is the imaging study of choice for evaluating abdominal pain or bleeding in pregnant patients in the first or second trimester. The goal of ED ultrasound is to establish the presence of an IUP, so as to rule out effectively an ectopic pregnancy. Ectopic pregnancy is the second leading cause overall of maternal mortality and the number one cause of maternal mortality during the first trimester.

14. **How early can an IUP be detected using ultrasound? What value of β-human chorionic gonadotropin (HCG) does this correspond to?**
    An IUP may be detectable at 5 weeks by transvaginal ultrasound at a β-HCG level of 1800 mIU/mL and at 6 weeks or greater with a β-HCG of 5000 mIU/mL using transabdominal ultrasound. The **discriminatory zone,** or level of β-HCG at which one would expect to see evidence of an IUP, depends on the institution.

15. **How sensitive is ultrasound for the evaluation of ectopic pregnancy?**
    Several studies have shown that 75–80% of patients have a diagnostic ultrasound (i.e., either an IUP or a demonstrable ectopic pregnancy). The problem is that in the remaining 20% of patients with nondiagnostic ultrasounds, nearly one fourth have ectopic pregnancies. This increase in ectopic pregnancy among patients with nondiagnostic ultrasound suggests that this group should have an aggressive workup, including an obstetric-gynecologic consultation in the ED.

    Braffman BH, Coleman BG, Ramchandani P, et al: Emergency department screening for ectopic pregnancy: A prospective US study. Radiology 190:797–802, 1994.

16. **Describe the pitfalls in pelvic ultrasonography.**

For emergency physicians, the goal of pelvic ultrasonography is to determine whether an IUP is present. It is not clear how well emergency physicians evaluate the adnexa, pelvic free fluid, or ovaries. Cornual pregnancies may be mistaken for an IUP, with an attendant risk of rupture and hemorrhage. The question of heterotopic pregnancies (i.e., simultaneous IUP and ectopic pregnancy) must be considered. In populations without risk factors for ectopic pregnancy, the risk of a heterotopic gestation is approximately 1 in 30,000 pregnancies. The incidence increases markedly, however, in patients with preexisting pelvic inflammatory disease or scarring and is greatest for patients receiving medical fertility assistance, in whom the incidence is estimated to be 1 in 100 to 1 in 400 pregnancies. A pseudosac can be seen in 20% of ectopic pregnancies. It is formed in response to the β-HCG produced by the abnormal pregnancy. It consists of a single-ringed structure in the endometrial cavity, and it can be mistaken for a true gestational sac, which consists of **two** concentric rings.

17. **What other abdominal structures can be evaluated by emergency ultrasound?**

Evaluation of the abdominal aorta can be useful in elderly patients who present with a pulsatile abdominal mass, nontraumatic abdominal pain or flank pain, hypotension of unknown cause, or unexplained pulseless electrical activity. AAA is manifested by aortic diameter greater than 3 cm with most symptomatic aneurysms being greater than 5 cm (Fig. 5-5). Studies by radiologists and emergency physicians showed sensitivity and specificity of 100% for the detection of AAA. Studies showed a 90% correlation of ultrasound-determined aortic diameter to pathologic specimens.

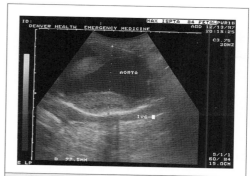

Figure 5-5. Long-axis view of a 7.75-cm diameter abdominal aortic aneurysm.

Kuhn M, Bonnin RL, Davey MJ, et al: Emergency department ultrasound scanning for abdominal aortic aneurysm: Accessible, accurate and advantageous. Ann Emerg Med 36:219–223, 2000.

18. **What is the significance of increased aortic diameter?**

Longitudinal studies have shown that patients with AAA have an increase in aortic diameter of approximately 0.5 cm/year. Patients with an aortic diameter of greater than 5 cm have a 25% chance of rupture within 5 years, with larger aneurysms having a greater chance of rupture. Aneurysms that rupture have a mortality of greater than 80%, so ultrasound is an important tool in the detection of AAA.

19. **Describe the uses of cardiac ultrasonography in the ED.**

There are two primary indications for cardiac ultrasonography in the ED. It may be used during the trauma examination to detect pericardial effusions in patients thought to have mechanisms of injury or clinical presentations consistent with pericardial tamponade or cardiac rupture. Detection of nontraumatic pericardial effusions is also possible (i.e., malignancy, uremic, rheumatologic). The other major indication is for the evaluation of patients presenting in cardiac arrest. Contractility can be assessed in patients presenting in cardiac arrest when there is a question of pulseless electrical activity. When patients have no evidence of cardiac contractility and other reversible causes of pulseless electrical activity have been ruled out, strong consideration should be given to terminating the resuscitation.

20. How can ultrasound be used to evaluate flank pain?
Ultrasound has been used to identify hydronephrosis and urinary calculi. Hydronephrosis is dilation of the renal pelvis and ureter caused by distal obstruction of the collecting system. Urinary calculi can be seen at any point from the renal pelvis to the ureteral-vesicular junction and appear as hyperechoic, round structures with distal attenuation shadows.

KEY POINTS: PRIMARY INDICATIONS FOR EMERGENCY ULTRASOUND

1. Blunt abdominal trauma

2. Suspected pericardial effusion/tamponade

3. Suspected ectopic pregnancy

4. Suspected AAA

5. Suspected gallbladder disease

6. Ultrasound-guided central access

7. Suspected renal colic

21. What is the role of ultrasound in the evaluation of patients with flank pain?
The results of studies have been discouraging. By itself, ultrasound is only 64–75% sensitive for the identification of renal calculi and even less sensitive for the evaluation of acute hydronephrosis. Studies that combined kidney, ureter, and bladder radiographs and ultrasound in well-hydrated patients showed improved ability to identify kidney stones and hydronephrosis. In the end, a noncontrast CT is a far superior imaging tool for the patients presenting with suspected renal colic.

22. What are some future applications for emergency ultrasound?
The uses for emergency ultrasound continue to be elucidated. For instance, one of the fastest-growing applications is to guided invasive procedures. This is not confined with vascular access but also other procedures such as localization and drainage of abscesses, lumbar puncture, placement of an intravenous pacer wire, or suprapubic bladder aspiration, to name a few. Other tremendously useful applications are the evaluation of patients in cardiac arrest, undifferentiated hypotension or shock, suspected deep venous thrombosis, and testicular torsion.

23. Has the political environment changed with respect to emergency physicians using ultrasound?
Yes, a lot has changed in recent years. Ultrasound use by emergency physicians has gone from a novelty experience to something that is tested on emergency medicine specialty boards and the national inservice exam, taught in the vast majority, if not all residency programs, and used in a widespread fashion in clinical practice. As such, the question is no longer whether or not it will be used by emergency physicians, but rather how it can be used to best improve the care of ED patients.

CHAPTER 6

GERIATRIC EMERGENCY MEDICINE

Kenneth C. Jackimczyk, MD

1. Why dedicate a chapter to geriatric emergency medicine?

Elderly persons are a rapidly growing segment of the population. In 2004, approximately 36 million people in the United States were older than age 65. By the year 2030, this number is expected to double, and over the next 20 years the number of individuals older than age 85 will grow three times faster than the general population.

Geriatric patients have unique medical and social characteristics. Patients older than 65 years account for 15% of all emergency department (ED) visits. Elderly patients frequently arrive in ambulances, stay in the ED longer, require more diagnostic studies, and have a higher admission rate than younger patients.

Administration on Aging: Older Americans in 2004: Key Indicators of Well Being. Available at www.aoa.dhhs.org

Meldon SW, Ma OJ, Woolard R (eds): Geriatric Emergency Medicine. New York, McGraw-Hill, 2004.

2. What important physiologic changes occur with aging?

- Musculoskeletal: Loss of muscle strength, impaired mobility, decreased bone mass
- Cardiovascular: Decreased cardiac output, increased systolic blood pressure
- Pulmonary: Increased lung compliance, decreased functional reserve
- HEENT: Impaired hearing and vision
- Renal: Decreased renal blood flow and glomerular filtration rate (GFR)
- Immune system: Decreased cellular immunity
- Dermatologic: Impaired thermoregulation

3. List the top 10 reasons elderly patients come to the ED.

1. Chest pain
2. Trauma
3. Pneumonia
4. Congestive heart failure
5. Abdominal pain
6. Electrolyte imbalance or dehydration
7. Stroke
8. Diabetes
9. Change in mental status
10. Sepsis

KEY POINTS: PRINCIPLES OF GERIATRIC EMERGENCY MEDICINE

1. Vital signs can be normal in the elderly patient with serious illness.

2. Adverse medication reactions are common in elderly patients.

3. Atypical presentations of serious diseases are more common.

4. **How can emergency medical services (EMS) personnel facilitate the care of elderly patients?**

Elderly patients account for more than one third of EMS transports to the ED. EMS personnel can obtain information from family or health care workers at the scene regarding the patient's social and physical environment, his or her baseline functional and mental status, and the reason for EMS activation. Ambulance personnel should obtain lists of medications the patient is using and any documentation regarding living wills or advance directives.

5. **What is the significance of fever in elderly patients?**

Elderly patients presenting with fever have a significant risk of bacteremia. Conversely, because of their blunted fever response, bacteremic elderly patients may not be febrile. Don't be lulled into complacency by a lack of fever in an ill-appearing elderly patient.

6. **What are the four types of elder abuse?**
   1. **Physical abuse:** Nonaccidental force that results in bodily injury, pain, or impairment (e.g., hitting, biting, slapping, sexual assault, burns, or unreasonable restraint [physical, chemical])
   2. **Psychological abuse:** An act carried out with the intent of causing emotional pain or injury (e.g., threats to abandon, institutionalize, or harm physically)
   3. **Exploitation:** Caretaker use of the resources of an elder for monetary or personal profit (e.g., stealing Social Security checks or retirement checks or coercion to change wills or other legal documents)
   4. **Neglect:** Failure of the caretaker to provide the services necessary to avoid physical harm, mental anguish, or mental illness. This neglect can be *intentional* (e.g., willfully withholding food or medicine, abandonment for prolonged periods, or failure to provide proper hygiene) or *unintentional* (e.g., caretaker forgets to administer medicine or food or is physically unable to provide services for the patient)

   Kleinschmidt KC. Elder abuse: A review. Ann Emerg Med 30:463–472, 1997.

7. **What red flags in the history should alert the physician to the possibility of elder abuse?**
   - Delay in presentation with injury
   - Discrepancies in history between patient and caregiver
   - Vague or implausible explanation for injury
   - Repetitive injuries
   - Missed appointments and noncompliance with medications
   - Frequent ED visits for a chronic illness (despite a clear and previously defined medical plan)
   - No caregiver accompanying an impaired patient to the ED

8. **What red flags in the physical examination should alert the physician to the possibility of elder abuse?**
   - Subdued, oversedated, or withdrawn behavior
   - Unkempt or soiled appearance
   - Poor nutrition or dehydration
   - Multiple or unexplained bruises or cuts
   - Gross decubiti or pressure sores
   - Burns or bites
   - Rectal or vaginal bruises or tears
   - Occult fracture

9. **Why is it important to know the elderly patient's current medications?**

Adverse drug related events are a significant cause of morbidity in elderly patients and are the most common cause of iatrogenic illness in elderly patients. The average elderly person uses more than four prescription drugs and more than two over-the-counter medications daily. These numbers are even higher for institutionalized patients. Adverse reactions to medications occur twice as often in elderly patients and are directly proportional to the number of medications being taken.

Hohl CM, Dankoff J, Colacone A, et al: Polypharmacy: Adverse drug-related events and potential adverse drug interactions in elderly patients presenting to an emergency department. Ann Emerg Med 38:666–671, 2001.

10. **What presenting complaints should lead me to suspect that the patient is experiencing an adverse reaction to medications?**
    - Altered level of consciousness
    - Weakness
    - Dizziness
    - Syncope

11. **Should I worry if a geriatric trauma victim has normal vital signs with apparently minor injuries?**
    Yes. Elderly patients have the highest trauma mortality rate of any age group. Geriatric patients have a blunted tachycardic response to injury. A "normal" blood pressure of 120/80 mmHg may represent relative hypotension in the elderly hypertensive patient. The elderly patient's diminished cardiovascular reserve, the increased susceptibility to fractures, and the presence of comorbid conditions such as coronary artery disease can result in significant morbidity, even with injuries that appear to be minor. Normal vital signs or a low injury severity score should never put the physician at ease.

D'Andrea CC: Geriatric trauma. In Ferrera PC, Colucciello SA, Marx JA, et al. (eds): Trauma Management: An Emergency Medicine Approach. St. Louis, Mosby, 2001, pp 533–545.

12. **Which presentations in geriatric trauma are associated with an extremely high mortality rate?**
    - Automobile-pedestrian accidents (>50% mortality)
    - Presenting systolic blood pressure less than 130 mmHg
    - Acidosis (pH <7.35)
    - Multiple fractures
    - Head injury (67% of unconscious elderly trauma patients die)
    - Pelvic fractures

Mandavia D: Geriatric trauma. Emerg Med Clin North Am 16:257–274, 1998.

13. **Aren't falls a fact of life in elderly Patients?**
    No. Any fall in an elderly patient should raise concern. Ten to 15% of geriatric falls result in serious injury, and 50% of hospitalized patients die within 1 year of their fall.

14. **What is different about evaluating the elderly patient after a fall?**
    It is essential to assess the *cause* of the fall as well as the *injuries* that have occurred. Falls may result from either physiologic or environmental factors. Physiologic factors include muscle weakness, gait disorders, visual impairment, and syncope. Environmental disorders include dark hallways, loose rugs, and low-lying tables. The evaluation for syncope should focus on acute cardiovascular causes (dysrhythmias, myocardial infarction), neurologic events, hypovolemia, and adverse reactions to medications.

KEY POINTS: FALLS IN GERIATRIC PATIENTS

1. Falls in elderly patients are a serious problem.

2. Check for both physiologic and environmental causes of the fall.

3. Consider syncope as the cause of the fall.

15. **Don't elderly patients always have abnormal laboratory values?**

No. In contrast to pediatric patients, most laboratory values in elderly patients do not require different reference ranges from traditional adult values. The fact that the patient is old should not be used to justify abnormal laboratory values. There are, however, some exceptions in patients older than age 65:

- Elevated serum alkaline phosphatase (may be 2.5 times greater than the normal)
- Elevated fasting blood glucose (135 to 150 mg/dL)
- Elevated erythrocyte sedimentation rate (40 mm/hour)
- Decreased hemoglobin (11.0 g/dL in women or 11.5 g/dL in men)
- Elevated blood urea nitrogen (28 to 35 mg/dL)

Sanders AB: Emergency Care of the Elder Person. St. Louis, Beverly Cracom Publications, 1996.

16. **Can procedural sedation be performed safely in the geriatric patient?**

Yes, but the physician must be aware of the altered pharmacokinetics and pharmacodynamics in elderly patients. As the body ages, there is a reduction in lean body mass and total body water and an increase in total body fat. There also is a decrease in renal and hepatic blood flow. This has an effect on the metabolism and the distribution of medications administered to an elderly patient. Elderly patients have increased central nervous system sensitivity to analgesic and sedative medications. Remember: *start low and go slow.*

17. **Should I be concerned about atypical presentations of acute myocardial infarction (AMI) in elderly patients?**

Yes. AMI is the leading cause of death in elderly patients. Half of all AMIs occur in elderly patients and result in 80% of all deaths due to AMI. Nearly 40% of elderly patients diagnosed with AMI did not complain of chest pain on presentation, and, similarly, 50% had no evidence of ischemia or infarct on their presenting electrocardiogram (ECG). For these reasons, it is imperative that the ED physician know the atypical presentations of AMI in elderly patients. The mnemonic **GRANDFATHERS** refers to atypical presentations of AMI in elderly patients:

General malaise	**F**alls or **F**lu symptoms
Refers to a gastrointestinal complaint	**A**typical chest pain
Altered mental status	**T**rouble walking
Neurologic deficits	**H**ypotension
Dyspnea	**E**xhaustion
	Reverse in functional status
	Syncope or presyncope

18. **Should I resuscitate the elderly patient in cardiac arrest?**

Yes. Resuscitation studies document no difference in the percentage of successful outcomes across the age spectrum, and elderly patients who survive are no more likely to sustain irreversible brain injury than younger patients. Unless there is a well-defined advance directive, there should be no discrimination based on age in resuscitating elderly patients in cardiac arrest.

Gazmuri RJ. Outcome after cardiopulmonary resuscitation: Is age a factor. Crit Care Med 27:2295–2296, 1999.

19. **Is it safe to use thrombolytics in the elderly patient?**

Yes. Despite the increased incidence of intracerebral hemorrhage in geriatric patients, most studies show benefits to using thrombolytics in elderly patients.

20. **How does my approach to acute abdominal pain change in elderly patients?**
Acute abdominal pain in elderly patients is a serious complaint. More than half of geriatric patients with acute abdominal pain will require admission. Delay in presentation and the decreased pain perception associated with aging make perforation more likely. Atypical presentations of intra-abdominal diseases are more common in elderly patients. Pay attention to vital signs, but do not be lulled into a false sense of security if the vital signs are normal. Keep a broad differential diagnosis and consider the common disorders such as appendicitis and cholecystitis but also remember diseases specific to older patients, such as diverticulitis, volvulus, mesenteric ischemia, abdominal aortic aneurysm, and carcinomas. Do not forget extra-abdominal sources, such as pneumonia or AMI. Do not delay surgical consultation waiting for laboratory results or radiographs.

21. **Which is more serious, dementia or delirium?**
Delirium. Delirium is considered a medical emergency. A change in mental status is a common presentation to the ED for many elderly patients. It is also common for patients already to have an underlying dementia. To attribute a change in mental status to worsening dementia is a serious error because delirium is reversible and carries with it a higher mortality.

O'Keefe KP: Elderly patients with altered mental status. Emerg Med Clin North Am 16:701–715, 1998.

22. **How do I differentiate between delirium and dementia?**
See Table 6-1.

TABLE 6-1. DIFFERENTIATION BETWEEN DELIRIUM AND DEMENTIA	
Delirium	**Dementia**
Acute in onset	Insidious in onset
Decreased level of consciousness	Clear consciousness
Waxes and wanes	Progressive decline
Reversible cause	Usually irreversible cause
Irregular sleep-wake pattern	Regular sleep-wake pattern

23. **What special concerns are there in discharging elderly patients?**
- **Cognitive function:** Can the patient still live independently and self-administer medications?
- **Physical function:** Can the patient perform the activities of daily living? Does the patient require assistance devices such as wheelchairs?
- **Physical environment:** Can the patient safely return with his or her current cognitive or functional status? Did the current environment contribute to the ED presentation?
- **Social environment:** Will the caregiver or spouse be able to care for the patient? Is health care supervision available?
- **Resources:** Is a telephone available? Is money available for medicine or follow-up appointments? Is there transportation to get to a follow-up appointment?

CHAPTER 7

SAFETY IN EMERGENCY MEDICINE

Robert L. Wears, MD, MS, and Patrick G. Croskerry, MD, PhD

PATIENT SAFETY

1. **The emergency department (ED) has been described as a "natural laboratory" for the study of safety. What makes it so?**

   The typical work conditions in EDs detract from optimal human performance. These might be divided into two types: failure-producing conditions (FPCs) and violation-producing conditions (VPCs). The former lead to what in folk wisdom is called "human error," and the latter are conditions that lead people to deviate from formal procedures.

2. **Define some basic safety terms.**

   An **error** is a term of historical interest only. It was originally defined as the failure of a planned action to be completed as intended (i.e., error of execution) or the use of a wrong plan to achieve an aim (i.e., error of planning). The concept of error has not proven useful in creating safer systems of care and in fact may be harmful, because of its slipperiness and the pejorative baggage that it carries.

   Active faults are those whose effects are seen immediately. They are most often associated with those who perform on the front line (the ED is as front line as it gets).

   A **latent fault** is one whose adverse consequences may lie dormant for some time, and only becoming evident when it combines with other factors to breach the system's defenses. Responsibility for latent faults can often be laid at the feet of those who designed or manage the system.

   Slips describe attentional or perceptual failures in the execution of an observable action sequence. Covert internal events (generally associated with memory failures) leading to a failure of execution are referred to as *lapses*. Both slips and lapses are actions that deviate from an intended plan.

   A **mistake** is a deficiency or failure in either the judgment or inferential process involved in the selection of an objective, or in the specification of the means to achieve it, irrespective of whether or not the actions directed by this decision-scheme run according to plan.

   An **incident** or **near miss** is a failure in some aspect of care that is either caught in time, mitigated, or fortunately has no effect on the patient.

   An **accident** or **adverse event** is an injury caused by medical management rather than the underlying condition of the patient. Both incidents and accidents are typically judged according to their preventability, but this is a fraught concept.

   Negligent adverse events represent a subset of preventable adverse events that satisfy legal criteria used in determining negligence (i.e., whether or not the care provided failed to meet the standard of care reasonably expected of an average physician qualified to take care of the patients in question).

   Leape LL: Error in medicine. JAMA 272:1851–1857, 1994.
   Reason J: Managing the Risks of Organizational Accidents. Aldershot, UK, Ashgate Publishing, 1997.

3. **Why don't we use the term *error* anymore?**

Error is a folk model for explaining performance. Errors are mental constructs that are developed after the fact to explain outcomes. They are like optical illusions, simultaneously convincing and misleading. If we could make health care safer but still committed errors, we would be pleased, and if we eliminated errors but still had the same burden of adverse events we would not. The problem is not error; the problem is harm.

Berwick DM: Patient safety: Lessons from a novice. Focus Patient Safety 4(3):3, 2001.
Wears RL: Beyond error. Acad Emerg Med 7:1175–1176, 2000.
Woods DD, Cook RI: Nine steps to move forward from error. Cogn Technol Work 4:137–144, 2002.

4. **I've heard the term *iatrogenic*. Isn't that when physicians make mistakes?**

Yes. The term *iatrogenic* was originally used to describe "disorders induced in the patient by autosuggestion based on the physician's examination, manner, or discussion" but later gained a broader definition as "the creation of additional problems or complications resulting from treatment by a physician or surgeon" (Dorland's Medical Dictionary, 25th ed, 1974). Recently, it has come to be used in a more general sense to describe adverse outcomes that result from a patient's treatment within the health care system. A more appropriate term to describe such error is *comiogenic*, proposed by Sharpe and Faden (1998). It has its origin in the Greek root *komein* "to take care of," familiar to us in the term *nosocomial*, which describes disease (Gr. *nosos*) that originates in the hospital. This new term has the advantage of embracing the diverse sources of harm that can occur to patients in health care systems.

Sharpe VA, Faden AI. Medical Harm: Historical, Conceptual and Ethical Dimensions of Iatrogenic Illness. New York: Cambridge University Press; 1998.

5. **What's the breakdown of safety problems in the ED?**

We really don't know, as there haven't been any systematic studies to date. Most of what is known comes from incidental observations made in the major studies on hospitalized patients who came through the ED, a few ED studies, and anecdotal observations. It appears that the incident rate, especially of slips and lapses, is probably quite high but that the majority of these are corrected before they result in an adverse outcome. One thing appears clear: The most costly and deadly problems generally result from mistakes associated with delayed or missed diagnoses.

6. **Am I likely to survive a career in emergency medicine (EM) without being involved in a serious adverse event?**

No. When you work in a jungle, you get bitten by snakes.

7. **What's the ratio of detected to undetected failures?**

About 1:50.

Kohn LT, Corrigan JM, Donaldson MS (eds): To Err is Human: Building a Safer Health System. Washington, DC, National Academy Press, 1999.

8. **What proportion of adverse events are preventable?**

About 70%.

Kohn LT, Corrigan JM, Donaldson MS, eds. To Err is Human: Building a Safer Health System. Washington, DC, National Academy Press, 1999.

9. **What are FPCs? Give examples in the ED.**

An FPC is any factor or condition that increases the probability of failure in a given system. There is no other area of medicine in which this combination of FPCs exists. If you hadn't already realized it, you have chosen a career in one of the most difficult areas of medicine.

- Diagnostic uncertainty
- High decision density
- High cognitive load

- Novel or infrequently occurring situations
- Time limitations for detection and correction of error
- Low signal-to-noise ratio
- Overcrowding/channel capacity overload (**R**esource **A**vailability **C**ontinuous **Q**uality **I**mprovement **T**rade-**O**ff [RACQITO])
- Mismatch between real and perceived risk
- Poor feedback
- Poor quality of person-to-person information transfer
- Experience/training/education limitations
- Disruption of circadian rhythms by shift work
- Compromised task-pacing through interruptions/interventions
- High physical and emotional stress levels

10. **Most of these look self-evident, but what is meant by the low signal-to-noise ratio FPC?**

    Signals are critical pieces of information that must not be missed. No signal is received in isolation. All signals are accompanied by noise, which consists of distracting stimuli or pieces of information that reduce the likelihood of detecting the signal. A low signal-to-noise ratio occurs when the base-rate or incidence of the serious condition or diagnosis is low (e.g., subarachnoid hemorrhage) and well exceeded by the more common and usually benign diagnoses (tension and migraine headaches). The major problem in detection is that the signs and symptoms of both the signal and the noise can often be very similar to each other. Unfortunately, low signal-to-noise ratios exist for all serious conditions that present in the ED (e.g., abdominal aortic aneurysm as a cause of abdominal pain, pulmonary embolus as a cause of dyspnea, ectopic pregnancy as a cause of syncope, spinal column infection as a cause of low back pain, aortic dissection as a cause of chest pain).

11. **What is the significance of the high cognitive load FPC?**

    Cognitive load refers to the amount of thinking activity that an emergency physician must deal with at a given moment in time. It requires varying degrees of memory, concentration, processing, and problem solving. Not infrequently, physicians are responsible for a variety of patients with a variety of illnesses, with a variety of acuities. It is akin to a juggler maintaining a number of objects in the air at the same time. In no other branch of medicine is cognitive load so high and the burden of switching cognitive frames so great.

12. **How can we reduce cognitive load?**

    In an ideal world, we should not be put in situations in which cognitive loading is excessive because, inevitably, this will lead to failure. However, the pace of the ED is sometimes difficult to predict, and there will be times when volume and acuity reach dangerous levels no matter how well one has prepared. Under these conditions, any strategy or device that reduces the amount of cognitive work and cognitive time will reduce cognitive load. Appropriate designation and delegation of tasks within the caregiver team distributes the cognitive load and reduces the individual burden. Other examples are as follows:

    - Mnemonics
    - Hand-held computers
    - Algorithms
    - Decision rules
    - Clinical practice guidelines/pathways
    - Broselow-Luten pediatric resuscitation color-coding system

13. **Don't all these aids lead to "medicine by numbers" and reduce my autonomy?**

    The practice of medicine is more complex than ever, and we need all the cognitive help we can get. There is ample room left for autonomy and clinical judgment. In addition, these aids can never be made specific enough to fit all clinical circumstances, so judgment in their application is still required.

14. How does the poor feedback FPC cause failures?

The efficient performance of any system depends on timely and reliable feedback. Good feedback results in good calibration, and physicians are no exception. In the absence of feedback, emergency physicians will assume their diagnoses and management are acceptable and there is no need to change behavior or recalibrate. The reliability and timeliness of feedback in the ED are generally poor. Whether we admit patients to the hospital or discharge them to outpatient care, we rarely know the consequences of our actions.

15. What is RACQITO?

It refers to conditions under which the vital signs of the ED become unstable. It is a tipping point at which a trade-off begins between the resources available to the ED and the ability of the people working there to maintain continuous quality improvement of care. Under conditions of RACQITO, the failure rate goes up and the quality of patient care declines.

16. What are VPCs? Give examples in the ED.

VPCs are factors that lead clinicians to deviate from formal procedures or from other customs of good practice. They are associated with individual performance characteristics, having their origins in gender, cultural (local and general), and personality traits. Some examples are as follows:

- Underconfidence
- Overconfidence
- Perceived requirement to follow authority gradient
- Safety procedure compliance seen as an inconvenience
- Maladaptive group pressures
- Maladaptive copying behavior
- Risk-taking behavior
- Individual and/or group normalization of deviance
- Production pressure

In addition, some sorts of violations (*necessary violations*) are present in a complex system such as the ED. These are violations that are required to get the work done or meet production goals. For example, "working to rule," that is, refusing to engage in necessary violations, is a common job action strategy that can bring production to a halt.

17. What is normalization of deviance?

First, the "deviance" refers to the presence of individual or combinations of FPCs and VPCs. By definition, their very presence is a deviation from a safe environment. Usually, they are identified and the appropriate corrections made to restore safety. In some EDs, however, insufficient resources or other limiting factors lead to persistence of these conditions. Eventually, people simply get used to working under these conditions; that is, the deviance becomes normalized, and a chronic state of RACQITO is established. An example of this is inadequate ED physician or nurse staffing for a given workload and acuity.

18. What's the difference between safety management and continuous quality improvement (CQI)?

Safety seems to be a special case of quality. There is a great deal of overlap, but there are also significant differences.

19. What are the components of safety management?

The three main components of safety management are *reduction, containment,* and *mitigation.* Ideally, we would like to reduce the total number of failures; barring that, we would like to contain the failures that still occur so they do not impact on patients (or staff); barring that, we would like to mitigate the effects of those failures that do impact on patients (or staff).

20. **Give examples of strategies for safety management in the ED.**
    - Designing good work environments using human factors engineering (HFE) principles
    - Improved detection and assessment of latent faults
    - Improved detection and reporting systems for active failures
    - Discovery, assessment, and elimination of specific FPCs
    - Cultural and individual awareness training to reduce VPCs
    - Recognizing RACQITO and the conditions that produce it
    - Training in teamwork behaviors in the ED
    - Improved response and support for individuals when adverse outcomes occur

21. **What does the expression "geography is destiny" mean in the ED?**
    It refers to the triage process in the ED, and the tendency to be treated according to where, or in whose territory, the patient happens to be. First, the triage system of EDs operates by trying to place the right patient in the right room. Thus, eye complaints go to the eye room, cardiac complaints into the cardiac room, and so forth. Physicians and nurses tend to "anchor" on where the patient is initially placed (see following), which can be problematic and lead to error when the presenting symptoms are misleading (e.g., a complaint of constipation might be a dissecting abdominal aortic aneurysm). Thus, we need to maintain a state of willingness to undo geographical cues. Second, it refers to the natural tendency of experts to see particular problems within their own frame of reference. Often, the process of perception depends less on what is before our eyes and more on what we expect to see. If one walks around with a hammer, everything begins to look like a nail. Right-sided abdominal pain in a female may look like appendicitis to the surgeon, renal colic to the urologist, pelvic inflammatory disease to the gynecologist, and somatization to the psychiatrist. Thus, when we send patients down particular paths, we may be committing them to particular destinies. Experts are best engaged at the point at which the problem has become fairly well defined, and, until it is, the ED physician remains the best source of expertise. We should remember, too, that a consult is a consult and not a transfer of care.

22. **What proportion of failures in the ED are due to negligence?**
    Relatively low—probably less than 5%. It is virtually meaningless to label bad outcomes as being the result of "bad apples." Human activity characterizes virtually all aspects of ED function, and whenever we see failure and its consequences, it will usually have been mediated by humans. Inevitably, physicians, nurses, technicians, and others will be the human vector by which the failure makes its appearance. This association of humans with failure leads to a natural tendency to blame people when failures occur. This tendency is referred to as *fundamental attribution error.*

23. **What is fundamental attribution error?**
    It's a term used by psychologists to describe our tendency to attribute blame to people when things go wrong. For example, if we see someone fall over we might characterize him or her as careless, clumsy, or accident-prone, that is, we attribute the witnessed event to a failing or dispositional qualities in that person. However, it might be the case that the person fell over because the floor was slippery and he or she was on the way to urgently assist someone. In this case, less visible situational factors might have been more responsible for the outcome. This doesn't mean there are not people out there who are careless and clumsy, but rather we should be more willing to consider situational factors when seeking explanations for why things go wrong. Taking this to an extreme, some believe there should be no such term as *error* because, ultimately, we might explain all outcomes by situational factors. This takes us close to causal determinism and the so-called *illusion of free will.* Do we, in fact, enjoy any real

control over what we do? On a less philosophical note, it is not uncommon to hear some emergency care providers abnegating responsibility for poor quality of care by virtue of the system and conditions under which they are obliged to work and over which they have limited control.

Dekker S: The Field Guide to Human Error Investigations. Aldershot, UK, Ashgate, 2002.

Henriksen K, Kaplan H: Hindsight bias, outcome knowledge and adaptive learning. Qual Saf Health Care 12(Suppl 2):ii46–ii50, 2003.

24. **Are psychiatric patients especially vulnerable to failure in the ED?**
Yes. In fact, the earliest reports of failures in the ED related to the management of psychiatric patients. Historically, we have failed to provide them with adequate medical clearance; we have underestimated their concurrent physical illness, and we have made attribution errors. Some studies have suggested the attitudes of ED personnel can actually increase the risk of suicide in vulnerable patients. Part of the problem is that the psychiatric patient in the ED does not fit the type of "model" patient that we like to see (Table 7-1).

TABLE 7-1. CONTRASTING FEATURES OF PSYCHIATRIC AND NONPSYCHIATRIC PATIENTS

Feature	Nonpsychiatric Patient	Psychiatric Patient
Physical illness	Present	Absent
Behavior	Passive, compliant	Passive/aggressive, noncompliant
Attitude of patient	Grateful/appreciative	Neutral, ungrateful/resentful
Diagnosis	Mostly objective	Mostly subjective
Work-up	Relatively fast	Usually slow
Lab/imaging studies	Contributory	Noncontributory
Management	Relatively clear	Difficult/deferred
Endpoint	Often definitive	Poor, revolving
Compliance	Usually good	Usually poor
Attitude of staff	Good, supportive	Often unsupportive

25. **Do we make attribution errors in our perception of ourselves?**
Yes. There is probably no one harder on physicians than physicians themselves. When we perceive ourselves as having "committed" an error, our reaction is often inappropriate, being overly harsh and punitive. However, by increasing our awareness and understanding of the contextual nature of these failures, we can develop a more appropriate response to it when it occurs.

26. **This begins to sound like a psychology course. I thought I was in EM.**
It's true that many of the terms that have come into usage in the new science of Safety in Health Care have their origin in the discipline of psychology. This is no accident! Much of the groundwork in this area was done by psychologists, ergonomists, sociologists, engineers, and others with a special interest in the area of human performance. One of the earliest commentators on error was James Sully, a professor of Mind and Logic at University College, London in the late 19th century. More recently, another professor at University College, the psychologist Charles Vincent, has made significant contributions to our understanding of accidents and incidents in Medicine. The father of modern approaches to Human Error is James Reason, for many years a professor of Psychology at Manchester University in England.

27. What are the three major categories of safety problems in the ED?
Procedural, affective, and cognitive.

KEY POINTS: SAFETY IN EMERGENCY MEDICINE

1. *Error* is a term of historical interest only; it is an illusion created by hindsight bias.

2. Performance failures have their roots in the context of work and how it interacts with the human worker; the only malleable element is the context of work.

3. Special skills in psychology and engineering are required to understand and successfully manage safety problems.

28. Give examples.
Procedural failures are those that occur during the performance of a procedure. They involve some sort of psychomotor failure through a breakdown in or between motor function and visual and touch sensory modalities. They are often highly visible; their immediate consequences are apparent, and they are usually improvable by training and practice. Some examples are esophageal intubation, causing a pneumothorax putting in a central line, getting a venous sample while attempting an arterial blood gas, improper application of a cast, poor suturing technique, causing further injury while reducing a dislocation, injuring internal organs putting in a chest tube, and so forth. High-fidelity simulation techniques offer much promise in reducing procedural failures.

Affective problems occur when the physician's affective state influences the quality and validity of clinical decision making. This is usually occult, and physicians themselves may be unaware of the influence of their own affective state on decision making. The affective state can be independent of or related to patients in their care. An example of an independent instance would be if the physician was experiencing a temporary mood disruption or even a depressed or hypomanic state. This might result in the quality of decisions for all patients being compromised. Related instances, in contrast, occur when the physician develops feelings, either positive or negative, toward a specific patient or specific groups of patients. This is referred to as countertransference. *Negative countertransference* occurs when the physician develops negative feelings toward a patient, often on the basis of significant exemplars in the physician's past; that is, the patient reminds the physician of a previous patient, class of patient, or some other figure with whom the physician has had a bad experience. As a result, the quality of decision making and care may be compromised. Patients with borderline personality disorder have an unusual capacity for generating negative countertransference in their caregivers. *Positive countertransference* can also compromise decision making and management. An example would be overinvestigating a trivial complaint in a patient (through concern about not missing something significant) toward whom the physician has strong positive feelings. The *chagrin factor* is another example when physicians modify their investigations so that they do not expose themselves, or the patient, to the chagrin that might result from turning up an undesirable finding.

Cognition is involved in all human behavior, from the simple *skill-based* levels, through the higher order, *rule-based* behaviors, to the most complex level of cognition that is involved in *knowledge-based* behavior (Table 7-2). The execution of a well-rehearsed, automatic motor skill (e.g., intubation), requires little cognitive input other than simple visual and touch monitoring. An increased level of cognitive input is clearly needed for rule-based behaviors, but even complex medical acts, such as those directed by advanced cardiac life support (ACLS) algorithms, can be performed with minimum cognitive involvement. However, knowledge-based

Level	Activity
TABLE 7-2. THE COMPLEXITY OF COGNITIVE BEHAVIOR IN THE ED	
Skill-Based	Wound repair
	Dislocation reduction
	Intubation
Rule-Based	Radiographic decision rules
	Clinical practice guidelines
	Algorithms
Knowledge-Based	Clinical decision making
	Management decisions
	Diagnostic reasoning

cognitive behavior involves interpreting and understanding novel situations and problems within the context of specific domain knowledge (e.g., integrating the presenting complaint, past medical history, physical examination, and laboratory findings in a patient with syncope). There is clearly some overlap in cognitive complexity between different levels. As experience accumulates, more and more behaviors can be relegated to lower levels of cognitive involvement. Thus, paradoxically, novices operate at the knowledge-based level almost all the time, whereas experts operate at the skill-based level most of the time.

Cognitive failures can occur at any level in this hierarchy of thinking processes. Not surprisingly, it is mostly at the highest level, knowledge-based behavior. The incidence of cognitive failure increases under conditions of uncertainty, especially when thinking is hurried or pressured and when heuristics are used. Interestingly, cognitive failures, when viewed in retrospect, are almost always judged preventable. This undoubtedly says more about the person making the judgment than it does about the actor(s) involved in the failure.

Croskerry P: The cognitive imperative: Thinking about how we think. Acad Emerg Med 7:1223–1231, 2000.

29. What are heuristics?

Heuristics are strategies for thinking. The term usually refers to strategies that build economy and abbreviation into the thinking process. Essentially, a well-established heuristic is a disposition or cognitive bias to respond in a particular way to a particular situation. For the most part, they are very useful to us in the ED, where we are often looking for short cuts. Occasionally, however, they can get us into trouble.

30. Give some examples of cognitive biases.

There are probably a couple of dozen cognitive biases. Many of them derive from five archetypal heuristics: *representativeness, availability, anchoring, confirmation,* and *satisficing.*

31. What is representativeness?

Representativeness is a subjective assessment or judgment of how similar a particular example is to its parent population. For example, patients who are experiencing angina will classically present with gradual onset of a visceral quality of retrosternal pain, which may radiate to the arm, shoulder, neck, or jaw; lasts 5–15 minutes; and may be associated with nausea, diaphoresis, and dyspnea. These symptoms and signs are generally held to be representative of the class of patients with angina. However, some patients (geriatric, diabetic, female) are more likely to present with atypical symptoms. The more unrepresentative the patient's presentation is, the greater the chances of the diagnosis being delayed or missed altogether. Because of unrepresentativeness, young patients are also more likely to experience a failed diagnosis.

Representativeness error accounts for a significant proportion of patients with chest pain caused by acute myocardial infarction (AMI) being sent home from the ED. Insufficient experience or training increases the likelihood of making the representativeness error. Unfortunately, most medical textbooks tend to describe prototypical disease, and, therefore, students are unwittingly trained to look for representativeness or prototypical manifestations of disease.

32. What is availability?

In the normal course of thinking, some memories will be more available to us than others. For example, if an emergency physician saw a patient a week ago who presented with a headache that turned out to be a subarachnoid hemorrhage, the image of that patient and the association of headache with subarachnoid hemorrhage are more available or recent than, say, a headache that was seen a year ago. Thus, the physician may have a greater tendency to look for a subarachnoid hemorrhage than would otherwise be dictated by the presentation of a particular patient. Availability might similarly be increased by a colleague's description of a clinical encounter, a recent presentation of a case at rounds, or if the physician had recently read a review of a particular disease. Availability would be *decreased* by long intervals since encountering, or never having previously seen, a particular disease (out of sight, out of mind). Availability is not solely determined by recency of experience. It also depends on the salience and emotional valence of previous encounters. For example, if the physician had a particularly vivid experience 10 years ago, missing an AMI in a young person, thenceforth the physician might be over-cautious in managing all patients with chest pain, which might result in a bias toward overconsultation and poor utilization of resources. Thus, availability influences decision making and can lead to both overdiagnosing and underdiagnosing. The latter, when physicians are in the out of sight, out of mind mode, can result in serious misses.

33. What is anchoring?

Anchoring can give rise to particularly difficult failures in the ED. These occur when paramedics, nurses, or physicians attach, commit, or anchor to a particular diagnosis very early on in the presentation. This usually occurs because certain sign and symptom patterns may strongly suggest a particular diagnosis, which is adopted without giving sufficient consideration to other possibilities on the differential. For example, consider a 60-year-old male with a history of renal stones presenting with flank pain, nausea and vomiting, and hematuria. The obvious diagnosis is ureteral colic, and inexperienced nurses and physicians will anchor on this. For the vast majority of cases, the anchor will serve them well, but occasionally an aortic dissection will be missed, with sometimes fatal consequences. The order in which information is obtained strongly influences anchoring, with initial information being given greater importance than that gathered later. Anchoring is very difficult to recognize in oneself; perhaps the only sure way out of it is to have a new set of eyes look at the problem (such as often occurs at change of shift).

34. What is confirmation bias?

It is the tendency to look for evidence or information that can be used to bolster a hypothesis that has already been adopted (i.e., to look for things that rule in a diagnosis); it also includes the tendency to fail to perceive evidence that might be disconfirming to the current world-view. Consider a patient who presents to the ED with a headache and fever and the physician hypothesizes that the headache has a benign origin associated with a flulike syndrome. In the course of physical examination, the physician finds neck stiffness, which he or she attributes to myalgia and tension of the neck muscles. This is confirmation bias; the physician is fitting a significant finding (in this context of headache and fever) into the preformed diagnosis of a flulike illness. Instead, a far more powerful strategy would be to look for disconfirming evidence that rejects a working hypothesis. In this case, a lumbar puncture would quickly settle the issue and rule out meningitis. If anchoring occurs early on in a presentation, and the clinician tends to work with a strong confirmation bias, the boat may be missed completely.

35. **What is search satisficing?**

This is an example of another cognitive bias, one that probably has its origin in both the representativeness and anchoring heuristics. Essentially, it refers to the tendency to call off a search once something has been found. It is illustrated by the question: "What is the most commonly missed fracture in the ED?" The answer is not C7, the scaphoid, or Lisfranc (all occasionally missed), but *the second fracture*, because we have a tendency to satisfy ourselves when we find the first fracture and call off the search for others. Search satisficing errors similarly arise when we call off the search for additional foreign bodies, concurrent diagnoses, coingestants in a poisoning, and so forth.

CHAPTER 8

HOW TO CRITICALLY REVIEW EMERGENCY MEDICINE LITERATURE

Debra Houry, MD, MPH

1. **Can I skip this chapter if I don't plan to do research?**
   No! Reading the medical literature carefully and incorporating it into clinical practice are important for all physicians.

2. **Why should I read medical journals?**
   - To learn the clinical features and management of diseases seen in practice
   - To determine whether a new or existing diagnostic test or treatment would be beneficial for your patients
   - To stay abreast of recent medical developments and issues

3. **How do I determine what articles to read?**
   See Fig. 8-1.

4. **Which study design is the best?**
   Randomized controlled trials are considered the strongest studies. Patients are randomly assigned to treatment groups, limiting selection bias. These studies are uncommon in the emergency medicine literature and often require large study populations. Other study designs may be more appropriate, such as in instances when performing a randomized trial would be unethical (withholding a life-saving treatment or exposing patients deliberately to harm).

5. **Are there any other types of study designs I should be familiar with?**
   Yes, cohort, case-control, and case series studies. **Cohort studies** divide groups by exposure status and prospectively follow the groups over time to determine who develops the disease. These studies are used to calculate the relative risks of various exposures. **Case-control studies** retrospectively compare cases (individuals with the disease) with controls (individuals without the disease) to determine the frequency of exposures. These research studies are subject to recall bias but can be used to determine odds ratios. **Case series** report characteristics of patients with a particular disease and can be valuable when looking at rare diseases or outcomes (human immunodeficiency virus [HIV] first was reported as a case series of *Pneumocystis carinii* pneumonia in homosexual populations).

6. **What is blinding? Why is it important?**
   A technique in which patients, physicians, researchers, and anyone else involved in the research study are unaware of whether patients are in the experimental or control group. This helps eliminate potential bias, unequal distribution of groups, differential administration of interventions, and distorted results and outcome assessments.

7. **Do sample size and power matter?**
   Power is the probability that the study will detect a treatment effect between the two experimental groups. The smaller the size of the treatment effect being studied, the larger the sample size should be. Many studies do not have a large enough sample size to detect a statistically significant difference and may report negative results when a significant difference

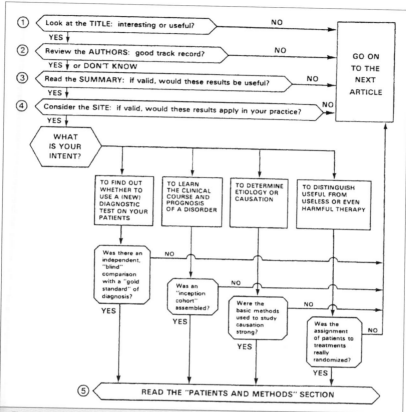

Figure 8-1. Determining which articles to read. (From Sackett DL: How to read clinical journals: 1. Why to read them and how to start reading them critically. Can Med Assoc J 124:555–558, 1981, with permission.)

may have been detected in an appropriate sample size. Without adequate power, the study results may be inconclusive.

8. **What does "number needed to treat" mean?**
This is the number of patients who would have to receive the treatment for just one patient to benefit from the treatment. For example, if the number needed to treat is 100, then 100 patients would need to have the treatment for 1 person to benefit from it. A lower number needed to treat is obviously better, but if the benefit is preventing mortality, a larger value may be acceptable. You can calculate the number needed to treat by dividing 1 by the absolute risk reduction proportion.

9. **What should I look for when evaluating a chart review study?**
1. Trained chart abstractors
2. Explicit criteria for case selection and exclusion
3. Defined study variables
4. Standardized abstraction forms for data collection

5. Periodic meetings among researchers to resolve abstraction disputes
6. Monitored performance of abstractors
7. Blinded chart reviewers
8. Measures of interrater agreement

10. **What does a *p* value refer to?**
The probability that the results of a study or the differences between study subsets occurred by chance. The most commonly used value, $p < .05$, means that there is less than a 5% probability that the study results occurred by chance. This is statistically significant but not necessarily clinically significant. A decrease by 1 minute in overall emergency department (ED) length of stay may be statistically significant ($p < .05$), but a 1-minute reduction in overall length of stay likely has no clinical relevance for physicians or patients.

11. **How do I interpret confidence intervals?**
A confidence interval is the expected range of results in the study population. A 95% confidence interval means that you would expect 95% of your results to fall within the specified range. A smaller range of values or less variance usually is found with larger sample sizes. A wide confidence interval could mean that some of the study results may not be clinically significant. Look at the upper and lower boundaries of the confidence interval and determine if both values still would hold clinical significance for you. If only the upper boundary value would have significance, there may not be an overall clinical benefit.

12. **Does it matter who sponsors a study?**
Yes. Any direct involvement in a study by a sponsor, particularly one with a financial interest in the outcomes of the research (e.g., pharmaceutical industry), has the potential to influence the study. Sponsors should not have any input into study design, data collection, or method of reporting the results. Unfortunately, many research studies do not adhere to these standards. Disclosure of financial support is important and should alert the reader that there is the potential for introduction of bias into the study. Industry-sponsored studies may provide valuable information but must be reviewed carefully.

KEY POINTS: CRITICAL REVIEW OF EMERGENCY MEDICINE LITERATURE

1. Randomized controlled trials are the best studies, but other studies may also be valid.

2. A $p < .05$ is statistically significant.

3. A smaller confidence interval is better.

4. Sponsorship may influence how results are presented.

13. **Should I read reviews on clinical topics?**
This depends on many factors:
- Are you looking for basic knowledge or understanding of a disease process? If so, a clinical review may be sufficient and can provide the foundation for you to continue your reading on the topic.
- Are you looking for the latest information? Clinical reviews may be outdated by the time of publication because the literature on which they are based was written before the review.
- Is it a narrative or systematic review? In narrative reviews, the author selects the articles to include in the review and summarizes the topic based in part on his or her experience. In a

systematic review, the author identifies articles through a search and includes or excludes the articles based on predefined criteria and summarizes the topic based on strength of the evidence from the included articles.

14. How do I practice evidence-based medicine?

Critically reviewing the medical literature and applying the best evidence to your practice is evidence-based medicine. After reading this chapter, you should be able to read research studies and determine the strength of the studies and their findings.

15. What are some of the statistical terms I should be familiar with?
- **Relative risk:** The risk of developing a disease after an exposure compared with individuals without an exposure: $A/(A + B) \div C/(C + D)$
- **Odds ratio:** The odds of developing a disease after an exposure compared with those without an exposure: $(AD)/(BC)$
- **Sensitivity:** The proportion of people with a positive test result who truly have the disease: $A/(A + C)$
- **Specificity:** The proportion of people with a negative test result who do not have the disease: $D/(B + D)$
- **Positive predictive value:** The likelihood that a person with a positive test result actually has the disease: $A/(A + B)$
- **Negative predictive value:** The likelihood that a person with a negative test result does not have the disease: $D/(C + D)$

See Fig. 8-2 for reference.

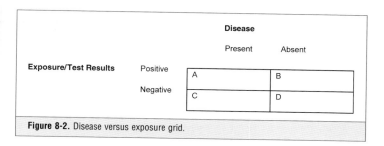

Figure 8-2. Disease versus exposure grid.

BIBLIOGRAPHY

1. Barratt A, Wyer PC, Hatala R, et al: Tips for learners of evidence-based medicine: 1. Relative risk reduction, absolute risk reduction, and number needed to treat. Can Med Assoc J 171:353–358, 2004.

2. Davidoff F, DeAngelis CD, Drazen JM, et al: Sponsorship, authorship, and accountability. JAMA 286:1232–1234, 2001.

3. Gallagher EJ: P<0.05: Threshold for decerebrate genuflection. Acad Emerg Med 6:1084–1087, 1999.

4. Gilbert EH, Lowenstein SR, Koziol-McLain J, et al: Chart reviews in emergency medicine: Where are the methods? Ann Emerg Med 27:305–308, 1996.

5. Jones JB: Research fundamentals: Statistical considerations in research design: A simple person's approach. Acad Emerg Med 7:194–199, 2000.

6. Sackett DL: How to read clinical journals: Why to read them and how to start reading them critically. Can Med Assoc J 124:555–558, 1981.

ALTERED MENTAL STATUS AND COMA

Kenneth C. Jackimczyk, MD

CHAPTER 9

1. What is coma? What terms should be used to describe altered sensorium?

A depressed mental state in which verbal and physical stimuli cannot elicit useful responses. Other terms, such as *lethargic, stuporous,* or *obtunded,* mean different things to different observers and should be avoided. You may be "alert but confused" as you read this chapter. It is best to describe the mental functions the patient can perform (e.g., the patient is oriented to person, place, and time; knows the name of the President; and can count backward from 10).

2. What causes coma?

Mental alertness is maintained by the cerebral hemispheres in conjunction with the reticular activating system. Coma can be produced by diffuse disease of both cerebral hemispheres (usually a metabolic problem), disease in the brain stem that damages the reticular activating system, or a structural central nervous system (CNS) lesion that compresses the reticular activating system. Less than 20% of patients have a structural cause for their coma.

3. How can I remember the causes of coma and altered mental status?

TIPS-vowels—that is, TIPS-AEIOU.

TIPS

T = **T**rauma, temperature

I = **I**nfection (CNS and systemic)

P = **P**sychiatric

S = **S**pace-occupying lesions, stroke, subarachnoid hemorrhage, shock

VOWELS

A = **A**lcohol and other drugs

E = **E**pilepsy, **e**lectrolytes

I = **I**nsulin (diabetes)

O = **O**xygen (lack of), **o**piates

U = **U**remia

4. What important historical facts should be obtained from the patient with altered mental status or coma?

This seems like a stupid question because the patient with altered consciousness cannot give you a reliable history, and the comatose patient cannot give any history at all! You should carefully question prehospital personnel and attempt to contact the patient's friends or family. Ask about the onset of symptoms (acute or gradual), recent neurologic symptoms (headache, seizure, or focal neurologic abnormalities), drug or alcohol abuse, recent trauma, prior psychiatric problems, and past medical history (neurologic disorders, diabetes, renal failure, liver failure, or cardiac disease). If you are having trouble getting historical information, search the patient's belongings for pill bottles, check the patient's wallet for telephone numbers or names of friends, and review previous medical records.

5. How can I perform a brief, directed physical examination on a patient with altered consciousness?

The goal of the physical examination is to differentiate structural focal CNS problems from diffuse metabolic processes. Pay special attention to vital signs, general appearance, mental status, eye findings, and the motor examination. Vital signs and eye findings are discussed elsewhere in this chapter.

The **general appearance** should be noted before examining the patient. Are there signs of trauma? Is there symmetry of spontaneous movements?

Motor examination is done to determine the symmetry of motor tone or strength and response of deep tendon reflexes.

Huff JS: Altered mental status and coma. In Tintinalli JE, Kelen JD, Stapczynski JS (eds): Emergency Medicine: A Comprehensive Study Guide, 6th ed. New York, McGraw-Hill, 2004, pp 1390–1397.

6. How do I evaluate the patient's mental status?

Mental status can be assessed quickly. Ask four sets of progressively more difficult questions: (1) orientation to person, place, and time; (2) name the President of the United States; (3) count backward from 10 (if done correctly, ask for serial 3s or 7s); and (4) recent recall of three unrelated objects.

7. What is the Glasgow Coma Scale?

A simple scoring system used in trauma patients to define the level of consciousness. It is useful for standardizing assessments among multiple observers and for monitoring changes in the degree of coma. The score is determined by eliciting the best response obtained from the patient in three categories (Table 9-1). It is not sensitive enough to detect subtle alterations of consciousness in the noncomatose patient.

TABLE 9-1. GLASGOW COMA SCALE		
Observation		**Points**
Eye opening	Spontaneous	4
	To verbal command	3
	To pain	2
	No response	1
Best verbal response	Oriented/converses	5
	Confused conversation	4
	Inappropriate words	3
	Incomprehensible sounds	2
	No response	1
Best motor response	Obeys	6
	Localizes pain	5
	Flexion withdrawal	4
	Decorticate posture	3
	Decerebrate posture	2
	No response	1
Total points		**3–15**

8. How important is measuring the temperature of the comatose patient?

Vital signs often provide clues to the cause of coma. A core temperature must be obtained. An elevated temperature should lead you to investigate the possibility of meningitis, sepsis, heat stroke, or hyperthyroidism. Hypothermia can result from environmental exposure, hypoglycemia, or, rarely, addisonian crisis. Do not assume that an abnormal temperature has a neurogenic cause until you eliminate other causes.

9. **What is the significance of other vital signs?**
   - Check the **cardiac** monitor. Bradycardia or arrhythmias can alter cerebral perfusion and cause altered sensorium.
   - Carefully count **respirations.** Tachypnea may indicate the presence of hypoxemia or a metabolic acidosis, and diminished respiratory efforts may require assisted ventilation.
   - Check the **blood pressure.** Do not assume that hypotension has a CNS cause. Look for hypovolemia or sepsis as a cause for hypotension, but remember that adults (in contrast to infants) cannot become hypovolemic from intracranial bleeding alone. Hypertension may be a result of increased intracranial pressure, but uncontrolled hypertension also may cause encephalopathy and coma.
   - Do not forget to obtain the fifth vital sign—measurement of **oxygen saturation** with a pulse oximeter.

10. **What is Cushing's reflex?**
    An alteration of vital signs—increased blood pressure and decreased pulse—secondary to increased intracranial pressure.

11. **Define decorticate and decerebrate posturing.**
    Posturing may be seen with noxious stimulation in a comatose patient with severe brain injury.
    - **Decorticate posturing** is hyperextension of the legs with flexion of the arms at the elbows. Decorticate posturing results from damage to the descending motor pathways above the central midbrain.
    - **Decerebrate posturing** is hyperextension of the upper and lower extremities; this is a graver sign. Decerebrate posturing reflects damage to the midbrain and upper pons. If you have trouble remembering which position is which, think of the upper extremities in flexion with the hands over the heart (*cor*) in de-*cor*-ticate posturing.

12. **What information can be obtained from the eye examination of the comatose patient?**
    The eyes should be examined for **position, reactivity,** and **reflexes.** When the eyelids are opened, note the **position** of the eyes. If the eyes flutter upward, exposing only the sclera, suspect psychogenic coma. If the eyes exhibit bilateral roving movements that cross the midline, you know that the brain stem is intact. Pupil **reactivity** is the best test to differentiate metabolic coma from coma caused by a structural lesion because it is relatively resistant to metabolic insult and usually is preserved in a metabolic coma. Pupil reactivity may be subtle, necessitating use of a bright light in a dark room.

13. **How do I test the eye reflexes?**
    Testing of the eye **reflexes** is the best method for determining the status of the brain stem. Two methods can be used: (1) oculocephalic (doll's eyes) or (2) oculovestibular (cold calorics). Oculocephalic testing requires rapid twisting of the neck, which is a bad idea in the unconscious patient because occult cervical spine trauma may be present. Oculovestibular testing is easy to do and can be done without manipulating the neck. The ear canal is irrigated with 50 mL of ice water. A normal awake patient has two competing eye movements: rapid nystagmus away from the irrigated ear and slow tonic deviation toward the cold stimulus. Remember the mnemonic **COWS** (**C**old **O**pposite, **W**arm **S**ame), which refers to the direction of the fast component. (See Fig. 9-1.)

14. **How do I interpret the eye reflexes?**
    A patient with psychogenic coma has normal reflexes and exhibits rapid nystagmus. A comatose patient with an intact brain stem lacks the nystagmus phase, and the eyes deviate slowly toward

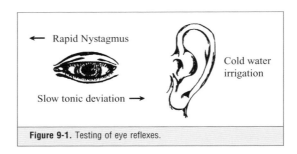

Figure 9-1. Testing of eye reflexes.

the irrigated ear. If the eyes do anything else (usually not a good sign), refer to a neurology text to determine the exact location of the lesion.

Wolfe R, Brown D: Coma and depressed level of consciousness. In Rosen P, Barkin RM (eds): Emergency Medicine: Concepts and Clinical Practice, 5th ed. St. Louis, Mosby, 2002, pp 137–144.

15. **I want to impress the attending physicians. Do you have any tips on physical examination that will let me assume my rightful position as star student?**
   - If a confused patient is suspected of being postictal, look in the mouth. A tongue laceration supports the diagnosis of a seizure.
   - Put on gloves and inspect the scalp. Occult trauma is often overlooked, and you may find a laceration or dried blood. An old scar on the scalp may tip you off to a post-traumatic seizure disorder.
   - Do not be fooled by a *positive blink test* in a patient with suspected psychogenic coma. When you rapidly flick your hand at a comatose patient who has open eyes, air movement may stimulate a corneal reflex in a patient who is truly comatose.
   - Do not be misled by the odor of alcohol. Alcohol has almost no detectable odor, which is why alcoholics drink vodka at work. Other spirited liquors such as brandy have a strong odor. The comatose executive who "smells drunk" may have had a sudden subarachnoid hemorrhage and spilled brandy on his or her shirt.

16. **Which plain radiographs should be obtained in the comatose patient?**
   A cervical spine series (or cervical spine computed tomography [CT]) must be obtained in any comatose patient with suspected trauma because physical examination is unreliable. A chest radiograph may be helpful if hypoxemia or pulmonary infection is suspected.

17. **Which diagnostic tests should be obtained in the patient with a significantly altered level of consciousness?**
   Obtain a rapid blood glucose (Dextrostix), and correct hypoglycemia if it is found. If alcohol intoxication is suspected, determine the alcohol level with either a Breathalyzer or serum blood alcohol. If the pupils are constricted or if narcotic ingestion is suspected, intravenous naloxone should be given. If hypoglycemia or alcohol intoxication is not found to be the cause of the patient's confusion, further tests are warranted. A complete blood count, electrolytes, blood urea nitrogen, glucose, and oxygen saturation should be obtained. Toxicologic screens may be done in a patient with a suspected ingestion, but they are expensive and do not detect routinely every possible ingested substance. Liver function tests, ammonia level, calcium level, carboxyhemoglobin level, and thyroid function studies may be helpful in selected patients.

18. **When should I order a CT scan?**
   Although CT scans have revolutionized the practice of neurology, they are not indicated in every comatose patient. A good history, physical examination, and a few simple laboratory tests are

adequate in many cases seen in the emergency department (ED) because drug and alcohol abuse are common. If a structural lesion is suspected, however, a CT scan should be ordered immediately. If the condition of a patient with a suspected metabolic coma worsens or does not improve after a brief period of observation, a CT scan should be obtained.

19. **When should a lumbar puncture (LP) be done?**

The indications and timing of LP depend on two questions: (1) Is CNS infection suspected? (2) Is there a suspicion of a structural lesion causing increased intracranial pressure? (See Fig. 9-2.)

Edlow JA, Caplan LR: Avoiding pitfalls in the diagnosis of subarachnoid hemorrhage. N Engl J Med 342:29–36, 2000.

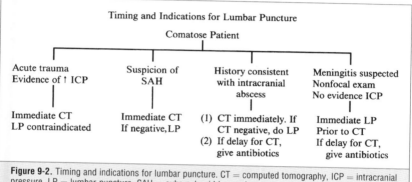

Figure 9-2. Timing and indications for lumbar puncture. CT = computed tomography, ICP = intracranial pressure, LP = lumbar puncture, SAH = subarachnoid hemorrhage.

20. **Okay. I have made the diagnosis of coma. What are my initial treatment priorities?**

Emergency medicine requires simultaneous assessment and treatment. A brilliant diagnosis is useless in a dead patient. Start with the **ABCs**: airway, breathing, circulation and cervical spine. Intubate patients with apnea or labored respirations, patients who are likely to aspirate, and any patient who is thought to have increased intracranial pressure. Maintain cervical spine precautions until the possibility of trauma has been excluded. Hypotension should be corrected so that cerebral perfusion pressure can be maintained.

KEY POINTS: ALTERED MENTAL STATUS AND COMA

1. Goal of physical exam is to differentiate structural from metabolic cause.

2. Focus on vital signs, mental status, and motor exam.

3. Check a rapid blood glucose on every comatose patient.

4. Immediately intubate the comatose patient if increased intracranial pressure is suspected.

21. **I've addressed the ABCs. What do I do next?**

Check a Dextrostix; if the glucose is low, treat hypoglycemia with D50W. It is better to do a rapid blood glucose determination rather than to give glucose empirically. Next, give 100 mg of thiamine, and if opioid use is suspected, give 2 mg of naloxone intravenously. Empirical administration of flumazenil (benzodiazepine antagonist) or physostigmine (reverses anticholinergic agents) is not routinely indicated in comatose patients. Antibiotic administration is considered in all febrile patients with coma of unknown origin. In suspected drug overdose, activated charcoal, 1 gm/kg, may be instilled via nasogastric tube. A comatose patient with increased intracranial pressure should be intubated and mechanically ventilated. Mannitol, 0.5 to 1 gm/kg intravenously, should be considered.

Hoffman RS, Goldfrank LR: The poisoned patient with altered consciousness: Controversies in the use of a coma cocktail. JAMA 274:562–569, 1995.

22. **I think my patient is faking it. How can I tell if this is psychogenic coma?**
First, be grateful. A patient in psychogenic coma is better than one who is angry and combative. Approach the patient incorrectly, and you can awaken the patient to a hostile alert state.

Do a careful neurologic examination. Open the eyelids. If the eyes deviate upward and only the sclera show (Bell's phenomenon), you should suspect psychogenic coma. When the eyelids are opened in a patient with true coma, the lids close slowly and incompletely. It is difficult to fake this movement. Lift the arm and drop it toward the face; if the face is avoided, this is most likely psychogenic coma. If this does not work, you may want to check some simple laboratory tests, including a Dextrostix. If the patient remains comatose, irritating but nonpainful stimuli, such as tickling the feet with a cotton swab, may elicit a response. Remember that this test is not a test of wills between you and the patient. There is no indication for repeated painful stimulation because it can make the patient angry and ruin attempts at therapeutic intervention.

If all else fails, perform cold caloric testing. The presence of nystagmus confirms the diagnosis of psychogenic coma. What do you do then? It is time to pick up a copy of *Psychiatry Secrets*.

CHAPTER 10

FEVER

Diane M. Birnbaumer, MD, and Ryan P. Lamb, MD

Give me the power to produce fever and I'll cure all disease.
—Parmenides, 500 BC

Humanity has but three great enemies: fever, famine, and war: of these, by far the greatest, by far the most terrible, is fever.

—Sir William Osler

1. **What is fever?**
A true fever is caused by elevation of the hypothalamic set point. This causes the body to attempt to generate heat (e.g., by shivering) to elevate the body's core temperature. In contrast, hyperthermia results in an elevated temperature without altering the set point, so the body attempts to cool itself to achieve a normal temperature. Some examples of hyperthemia include heat stroke, hyperthyroidism, burns, and malignant hyperthermia.

2. **Is fever a common chief complaint in the emergency department (ED)?**
Yes. Fever accounts for 4.8% of all adult and 20% to 40% of all pediatric visits to the ED.

   McCaig LF, Burt CW: National Hospital Ambulatory Medical Care Survey: 2002 Emergency Department Summary. www.cdc.gov/nchs/data/ad/ad340.pdf.

3. **Is a fever good for anything, or is it just to make me feel miserable?**
As you can see from the previous quotes, this is a matter of debate that has been ongoing for more than 2500 years. Today, many investigators believe that fever is beneficial in fighting disease. Decades ago, before the discovery of antibiotics, experimentation revealed that syphilis could be cured by inducing fevers by infecting a patient with malaria. (Although successful, unless you want a letter from a lawyer, you probably shouldn't use that form of treatment.) Higher temperatures increase the activity of neutrophils and lymphocytes and decrease the levels of serum iron, a substrate that many bacteria need to reproduce. Other studies, however, indicate that fever may actually be detrimental in patients with tetanus, streptococci, and pneumococci.

4. **What temperature constitutes a fever?**
It varies depending on the patient:
   - In adults, a temperature of 38.3°C (100.9°F) is considered a fever.
   - Certain patient populations may be exceptions, and this should be taken into account (e.g., the elderly, intravenous drug users, and immunocompromised patients). These patients may not be able to mount a temperature high enough to constitute a fever by the previous definition.
   - A temperature of 41.5°C (106.7°F) usually represents hyperthermia and not a true fever, especially in adults.

5. **Does it matter which method I use to take a temperature?**
Yes. Rectal temperatures are considered the most accurate representation of core temperatures. Oral, axillary, and tympanic temperature measurements are frequently inaccurate. There is not a correction factor for these alternate modalities that provides a reliable assessment of the core

temperature. When an accurate temperature measurement is crucial to the patient's care, a rectal temperature measurement is necessary.

Craig JV, Lancaster GA, Taylor S, et al: Infrared ear thermometry compared with rectal thermometry in children: a systemic review. Lancet 360:603–609, 2002.

Craig, J.V., Lancaster GA, Williamson GR, et al: Temperature measured at the axilla compared with rectum in children and young people: systemic review. BMJ 320:1174–1178, 2000.

6. **What about subjective fevers? Can mothers accurately judge whether their child has a fever without using a thermometer?**
   Trust mothers—they know. Depending on the study, mothers are accurate in assessing the presence or absence of a fever 50% to 80% of the time. They seem to be more accurate at detecting when the child is febrile than they are at determining that the child is afebrile. Most pediatricians feel that fevers reported by mothers are probably real and need to be taken seriously.

   Graneto JW, Soglin DF: Maternal screening of childhood fever by palpation. Pediatr Emerg Care 12:183–184, 1996.

7. **Does the degree of fever indicate the severity of the illness?**
   No. There is no degree of fever that has been clearly associated with a specific risk of infection in patients, although, prior to the widespread use of the *Haemophilus influenzae* vaccine, temperatures over $41.1°C$ were associated with a higher incidence of serious bacterial illness in children. In pediatric medical decision making, the temperature should be used as only one piece of information in conjunction with many other factors.

8. **Can a fever be dismissed if it responds to antipyretics?**
   No. Acetaminophen is treating the fever not the illness causing the fever. Temperature decline in response to acetaminophen, aspirin, or ibuprofen is seen in patients with both serious and benign causes of fever.

9. **Are there causes of fever other than infection?**
   Yes. Although infections are definitely the most common causes of fever, there are numerous other causes. Neoplastic diseases (e.g., leukemia, lymphoma, solid tumors) and collagen vascular diseases (e.g., giant cell arteritis, polyarteritis nodosa, systemic lupus erythematosus, rheumatoid arthritis) are the second and third most common causes of fever. Other causes include central nervous system lesions (e.g., stroke, intracranial bleed, trauma), factitious fever, drugs, and environmental heat exposure.

10. **Which drugs can cause fevers?**
    Although any drug is capable of producing a *drug fever,* the most common are listed in Table 10-1. Of these, penicillin and penicillin analogs are the most frequent causative agents. The fever usually begins 7–10 days after initiation of drug therapy. There is an associated rash or eosinophilia in about 20% of cases. In addition to drug fevers, cocaine, amphetamines, tricyclic antidepressants, and aspirin may produce fevers after an acute ingestion, particularly in an overdose. Drug fever should always be a diagnosis of exclusion.

11. **What is an FUO?**
    No, not a UFO, an FUO. FUO, or **fever of unknown origin,** is defined as a fever greater than $38.3°C$ ($100.9°F$), documented on several occasions during a period longer than 3 weeks, with an uncertain diagnosis after 1 week of evaluation in the hospital. If the patient presents for an initial evaluation of a fever, it is not a FUO. The most common cause of FUO is occult infection and malignancy, each accounting for approximately 30% of cases.

TABLE 10-1. DRUGS COMMONLY ASSOCIATED WITH "DRUG FEVERS"

Antibiotics
INH
Nitrofurantoin
Penicillins, cephalosporins
Rifampin
Sulfonamides
Anticancer drugs
Bleomycin
Streptozocin
Cardiac drugs
Hydralazine
Methyldopa
Nifedipine
Phenytoin
Procainamide
Quinidine
Anticonvulsants
Phenytoin
Carbamazepine
NSAIDs
Ibuprofen
Salicylates
Others
Barbiturates
Cimetidine
Iodides

INH = isoniazid, NSAIDs = nonsteroidal anti-inflammatory drugs.

12. **How do I evaluate a patient with a fever?**
A thorough **history** and **physical examination** are paramount. Pay particular attention to associated symptoms (e.g., cough, shortness of breath, pain, dysuria), duration of fever, ill contacts, history or risk of immunocompromise (e.g., acquired immunodeficiency syndrome [AIDS], diabetes, elderly, asplenic), travel, and current medications. In the physical examination, note the general appearance of the patient (Does the patient look "sick" or "well"?). Pay particular attention to subtleties, such as mild mental status changes or rashes that might be indicative of more serious systemic diseases. Examine the patient for more occult sites of infection such as the nose/sinuses and rectum (prostatitis, perirectal abscess) and consider performing a pelvic examination. Leave no stone unturned when working up fever.

KEY POINTS: FEVER

1. Increased temperature may be indicative of either a fever or hyperthermia due to another cause, such as heat illness, particularly in times of increased ambient temperatures.

2. Response (or lack thereof) to antipyretics does not differentiate serious from more benign causes of fever.

3. The degree of temperature elevation is not predictive of serious illness.

4. In patients with fever, measuring a white blood cell count or band count is rarely useful in differentiating bacterial versus viral illness.

5. Evaluation of the patient presenting with fever should be individualized and based on the patient's presentation not just on the presence of a fever.

13. What about the vital signs?

Why do you think they call them "vital"? Most importantly, vital signs help assess the degree of the patient's illness and provide guidance for workup and treatment of a febrile illness. Patients with fever often have increased pulse and respirations, but it is important to look at the magnitude of the increase. The pulse should increase about 10 bpm for each $0.6°C$ ($1°F$) increase in temperature. A **pulse-temperature dissociation** occurs when the patient has a fever but a heart rate that is lower than would be expected for the degree of fever. This dissociation occurs in typhoid, malaria, legionnaires' disease, and mycoplasma. In early septic shock, tachycardia that is inappropriate for the degree of fever is often seen. Tachypnea out of proportion to fever is characteristic of pneumonia and gram-negative bacteremia. Hypotension, particularly paired with tachycardia, raises the concern of sepsis.

14. What laboratory tests should I order? How about radiographs?

There are no laboratory tests or radiographs that are always needed for every patient. It varies greatly depending on the patient. Usually the history and physical exam will direct you toward which tests to get. Clinical judgment guides the need for diagnostic studies (e.g., in a patient who has recently received chemotherapy and presents with a fever, a white blood cell [WBC] count is needed to check for neutropenia).

15. How valuable is the WBC count?

The absolute WBC and band count are neither sensitive nor specific and, if measured at all, should be interpreted in light of the patient's clinical picture. Some patients may present with serious infections but have a normal WBC count and differential, such as the elderly or the immunocompromised. Low WBC counts may be indicative of immunocompromise, viral illnesses, or septicemia. Conversely, an elevated WBC count may be seen in nonbacterial illnesses, such as a viral syndrome, dehydration, or a sympathomimetic overdose.

16. What about antibiotics? Should everyone with a fever get antibiotics?

Absolutely not. Antibiotic use should be based on the patient's specific presentation and diagnosis after a thorough history and physical examination and directed laboratory and ancillary tests. Most clinicians advocate giving appropriate antibiotics immediately to any patient who appears toxic or has suspected bacterial meningitis, without delaying for results of ancillary test or culture results. Other patients who should be considered for early antibiotics are immunocompromised patients (e.g., neutropenic patients, transplant patients, AIDS patients) and elderly patients.

17. **So what's the bottom line on fever?**
Solving the medical mystery of a patient's fever is challenging. The keys are the history, physical, general appearance, and vital signs of the patient. For each of these key points, certain patient populations have limitations in providing the clinician with enough information (e.g., a healthy child with lots of cardiopulmonary reserve can look great and suddenly decompensate; a patient with an altered sensorium cannot provide a good history; elderly patients may not mount a fever even with a life-threatening infection). Each febrile patient must be evaluated on a case-by-case basis.

18. **How do I approach a child younger than 3 years with a fever?**
See Chapter 59.

CONTROVERSY

19. **If my patient is febrile, should I always attempt to lower the temperature?**
This is controversial. Fever may actually be beneficial in fighting some infections. Antipyretics may mask a fever and delay a proper work-up and treatment of a patient. However, most physicians use antipyretics for patients who are uncomfortable because of fever. You should consider using antipyretics in pregnant women, children at risk for febrile seizures, and patients with preexisting cardiac compromise who would not tolerate the increased metabolic demands of a fever. If the temperature is above 41.5°C (106.7°F), rapid cooling measures should be used, and the diagnosis and evaluation for hyperthermia (in particular, heat illness) should be considered.

CHAPTER 11

CHEST PAIN

Timothy Janz, MD, and James E. Brown, MD

1. **Why is the cause of chest pain often difficult to determine in the emergency department (ED)?**
   - Various disease processes in a variety of organs may result in chest pain.
   - The severity of the pain is often unrelated to its life-threatening potential.
   - The location of the pain as perceived by the patient frequently does not correspond with its source.
   - Physical findings, laboratory assays, and radiologic studies are often nondiagnostic in the ED.
   - More than one disease process may be present.
   - The causes of acute chest pain often can be dynamic processes.

2. **Why is the location of chest pain not diagnostic of its cause?**
   Somatic fibers from the dermis are numerous and enter the spinal cord at a single level, resulting in sharp, localized pain. Visceral afferent fibers from internal organs of the thorax and upper abdomen are less numerous. They enter the spinal cord at multiple levels from T1 to T6, resulting in a pain that is dull, aching, and poorly localized. Connections between the visceral and somatic fibers may result in the visceral pain being perceived as originating from somatic locations, such as the shoulder, arm, neck, or jaw.

   Hamilton GC, Malone S, Janz TG: Chest pain. In Hamilton GC, Sanders AB, Strange GR, Trott AT (eds): Emergency Medicine An Approach to Clinical Problem-Solving, 2nd ed. Philadelphia, W.B. Saunders, 2003, pp 131–153.

3. **List life-threatening causes of acute chest pain that must be considered first when evaluating a patient in the ED.**
   - Myocardial infarction
   - Aortic dissection
   - Unstable angina
   - Pulmonary embolism (PE)
   - Pneumothorax
   - Acute pericarditis
   - Esophageal rupture

   Brown JE, Hamilton GC: Chest pain. In Marx JA, Hockberger RS, Walls RM, et al (eds): Rosen's Emergency Medicine: Concepts and Clinical Practice, 6th ed. St. Louis Mosby, 2002, pp 183–192.

4. **List some other conditions that may present as chest pain.**
   - Stable angina
   - Valvular heart disease
   - Pneumonia
   - Pleurisy
   - Reflux esophagitis
   - Esophageal spasm
   - Thoracic outlet syndrome
   - Musculoskeletal pain
   - Peptic ulcer disease
   - Cholecystitis
   - Pancreatitis
   - Herpes zoster
   - Anxiety
   - Hyperventilation
   - Sickle cell anemia
   - Cocaine use

5. **What is the best initial approach to patients presenting with chest pain?**
With few exceptions, all patients with acute chest pain should be approached with the assumption that a life-threatening cause is present. Before any diagnostic studies are undertaken, supplemental oxygen, intravenous access, and cardiac monitoring should be initiated (Fig. 11-1).

Hamilton GC, Malone S, Janz TG: Chest pain. In Hamilton GC, Sanders AB, Strange GR, Trott AT (eds): Emergency Medicine An Approach to Clinical Problem-Solving, 2nd ed. Philadelphia, W.B. Saunders, 2003, pp 131–153.

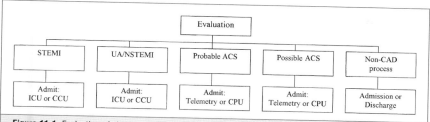

Figure 11-1. Evaluation of chest pain. STEMI = ST segment elevation myocardial infarction, NSTEMI = non-ST segment elevation myocardial infarction, UA = unstable angina, ACS = acute coronary syndrome, CAD = coronary artery disease, ICU = intensive care unit, CCU = coronary care unit, CPU = chest pain observation unit.

6. **How do I begin to assess the patient with chest pain?**
An accurate history is the most important component of the evaluation. Factors to be considered include onset, character and quality, severity, location, pattern of radiation, duration of pain, and associated symptoms. Precipitating factors, such as exertion, movement, or inspiration, and relieving factors, such as rest, nitroglycerin, or body position, may provide clues to the origin of the pain (Table 11-1).

Jones ID, Slovis CM: Emergency department evaluation for the chest pain patient. Emerg Med Clin North Am 19:269–282, 2001.

7. **What are the major risk factors associated with ischemic heart disease, PE, and aortic dissection?**
The risk factors associated with ischemic heart disease are age older than 40 years, male gender, a family history of ischemic heart disease, cigarette smoking, hypercholesterolemia, hypertension, and diabetes mellitus. Of patients with PE, 80–90% have one or more risk factors related to Virchow's triad, including intimal damage to a blood vessel (trauma or surgery), venous stasis (immobility), or hypercoagulability (malignancy, coagulation disorders, or inflammatory conditions). One of the most significant risk factors for PE is a previous venous thromboembolism. Hypertension is the major risk factor in approximately 90% of patients with aortic dissection.

Antman EM, Anbe DT, Armstrong PW, et al: ACC/AHA guidelines for the management of patients with ST-elevation myocardial infarction—executive summary. Circulation 110:588–636, 2004.
Diop D, Aghababian RV: Definition, classification, and pathophysiology of acute coronary ischemic syndromes. Emerg Med Clin North Am 19:259–268, 2001.
Klompas M: Does this patient have an acute thoracic aortic dissection? JAMA 287:2262–2272, 2002.

8. **Is radiating chest pain significant?**
Radiating chest pain is suggestive but not diagnostic of cardiac ischemia. Visceral pain, including aortic, esophageal, gastric, and pulmonary processes, may present with radiation of pain to the neck, shoulder, or arm. Chest pain that radiates to the arm or neck increases the likelihood of acute coronary syndrome. Approximately two thirds of patients with chest pain that

TABLE 11-1. CLASSIC PATTERNS OF CHEST PAIN

Etiology	Quality	Location	Radiation	Duraton	Associated Symptoms	Onset
Myocardial infarction	Visceral	Retrosternal	Neck, jaw, shoulder, arm	>15 min	Nausea, vomiting, diaphoresis, dyspnea	Variable
Angina	Visceral	Retrosternal	Neck, jaw, shoulder, arm	5–15 min	Nausea, diaphoresis, dyspnea	Gradual
Aortic dissection	Severe, tearing	Retrosternal	Interscapular	Constant	Nausea, dyspnea, diaphoresis	Sudden
Pulmonary embolism	Pleuritic	Lateral		Constant	Dyspnea, apprehension	Sudden
Pneumothorax	Pleuritic	Lateral	Neck, back	Constant	Dyspnea	Sudden
Pericarditis	Sharp, stabbing	Retrosternal	Neck, back shoulder, arm	Constant	Dyspnea, dysphagia	Variable
Esophageal rupture	Boring	Retrosternal, epigastric	Posterior thorax	Constant	Diaphoresis, dyspnea (late)	Sudden
Esophagitis	Aching, boring	Retrosternal	Interscapular	Minutes to hours	Dysphagia	Variable
Esophageal spasm	Visceral	Retrosternal	Interscapular	Minutes to hours	Dysphagia	Variable
Musculoskeletal	Sharp, aching, superficial	Localized		Variable	Dyspnea	Variable

radiates to the neck, jaw, or arms have a final diagnosis of acute coronary syndrome. Chest pain radiating to both arms increases the likelihood of acute coronary syndrome sevenfold.

Hamilton GC, Malone S, Janz TG: Chest pain. In Hamilton GC, Sanders AB, Strange GR, Trott AT (eds): Emergency Medicine An Approach to Clinical Problem-Solving, 2nd ed. Philadelphia, W.B. Saunders, 2003, pp 131–153.

9. **How does the patient's appearance correlate with the origin of chest pain?**
Catastrophic illnesses often result in anxiety, diaphoresis, and an ill appearance. Splinting may be caused by PE, pleurisy, pneumothorax, pneumonia, or musculoskeletal chest pain. Levine's sign, which consists of a patient placing a clenched fist over the sternum to describe the pain, is frequently associated with ischemic heart disease. Kussmaul's sign is a paradoxical filling of the neck veins during inspiration, which suggests a right ventricular infarction, PE, or pericarditis with associated cardiac tamponade.

Jones ID, Slovis CM: Emergency department evaluation for the chest pain patient. Emerg Med Clin North Am 19:269–282, 2001.

10. **How are vital signs helpful?**
A blood pressure difference of more than 20 mmHg between the upper extremities or a loss or reduction of lower extremity pulses is very suggestive of an aortic dissection. The presence of tachycardia should raise the suspicion of serious pathology or severe pain. Tachypnea may be caused by the PE, pneumonia, or pneumothorax, or may be secondary to pain. An elevated temperature usually indicates an inflammatory or infectious process, such as pericarditis or pneumonia. However, fever can also be associated with acute myocardial infarction and PE.

11. **Which physical examination findings may help differentiate the causes of acute chest pain?**
Isolated physical findings are rarely diagnostic of the origin of chest pain, but when used in context with the history, they may be extremely valuable. Palpation may reveal localized tenderness and reproduce musculoskeletal pain, but 5–10% of patients with acute coronary syndrome have chest pain and associated palpable chest tenderness. Cardiac auscultation may reveal a new murmur of aortic insufficiency suggestive of aortic dissection or a new murmur of mitral regurgitation secondary to papillary muscle dysfunction from acute coronary syndrome. A third or fourth heart sound increases the likelihood of acute coronary syndrome. A pericardial friction rub is diagnostic of pericarditis. Mediastinal air from an esophageal or bronchial rupture results in a crunching sound called *Hamman's sign*. Decreased breath sounds or hyperresonance may indicate a pneumothorax. Localized rales suggest pulmonary pathology as the cause of the chest pain. Patients with unilateral leg swelling, pitting edema of one leg, tenderness over the deep venous system, or calf swelling are likely to have PE as the cause of their chest pain.

Goodacre S, Locker T, Morris F, et al: How useful are clinical features in the diagnosis of acute, undifferentiated chest pain? Acad Emerg Med 9:203–208, 2002.

12. **How is the electrocardiogram (ECG) helpful in the evaluation of chest pain?**
The ECG findings most often associated with acute coronary syndrome are ST segment elevation, ST segment depression, inverted T waves, and new bundle branch blocks. Initially, the ECG may be normal in 20–50% of ED patients who are later diagnosed as having had an acute myocardial infarction. Comparison with previous ECGs may reveal subtle but significant changes. In pericarditis, the initial ECG changes may consist of diffuse ST elevation with depression of the PR segment. The ECG associated with a PE often demonstrates a normal sinus rhythm. The most common ECG findings associated with acute PE are sinus tachycardia or nonspecific ST-T wave abnormalities in the right precordial leads. Right heart strain secondary to a PE will result in a peaked P wave, right axis deviation, or a prominent S wave in

lead I; a Q wave in lead III; and a new T-wave inversion in lead III (S1 Q3 T3 pattern); however, these classic ECG changes associated with PE occur infrequently.

Savonitto S, Ardissino D, Grauger CB, et al: Prognostic value of the admission electrocardiogram in acute coronary syndromes. JAMA 281:707–713, 1999.

Smith SW, Whitman W: Acute coronary syndromes: Acute myocardial infarction and ischemia. In Chan TC, Brady WJ, Harrigan RA, et al. (eds): ECG in Emergency Medicine and Acute Care, Philadelphia, Elsevier, 2005.

13. **What abnormalities appear on the chest radiograph in diseases causing chest pain?**
The chest x-ray films of patients presenting with chest pain are frequently normal but may be diagnostic, as in a pneumothorax. Aortic dissection may show a widened mediastinum or a 4–5 mm or greater separation between the calcified intima and the lateral edge of the aortic knob. PE may show nonspecific signs such as atelectasis or an elevated hemidiaphragm. Rare signs include Hampton's hump, a wedge-shaped, pleural-based infiltrate representing an area of infarction, and Westermark's sign, which is an absence of pulmonary shadows distal to a central embolism. Pneumonia typically produces one or more areas of pulmonary consolidation, which may show atelectasis and be accompanied by pleural effusion and cavitation. Esophageal rupture classically can be associated with subcutaneous emphysema, pneumomediastinum, left-sided pleural effusion, or left-sided pneumothorax.

Ioaunides JP, Salem D, Chew PW, Lau J: Accuracy of imaging technologies in the diagnosis of acute cardiac ischemia in the emergency department. Ann Emerg Med 37:471–477, 2001.

14. **Are cardiac enzymes useful in the evaluation of chest pain in the ED?**
Serial measurements documenting a rise of troponin I, troponin T, and creatine kinase MB (CK-MB) can confirm the diagnosis of myocardial infarction. However, single determinations in the ED are frequently nondiagnostic because 3–4 hours may be required prior to elevation in the troponins or CK-MB level. Myoglobin may be detected within 2 hours after the onset of a myocardial infarction. Although the sensitivity of myoglobin approaches 90% in 4–6 hours, it is not specific for cardiac injury. Troponins are the biochemical markers of choice. They are highly specific of myocardial injury, rise at 4–6 hours, remain elevated for up to 10 days, and are more specific than CK-MB. Although troponins provide improved specificity compared with other biochemical markers for acute myocardial infarction, there are clinical processes that can be associated with elevated values. In the ED, the most important differential diagnoses of chest pain with troponin elevation are acute PE and myocarditis. Troponin elevations associated with acute PE typically occur with large emboli and are the result of acute right heart strain and overload.

Balk EM, Ioannidis JP, Salem D, et al: Accuracy of biomarkers to diagnose acute cardiac ischemia in the ED: A meta-analysis. Ann Emerg Med 37:478–494, 2001.

Hamm CW, Giannitsis E, Katus HA: Cardiac troponin elevations in patients without acute coronary syndrome. Circulation 106:2871–2872, 2002.

Kontos MC, Shah R, Fritz LM, et al: Implication of different cardiac troponin I levels for clinical outcomes and prognosis of acute chest pain patients. J Am Coll Cardiol 43:958–965, 2004.

15. **Are there any bedside tests that may help to identify the origin of acute chest pain?**
Several bedside tests may be helpful, but they are rarely diagnostic in themselves. Relief with nitroglycerin occurs in both angina and esophageal spasm, whereas acute myocardial infarction and unstable angina (acute coronary syndromes) may remain unrelieved. Antacids or *GI cocktails,* consisting of viscous lidocaine and an antacid, frequently resolve esophageal pain but also relieve pain in 7% of patients with angina. The use of antacids as a diagnostic test should be avoided. Pain from pericarditis is frequently worse in the supine position and relieved when leaning forward. Pain from esophageal disease is worsened with changes in position such as leaning forward or lying down. Musculoskeletal pain is also worsened with movement.

16. **Are there any other useful radiologic studies?**
    Aortic dissection may be diagnosed by a thoracic arteriogram, a rapid-sequence computed tomography (CT) scan, or by a transesophageal echocardiogram. A suspected PE may be confirmed by a ventilation-perfusion scan, spiral CT scan of the thorax, or pulmonary angiography. Esophageal rupture may be diagnosed by an esophagogram with a water-soluble contrast material.

    Ioanides JP, Salem D, Chew PW, Lau J: Accuracy of imaging technologies in the diagnosis of acute cardiac ischemia in the emergency department. Ann Emerg Med 37:471–477, 2001.

    Henrikson CA, Howell EE, Bush DE, et al: Chest pain relief by nitroglycerin does not predict active coronary artery disease. Ann Intern Med 139:979–986, 2003.

17. **What special considerations must be taken into account when evaluating chest pain in geriatric, diabetic, or female patients?**
    Although the sources of chest pain in the elderly do not differ significantly from the general population, the presenting symptoms are often atypical. Instead of chest pain, ischemic heart disease may manifest as sudden progressive dyspnea, abdominal or epigastric fullness, extreme fatigue, confusion, or syncope. Patients with diabetes mellitus may have altered pain perception, resulting in an atypical presentation similar to that of the elderly. The risk of coronary heart disease in women increases with menopause, particularly in those women not using estrogen therapy. Women with ischemic heart disease present in atypical patterns more frequently than men. This is because of the higher prevalence of less common causes of ischemia such as vasospastic and microvascular angina.

    Hamilton GC, Malone S, Janz TG: Chest pain. In Hamilton GC, Sanders AB, Strange GR, Trott AT (eds): Emergency Medicine An Approach to Clinical Problem-Solving, 2nd ed. Philadelphia, W.B. Saunders, 2003, pp 131–153.

    Lee PY, Alexander KP, Hammill BG, et al: Representation of elderly persons and women in published randomized trials of acute coronary syndromes. JAMA 286:708–713.

KEY POINTS: CHEST PAIN

1. The primary goal of the evaluation of acute chest pain is the inclusion or exclusion of a life-threatening disease process.

2. A thorough history is the most important diagnostic tool in the evaluation of chest pain.

3. Acute chest pain associated with radiation to the arms, neck, or jaw is often caused by acute coronary syndromes.

4. In the evaluation of chest pain, the electrocardiogram and cardiac enzymes are only helpful if they demonstrate positive findings.

5. Chest pain in elderly and diabetic patients is caused by common diseases but often presents in atypical fashion.

18. **Approximately 4% of patients with chest pain caused by acute myocardial infarction are discharged to home. What factors have been associated with failure to make the diagnosis?**
    - Patient younger than typically seen
    - Failure to obtain an accurate history
    - Incorrect interpretation of the ECG
    - Failure to recognize atypical presentations
    - Hesitance to admit patients with vague symptoms

- Reliance on laboratory assays such as cardiac enzymes
- Insufficient experience or training

Pope JH, Aufderheide TP, Ruthazer R, et al: Missed diagnosis of acute cardiac ischemia in the emergency department. N Engl J Med 342:1163–1170, 2000.

Rusnak RA, Stair TO, Hansen K, Fastow JS: Litigation against the emergency physician: Common features in cases of missed myocardial infarction. Ann Emerg Med 18:1029–1034, 1989.

BIBLIOGRAPHY

1. American Heart Association: www.americanheart.org
2. Gibler WB, Cannon CP, Blomkalns AL, et al: Practical implementation of the guidelines for unstable angina/non-ST-segment elevation myocardial infarction in the ED. Circulation 111:2699–2710, 2005.
3. Lee TH, Goldman L: Evaluation of the patient with acute chest pain. N Engl J Med 342:1187–1195, 2000.

CHAPTER 12

ABDOMINAL PAIN

Rick A. McPheeters, DO, and Thomas B. Purcell, MD

1. **What is the difference between visceral and somatic pain? How is this of practical importance?**

   Evolving patterns of pain frequently reveal the source and give an idea of the extent to which the process has advanced. Early, the patient may describe a deep-seated, dull pain (**visceral pain**) emanating from hollow viscera or the capsule of solid organs. This pain is poorly localized but generally falls somewhere along the midline of the abdomen. Later, as inflammation progresses to the parietal peritoneum, the pain becomes better localized, lateralized over the involved organ, sharper in intensity (**somatic** or **parietal pain**), and constant. Visceral pain that is superseded by somatic pain frequently signals the need for surgical intervention. A clear understanding of the process enables the clinician to identify more precisely the cause and rate of progression of pathology.

   Fischer JE, Nussbaum MS, Chance WT, Luchette F: Manifestations of gastrointestinal disease. In Schwartz SI, Shires GT, Spencer FC, et al (eds): Principles of Surgery, 7th ed. New York, McGraw-Hill, 1999, pp 1033–1079.

2. **What is the difference between localized and generalized peritonitis?**

   As the peritoneum adjacent to a diseased organ becomes inflamed, palpation or any abdominal movement causes stretching of the sensitized peritoneum and, consequently, pain localized at that site (localized peritonitis). If irritating material (pus, blood, gastric contents) spills into the peritoneal cavity, the entire peritoneal surface may become sensitive to stretch or motion, and any movement or palpation may provoke pain at any or all points within the abdominal cavity (generalized peritonitis).

3. **What are the common areas of referred pain associated with abdominal pain?**

   See Fig. 12-1.

4. **Which tests for peritoneal irritation are best?**

   Rebound tenderness is the traditional physical examination finding for peritonitis. In a patient with likely generalized peritonitis (obvious distress, an excruciating pain every time the ambulance hits a bump), the standard tests for rebound tenderness are unnecessarily harsh. Asking the patient to cough generally supplies adequate peritoneal motion to give a positive test. When in every respect the examination is normal, one highly sensitive test for peritoneal irritation is the heel-drop jarring (Markle) test. The patient is asked to stand, rise up on tiptoe with knees straight, and forcibly drop down on both heels with an audible thump. Among patients with appendicitis, this test was found to be 74% sensitive, compared with 64% for the standard rebound test.

   Markle GB: Heel-drop jarring test for appendicitis [letter]. Arch Surg 120:243, 1985.

5. **Why is it important to establish the temporal relationship of pain to vomiting?**

   Generally, pain preceding vomiting is suggestive of a surgical process, whereas vomiting before onset of pain is more typical of a nonsurgical condition. Epigastric pain that is relieved by vomiting suggests intragastric pathology or gastric outlet obstruction.

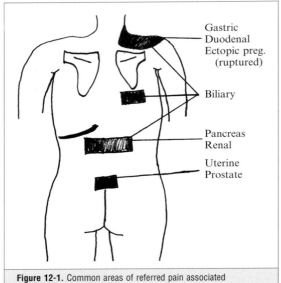

Figure 12-1. Common areas of referred pain associated with abdominal pain.

6. **What is the relationship of peritoneal inflammation to loss of appetite?**
Anorexia, nausea, and vomiting are directly proportional to the severity and extent of peritoneal irritation. The presence of appetite does not rule out a surgically significant inflammatory process, such as appendicitis. A retrocecal appendicitis with limited peritoneal irritation may be associated with minimal gastrointestinal (GI) upset, and one third of all patients with acute appendicitis do not report anorexia on initial presentation.

Rothrock SG, Green SM, Dobson M, et al: Misdiagnosis of appendicitis in nonpregnant women of childbearing age. J Emerg Med 13:1–8, 1995.
Wagner JM, McKinney WP, Carpenter JL: Does this patient have appendicitis? JAMA 276:1589–1594, 1996.

7. **Discuss the pitfalls in evaluating elderly patients with acute abdominal pain.**
Advanced age may and often does blunt the manifestations of acute abdominal disease. Pain may be less severe; fever often is less pronounced, and signs of peritoneal inflammation, such as muscular guarding and rebound tenderness, may be diminished or absent. Elevation of the white blood cell (WBC) count is also less sensitive. Cholecystitis, intestinal obstruction, and appendicitis are the most common causes for acute surgical abdomen in the elderly. Because of atypical clinical presentations, additional screening tests, such as amylase, liver function studies, and alkaline phosphatase, and the liberal use of ultrasound or computed tomography (CT) scan may be useful in this age group.

8. **What other factors should be sought in the history that may alter significantly the presentation of patients with abdominal pain?**
Symptoms and physical findings in patients with schizophrenia and diabetes may be muted significantly. The prior use of narcotics, steroids, or antibiotics may alter signs and laboratory results substantially.

Bickerstaff LK, Harris SC, Leggett RS, et al: Pain insensitivity in schizophrenic patients. Arch Surg 123:49–51,1988.

9. **What is the significance of obstipation?**

Obstipation—the inability to pass either stool or flatus—for more than 8 hours despite a perceived need is highly suggestive of intestinal obstruction.

10. **What vital sign is associated most closely with the degree of peritonitis?**

Tachycardia is virtually universal with advancing peritonitis. The initial pulse is less important than serial observations. An unexplained rise in pulse may be an early clue that early surgical exploration is indicated. However, this response may be blunted or absent in elderly patients.

11. **Does the duration of abdominal pain help in categorizing cause?**

Severe abdominal pain that persists for 6 or more hours is likely to be caused by surgically correctable problems. Patients with pain of more than 48 hours' duration have a significantly lower incidence of surgical disease than do patients with pain of shorter duration.

12. **Name the two most commonly missed surgical causes of abdominal pain.**

Appendicitis and acute intestinal obstruction.

13. **Is there a place for narcotic analgesics in the management of acute abdominal pain of uncertain cause?**

For fear of masking vital symptoms or physical findings, old, conventional surgical wisdom proscribes the use of narcotic analgesics until a firm diagnosis is established. Increasingly, however, studies have demonstrated that pain medication may be given to selected patients with stable vital signs because the analgesic effect may be reversed readily at any time by the administration of naloxone. Pace and Burke, in a prospective, double-blind study of 71 patients with acute abdominal pain, found that pain control with morphine had no deleterious effect on preoperative diagnostic accuracy. Although inconclusive, a growing body of data suggests that evaluation of acute abdominal disease may be facilitated when severe pain has been controlled and the patient can cooperate more fully.

McHale PM, LoVecchio F: Narcotic analgesia in the acute abdomen—A review of prospective trials. Eur J Emerg Med 8:131–136, 2001.

Pace S, Burke TF: Intravenous morphine for early pain relief in patients with acute abdominal pain. Acad Emerg Med 3:1086–1092, 1996.

14. **Which are the most useful preliminary laboratory tests to order?**

A complete blood count with differential and urinalysis generally are recommended. The initial hematocrit helps to define antecedent anemia. An elevated WBC count suggests significant pathology but is nonspecific. Elevated urinary specific gravity reflects dehydration, and an increased urinary bilirubin in the absence of urobilinogen points toward total obstruction of the common bile duct. Pyuria, hematuria, and a positive dipstick for glucose and ketones may reveal nonsurgical causes for abdominal pain. For patients with epigastric or right upper quadrant pain, lipase and liver function studies are advised. Any woman with childbearing capability should receive a pregnancy test. Serum electrolytes, glucose, blood urea nitrogen, and creatinine are indicated if there is clinical dehydration or other reason to suspect abnormality such as renal failure, diabetes, or a metabolic acidosis.

15. **Are radiographs always indicated?**

No. Plain films of the abdomen have the highest yield when used in the evaluation of patients with suspected bowel obstruction, intussusception, ileus, and free air secondary to a perforated viscus. They have much less utility in detecting intraabdominal mass, renal calculi, diverticulitis, gallbladder disease, and abdominal aortic aneurysms. If these disorders are suspected, other studies such as ultrasound or abdominal CT are more appropriate. Conversely, among patients with uncomplicated peptic ulcer disease or massive hematemesis, pain present for more than

1 week, strangulated abdominal wall hernias, or other obvious clinical indications for laparotomy, plain radiographs add little.

Greene CS: Indications for plain radiography in the emergency department. Ann Emerg Med 15:257–260, 1986.

16. **Which plain films are most useful?**
Traditional teaching holds that plain abdominal films should include a supine view plus either an upright view or a left lateral decubitus view (if unable to stand). The **supine view of the abdomen** is the most informative and worthwhile abdominal film. The upright film is superior for visualizing air-fluid levels associated with ileus, obstruction, or biliary air. The **erect chest radiograph** is most sensitive for detection of free intraperitoneal air and may show basal pneumonia, ruptured esophagus, elevated hemidiaphragm, air-fluid levels associated with subdiaphragmatic or hepatic abscess, pleural effusion, and pneumothorax. In the evaluation of patients with abdominal pain, the upright chest film, taken alone, has been shown to be more useful than films of the abdomen itself.

17. **Are air-fluid levels within the intestine always abnormal?**
No. It is commonly taught that air-fluid levels when seen on an upright abdominal film are *pathognomonic* for small bowel obstruction. A study of 300 normal patients by Gammill and Nice showed, however, that the average number of air-fluid levels was four per patient, with some films showing 20. Although typically less than 2.5 cm in length, some were 10 cm. Most of the air-fluid levels were found in the large bowel; only 14 of 300 normal patients studied showed air-fluid levels in the small bowel. The authors suggested that before air-fluid levels are used as the sole criterion for the diagnosis of paralytic ileus or mechanical obstruction, one should see more than two air-fluid levels within dilated loops of the small bowel.

Gammill SL, Nice CM: Air fluid levels: Their occurrence in normal patients and their role in the analysis of ileus. Surgery 71:771–780, 1972.

18. **A 7-year-old child presents with acute abdominal pain with a history of several similar bouts over the past 5 months. Physical examination is unremarkable. What is the most likely cause?**
In children older than age 5, abdominal pain that is intermittent and of more than 3 months' duration is **functional** in greater than 95% of cases, especially in the absence of objective findings such as fever, delayed growth patterns, anemia, GI bleeding, or lateralizing pain and tenderness.

KEY POINTS: COMMON DISEASES THAT CAN SIMULATE ACUTE ABDOMEN

1. Diabetic ketoacidosis

2. Food poisoning

3. Pneumonia

4. Pelvic inflammatory disease

19. **A patient with severe abdominal pain is found to be in diabetic ketoacidosis (DKA). How do I decide whether the abdominal pain is a manifestation of the DKA or whether a surgical condition has precipitated DKA?**
Patients with established DKA often present to the emergency department (ED) with severe abdominal pain. Although the precise mechanism of abdominal pain and ileus in patients with

DKA is not well understood, hypovolemia, hypotension, and a total body potassium deficit probably contribute. An acute surgical lesion may initiate DKA; nevertheless, most patients in DKA have no such pathology. Abdominal symptoms characteristically resolve as medical treatment restores the patient to biochemical homeostasis. Treatment of the DKA must precede any surgical intervention because of the extremely high intraoperative mortality among patients not so stabilized. If symptoms persist despite adequate correction of DKA, then an underlying surgical pathology becomes more likely.

20. **Is a rectal exam necessary in the patient with suspected acute appendicitis?**
The literature is inconsistent as to its usefulness in aiding the diagnosis; however, failure to perform a rectal exam is cited frequently in successful malpractice claims. Some other diseases may be effectively diagnosed only by rectal exam (e.g., prostatitis, occult GI bleed).

Craig S: Acute appendicitis. eMedicine 2005. www.emedicine.com/emerg/topic41.htm

WEBSITE

e-Medicine: www.emedicine.com

BIBLIOGRAPHY

1. American College of Emergency Physicians (ACEP): Clinical policy: Critical issues for the initial evaluation and management of patients presenting with a chief complaint of nontraumatic acute abdominal pain. Ann Emerg Med 36:406–415, 2000.

2. Brewer RJ, Golden GT, Hitch DC, et al: Abdominal pain: An analysis of 1,000 consecutive cases in a university hospital emergency room. Am J Surg 131:219–233, 1976.

3. Jaffe BM, Berger DH: The appendix. In Brunicardi CF, Anderson DK, Billiar TR, et al (eds): Schwartz's Principles of Surgery, 8th ed. New York, McGraw-Hill, 2005, pp 1119–1137.

4. Parker LJ, Vukov LF, Wollan PC: Emergency department evaluation of geriatric patients with acute cholecystitis. Acad Emerg Med 4:51–55, 1997.

5. Silen W: Cope's Early Diagnosis of the Acute Abdomen, 21st ed. New York, Oxford University Press, 2005.

CHAPTER 13

NAUSEA AND VOMITING

Juliana Karp, MD

1. **Vomiting? Do I really need to read this chapter when there are so many more interesting chapters in this book?**

   Yes! One of the most common and harmful mistakes made in the emergency department (ED) is assuming that nausea and vomiting are the result of gastroenteritis without thinking of and ruling out more serious causes. In addition, vomiting is one of the most common presenting complaints in the ED.

2. **What causes vomiting?**

   The act of vomiting is a highly complex act involving a vomiting center in the medulla. This center may be excited in four ways:

   - Via vagal and sympathetic afferents from the peritoneum; gastrointestinal, biliary, and genitourinary tracts; pelvic organs; heart; pharynx; head; and vestibular apparatus
   - By impulses coming from sites higher in the central nervous system
   - Via the chemoreceptor trigger zone located in the floor of the fourth ventricle
   - Via the vestibular or vestibulocerebellar system (motion sickness and some medication-induced emesis)

3. **Can vomiting itself lead to potential complications?**

   Yes. Some of these are life threatening:

   - Esophageal perforation or Mallory-Weiss tear
   - Severe dehydration
   - Metabolic alkalosis
   - Severe electrolyte depletion (particularly sodium, potassium, and chloride ions)
   - Pulmonary aspiration
   - Esophageal or gastric bleeding

4. **List the common gastrointestinal disorders that cause vomiting.**

   - Gastroenteritis
   - Gastric outlet obstruction
   - Gastric retention
   - Alcoholic gastritis
   - Pancreatitis
   - Hepatitis
   - Small bowel obstruction
   - Appendicitis
   - Cholecystitis
   - Diabetic gastroparesis

KEY POINTS: CHARACTERISTICS OF GASTROENTERITIS

1. True abdominal or pelvic tenderness is not usually present in gastroenteritis.

2. Gastroenteritis usually consists of both vomiting and diarrhea.

3. Gastroenteritis is usually a self-limited disorder, but IV rehydration and electrolyte replacement may be necessary.

5. **Are there different gastrointestinal causes of vomiting in children?**
Yes, particularly during the first year of life. These include gastrointestinal atresia, malrotation, volvulus, Hirschsprung's disease, gastroesophageal reflux, pyloric stenosis, intussusception, and inguinal hernia. (Vomiting in children presents considerations not covered in this chapter. See Chapter 62.)

Davenport M: ABC of general surgery in children: Surgically correctable causes of vomiting in infancy. BMJ 312:236–239, 1996.
Fuchs S, Jaffe D: Vomiting. Pediatr Emerg Care 6:162–170, 1990.

6. **List the common causes of vomiting other than gastrointestinal disorders.**
   - Infections
   - Pneumonia
   - Meningitis
   - Sepsis
   - Metabolic disturbances (diabetic ketoacidosis, uremia, hypercalcemia)
   - Toxicologic (digoxin, theophylline, aspirin, iron)
   - Neurologic (hydrocephalus, cerebral edema)
   - Renal calculi
   - Ovarian or testicular torsion
   - Pregnancy
   - Ruptured ectopic pregnancy
   - Labyrinthitis
   - Myocardial ischemia

7. **Can the character of the vomit help you to make a diagnosis?**
Sometimes, especially with gastrointestinal disorders. In acute gastritis, vomit is usually stomach contents mixed with a little bile. In biliary or ureteral colic, the vomit is usually bilious. In sympathetic shock (acute torsion of abdominal or pelvic organ), it is common for the patient to retch frequently but vomit only a little. In intestinal obstruction, the character of vomit varies—first gastric contents, then bilious material, with progression to brown feculent material that is pathognomonic of distal small or large bowel obstruction. Vomiting of blood is a whole different story (see Chapter 32).

Silen W (ed): Cope's Early Diagnosis of the Acute Abdomen. New York, Oxford University Press, 2000.

8. **What else do I need to ask the patient?**
   - **Associated signs and symptoms,** such as pain, fever, jaundice, and bowel habits. Think of hepatitis or biliary obstruction with jaundice. Always remember that gastroenteritis is uncommon without diarrhea.
   - **Relationship of vomiting to meals.** Vomiting that occurs soon after a meal is common with gastric outlet obstruction from peptic ulcer disease. Vomiting after a fatty meal is common

with cholecystitis. Vomiting of food eaten more than 6 hours earlier is seen with gastric retention.

- **Do not always focus on the gastrointestinal system.** Ask about medications and possible drug use, headache and other neurologic symptoms, and last menstrual period. Inquire about cardiac risk factors, especially in older patients.

9. **What do I look for on the physical examination?**
   Physical examination is helpful but can be unreliable. Look for signs of dehydration, particularly in children. Check for bowel sounds, which are increased in gastroenteritis and absent with obstruction or serious abdominal infections. Abdominal tenderness may be present in a variety of disorders, but a rigid abdomen points to peritonitis, a surgical emergency. Women of childbearing age with vomiting and abdominal or pelvic pain require a pelvic examination. Always remember the neurologic examination.

10. **Are laboratory tests indicated?**
    This question must be answered on an individual basis. In general, tests should be ordered based on the history and physical examination. Diabetics and elderly patients can "hide" serious infections and metabolic disturbances. Be careful with these patients.

11. **When should I order radiographs?**
    This must be judged on an individual basis. Abdominal radiography is usually nonspecific but may show free air with perforation of an abdominal viscus or dilated bowel with obstruction. A chest film can be useful in cases of protracted vomiting to rule out aspiration or pneumomediastinum. Lobar pneumonia with diaphragmatic irritation may cause vomiting with abdominal pain and few respiratory symptoms.

KEY POINTS: DIAGNOSIS OF THE VOMITING PATIENT

1. Always consider etiologies other than gastrointestinal disorders.

2. Take a thorough history, especially in the very young and elderly.

3. Always consider accidental ingestions in children and medication side effects or toxicities in adults.

4. Laboratory testing and radiographs are seldom useful in gastroenteritis but may be helpful to identify other causes of vomiting.

12. **How should I treat the vomiting patient?**
    1. Always remember to **protect the airway.** Patients with altered mental status should be placed on their side to prevent aspiration. Intubate early when necessary.
    2. **Intravenous (IV) fluids** usually are indicated for rehydration; normal saline or lactated Ringer's solution is preferred.
    3. **Nasogastric suction** can be therapeutic and diagnostic and is always indicated when there is a suspicion of a gastrointestinal bleed or small bowel obstruction.
    4. **Medications** to relieve nausea and vomiting must be used judiciously, especially in patients with altered mental status, hypotension, or uncertain diagnosis.
    5. Determine and, if possible, treat the underlying cause.

13. **What medications should I use?**
    See Table 13-1.

TABLE 13-1. ANTIEMETIC MEDICATIONS

Generic Name	Trade Name	Indication	Dose
Palonosetron	Aloxi	Vomiting with chemotherapy	0.25 mg IV prior to chemotherapy
Meclizine	Antivert	Vertigo and motion sickness	25 mg PO q.i.d.
Dolasetron mesylate	Anzemet	Vomiting associated with anesthesia or chemotherapy	12.5–100 mg PO or IV single dose
Hydroxyzine	Atarax	Nausea, vomiting, anxiety	25–100 mg PO or IM t.i.d. or q.i.d.
Diphenhydramine	Benadryl	Motion sickness	25–50 mg PO or IV q.i.d.
Prochlorperazine	Compazine	Nausea, vomiting, anxiety	10 mg PO, IM, or IV q.i.d. 25 mg PR b.i.d.
Aprepitant	Emend	Nausea and vomiting, with chemotherapy	125 mg PO on day 1, 80 mg PO on days 2 and 3
Phosphorated carbohydrate	Emetrol	Nausea and vomiting,	1–2 tbs PO q 15 min (not to exceed 5 doses)
Droperidol mg	Inapsine	Nausea and vomiting	0.625–2.5 mg IV or 2.5 IM (black box warning: QT prolongation)
Granisetron	Kytril	Nausea and vomiting with chemotherapy	10 μg/kg IV or 1 mg PO b.i.d. (only on day of chemotherapy)
Dronabinol	Marinol	Refractory nausea and vomiting with chemotherapy	5 mg PO t.i.d. or q.i.d.
Promethazine	Phenergan	Nausea vomiting, motion sickness, anxiety	12.5–50 mg PO, PR or IV q.i.d. (black box warning: children younger than 2 y/o)
Metoclopramide	Reglan	Nausea, vomiting, gastroesophageal reflux, gastroparesis	5–10 mg PO or IV dosage varies
Chlorpromazine	Thorazine	Nausea, vomiting, anxiety	10–25 mg PO q.i.d. 25 mg IM q.i.d. 100 mg PR q.i.d.
Trimethobenzamide	Tigan	Nausea and vomiting	250 mg PO t.i.d. or q.i.d. 200 mg PR t.i.d. or q.i.d. 200 mg IM t.i.d. or q.i.d.

Continued

TABLE 13-1. ANTIEMETIC MEDICATIONS—CONT'D

Generic Name	Trade Name	Indication	Dose
Scopolamine	Transderm Scop	Nausea, vomiting, motion sickness	1 patch q 3 days
Hydroxyzine pamoate	Vistaril	Nausea, vomiting, anxiety	25–100 mg PO or IM t.i.d. or q.i.d.
Ondansetron	Zofran	Nausea and vomiting with chemotherapy	Dosage varies

b.i.d. = twice a day, IM = intramuscular, IV = intravascular, PO = per os, PR = per rectum, q.i.d. = four times a day, t.i.d. = three times a day.

WEBSITES

1. Inapsine black box warning: www.fda.gov/medwatch/safety/2001/safety01.htm

2. Phenergan black box warning: www.fda.gov/medwatch/safety/2005/phenergan_deardoctorletter.pdf

BIBLIOGRAPHY

1. Ernst A: Prochlorperazine versus promethazine for uncomplicated nausea and vomiting in the emergency department: A randomized, double-blind clinical trial. Ann Emerg Med 36:89–94, 2000.

2. Harwood-Nuss AL, et al (ed): The Clinical Practice of Emergency Medicine, 4th ed. Philadelphia, Lippincott Williams & Wilkins, 2005.

3. Marx JA, Hockberger RS, Walls RM (eds): Rosen's Emergency Medicine: Concepts and Clinical Practice, 5th ed. St. Louis, Mosby, 2002.

CHAPTER 14

HEADACHE

Wyatt W. Decker, MD, and Luis H. Haro, MD

1. **How common are headaches? How often do people see a physician for one?**
   Of the U.S. population, 70% report having had a headache, and 5% have seen a physician for one. Greater than 1% of all office and emergency department (ED) visits are for headaches.

2. **When someone has a headache, what exactly is it that hurts?**
   The brain, the pia and arachnoid mater, the skull, and the choroid plexus cannot feel pain. The structures in the head that can feel pain include the scalp; skin; vessels; scalp muscles; parts of the dura mater; dural arteries; intracerebral arteries; cranial nerves V, VI, and VII; and the cervical nerves. Irritation of any of these may result in a headache.

3. **Name the most common headaches for which patients seek treatment.**
   Muscle contraction (tension) and vascular (migraine) headaches have a much higher incidence and are most common. Although painful, these disorders do not have life-threatening sequelae.

   Locker R, Mason S, Rigby A: Headache management-Are we doing enough? An observational study of patients presenting with headache to the emergency department. Emerg Med J 21:327-332, 2004.

4. **What true emergencies may present as a headache?**
   Headaches that are true emergencies include intracranial bleeding (subarachnoid hemorrhage, subdural or epidural hematoma, intracranial hemorrhage), ischemic cerebrovascular accident (CVA), dissection of a carotid or vertebral artery, hypertensive encephalopathy, brain tumor, giant cell arteritis (temporal arteritis), vasculitis, central nervous system infections (meningitis and abscess), cavernous sinus disease, pseudotumor cerebri, and dural venous thrombosis.

   Field AG, Wang E: Evaluation of the patient with nontraumatic headache: An evidence based approach. Emerg Med Clin North Am 17:127-152, 1999.

5. **How do I approach a patient presenting to the ED with a headache?**
   In the ED, you must think first of headaches that have high morbidity and mortality and then of headache causes that are more common. If you don't, you may overlook serious pathology. To help sort out the serious headaches, several red flags should be kept in mind (Table 14-1).

   Freitag FG, Diamond M: Emergency treatment of headache. Med Clin North Am 75:749-761, 1991.
   Lipton RB, Bigal ME, Steiner TJ, et al: Classification of primary headaches. Neurology 63:427-435, 2004.

6. **Are there clinical clues to distinguish tension and migraine headaches from headaches caused by more ominous conditions?**
   Yes. Tension and migraine headaches tend to be recurrent and similar from one episode to the next. A headache that is described as a "first" or "worst" headache or even just different from prior headaches requires close evaluation. A sudden, severe onset, commonly described as "the worst headache I have ever had," is classic for a subarachnoid hemorrhage. Likewise, the dull, boring headache that is unremitting over days to weeks and awakens one from sleep causes concern for an intracranial mass lesion or depression. Although focal neurologic signs are often

TABLE 14-1.   RED FLAGS IN PATIENTS WITH HEADACHE

Headache Characteristics	Differential Diagnosis	Possible Work-Up
Headache begins after age 50	Mass lesion, temporal arteritis	Erythrocyte sedimentation rate, neuroimaging
Sudden onset of headache	Subarachnoid hemorrhage, pituitary apoplexy, hemorrhage into a mass lesion or vascular malformation, mass lesion (especially posterior fossa)	Neuroimaging, LP if CT is negative
Headaches increasing in frequency and severity	Mass lesion, subdural hematoma, medication overuse	Neuroimaging, drug screen
New-onset headache in patient who has risk factors for HIV, cancer	Meningitis (chronic or carcino matous), brain abscess (including toxoplasmosis), metastasis	Neuroimaging, LP if neuro imaging is negative
Headache with fever, meningismus, rash, or altered mentation	Meningitis, encephalitis, Lyme disease, systemic infection, collagen vascular disease	Neuroimaging, LP, serology
Focal neurologic symptoms or signs of disease (other than typical aura)	Mass lesion, vascular malformation, stroke, collagen vascular disease	Neuroimaging, collagen vascular evaluation (including antiphospholipid antibodies)
Papilledema	Mass lesion, pseudotumor, meningitis	Neuroimaging, LP
Headache after head trauma	Intracranial hemorrhage, sub dural hematoma, epidural hematomas, post-traumatic headache	Neuroimaging of brain, skull, and possibly cervical spine

CT = computed tomography, HIV = human immunodeficiency virus, LP = lumbar puncture.

present before the onset of a classic migraine, those that are atypical for the patient warrant concern. Associated fever requires evaluation for infection, tumor, or drug use.

7. **The most important aspect of evaluating a patient with a headache complaint is the history. List the essential questions to ask in evaluating a patient with a headache.**
   1. Have you ever had a headache similar to this one before?
   2. Is this headache different from the ones you've had before?

3. Have you had any recent head trauma?
4. What were you doing at the onset of the headache?
5. How did this headache start?
6. What treatment were you using at home?

Field AG, Wang E: Evaluation of the patient with nontraumatic headache: An evidence based approach. Emerg Med Clin North Am 17:127-152, 1999.

8. **Why are age and onset important in the history of a patient with a headache?**
   Headaches beginning after age 55 are much more likely to have a serious cause, such as a mass lesion, giant cell arteritis, or cerebrovascular disease. Knowing the age of onset of headaches also can aid in diagnosis. Migraines most commonly begin before age 30. Tension-type headaches usually begin before age 50. Headaches occurring in the peripartum period may be caused by cortical vein or sagittal sinus thrombosis. In general, if a patient has a long history of previous similar attacks, a serious cause is less likely. If a patient reports numerous identical attacks treated at home, it is important to understand why this particular one led to an ED visit.

9. **Does the physical examination add any information?**
   The history should give you a good idea of what the problem is. The physical findings may support or refute your hypothesis. Vital signs are important. A fever may reflect infection. Hypertension may cause headache. Abnormal pulse or respiration may be due to infection or toxins. All vital signs may be altered, however, in the face of severe pain. On the head examination, palpate temporal arteries, sinuses, temporomandibular joints, and the scalp for tenderness. Check for nuchal rigidity and photophobia. Perform a focused or complete neurologic examination as indicated by the patient's history and general physical examination.

10. **How do I evaluate a patient who presents with a new sudden onset of a severe headache? What should be in my differential diagnosis?**
    See Table 14-2.

11. **What is the sensitivity of a noncontrast head Computed Tomography (CT) for detection of a subarachnoid hemorrhage?**
    Historically, 10–15% of subarachnoid hemorrhages were not seen on CT scans of the brain. Advances in imaging technology have led to improved accuracy of this study, however, and currently approximately 95% of subarachnoid hemorrhages are detected on CT scans of the head if done within 24 hours of the onset of symptoms. A lumbar puncture (LP) needs to be done to rule out subarachnoid hemorrhage in a patient with a normal CT scan with near 100% sensitivity.

Fontanarosa PB: Recognition of subarachnoid hemorrhage. Ann Emerg Med 18:1199-1205, 1989.

12. **How do I differentiate between a traumatic tap and a subarachnoid bleed?**
    By comparing the red blood cell counts in tube 1 and tube 3 or 4. With a traumatic tap, the blood should clear as it is collected, and an early tube is expected to have more cells than a later one. Xanthochromia, or heme pigment tinting, is always present if blood has been in the cerebrospinal fluid for 12 hours or longer and confirms an intracranial bleed.

13. **What are migraine headaches?**
    Although people may refer to any severe headache as a migraine, a migraine is a specific type of headache. True migraines are familial and affect women twice as often as men. The first headache usually occurs in an individual in their teens or 20s. Headaches typically are described as unilateral, severe, and throbbing and commonly are associated with photophobia and nausea. The headache may be nonthrobbing, however. Variations on all of the symptoms occur, but each patient tends to experience a similar constellation of symptoms with each headache.

TABLE 14-2. DIFFERENTIAL DIAGNOSIS AND WORK-UP FOR ACUTE, SEVERE HEADACHE

Pathologic Process	Clinical Characteristics	Work-Up
Subarachnoid hemorrhage	Headache worst of life Headache abrupt, effort related Normal neurologic examination to focal deficit or coma	CT; if normal, do LP
Vascular intracranial dissection (carotid, vertebral, or middle cerebral artery)	History of trauma, Marfan's syndrome, collagen disorders Carotid Ipsilateral headache Horner's syndrome CVA Vertebral Occipital-nuchal headache and posterior circulation CVA	Magnetic resonance angiography preferred Vascular ultrasound and conventional angiography if MRI not an option
Intracerebral hemorrhage	History of hypertension History of brain tumor Severe headache with signs of elevated intracranial pressure and depressed mental status	CT
Cerebral venous thrombosis (superior sagittal sinus or transverse sinus)	Postpartum, hypercoagulable states, and abrupt, dull, constant headache Sixth nerve palsy, seizures Signs of raised intracranial pressure	MRI, magnetic resonance venography, or conventional angiography
Pituitary apoplexy	Abrupt severe headache, progressive visual loss with subsequent signs of pituitary insufficiency	CT with coronal views of the pituitary

CT = computed tomography, CVA = cerebrovascular accident, LP = lumbar puncture, MRI = magnetic resonance imaging.

14. **What specific entities must be considered in patients with a headache and a history of immunosuppression?**
   In a patient known to have cancer, brain metastases or infections related to immunosuppression are more likely. In patients who are seropositive for human immunodeficiency virus (HIV),

opportunistic infections, such as cryptococcal meningitis or toxoplasmosis, brain abscess, and primary lymphoma of the central nervous system should be considered.

15. **What is special about a new-onset headache in a patient older than 55 with general malaise?**

    Temporal arteritis is a systemic arterial vasculitis that is rare before age 50 and dramatically increases in incidence afterward. Also known as *giant cell arteritis,* temporal arteritis should be suspected in any patient older than age 50 who has a new-onset headache or a change in an established pattern of headache. It is associated with localized scalp tenderness (anywhere in the scalp), malaise, myalgias, arthralgias, polymyalgia rheumatica, low-grade fevers, or other constitutional symptoms. Untreated, temporal arteritis can result in visual loss or stroke. Jaw claudication, if present, is strongly suggestive of the disorder. Erythrocyte sedimentation rate is greater than 50 mm/hour, and biopsy is required to establish the diagnosis. Treatment should be initiated promptly based on the clinical presumption and results of the erythrocyte sedimentation rate and not delayed by biopsy. The initial doses of prednisone range from 60 to 80 mg daily.

    Younge BR, Cook BE, Bartley GB, et al: Initiation of glucocorticoid therapy: Before or after temporal artery biopsy? Mayo Clin Proc 79:483-491, 2004.

16. **What is a sentinel bleed?**

    Approximately 50% of patients who have subarachnoid hemorrhage experience a warning or sentinel hemorrhage before their catastrophic bleed. This warning hemorrhage tends to occur days to months before the major event and is characterized by a headache of unusual severity and location that is similar to but less intense than that occurring with the major bleed. These headaches caused by sentinel hemorrhages tend to resolve over 1 or 2 days but may last for 2 weeks. Sentinel hemorrhages are associated with nausea and vomiting in approximately 20% of subarachnoid hemorrhage patients, neck stiffness or neck pain in 30%, visual disturbances in 15%, and motor or sensory abnormalities in 15–20%. The warning headaches of sentinel hemorrhages are so atypical and alarming that 40–75% of the patients seek medical attention. Commonly, these headaches are misdiagnosed as migraine, sinusitis, or tension-type headache, however, and the patients are discharged from medical care.

17. **How do I treat a migraine headache?**

    Patients who are unable to control their headache at home often present to the ED for better pain control or supportive therapy. The choice of treatment is based on case presentation, prior medications used, time elapsed since onset, patient's prior response to therapy, existence of comorbid conditions, and severity of the current attack (Table 14-3).

18. **How are cluster headaches different from migraines? How are they treated?**

    These are nonfamilial headaches predominantly affecting men. Excruciating unilateral pain lasting 30–90 minutes occurs multiple times a day for weeks, followed by a pain-free interval. During the attacks, autonomic signs of rhinorrhea and lacrimation frequently occur on the same side of the face. Attacks may be induced by smoking or alcohol. In the ED, oxygen relieves 90% of cluster headaches within 15 minutes. Other treatments include corticosteroids, calcium channel blockers, lithium, and methysergide.

19. **How do I treat tension headaches?**

    When other causes of headache have been investigated, treatment starts with reassurance and education. Because these headaches are usually chronic, they should be treated with nonaddictive analgesics. Biofeedback and acupuncture may be beneficial. All patients with this diagnosis should be screened for mood disorders because depression is a common cause of tension headaches.

TABLE 14-3. SELECTED MEDICATIONS FOR ACUTE MIGRAINE ATTACKS

Medication	Dose and Route*	Comments
Mild to moderate		
Acetaminophen	500–1000 mg	
Aspirin	650–1000 mg	GI upset
Ibuprofen	600–800 mg	GI upset
Naproxen sodium	275–550 mg	GI upset
Indomethacin	50 mg rectal suppository	
Moderate to severe		
Dihydroergotamine	1 mg IV or IM	May be repeated in 1 hr but not if triptans used already. Contraindicated in HTN, PVD, CAD, and pregnancy
Sumatriptan	6 mg SQ	May be repeated in 1 hr but not if ergots used already. Contraindicated in HTN, PVD, CAD, and pregnancy
Metoclopramide	10 mg IV or IM	Sedation and dystonic reaction
Prochlorperazine	10 mg IV or IM	Sedation and dystonic reaction
Ketorolac	30–60 mg IM or at risk for renal failure 15–30 mg IV	GI upset; caution in elderly and patients
Meperidine	25–100 mg IV or IM treatment modalities	Opioids less efficacious than other medications
Butorphanol	2 mg IV treatment modalities	Opioids less efficacious than other medications
Refractory attack, status migrainosus		
Dihydroergotamine	1 mg IV	Use in conjunction with antiemetic
Steroids	Various regimens	Controversial; based on anecdotal evidence

CAD = coronary artery disease, GI = gastrointestinal, HTN = hypertension, IM = intramuscular, IV = intravascular, PVD = peripheral vascular disease, SQ = subcutaneous.
*Assumes average-size adult patient.

20. **Which toxin may bring in entire families complaining of headache?**
   Improperly vented exhaust from stoves, furnaces, and automobiles may cause exposure to carbon monoxide. This colorless, odorless gas binds hemoglobin in preference to oxygen. Family members complain of recurring headache, dizziness, and nausea that are worst on awakening in the morning and improve after leaving the home. The treatment is high-flow oxygen for mild cases and hyperbaric oxygen for severe cases. Investigation of the source must not be overlooked.

21. **What special diagnostic considerations must be given to a patient with Acquired immunodeficiency syndrome (AIDS) and headache?**

Headache is a frequent complaint among AIDS patients, occurring in 11–55% of patients and may occur in many AIDS-related conditions. Aseptic meningitis associated with lymphocytic pleocytosis is seen in patients at the time of seroconversion. During acute HIV infections, patients may describe headache in association with fever, lymphadenopathy, sore throat, and myalgias. *Toxoplasma gondii* produces multiple brain abscesses and bilateral, persistent headaches. The diagnosis of toxoplasmosis is made by CT, magnetic resonance imaging (MRI), or brain biopsy. Other central nervous system lesions include B-cell lymphoma and progressive multifocal leukoencephalopathy. Cryptococcal meningitis is a common cause of headache in AIDS patients, occurring in 10% of patients. Meningitis is characterized by fever, headache, and nausea. The presence of meningismus or mental status changes is uncommon. Patients who have HIV and who present to the ED with persistent headache usually require neuroimaging, and if imaging is normal, LP should be done.

22. **What rapidly progressive infectious entity presents with fever, altered mental status, history of headache, and on physical examination no signs of meningismus?**

Herpes simplex encephalitis, the most common form of sporadic encephalitis. This is a necrotizing, hemorrhagic illness that results in brain destruction that mandates early aggressive treatment with antiviral therapy. LP with polymerase chain reaction and gadolinium-enhanced MRI are the diagnostic methods of choice.

23. **Describe the presentation of idiopathic intracranial hypertension. What is the complication if not treated appropriately?**

Formerly known as *benign intracranial hypertension* or *pseudotumor cerebri*, this entity presents classically in obese young women with recurrent headaches that are constant or intermittent and that may present with bilateral papilledema. Transient pulsatile tinnitus and visual phenomena are common. Occasionally, sixth nerve palsy may be seen in the physical examination. Usually CT is done to rule out a mass lesion, and if negative, LP is done; this not only is diagnostic but also commonly therapeutic. High opening pressure (25 to 40 cm H_2O) and a suggestive clinical scenario are diagnostic. Without treatment, there is a risk of visual loss. Treatment is with serial LPs, acetazolamide, and diuretics such as furosemide. Optic nerve fenestration is indicated in refractory cases.

KEY POINTS: HEADACHE

1. A response to analgesics does *not* exclude life-threatening causes of headache.

2. Current CT head scan identifies 95%, or 19 in 20, subarachnoid hemorrhages. LP is needed if subarachnoid hemorrhage (SAH) is a serious possibility.

3. HIV-positive patients presenting with headache should have a CT head with contrast to exclude opportunistic infections including toxoplasmosis.

4. A careful history and physical examination, including neurologic function, will identify most patients with life-threatening causes of other headache.

24. **Which cranial nerves pass through the cavernous sinus?**

Cranial nerves III, IV, V1 and V_{1-2}. Cavernous sinus disease may present as only a retro-orbital headache. An abnormality of any of the nerves passing through the cavernous sinus is suggestive of the diagnosis, however, and warrants further evaluation.

25. **How common are headaches in children?**

By age 7, 35% of children have reported infrequent headaches; 2.5% have reported frequent nonmigraine headaches, and 1.4% have been diagnosed with migraine. By age 15, more than 50% have reported infrequent headaches; 15% have reported frequent nonmigraine headaches, and 5% have been diagnosed with migraine. Treatment can start with acetaminophen or ibuprofen. Ruling out significant pathology is crucial in children. Subarachnoid hemorrhage, primary cerebral tumors, CVAs, metabolic conditions, and toxicologic causes should be considered.

26. **What is a blood patch?**

One third of patients experience headaches within hours of a diagnostic LP. This can occur secondary to the leakage of cerebrospinal fluid from the dural rent that results in dilation of intracranial vessels and traction. Headache is usually worse when the patient sits up and gets better with bed rest. Treatment includes bed rest and analgesia. If all conservative methods fail, autologous blood clot is used, the so-called blood patch. Blood is drawn from the patient and injected into the soft tissue at the site of the LP (using smaller needle diameter for the LP decreases the incidence of spinal headache).

27. **My 23-year-old patient with a history of migraines presents with a typical attack. She suggests the probability of a misdiagnosis and asks about the possibility of a brain tumor as the reason for her recurrent headaches. What can you tell her?**

The most common presenting symptoms of patients with primary brain tumors in the ED are headache (56%), altered mental status (51%), nausea or vomiting (37%), seizures (37%), and visual changes (23%). On physical examination, motor weakness is present in 37%; ataxia, papilledema, and cranial nerve palsies are present in 20–30%. The absence of any of these signs and symptoms beyond a headache does not eliminate completely the possibility of a brain tumor. In the absence of these findings and a typical migraine attack, the likelihood of a brain tumor is extremely low.

Snyder H, Robinson K, Shah D, et al: Signs and symptoms of patients with brain tumors presenting to the emergency department. J Emerg Med 11:253-258, 1993.

BIBLIOGRAPHY

1. Durand ML, Calderwood SB, Weber DJ, et al: Acute bacterial meningitis in adults: A review of 493 episodes. N Engl J Med 328:21–28, 1993.

2. Field AG, Wang E: Evaluation of the patient with nontraumatic headache: An evidence based approach. Emerg Med Clin North Am 17:127–152, 1999.

3. Fontanarosa PB: Recognition of subarachnoid hemorrhage. Ann Emerg Med 18:1199–1205, 1989.

4. Forsyth PA, Posner JB: Headaches in patients with brain tumors: A study of 111 patients. Neurology 43:1678–1683, 1993.

5. Freitag FG, Diamond M: Emergency treatment of headache. Med Clin North Am 75:749–761, 1991.

6. Henry GL: Headache. In Rosen P, Barkin RM (eds): Emergency Medicine: Concepts and Clinical Practice, 4th ed. St. Louis, Mosby, 1999, pp 2119–2131.

7. Linder SL, Winner P: Pediatric headache. Med Clin North Am 85:1037–1053, 2001.

8. Newman LC, Lipton RB: Emergency department evaluation of headache. Neurol Clin 16:285–303, 1998.

9. Snyder H, Robinson K, Shah D, et al: Signs and symptoms of patients with brain tumors presenting to the emergency department. J Emerg Med 11:253–258, 1993.

10. Ward TN, Levin M, Phillips JM: Evaluation and management of headache in the emergency department. Med Clin North Am 85:971–985, 2001.

CHAPTER 15

SYNCOPE, VERTIGO, AND DIZZINESS

William F. Young, Jr, MD

1. **Must I pick up this next patient with a complaint of dizziness?**

   Yes, and be prepared to see many more because up to 25% of patients include some element of dizziness in their primary complaint, and it is the most common complaint in patients older than 75 years.

2. **How do I approach this vague and ill-defined problem?**

   Is the patient using "dizzy" to describe a sensation of vertigo (the illusion of motion), lightheadedness (presyncope or frank syncope), or disequilibrium (imbalance)? Vertigo is the feeling you get when (usually, as a child) you spin around until you cannot stand up. Most patients can also recall having gotten up too fast from a supine position and feeling the "head rush" of lightheadedness. Those with disequilibrium often describe imbalance while walking, especially in the dark. Try to let the patient compare his or her current symptoms to these common experiences we all have felt.

3. **What is vertigo?**

   Vertigo is a great must-see Hitchcock film that stars Jimmy Stewart and involves murder, suicide, San Francisco, and a flawed hero. You can see it later after you read this chapter.

4. **How does one know his or her position in space?**

   We use a combination of visual clues (the horizon looks level), sensory input (proprioception says all my weight is on my feet), and vestibular (the "bubble level" in my inner ear says I'm level and still) input to determine our spatial orientation in space. When they don't agree, we feel dizzy.

5. **How does the vestibular system work?**

   The semicircular canals use the principle of liquid inertia to determine angular acceleration. The canals, oriented in three planes, are filled with a fluid, endolymph. When the head turns, the fluid tends to remain in the same place in space while the canal moves around it. Hair cells in the ampulla bend in response to this relative movement and send impulses via cranial nerve VIII to multiple radiations in the brain stem, cerebellum, and cerebrum.

6. **If the patient has vertigo, why is it important to distinguish between peripheral and central causes?**

   Although peripheral vertigo accounts for about 80% of the causes of true vertigo, central causes include more malignant etiologies, such as cerebellar infarction/bleeding, vertebrobasilar stroke, and brain stem lesions.

7. **What causes peripheral vertigo?**

   Benign paroxysmal positional vertigo (BPPV), Ménière's disease, and labyrinthitis are the major causes, followed by external auditory canal occlusion, otitis media, and perilymphatic fistula from trauma.

8. **What are the characteristics of peripheral vertigo?**

   DR FLIP. This mnemonic also reminds you that the Epley maneuver (later), which flips the patient, helps some causes of peripheral vertigo.

- **D** = **D**eafness (unilateral hearing loss is common)
- **R** = **R**inging in the ears (tinnitus)
- **F** = **F**atigable on repeated testing
- **L** = **L**atency after Dix-Hallpike maneuver
- **I** = **I**ntense symptoms (nausea)
- **P** = **P**ositional in nature

9. **What causes central vertigo?**
Bad stuff. Vertebrobasilar ischemia, multiple sclerosis, cerebellar infarction /hemorrhage, basilar migraine, and cerebellopontine angle mass lesions.

10. **What are the characteristics of central vertigo?**
CVA:
- **C** = **C**ranial nerve deficits
- **V** = **V**ertical nystagmus (never seen in peripheral vertigo except during Dix-Hallpike maneuver)
- **A** = **A**taxia (with severe gait impairment)

11. **How do I differentiate between vertigo and postural hypotension?**
Both conditions can cause dizziness with position change, nausea, vomiting, and diaphoresis, but the sensation of movement (vertigo) is absent in postural hypotension. Dizziness occurring without a postural change, such as rolling over in bed, is usually vertigo.

12. **What are the key points for each of the causes of peripheral vertigo?**
BPPV is the most common (50%), is most acute in onset (minutes), is due to debris in the posterior semicircular canal, and responds to the Epley maneuver. Labyrinthitis is less common (25%), occurs over days, and is probably associated with a viral infection and responds to corticosteroids. Ménière's is least common (10%), is less acute in onset (hours), is associated with hearing loss, tinnitus, and increased endolymph volume; and may respond to diuretics and antihistamines.

Barton J, Branch WT: Approach to the patient with vertigo. UpToDate Online Nov 2004. www.uptodate.com

13. **What targeted bedside tests aid in the diagnosis of vertigo?**
Examine the eyes for ocular palsies and nystagmus. Examine the ears for infection, perforation, and hearing function. Perform a full neurologic exam including cranial nerves, gait, stance, and cerebellar function. Perform the Dix-Hallpike and Epley maneuvers.

14. **How is nystagmus evaluated in the work-up of vertigo?**
Asymmetric impulses from the semicircular canals cause the eyes to drift toward the diseased side and "correct" with the fast component of nystagmus to the opposite normal side. In peripheral lesions, the nystagmus occurs when looking straight ahead but worsens when looking to the normal ear. When testing nystagmus, don't have the patient fix on your finger because this inhibits the nystagmus.

15. **What is the Dix-Hallpike maneuver?**
This diagnostic maneuver involves moving the patient rapidly from a sitting position with the head turned 45 degrees to the right (or left if testing that side) to a position with the head hanging down in a supine right (or left) ear down position with the chin pointed upward. Nystagmus, often toward the dependent eye or forehead, is characteristically associated with a delay of a few seconds and fatigable symptoms of vertigo on repetition. BPPV is confirmed with a positive test.

Pigott DC, Rosko CJ: The dizzy patient: An evidence-based diagnostic and treatment strategy. Emergency Medicine Practice Vol. 3 No. 3 March 2001. http://ebmedpractice.net/

16. **What is the Epley maneuver?**

The Epley maneuver is an attempt to physically move debris in the posterior semicircular canal into the utricle to improve symptoms in a patient with BPPV. It is successful about half the time. The technique is well described elsewhere with pictures but essentially involves performing the Dix-Hallpike maneuver, then turning the head to the opposite side while still supine and flipping over in the same direction to almost a prone position.

Furman JM, Cass SP: Benign paroxysmal positional vertigo. N Engl J Med 341:1590-1596, 1999.

17. **How does a patient with acoustic neuroma present?**

Patients with this rare cause of vertigo usually present with mild fluctuating central vertigo, progressive unilateral hearing loss, and tinnitus. Cranial nerve V and VII defects occur later. Audiometry and magnetic resonance imaging (MRI) are the tests of choice.

Barton J, Branch WT: Approach to the patient with vertigo. UpToDate Online Nov 2004. www.uptodate.com

18. **How do I treat peripheral (and central) vertigo?**

Treat peripheral vertigo with maneuvers and short-term vestibular suppressants. Acute labyrinthitis benefits from methylprednisolone in a 22-day taper. BPPV benefits from the Epley maneuver. Nonspecific vestibular suppressants include anticholinergics (e.g., scopolamine transdermal), antihistamines (meclizine 25–50 mg PO q 6 hr, dimenhydrinate 50 mg PO q 4–6 hr and diphenhydramine 25–50 mg PO q 4–6 hr) and benzodiazepines (diazepam 5–10 mg PO q 6 hr). Central vertigo requires evaluation by neurology or neurosurgery.

Strupp M, Zingler VC, Arbusow V, et al: Methylprednisolone, valacyclovir, or the combination for vestibular neuritis. N Engl J Med 351:354-361, 2004.

19. **What is syncope?**

A sudden temporary loss of consciousness with the inability to maintain postural tone. Because it is a symptom and not a disease, there are a wide variety of benign and life-threatening causes. Coma, head trauma, shock, and seizures may mimic syncope.

20. **What are the odds of determining the cause of a syncopal episode?**

Despite extensive and expensive work-ups, no cause is found in about 50% of cases. The three major categories of causes are summarized by the mnemonics HEAD, HEART, and VESSELS.

KEY POINTS: CAUSES OF SYNCOPE

1. HEAD (**h**ypoxemia and **h**ypoglycemia, **e**pilepsy, **a**nxiety, **d**ysfunctional brain stem)

2. HEART (**h**eart attack, **e**mbolism of pulmonary artery, **a**ortic obstruction, **r**hythm disturbance, **t**achydysrhythmia)

3. VESSELS (**v**asovagal, **e**ctopic, **s**ituational, **s**ubclavian steal, ENT, **l**ow systemic vascular resistance, **s**ensitive carotid sinus)

21. **Discuss the HEAD causes of syncope.**
    - **H** = **H**ypoxemia, **h**ypoglycemia
    - **E** = **E**pilepsy
    - **A** = **A**nxiety
    - **D** = **D**ysfunctional brain stem, vertebrobasilar ischemia, subarachnoid hemorrhage (SAH)

22. **Discuss the cardiovascular (HEART) causes of syncope.**
    - **H** = **H**eart attack (myocardial ischemia)
    - **E** = Pulmonary **e**mbolism
    - **A** = **A**orta (aortic obstructions caused by hypertrophic obstructive cardiomyopathy, aortic stenosis, and atrial myxoma)
    - **R** = **R**hythm disturbances such as sick sinus syndrome
    - **T** = **T**achyarrhythmias (ventricular tachycardia accounts for nearly 50% of the cardiac causes of syncope followed by sick sinus syndrome, bradycardia, and conduction blocks)

23. **What about the vascular (VESSELS) causes of syncope?**
    - **V** = **V**asovagal
    - **E** = **E**ctopic (reminds you of hypovolemia, ruptured abdominal aortic aneurysm [AAA])
    - **S** = **S**ituational (micturition, defecation, cough, Valsalva maneuver, although these may be caused by arrhythmias or vasovagal reactions)
    - **S** = **S**ubclavian steal (may cause syncope by loss of posterior cerebral circulation)
    - **E** = **E**NT (glossopharyngeal neuralgia, as from choking on a pretzel)
    - **L** = **L**ow systemic vascular resistance (drugs, Addison's, diabetic autonomic dysfunction, as in diabetes; medication-induced syncope)
    - **S** = **S**ensitive carotid sinus (accounts for only 4% of syncopal episodes)

24. **Summarize the initial concerns when treating a patient with syncope.**
    Most patients with syncope rapidly return to a normal mental status and have stable vital signs. There are treatment priorities, however.
    1. Obtain vital signs and evaluate and treat for immediate life threats (the ABCs [airway, breathing, circulation]).
    2. Oxygen, intravenous access, and cardiac and blood pressure monitoring should be initiated on patients who have abnormal vital signs, a persistent altered level of consciousness, chest pain, dyspnea, abdominal pain, or a significant history of cardiac disease.
    3. Assess for any trauma secondary to fall. Elderly patients are more likely to suffer head trauma secondary to syncope, and this may be a greater life threat initially than the cause of the syncope.

25. **Okay, I've ruled out the immediate life threats. Now what to I do?**
    Obtain a detailed history, do a directed physical examination, and obtain an electrocardiogram (ECG) on most patients. Then do a risk assessment and selectively obtain specific tests to determine whether admission is indicated.

26. **What components of the history are most important?**
    The diagnosis or the etiology of syncope is most often made from a careful, detailed history. The most important historical clue is the patient's recollection of the events just before the syncope. An abrupt onset of loss of consciousness with a brief (< 5 seconds) prodrome is a strong indicator of a cardiac cause, especially a rhythm disturbance. Similarly, syncope associated with exercise or while reclining or recumbent is associated with cardiac obstructive causes or arrhythmias. Patients who have vasovagal syncope often have premonitory symptoms of dizziness, yawning, nausea, and diaphoresis, and the event is during a period of some psychosocial stress. Clues to hypovolemia include thirst, postural dizziness, decreased oral intake, melena, or unusually heavy vaginal bleeding. Syncope after micturition, cough, head turning, defecation, swallowing, or meals suggests situational syncope. Previous episodes of syncope, upper extremity exertion (e.g., subclavian steal syndrome), and the presence of cardiac risk factors should be determined. A family history of sudden death may suggest long QT syndrome. Many medications can cause syncope, so determine all of the patient's current medications, especially when treating the elderly. Using a program to examine for drug interactions might reveal unexpected drug interactions (e.g., sildenafil [Viagra] and nitrates).

27. **How do I know it was not a seizure?**

Victims of arrhythmias and vasovagal faints often exhibit myoclonic jerks that many bystanders interpret as a seizure, so ask for specifics. A witness is invaluable but sometimes not available. Recovery from syncope is usually rapid, whereas a victim of a seizure awakens slowly with prolonged confusion or postictal state. Both may have trauma. The absence of an anion gap on blood drawn within 30 minutes of the event or no postictal state argues against a major motor seizure. Lateral tongue biting is highly specific for a major motor seizure.

Benbadis SR, Wolgamuth BR, Goren H, et al. Value of tongue biting in the diagnosis of seizures. Arch Intern Med 155:2346-2349, 1995.

28. **What is a directed physical examination?**

Be a detective, using HEAD, HEART, and VESSELS as a guide. Assume the patient with abrupt effort or exercise syncope has aortic stenosis or hypertrophic cardiomyopathy, and look for narrow pulse pressure, systolic murmur, or change in murmur with Valsalva. The presence of congestive heart failure places the patient at high risk. Examine the head carefully for trauma, bruits, and focal neurologic signs. Check blood pressure in both arms looking for subclavian steal. Search for occult blood loss or autonomic insufficiency. A complete neurologic examination is imperative in patients with possible HEAD causes of syncope.

29. **What tests are needed to assist in diagnosis?**

In most cases, none, except the ECG. A detailed history, a physical examination, and an ECG are sufficient to make the diagnosis in 50% of patients with syncope. The addition of a specific confirmatory test (e.g., echocardiography) is recommended for suspected cardiomyopathy.

30. **What about laboratory testing?**

In general, routine laboratory tests are of no help and should be ordered only if indicated by the history and physical examination.

31. **Who needs an ECG? What am I looking for?**

Most guidelines suggest that all patients with syncope should have an ECG because it is not invasive, may be diagnostic of a problem such as Brugada syndrome or long QT, and helps to risk stratify. Check for markers of cardiac disease, such as ischemia, infarction, arrhythmias, pre-excitation, long QT intervals, and conduction abnormalities. Left ventricular hypertrophy may be a clue to aortic stenosis, hypertension, or cardiomyopathy.

32. **If the basic evaluation is not diagnostic, who should receive further testing?**

In patients with unexplained syncope who have suspected organic heart disease or sudden syncope or who are older than age 65, consideration should be given to echocardiography and exercise treadmill testing. Holter or loop ECG monitoring also may be helpful.

33. **How useful is outpatient cardiac monitoring?**

Holter monitors continuously record data over a 24-hour period, which can be correlated to symptoms provided by a patient log. This brief window of monitoring finds about 4% of arrhythmias associated with symptoms and excludes arrhythmias as a cause of symptoms in another 15%. Extending the monitoring to 72 hours does not improve the yield. Loop ECG provides patient-activated recording of cardiac rhythm for 4 minutes before activation. These are useful in compliant patients with frequent episodes.

34. **What factors help to assign a patient to a high-risk or low-risk group?**

Studies attempting to determine high-yield risk factors such as the San Francisco syncope rule (CHESS: **c**ongestive heart failure, **h**ematocrit < 30, **E**CG abnormality, **s**hortness of breath, and **s**ystolic blood pressure [BP] < 90 mmHg), Geneva-Pittsburgh (age > 65, history of congestive heart failure [CHF], and abnormal ECG), and OESIL risk score from the European Society of Cardiology (age > 65, cardiovascular disease history, syncope without prodrome, and abnormal ECG) have been promising but are still in the validation phase of development. Consistent high-risk groups include older patients, patients with congestive heart failure, and those with an abnormal ECG.

Colivicchi F, Ammirati F, Melina D, et al: Development and prospective validation of a risk stratification system for patients with syncope in the emergency department: The OESIL risk score. Eur Heart J 24:811-819, 2003.

Quinn JV, Stiell IG, McDermott D, et al: Derivation of the San Francisco Syncope Rule to predict patients with short-term serious outcomes. Ann Emerg Med 43:224-232, 2003.

Sarasin FP, Hanusa BH, Perneger T, et al: A risk score to predict arrhythmias in patients with unexplained syncope. Acad Emerg Med 10:1312-1317, 2003.

35. Who is the best candidate for electrophysiologic studies?
A patient with structural heart disease with recurrent unexplained syncope because the diagnostic yield is reasonable and the treatment of the discovered abnormalities is often successful.

36. Are orthostatic vital signs helpful in the evaluation of syncope?
Yes and no. Orthostatic hypotension (defined as a blood pressure drop of 20 mm Hg on standing for 3–4 minutes) is associated with volume loss or autonomic insufficiency and an increased risk of fall and syncope. The European Society of Cardiology guidelines (www. escardio.org) recommend orthostatic vital signs as an essential evaluation tool. However, parameters for orthostatic hypotension are neither sensitive nor specific enough to warrant their use. A blood pressure drop of 20 mmHg has only 29% sensitivity and 81% specificity for 5% or greater fluid deficit. Of normal euvolemic patients older than 65 years, more than 25% falsely test positive. Reproduction of symptoms is a better predictor than any number change.

37. Are there guidelines for the evaluation of syncope?
Yes. American College of Emergency Physicians (ACEP): Clinical policy: Critical issues in the evaluation and management of patients presenting with syncope. Ann Emerg Med 37:771–776, 2001 and Brignole M, Alboni P, Benditt DG, et al: Guidelines on management (diagnosis and treatment) of syncope—Update 2004. Europace 6:467–537, 2004.

CHAPTER 16

SEIZURES

Kent N. Hall, MD

1. **What is a seizure? Why are seizures important to me?**

   A seizure is an episode of abnormal brain function caused by an aberrant electrical discharge from the brain. This electrical discharge may, or may not, result in characteristic muscle activity that is recognized as "seizure activity." In addition to tonic-clonic muscle activity, generalized seizures may also manifest as staring episodes, lip smacking or other minor motor activity, or complete disruption of muscle tone ("drop attacks"). Generalized seizures are often followed by a "postictal phase" characterized by confusion and/or lethargy. This phase usually lasts for 5–15 minutes, although it may last longer.

   The recognition and appropriate management of seizures are critically important to the patient and the emergency physician. Prolonged aberrant electrical activity in the brain causes neuronal destruction. This destruction is not due to build-up of metabolic by-products but is actually directly related to the electrical activity itself. For an unknown reason, the hippocampus is particularly sensitive to the damage from this electrical activity.

2. **How are seizures classified?**

   Seizures are classified according to the amount of brain involved in the abnormal electrical activity, its resulting physical manifestation, and its underlying cause. Overall, seizures are divided into two groups, generalized and focal (Table 16-1). Generalized seizures affect a large volume of brain tissue in the abnormal electrical activity, whereas focal seizures involve a specific brain area. Because of this, the manifestations of focal seizures, whether simple or complex, may lead to bizarre manifestations including hallucinations, memory disturbance, visceral symptoms (abdominal symptoms), and perceptual distortions. This has often resulted in the patient with partial seizures being misdiagnosed as having psychiatric disturbances.

   Often the emergency physician is presented with a patient who is not actively seizing but has "had a seizure." In this case, it is important to evaluate for secondary signs of seizure activity. These include bowel or bladder incontinence, biting of the tongue or buccal mucosa, and postictal confusion.

3. **What are the causes of seizures?**

   Seizures are abnormal electrical activity in the brain. **Primary seizures** are recurrent episodes without an underlying cause. This is classically referred to as epilepsy. **Secondary seizures** have a (usually non-neurologic) underlying condition. Table 16-2 lists the most common etiologies for secondary seizures.

4. **What is included in the differential diagnosis of seizure?**

   Anything that can cause a sudden disturbance of neurologic function may be mistaken for a seizure. Common processes that fall into this category include syncope, hyperventilation syndrome, migraines, movement disorders, and narcolepsy. Pseudoseizure is a special category and is discussed later.

5. **What should my priorities be in managing a patient who is actively seizing?**

   Start with the **ABCs.** Attention is always directed to the airway first. It is rare that a seizure patient needs to be intubated. Supplemental oxygen via nasal cannula should be given

TABLE 16-1. CLASSIFICATION OF SEIZURES

Type	Manifestations
Generalized	
Tonic-clonic (grand mal)	Loss of consciousness followed immediately by tonic contractions of muscles, then clonic contractions of muscles (jerking) that may last for several minutes. A period of disorientation (postictal period) occurs after the tonic-clonic activity.
Absence (petit mal)	Sudden loss of awareness with cessation of activity or body position control. The period usually lasts for seconds to minutes and is followed by a relatively short postictal phase.
Atonic (drop attacks)	Complete loss of postural control with falling to the ground, sometimes causing injury. It usually occurs in children.
Myoclonic	Brief, vigorous, spasmodic muscle contractions. These may affect the entire body or only specific areas.
Tonic	Prolonged muscle contraction. It occurs usually with associated deviation of the head and eyes in a particular direction.
Clonic	Repetitive jerking motions occur without any associated tonic muscle contraction.
Partial or focal	
Simple partial	Multiple patterns are possible depending on the area of the brain affected. If the motor cortex is involved, the patient will have contraction of the corresponding body area. If nonmotor areas of the brain are involved, the sensation may be paresthesias, hallucinations, and déjà vu.
Complex partial	Usually there is loss of ongoing motor activity with minor motor activity, such as lip smacking and walking aimlessly.
Partial with secondary generalization	Initial manifestations are the same as partial. However, the activity progresses to involve the entire body, with loss of postural control and possibly tonic-clonic muscle activity.

because of the increased oxygen demand caused by the generalized muscle activity. However, supplemental ventilation (bag-valve-mask) is rarely needed. Evaluation of the circulatory status can be readily accomplished by noting blood pressure, pulse, and capillary refill. Administration of crystalloids is usually all that is needed to correct hypotension. Check the temperature and administer antipyretics in appropriate doses when needed. Also, determination of the blood glucose and appropriate treatment should be included in this phase.

Airway protection can usually be accomplished by positioning the patient on his or her side. Suctioning of the patient's oral secretions will also help decrease the chance of aspiration. However, nothing should be put into the patient's mouth that might be bitten off (including fingers) and thus become an obstructing foreign body. *Gently* restraining the patient so he or she is not harmed is also important.

6. **What do I do if the patient doesn't stop seizing?**
Most seizures last for less than 2 minutes. When a seizure lasts longer, pharmacologic intervention is generally indicated. Benzodiazepines are the accepted first-line therapy.

TABLE 16-2. ETIOLOGIES OF SECONDARY SEIZURES

Metabolic

Hypoglycemia, hyperglycemia

Hyponatremia, hypernatremia

Hypocalcemia

Hypomagnesemia

Uremia

Hypothyroidism

Hepatic encephalopathy

High anion gap acidosis

Fever ("febrile seizures")

Infectious diseases

Meningitis

Encephalitis

Cerebral abscess

Cerebral parasitosis

HIV

Drugs/toxins (multiple)

Cocaine, lidocaine

Antidepressants

Theophylline

Alcohol withdrawal

Drug withdrawal

Structural

Trauma (recent and remote)

Intracranial hemorrhage

Vascular lesions

Mass lesions

Eclampsia

Hypertensive encephalopathy

HIV = human immunodeficiency virus.

The intravenous route is the preferred route of administration. Lorazepam is the conventional first choice because of theoretical issues related to duration of action. However, diazepam or midazolam may also be used. Diazepam may be administered intravenously, rectally, or intraosseously but is not recommended for intramuscular use because of uneven uptake. Midazolam may be administered rectally.

Once the seizure has ceased, anticonvulsants are used to keep it from recurring. Phenytoin is considered the first-line therapy. Table 16-3 shows the medications in this class along with their dosage and route of administration.

TABLE 16–3. ANTICONVULSANTS

Drug	Adult dose
Phenytoin	15–20 mg/kg IV at <50 mg/min
Fosphenytoin	15–20 mg PE/kg at 100–150 mg PE/min; may be given IM
Phenobarbital	20 mg/kg IV at 60–100 mg/min. May be given as IM loading dose
Valproate	10 mg/kg PR. Should be diluted 1:1 with water; slow onset of action
Pentobarbital	5 mg/kg IV at 25 mg/min, then titrate to EEG. Intubation required
Isoflurane	Via general endotracheal anesthesia

EEG = electroencephalogram, IM = intramuscular, IV = intravenous, PE = phenytoin sodium equivalents, PR = per rectum.

7. **What is status epilepticus? How is it managed?**
When seizures last longer than 5 minutes despite acute pharmacologic intervention or recur so frequently that normal mentation does not resume between the seizures, it is called "status epilepticus." In this case, immediate pharmacologic intervention is indicated. Table 16-4 gives an algorithm that can be used to manage the patient with status epilepticus.

Lowenstein DH, Alldredge BK: Status epilepticus. N Engl J Med 338:970, 1998.

TABLE 16–4. PROPOSED GUIDELINE FOR MANAGEMENT OF THE PATIENT WITH STATUS EPILEPTICUS

Time Frame	Measures
	Establish/maintain airway
	IV/oxygen/monitor
0–5 min	Dextrose, 0.5 gm/kg IV, if indicated
	Consider thiamine, 100 mg IV, and magnesium 1–2 gm IV for alcoholic or malnourished patients
	Lorazepam, 1 mg per min IV up to 0.1 mg/kg (or diazepam, 5 mg IV q 5 min up to 20 mg)
10–20 min	Phenytoin, 20 mg/kg IV at 50 mg/min, or fosphenytoin, 20 mg/kg PE IV at 150 mg/min
	Additional phenytoin, 5–10 mg/kg IV, or additional fosphenytoin, 5–10 mg/kg PE IV
	Phenobarbital up to 20 mg/kg IV at 50–75 mg/min IV
30 min	And/or
	General anesthesia with midazolam, 0.2 mg/kg slow IVP, then 0.75–10 μg/kg/min
	Or propofol, 1–2 mg/kg IV, then 1–15 mg/kg/hr
	Or pentobarbital, 10–15 mg/kg IV over 1 hr, then 0.5–1.0 mg/kg/hr

IV = intravenous, IVP = intravenous push, PE = phenytoin sodium equivalents.
Adapted from Lowenstein DH, Aldredge BK: Status epilepticus. N Engl J Med 338:970, 1998.

8. Is the history important?

The history if vitally important! The mnemonic **COLD** can be used to ensure you have covered the aspects of the seizure activity itself:

- **C** = **C**haracter: What type of seizure activity occurred?
- **O** = **O**nset: When did it start? What was the patient doing?
- **L** = **L**ocation: Where did the activity start?
- **D** = **D**uration: How long did it last?

In general, seizures start abruptly, are stereotyped (similar seizure activity recurs from attack to attack in an individual patient), are not provoked by environmental stimuli, are manifested by purposeless or inappropriate motor activity, and, except for petit mal seizures, are followed by a period of confusion or lethargy (the postictal phase). Other important historical aspects include the patient's past medical history (especially previous seizure history), alcohol use, toxic ingestions, current medications, any history of central nervous system (CNS) neoplasms, and history of recent or remote trauma.

9. In addition to the neurologic examination, what other parts of the physical examination are important?

A complete head-to-toe examination is important. In addition to looking for causes of the seizure, the physician should look for trauma caused by the seizure. The examination is often normal but occasionally may give clues to an underlying problem. Specifically, examination of the skin might reveal lesions from meningococcemia, other infectious problems, or stigmata of liver failure. Examine the head for trauma. If nuchal rigidity is found, meningitis or subarachnoid hemorrhage should be suspected. A heart murmur, especially if records indicate none was heard before, might indicate subacute bacterial endocarditis, with resultant embolization as the underlying cause of the seizure.

The neurologic examination is important. Focal neurologic findings, such as focal paresis after the seizure (Todd's paralysis), may indicate a focal cerebral lesion (tumor, abscess, cerebral contusion) as the cause of the seizure. Evaluation of the cranial nerves and the fundi can point to increased intracranial pressure.

10. What ancillary testing should I do in the patient with a history of seizures?

Extensive ancillary testing is reserved for the patient with new-onset seizure. For patients with a prior history of seizures who have an unprovoked attack, measurement of appropriate serum anticonvulsant levels is all that is required. The decision to proceed with further testing depends on the patient's history and physical findings at the time of presentation. If there is a question whether the patient had a major motor seizure, then measurement of the anion gap within 1 hour of the seizure might be of benefit.

A transiently (< 1 hour) raised anion gap is good evidence that a grand mal seizure has occurred. This is determined by blood samples drawn as close to the time of seizure as possible. Field blood samples are ideal for this study. If there is no anion gap acidosis, one may presume that the patient did not have a major motor seizure.

KEY POINTS: ANCILLARY TESTING IN PATIENTS WITH SEIZURES

1. Usually not indicated for patients with recurrent seizures unchanged from prior episodes

2. Should be limited to those tests designed to find underlying causes of seizures

3. Include blood chemistries (sodium, calcium, magnesium), blood sugar, appropriate drug screen, kidney function, and liver function

11. **And if the patient does not have a history of seizures?**

    If this is a new-onset seizure, ancillary tests are more important, although the yield is still quite low. A screen for metabolic derangements (sodium, calcium, glucose, magnesium, elevated blood urea nitrogen [BUN], or creatinine) is important. Toxicologic screens targeted at substances that are known to cause seizures (cocaine, lidocaine, antidepressants, theophyline, and stimulants are among the most common) should be obtained if clinically indicated.

12. **What about imaging studies?**

    In the patient with a first-time seizure, emergent neuroimaging is recommended for patients in whom a structural lesion is suspected. This includes patients with new focal deficits, persistent altered mental status, fever, recent head trauma, persistent headache, history of cancer, or presence of a coagulopathy or platelet disorder; patients who are on anticoagulation therapy; and patients who are human immunodeficiency virus (HIV) positive or otherwise immunosuppressed. Emergent neuroimaging should also be considered in the patient with first-time seizure who is older than 40 years or who has a partial seizure. Further recommendations are available at the American College of Emergency Physicians (ACEP) website.

    http://www.acep.org/webportal/PracticeResources/ClinicalPolicies

13. **What should be the disposition of the patient who presents with a seizure?**

    Patients who present with any of the following should be considered for emergent admission to the hospital for inpatient evaluation and therapy: persistent altered mental status, CNS infection, new focal abnormality, new intracranial lesion, underlying correctable medical problem (significant hypoxia, hypoglycemia, hyponatremia, dysrhythmia, significant alcohol withdrawal), acute head trauma, status epilepticus, and eclampsia. If the patient has a history of seizure and has a simple seizure and a subtherapeutic anticonvulsant level, then this should be addressed prior to discharge.

    Patients with new-onset seizures who have normal work-ups in the emergency department (ED) and are medically stable may be considered for discharge. In this case, contact with the patient's primary care physician or a consulting neurologist is important. Also important is instructing the patient on the possibility of another seizure and the advisability of avoiding working with hazardous machines, driving an auto, and climbing a ladder. Also, most states have laws that require reporting of a patient with seizures, if the patient has a driver's license.

KEY POINTS: EMERGENT NEUROIMAGING RECOMMENDATIONS FOR PATIENTS WITH SEIZURES

1. Emergent imaging for patients with new focal deficits, persistent altered mental status (with or without intoxication), fever, recent trauma, persistent headache, history of cancer, history of anticoagulation, or suspicion of acquired immunodeficiency syndrome (AIDS) and when timely follow-up cannot be ensured

2. Urgent imaging for patients who have completely recovered from their seizure and for whom no clear-cut cause has been identified to help identify a possible structural cause

3. Patients with first-time seizures who are older than 40 years or have partial-onset seizure

4. Patients with prior history of seizures who have a new seizure pattern or type or prolonged postictal confusion or worsening mental status

14. **Should I start the patient with a new seizure on antiepileptic medication prior to discharge?**

This decision is best made in consultation with the patient's primary care physician or neurologist. However, for patients with first-time seizures who meet discharge qualifications, it is common not to start them on anticonvulsants until seen in follow-up and further testing (i.e., electroencephalogram [EEG]) is completed.

15. **What is a pseudoseizure?**

Pseudoseizures are functional events that may mimic seizures in their motor activity or behavior. They are not caused by abnormal electrical discharges in the brain. In general, patients with pseudoseizures have underlying anxiety or hysterical/histrionic personality disorders. Pseudoseizures are difficult to diagnose in the ED. Some maneuvers that may be of benefit include suggesting to the patient that the seizure will stop soon or attempting to distract the patient with loud noises or bright lights during the "seizure" activity. Patients who show asynchronous extremity movements, forward thrusting movement of the pelvis, and eyes deviated toward the ground no matter what the head position are more likely to be having pseudoseizures. Simultaneous video and EEG monitoring can help to differentiate true seizures from pseudoseizures. In addition, a serum prolactin level drawn within 20 minutes of seizure activity should be elevated in the patient with true seizure. Unfortunately, neither of the previously mentioned modalities is routinely available in the ED.

CHAPTER 17

ANAPHYLAXIS

Vincent J. Markovchick, MD

1. **What is anaphylaxis?**
   A systemic immediate hypersensitivity reaction of multiple organ systems to an antigen-induced, IgE-mediated immunologic mediator release in previously sensitized individuals.

2. **What is an anaphylactoid reaction?**
   A potentially fatal syndrome clinically similar to anaphylaxis, which is not an IgE-mediated response and may follow a single first-time exposure to certain agents, such as radiopaque contrast media.

3. **Name the most common causes of anaphylaxis.**
   Ingestion, inhalation, or parenteral injection of antigens that sensitize predisposed individuals. Common antigens include drugs (e.g., penicillin), foods (shellfish, nuts, egg whites), insect stings (hymenoptera) and bites (snakes), diagnostic agents (ionic contrast media), and physical and environmental agents (latex, exercise, and cold). **Idiopathic anaphylaxis** is a diagnosis of exclusion that is made when no identifiable cause can be determined.

   Volcheck GW, Li JT: Exercise-induced uticariaurticaria and anaphylaxis. Mayo Clin Proc 72:140–147, 1997.

4. **List the common *target* organs.**
   - Skin (urticaria, angioedema)
   - Mucous membranes (edema)
   - Upper respiratory tract (edema and hypersecretions)
   - Lower respiratory tract (bronchoconstriction)
   - Cardiovascular system (vasodilation and cardiovascular collapse)

5. **What are the most common signs and symptoms?**
   The clinical presentation ranges from mild to life threatening. Mild manifestations that occur in most people include urticaria and angioedema. Life-threatening manifestations involve the respiratory and cardiovascular systems. Respiratory signs and symptoms include acute upper airway obstruction presenting with stridor or lower airway manifestations of bronchospasm with diffuse wheezing. Cardiovascular collapse presents in the form of syncope, hypotension, tachycardia, and arrhythmias.

6. **What is the role of diagnostic studies?**
   There is no role for diagnostic studies in anaphylaxis because diagnosis and treatment are based solely on clinical signs and symptoms. There is a role for skin testing either before administration of an antigen or in follow-up referral to determine exact allergens involved.

7. **What is the differential diagnosis?**
   Septic and cardiogenic shock, asthma, croup and epiglottitis, vasovagal syncope, and myocardial or any acute cardiovascular or respiratory collapse of unclear origin.

8. **What is the most common form of anaphylaxis, and how is it treated?**
   Urticaria, either simple or confluent, is the most benign and the most common clinical manifestation. This is thought to be due to a capillary leak mediated by histamine release. It may

be treated by the administration of antihistamines (orally, intramuscularly, or intravenously) or epinephrine (subcutaneously or intramuscularly).

9. **Summarize the initial treatment for life-threatening forms of anaphylaxis.**
   1. Upper airway obstruction with stridor and edema is treated with high-flow nebulized oxygen, racemic epinephrine, and intravenous (IV) epinephrine. If airway obstruction is severe or increases, perform endotracheal intubation or cricothyroidotomy.
   2. Acute bronchospasm is treated with epinephrine. Mild-to-moderate wheezing in patients with normal blood pressure may be treated with 0.01 mg/kg of 1:1000 epinephrine administered intramuscularly. If the patient is in severe respiratory distress or has a *quiet* chest, administer IV epinephrine via a drip infusion: 1 mg of epinephrine in 250 mL of D_5W at an initial rate of 1 µg/min with titration to desired effect. Bronchospasm refractory to epinephrine may respond to a nebulized beta agonist, such as albuterol sulfate or metaproterenol, in recommended doses.
   3. Cardiovascular collapse presenting with hypotension is treated with a constant infusion of epinephrine, titrating the rate to attain a systolic blood pressure of 100 mmHg or mean arterial pressure of 80 mmHg.
   4. For patients in full cardiac arrest, administer 1:10,000 epinephrine, 1 mg slow IV push or via endotracheal tube. Immediate endotracheal intubation or cricothyroidotomy should be performed.

KEY POINTS: ANAPHYLAXIS

1. Life-threatening target organs are the upper airway mucosa, bronchiole smooth muscle, and the cardiovascular system.

2. Hypotension is the indication for IV epinephrine.

3. Administer IV epinephrine as a drip, not as a bolus, in the noncardiac arrest situation.

10. **What are the adjuncts to initial epinephrine and airway management?**
    If intubation is unsuccessful and cricothyroidotomy is contraindicated, percutaneous transtracheal jet ventilation via needle cricothyroidotomy should be considered, especially in small children. IV diphenhydramine (1 mg/kg) should be given to all patients. Simultaneous administration of an H_2 blocker, such as cimetidine, 300 mg intravenously, may be helpful. Aerosolized bronchodilators, such as metaproterenol, are useful if bronchospasm is present. For refractory hypotension, pressors, such as norepinephrine or dopamine, may be administered. Glucagon, 1 mg intravenously every 5 minutes, may be helpful in *epinephrine-resistant* patients who are on long-term β-adrenergic blocking agents, such as propranolol. Corticosteroids have limited benefit because of the delayed onset of action, but they may be beneficial in patients with prolonged bronchospasm or hypotension.

    Muellman RL, Tran PT: Allergy, hypersensitivity and anaphylaxis. In Rosen P (ed): Emergency Medicine: Concepts and Clinical Practice, 5th ed. St. Louis, Mosby, 2002, pp 1619–1634.

11. **What are the complications of bolus IV epinephrine administration?**
    When epinephrine 1:10,000 is administered via IV push in patients who have an obtainable blood pressure or pulse, there is significant potential for overtreatment and the potentiation of hypertension, tachycardia, ischemic chest pain, acute myocardial infarction, and ventricular arrhythmias. Extreme care must be exercised in elderly patients and in patients with underlying coronary artery disease. It is much safer to give IV epinephrine by a controlled titratable drip infusion with continuous monitoring of cardiac rhythm and blood pressure.

    Horak A, Raine R, Opie LH, et al: Severe myocardial ischemia induced by intravenous adrenaline. BMJ 286:519, 1983.

12. **Is there a role for prophylactic treatment in anaphylaxis? How is this performed?**
     When the potential benefits of treatment or diagnosis outweigh the risks (e.g., administration of antivenom for life-threatening or limb-threatening snake bites), informed consent should be obtained if the patient is competent. Pretreatment with IV diphenhydramine (Benadryl) and corticosteroids should be carried out. An IV epinephrine infusion should be prepared. The patient should be in an intensive care unit (ICU) setting with continuous monitoring of blood pressure, cardiac rhythm, and oxygen saturation. Full intubation and cricothyroidotomy equipment should be at the bedside. Administration of the antigen (e.g., rattlesnake antivenom) should be started slowly with a physician at the bedside who is capable of immediately administering IV epinephrine and managing the airway. Nonionic contrast medium for diagnostic imaging studies should be given to patients with a history of anaphylaxis to ionic contrast material.

13. **What about steroids?**
     Because corticosteroids have an onset of action of approximately 4–6 hours after administration, they have limited or no benefit in the initial acute treatment of anaphylaxis. The administration of hydrocortisone (250 to 1000 mg intravenously) or methylprednisolone (125 to 250 mg intravenously), followed by a tapering dose over 7–10 days, is an acceptable regimen after the resolution of the initial anaphylactic episode.

14. **What is the disposition of a patient who initially responds to aggressive treatment?**
     Although most patients respond positively to early, aggressive treatment and may become asymptomatic, all patients with true anaphylactic reactions should be admitted to either an emergency department (ED) or hospital observation unit for 6–8 hours of observation. Patients who continue to have life-threatening symptoms (e.g., bronchospasm, hypotension, or upper airway obstruction) should be admitted to an ICU.

     Smit DeV, Cameron PA, Rainer TH: Anaphylaxis presentations to an emergency departmnentdepartment in Hong Kong: Iincidence and predictors of biphasic reactions. J Emerg Med 28:381–388, 2005.

15. **What is the prehospital or out-of-hospital treatment of anaphylaxis?**
     Patients who are known to be at high risk (e.g., previous anaphylactic reaction to hymenoptera) should be prescribed and educated in the self-administration of epinephrine into the muscles of the thigh with an autoinjector at the first sign of anaphylactic symptoms. Self-administration of oral diphenhydramine is indicated to treat mild reactions such as urticaria or concomitant with the administration of epinephrine.

16. **Is there an advantage of Intramuscular (IM) over subcutaneous epinepherine injection?**
     Yes, if injected into the thigh. A recent study has demonstrated higher peak plasma levels when epinephrine is injected into the muscles of the lateral thigh over injections subcutaneously or into the deltoid muscle.

     Simons, FER, Gu X, Simons KJ: Epinephrine absorption in aduultsadults: iIntramuscular versus subcutaneous injection. J Allergy Clin Immuno 108:871–873, 2001.

BIBLIOGRAPHY

1. Horak A, Raine R, Opie LH, et al: Severe myocardial ischemia induced by intravenous adrenaline. BMJ 286:519, 1983.
2. Lee ML: Glucagon in anaphylaxis (letter). J Allergy Clin Immunol 69:331, 1981.
3. Muellman RL, Tran PT: Allergy, hypersensitivity and anaphylaxis. In Rosen P (ed): Emergency Medicine: Concepts and Clinical Practice, 5th ed. St. Louis, Mosby, 2002, pp 1619–1634.

4. Runge JW, Martinex JC, Cavuti EM: Histamine antagonists in the treatment of acute allergic reactions. Ann Emerg Med 21237–242, 1992.
5. Simons FER, Gu X, Simons KJ: Epinephrine absorption in adults: Intramuscular versus subcutaneous injection. J Allergy Clin Immuno 108871–873, 2001.
6. Smit DeV, Cameron PA, Rainer TH: Anaphylaxis presentations to an emergency department in Hong Kong: Incidence and predictors of biphasic reactions. J Emerg Med 28381–388, 2005.
7. Volcheck GW, Li JT: Exercise-induced urticaria and anaphylaxis. Mayo Clin Proc 72140–147, 1997.

CHAPTER 18

LOW BACK PAIN

Gregg Miller, MD, and Robert Hockberger, MD

1. **Can I skip this chapter?**

   Not if you anticipate a career that involves caring for adults. Low back pain (LBP) is the second most common cause of physician visits, following upper respiratory symptoms. Approximately 70–85% of all people experience LBP during their lives. It is the most common cause of activity limitation in people younger than 45 years and the third most common cause in people older than 45 (after heart disease and arthritis). The cost of diagnosis, treatment, disability, lost productivity, and litigation due to LBP exceeds $50 billion annually, making it the third most expensive medical disorder in the United States, after heart disease and cancer.

   Anderson GBJ: Epidemiological features of chronic low-back pain. Lancet 354:581–585, 1999.

2. **What are the causes of LBP?**

   Roughly 97% of LBP cases are caused by mechanical spine disorders. Only 3% of cases are caused by nonmechanical spine disorders (especially spinal malignancy and infection) or visceral disease (particularly abdominal aortic aneurysm); however, these are medically significant causes of LBP that should not be missed in the emergency department (ED). (See Table 18-1.)

   Deyo RA, et al: Low back pain. N Engl J Med 344:363–370, 2001.

TABLE 18-1. DIFFERENTIAL DIAGNOSIS OF LBP		
Mechanical Spine Disorders	**Nonmechanical Spine Disorders**	**Visceral Disease**
Lumbar strain	**Malignancy**	**Abdominal Aortic**
Degenerative disk/facet disease	Multiple myeloma	**Aneurysm**
	Metastatic cancer	Pelvic organs
Herniated disk	Spinal column or cord cancer	PID
Spinal stenosis	Lymphoma	Prostatitis
Spondylolysis	**Infection**	Renal disease
Spondylolisthesis	Septic discitis	Pyelonephritis
Congenital spinal disease	Osteomyelitis	Nephrolithiasis
Traumatic fracture	Epidural abscess	Gastrointestinal disorders
Osteoporotic compression fracture	Shingles	Pancreatitis
	Inflammatory arthritis	Penetrating ulcer
		Cholecystitis

LBP = low back pain, PID = pelvic inflammatory disease.

3. **What should I ask when taking the patient's history?**

The goal of the history is to distinguish medically significant causes of LBP from the much more common mechanical spine disorders. **Spinal infection** should be suspected in children, immunocompromised patients, and intravenous drug users who present with localized spinal tenderness and fever (although only 50% of patients will have fever at the time of presentation). **Spinal malignancy** should be suspected in patients with a history of cancer or recent weight loss and in patients older than 50 years with progressive LBP lasting more than 1 month. **Occult spinal fracture** should be suspected in the elderly and in patients with known malignancy or osteoporosis (from steroid use or inactivity) who present with LBP of unclear cause. **Visceral causes** of LBP are usually distinguished by associated signs and symptoms.

Atlas SJ, Nardin RA: Evaluation and treatment of low back pain: An evidence-based approach to clinical care. Muscle Nerve 27:265–284, 2003.

4. **How should I focus my physical examination?**

Patients with signs or symptoms suggestive of visceral disease should receive a complete physical examination. All patients with LBP should get a complete neurologic exam, focusing on lower extremity strength, sensation, and reflexes. Mechanical spine disorders, with the exception of herniated lumbar disks or severe spondylolisthesis, should not compromise neurologic function. Rectal tone and sensation should be assessed if there is any concern for cord compression or sacral lesions. Localized spinal tenderness is suggestive of fracture, infection, or malignancy. Finally, a straight leg raise (SLR) test should be performed in patients with leg symptoms (see question 6). The differential diagnosis is summarized in Table 18-2.

Deyo RA, Rainville J, Kent DL: What can the history and physical examination tell us about low back pain? JAMA 268:760–765, 1992.

TABLE 18-2.	CLINICAL FEATURES OF LUMBAR DISK HERNIATION		
Disk	L4	L5	S1–2
Pain	Front of leg	Side of leg	Back of leg
Weakness	Knee extension	Great toe dorsiflexion	Foot plantarflexion
Sensory loss	Knee and medial foot	Side of calf, web of great toe	Back of calf and lateral foot
Reflex loss	Knee jerk	None	Ankle jerk

5. **What does it mean when a patient with LBP also has leg pain?**

Patients with LBP and leg pain (termed *sciatica*) may have one of two syndromes. Referred pain is caused by inflammation of the sciatic nerve. It is usually dull and poorly localized, does not radiate distal to the knee, and is not associated with a positive SLR test or neurologic impairment. Radicular pain is usually caused by nerve root impingement from a herniated lumbar disk or the narrowing of a vertebral foramen from spinal stenosis, but it may also occur with epidural metastases or abscesses in high-risk patients. It is sharp and well localized, frequently (but not always) radiates distal to the knee, invariably is associated with a positive SLR test, and may be associated with neurologic impairment.

6. **How do I perform an SLR test? How do I interpret the results?**

To perform an SLR test, have the patient lie supine while you slowly raise the involved leg (flexing the hip while keeping the knee extended) until the patient complains of discomfort. A positive SLR test occurs when leg elevation results in pain that radiates down the involved leg;

merely evoking pain confined to the low back or hamstrings does not count as a positive test. The SLR test is 80% sensitive but only 40% specific for a herniated disk; a crossed-SLR test, in which raising the uninvolved leg evokes pain radiating down the involved leg, is only 25% sensitive but 90% specific for disk herniation.

7. **Whom should I X-ray?**
   Lumbosacral spine radiographs should be obtained in patients suspected of having a spinal infection or malignancy, in persons exhibiting neurologic impairment, and when a spinal fracture is suspected (Table 18-3).

   Jarvik JJ, Hollingworth W, Heagerty P, et al: Diagnostic evaluation of low back pain with emphasis on imaging. Ann Intern Med 37:586–597, 2002.

TABLE 18-3. USE OF LS-SPINE X-RAY EXAMINATIONS IN EVALUATING LBP

Indication for X-Ray	Result Sought
Trauma	Fracture
Osteoporosis	Fracture
Corticosteroid use	Fracture, infection
Fever	Osteomyelitis
Injection drug use	Osteomyelitis
Unexplained weight loss	Metastases
History of cancer	Metastases
Midline spinal tenderness	Infection, fracture, cancer
Neurologic deficits	Infection, cancer, inflammatory arthritis
Older than 50 years	Infection, cancer, inflammatory arthritis
Failure of pain to resolve after 6 weeks	Infection, cancer, inflammatory arthritis
Unrelenting pain at rest	Infection, cancer, inflammatory arthritis

LBP = low back pain, LS = lumbosacral.

8. **In addition to X-rays, what other tests should I consider?**
   When spinal infection or malignancy is suspected, an erythrocyte sedimentation rate (ESR) should be obtained. An elevated ESR (usually greater than 60–80 mm/hr) should lead to further investigation, usually with a spinal computed tomography (CT) or magnetic resonance imaging (MRI). These tests should be obtained emergently in patients whenever there is evidence of acute neurologic compromise (e.g., loss of bowel or bladder function, motor weakness, or sensory changes).

   When acute neurologic compromise from lumbar disk herniation is suspected, emergent CT or MRI is indicated for patients exhibiting cauda equina syndrome or severe motor paralysis. Cauda equina syndrome presents as severe, often bilateral LBP associated with significant motor impairment and bowel or bladder dysfunction.

9. **What should I know about children who present with back pain?**

Back pain is rare in children. LBP that interferes with activities previously enjoyed by a child may be indicative of serious underlying pathology. Spondylolysis and spondylolisthesis due to sports are the most common causes of LBP in children (see later). Scoliosis does not usually cause back pain, but conditions that cause scoliosis (cancer, fracture, limb length discrepancy, infection, tumors) may cause pain. Although every attempt should be made to limit gonadal radiation in pediatric patients, children with LBP that is not clearly mechanical in nature should be imaged. An ESR may prove helpful when infection or malignancy is suspected.

King HA: Back pain in children. Orthop Clin North Am 30:467–474, 1999.

10. **Is there a difference between spondylosis, spondylolysis, and spondylolisthesis?**

Yes. The terminology is confusing. The prefix *spondylo-* means vertebrae. **Spondylosis** is a nonspecific term for degenerative spine disease. **Spondylolysis** implies severe degeneration with a resulting fracture of the pars interarticularis, which is the portion of the lateral mass of the vertebrae between the superior and inferior articular processes. When spondylolysis occurs bilaterally, anterior slippage of one vertebral body on another can occur, termed **spondylolisthesis**. Severe spondylolisthesis can cause neurologic impairment.

KEY POINTS: MEDICALLY SIGNIFICANT CAUSES OF LBP

1. Abdominal aortic aneurysm

2. Cauda equina syndrome

3. Lumbar disk herniation with severe neurologic compromise

4. Spinal malignancy

5. Spinal infection

11. **Who should be hospitalized for treatment?**

With the exception of previously discussed patients who require emergent CT or MRI, there are no standard indications for hospitalization. Patients with suspected disk herniation who are in significant physical distress or exhibit evidence of severe motor impairment of the lower extremities are often admitted for pain control and strict bed rest because failure to respond to aggressive conservative management may necessitate surgical intervention.

12. **How should patients be treated in the ED?**

Quickly. There is no need to await definitive diagnosis before providing pain relief. Oral or parenteral nonsteroidal anti-inflammatory drugs (NSAIDs) and a cold pack are first-line agents. Parenteral narcotics may be necessary to provide adequate analgesia.

13. **How should patients with musculoskeletal LBP be treated as outpatients?**

Most patients with mild-to-moderate discomfort do not require bed rest and actually do better if they continue with limited activity (i.e., no heavy lifting or prolonged sitting). Patients with severe discomfort may profit from bed rest for 2–3 days to rest injured muscles and ligaments. The period can extend to 7–10 days for patients with suspected disk herniation. A firm mattress is best. Most patients benefit from oral NSAIDs, but some require opioids to produce adequate analgesia during the first few days. Sedatives and muscle relaxants probably do little to relax injured muscles but, because of their sedating effects, may be helpful in improving patient compliance with instructions for bed rest.

http://www.cochrane.org/reviews/en/topics/51.html

14. **What aftercare instructions should I give my patients?**
Patients with suspected disk disease and patients with symptoms that don't improve within 1–2 weeks should be seen by a physician for follow-up evaluation. All patients should be instructed to return immediately if they develop worsening symptoms, particularly bowel or bladder dysfunction or progressive weakness.

15. **What happens to patients with LBP when they leave the ED?**
The prognosis for patients having a first episode of mechanical LBP is good: 70% are better by 1 week, 80% by 2 weeks, and 90% by 1 month. Most studies comparing medical management, chiropractic manipulation, and other treatment modalities rarely find significant differences in long-term outcome because almost everyone gets better no matter what you do. Patients who do not improve with conservative management may have significant medical disorders (inflammatory disorders, malignancy, infections, or disk disease) that were not apparent at the time of initial evaluation or, alternatively, may suffer from psychiatric disorders, drug dependence, or job dissatisfaction.

NONTRAUMATIC OCULAR EMERGENCIES

Daniel F. Danzl, MD

CHAPTER 19

1. **What are some of the unique issues regarding ophthalmologic pharmacology?**
   Topical agents may have systemic effects, so exercise caution when prescribing β-blockers, vasoconstrictors, and anticholinergics. Ointments have a longer duration of action but blur vision.

   Diagnostic medications include stains, such as fluorescein, that help identify corneal and conjunctival abnormalities, and topical anesthetics, which should never be dispensed. Nonsteroidal anti-inflammatory drugs, such as ketorolac or diclofenac, are useful for pain relief. Topical corticosteroids should generally be used after consultation with an ophthalmologist.

   Miotic eye drop bottles have green tops, and mydriatic/cycloplegic agents have red tops. Never allow Hemoccult drops (yellow or blue top) in an eye room because severe alkali burns have occurred.

2. **Name some of the considerations involving pupillary dilation.**
   Phenylephrine (2.5%) is a direct sympathomimetic and mydriatic. Dilation may last 4 hours, and patients with a shallow anterior chamber may develop acute glaucoma after leaving the emergency department (ED). Pupils generally do not require dilation in the ED. A panoptic ophthalmoscope provides a five times larger view of the undilated fundus. For short-term cycloplegia, consider tropicamide (1–6 hours) or 2–5% homatropine (1–2 days); never use atropine (1–3 weeks).

3. **What is conjunctivitis?**
   Inflammation of the bulbar and palpebral conjunctivae or mucous membranes. Viral conjunctivitis is usually bilateral with clear epiphora or tearing. A preauricular node suggests epidemic keratoconjunctivitis (adenovirus). Two common viral pathogens are herpes simplex, with dendritic ulcers, and herpes zoster, with involvement of the fifth cranial nerve.

   Bacterial conjunctivitis initially may be unilateral with purulent crusty drainage. Always consider an undiagnosed foreign body with unilateral conjunctivitis. *Chlamydia* or *Gonococcus* should be considered in neonates or adults with sexually transmitted diseases. Allergies may cause papillae under the lids, chemosis, and itching.

4. **How is conjunctivitis treated?**
   Common agents include aminoglycoside drops and sulfacetamide; the latter stings, which can decrease compliance. Erythromycin 0.5% is available only in ointment form. Reserve the topical fluoroquinolones for more severe infections and for contact lens wearers who are at risk for *Pseudomonas*. Avoid neomycin because hypersensitivity reactions are common.

5. **What is endophthalmitis?**
   Infection or inflammation within the globe. It usually is seen as a collection of pus in the anterior chamber (hypopyon) that resembles a dependent meniscus similar to the blood collection in a hyphema. Antecedent causes include corneal ulcers, direct inoculation or hematogenous spread, and conjunctivitis with organisms capable of penetrating the cornea (e.g., *Neisseria gonorrhoeae*, *Corynebacterium*, *Listeria*, *Haemophilus aegyptius*).

6. **What is the difference between periorbital and orbital cellulitis?**
   Periorbital (preseptal) cellulitis is soft tissue infection of anterior eye structures usually localized to the eyelids and conjunctivae. **Orbital cellulitis** is a more serious infection (behind the septum) that involves posterior eye structures. Both tend to be unilateral and may be preceded by trauma and upper respiratory, sinus, or dental infections. Orbital cellulitis is most often the result of direct spread from ethmoid sinusitis, whereas periorbital cellulitis usually is caused by hematogenous spread of bacteria.

7. **How do I differentiate clinically between periorbital and orbital cellulitis?**
   The two may be difficult to distinguish clinically, especially in children. **Periorbital cellulitis** tends to cause local eyelid symptoms and occasionally ocular discharge and may be associated with fever or leukocytosis. Visual acuity and pupillary reflexes are normal.

   Orbital cellulitis may present with all of the previous symptoms plus exophthalmos, fever, and pain with extraocular movements. Decreased visual acuity, loss of sensation over the ophthalmic and maxillary branches of the trigeminal nerve in V1 and V2 (division of cranial nerve V), and increased intraocular pressure are uncommon findings. Noncontrast computed tomography (CT) scanning of the orbit is liberally indicated with periorbital swelling when there is a possibility of postseptal infection.

8. **What is the common clinical presentation of cavernous sinus thrombosis?**
   Patients often progress from fever, headache, and chemosis to ophthalmoplegia, exophthalmos, and altered level of consciousness. Paralysis of cranial nerves III, IV, and VI usually is noted.

9. **What are some tricks to evaluate the red eye?**
   Topical application of anesthetic drops should decrease or eradicate pain secondary to an abrasion or conjunctivitis (not so with iritis or glaucoma). Redness at the corneal-scleral junction (perilimbic flush) suggests iritis or glaucoma. Shining a light into the normal eye should make the opposite eye hurt if the patient has iritis (because of consensual movement of the inflamed affected contralateral iris). In addition to the consensual pupillary reflex test, the accommodative test is suggestive, which is simply pain precipitated by accommodation. Pain with either maneuver suggests ciliary spasm.

10. **What typical findings help with the differential diagnosis of the red eye?**
    See Table 19-1.

TABLE 19-1. DIFFERENTIAL DIAGNOSIS OF THE RED EYE			
	Conjunctivitis	**Acute Iritis**	**Angle-Closure Glaucoma**
Incidence	Extremely common	Common	Uncommon
Discharge	Moderate to copious	Reflex epiphora	None
Vision	Normal	Slightly blurred	Very blurred (halos)
Pain	Gritty	Moderate	Severe
Conjunctival injection	Diffuse	Perilimbic	Perilimbic
Cornea	Clear	Keratotic precipitates	Steamy or hazy
Pupil size	Normal	Constricted	Dilated
Pupillary light response	Normal	Poor	Poor
Intraocular pressure	Normal	Normal	Elevated

11. **Describe the clinical presentation of iritis.**
Patients often present with perilimbic injection, ciliary spasm, and a constricted miotic pupil. Iritis can be bilateral and misdiagnosed as conjunctivitis. Check the anterior chamber for cells and flare and for keratotic precipitates (white cells) on the back of the cornea.

12. **What is acute angle-closure glaucoma?**
In a patient with a narrow anterior chamber angle, reduced illumination causes mydriasis; folds of the peripheral iris can block the angle, which prevents aqueous humor outflow. The rapid elevation of intraocular pressure causes optic atrophy if not treated promptly. The diagnosis may be delayed by the misleading systemic complaints of nausea, vomiting, and pain.

13. **How is iritis treated?**
Iritis is treated with systemic analgesics and a topical cycloplegic, not simply a mydriatic, to paralyze accommodation and dilate the iris. This prevents adhesions between the iris and the lens (posterior synechiae). Consider steroids in consultation with an ophthalmologist.

14. **How is acute angle-closure glaucoma treated?**
Acute glaucoma is treated with intravenous mannitol or glycerol to decrease intraocular pressure by osmotic diuresis, topical miotics (i.e., 2% pilocarpine or 0.5% timolol) to decrease pupil size and increase aqueous outflow, and acetazolamide intravenously to decrease aqueous production. Topical sympathomimetics such as apraclonidine also reduce aqueous humor production. Emergent ophthalmologic consultation is indicated.

15. **What is a subconjunctival hemorrhage?**
Subconjunctival hemorrhage occurs when a blood vessel ruptures under the conjunctiva. Without trauma, it often results from a Valsalva maneuver associated with coughing or vomiting. Reassure the patient that vision will not be affected and that the blood will be absorbed over 10–14 days. Patients on anticoagulants should have their international normalized ratio (INR) measured.

KEY POINTS: COMMON CAUSES OF AN APD

1. Central retinal artery occlusion
2. Central retinal vein occlusion
3. Optic neuritis
4. Retrobulbar neuritis

16. **What does the presence of an afferent pupillary defect (APD), also known as a marcus-gunn pupil, indicate?**
If the patient has an APD, it confirms damage in the retina or optic nerve. To perform the swinging flashlight test, swing the light after several seconds from the normal eye to the other eye. After a brief pupillary constriction in the abnormal eye, the redilation in response to light reflects afferent deprivation. Patients with an APD usually do not have a retinal detachment, macular or vitreous hemorrhage, glaucoma, trauma, or hysteria.

KEY POINTS: COMMON CAUSES OF ANISOCORIA

1. Horner's syndrome

2. Argyll-Robertson pupil

3. Adie's pupil

4. Post-traumatic or medication-induced mydriasis

5. Third nerve palsy

17. **In a patient with anisocoria, how does one determine which pupil is abnormal?**
Begin the examination in a darkened room; if there is more anisocoria in the light, the large pupil is failing to constrict and is abnormal. More anisocoria that develops going into the dark indicates that the miotic pupil is failing to dilate. Never just assume that the larger pupil is abnormal.

18. **What are common causes of a miotic pupil?**
The two most common are Horner's syndrome and an Argyll-Robertson pupil. The clinical manifestations of Horner's syndrome include ptosis, miosis, and anhydrosis (in a cold ED, check for dilated conjunctival vessels). Bronchogenic carcinoma, stroke, and brachial plexus pathology may present with Horner's syndrome.
  The Argyll-Robertson pupil is miotic, irregular, and displays light-near dissociation. The pupil constricts to accommodation but not to light. This finding is common with diabetes and syphilis. A common testing error is to hold and shine a penlight directly in front of the eye, which can cause the pupil to constrict from accommodation, not light.

19. **Is there another cause of light-near dissociation?**
The only other cause is Adie's pupil, which results from idiopathic parasympathetic denervation in the ciliary ganglion in the eye. The patient is often a young female with a mydriatic pupil that accommodates but does not react to light. Herpes zoster is another cause of Adie's pupil. There are no diseases that cause a pupil to react to light but fail to accommodate.

20. **How can I be certain that a patient with no history of eye trauma has a pupil dilated from a medication?**
If 1% pilocarpine fails to constrict the pupil, it is pharmacologically blocked, most commonly by phenylephrine, handling a scopolamine patch, or aerosolized anticholinergics.

21. **What are some other causes of a unilateral dilated pupil?**
This can be a normal finding or as a result of post-traumatic mydriasis or third nerve palsy.

22. **What are some common causes of nontraumatic loss of vision?**
See Table 19-2.

23. **Describe the presentation and treatment of central retinal artery and central retinal vein occlusion.**
Both occur in middle-aged atherosclerotic patients or elderly hypertensive patients and present as sudden painless loss of vision. Occlusion of the retinal artery or its branches results in a dilated nonreactive pupil with an APD on the affected side. The retina is pale with a cherry-red spot at the macula (macular blood supply is from the choroidal circulation). Occasionally,

TABLE 19-2.   COMMON CAUSES OF NONTRAUMATIC LOSS OF VISION

Transient monocular
Amaurosis fugax
Temporal arteritis
Migraine
Persistent monocular
Central retinal artery occlusion
Central retinal vein occlusion
Retinal detachment or hemorrhage
Vitreous or macular hemorrhage
Optic or retrobulbar neuritis
Internal carotid occlusion

Acute binocular
Migraine
Vertebral basilar insufficiency
Cerebrovascular disease
Toxins (methanol, salicylates, quinine, ergot)
Optic or retrobulbar neuritis
Hysteria
Malingering

amaurosis fugax precedes central retinal artery occlusion. The funduscopic examination of a central retinal vein occlusion is described as a "blood and thunder fundus" because of the presence of multiple large hemorrhages. Efforts to decrease intraocular pressure and dilate retinal vessels by increasing the pCO_2 (paper bag, carbogen), and globe massage are rarely useful acutely for arterial occlusions. Prognosis for both entities is poor.

24. **What are other causes of sudden painless monocular loss of vision?**
Suspect vitreous hemorrhage in diabetics with an obscured red reflex and retinal details. Nontraumatic retinal detachments are more common in patients with significant myopia. Patients often report seeing flashing lights. Most commonly, patients complain of seeing dark floating spots or floaters, which reflect benign vitreous separations and not a retinal detachment.

25. **How do optic neuritis and papilledema differ?**
Although these two processes appear similar on funduscopic examination, **optic neuritis** involves focal demyelination of the optic nerve, resulting in a hyperemic nerve head developing over hours to days. The average age of onset is in the 30s. An association with multiple sclerosis is common.

   Papilledema is swelling of the optic disc caused by increased intracranial pressure. It is usually bilateral but may be asymmetric and may be the result of brain abscess or tumor, intracranial bleeding, meningitis or encephalitis, hydrocephalus, severe hypertension, or pseudotumor cerebri. The earliest sign of papilledema is the loss of spontaneous venous pulsations. When difficult to appreciate, they can be elicited with ipsilateral jugular compression. (See Table 19-3.)

TABLE 19-3.   OPTIC NEURITIS VERSUS PAPILLEDEMA

	Optic Neuritis	Papilledema
Pupil reactivity	Slow	Normal
Visual acuity	Decreased	Normal
Pain	Present	Absent
Usual localization	Unilateral	Bilateral
Fundus	Blurred disc margins	Blurred disc margins

26. What are a couple of tricks to prove that a patient can see?
Induce nystagmus by spinning an opticokinetic drum, or simply hold a mirror in front of the eyes and slowly move it—tracking requires vision.

WEBSITES

1. http://webeyemd.com/default.htm

2. http://omni.ac.uk/browse/mesh/D005123.html

3. http://www.allhealthnet.com/Eye+Care/Conditions-Diseases/Ocular+Emergency/

CHAPTER 20

NONTRAUMATIC ENT EMERGENCIES

Danielle Raeburn, MD, and Katherine M. Bakes, MD

EPISTAXIS

1. **What are the most common causes of epistaxis?**

   Nosebleeds usually occur spontaneously often secondary to dry nasal mucosa or an infection. Infectious causes are most commonly viral or bacterial rhinitis or sinusitis. Minor local trauma from nose picking or direct blows to the nose are frequent causes. Less commonly detected sources include foreign bodies, tumors, coagulopathies, exposure to anticoagulant drugs such as aspirin or warfarin (Coumadin), and exposure to toxic or caustic materials such as cocaine. Nonsteroidal anti-inflammatory drug (NSAID) use does not appear to be associated with higher rates of epistaxis. Approximately 60% of people experience at least one nosebleed in their lifetime, and 6% of those seek medical attention for it.

   Shaw CB, Wax MK, Wetmore SJ: Epistaxis: A comparison of treatments. Otolaryngol Head Neck Surg 109:60–65, 1993.

   Sparacino LL: Epistaxis management: What's new and what's noteworthy. Lippincotts Prim Care Pract 4:498–507, 2000.

2. **Doesn't hypertension cause epistaxis?**

   Probably not as an acute event. The hypertensive patient who presents with a nosebleed typically has hypertension as a chronic condition and has developed atherosclerosis, which makes the blood vessels relatively fragile and more likely to be disrupted when exposed to any of the previously mentioned conditions. Recent studies suggest an association between hypertension and epistaxis, but proof of a direct relationship does not yet exist.

   Herkner H, Havel C, Mullner M, et al: Active epistaxis at ED presentation is associated with arterial hypertension. Am J Emerg Med 20:92–95, 2002.

   Lubianca Neto JF, Fuchs FD, et al: Is epistaxis evidence of end-organ damage in patients with hypertension? Laryngoscope 109:1111–1115, 1999.

3. **Does bleeding originate from any one particular source?**

   Approximately 90% of nosebleeds originate from the anterior portion of the nose, a rich vascular network on the anterior-inferior portion of the septum known as *Kiesselbach's plexus* or *Little's area*. The blood supply for most of this region is derived from the external carotid system. From a practical standpoint, a nosebleed with a source that can be seen directly or is controlled after proper placement of an anterior nasal pack is considered anterior. Posterior bleeds arise from a branch of the *sphenopalatine* artery and tend to be more difficult to control. Posterior bleeds usually occur in patients older than 50. The hemorrhage tends to be more severe, higher volume, and notable for the patient swallowing blood. Blood can be visualized in the posterior pharynx.

   Rosen's Emergency Medicine: Concepts and Clinical Practice, 5th ed. St. Louis, Mosby, 2002.

   Pfaff A, Moore GP: Otolaryngology. In Marx JH, Huckberger R, Walls R, et al (eds): Rosen's Emergency Medicine: Concepts and Clinical Practice, 5th ed. St. Louis, Mosby, 2002, pp 928–938.

4. **List the key questions to ask the patient.**

   1. Is there a prior history of nosebleeds?
   2. How about a past medical history of hypertension, excessive alcohol use, bleeding disorders, or other underlying conditions?

3. Was any trauma (even nose picking) involved?
4. On which side did the bleeding start?
5. Any recent sinus infections or surgeries?
6. How about warfarin or aspirin use?

Kucik CJ, Clenney T: Management of epistaxis. Am Fam Physician 71:305–f311, 2005.

5. **Summarize the key points to successful management of nosebleeds.**
   There are two key considerations. The first is that of **preparation.** Because epistaxis rarely presents as a life-threatening condition, there is time to assemble the necessary equipment and supplies for treatment (Table 20-1). While obtaining the history and quickly assessing ABCs, have the patient pinch the nose firmly (bilateral nasal ala compressing the septum) or place a nasal clamp on the patient with firm pressure on the septum. The examiner should wear disposable gloves, mask, and eye protection. The second key is to **identify the source** of the hemorrhage.

TABLE 20-1. SUPPLIES FOR THE TREATMENT OF NOSEBLEEDS

Examination	Stabilization	Treatment
Protective garb	Bayonet forceps	Silver nitrate cautery sticks
Head lamp or light	Cotton pledgets	Electrocautery (if available)
Nasal speculum	Lidocaine 4%	Gelfoam (or similar material)
Cotton swabs	Epinephrine 1:1000	Merocel sponge or nasal tampon
Fraser tip suction	Tetracaine 0.5%	½-inch petroleum-impregnated gauze
Emesis basin	Oxymetazoline hydrochloride (Afrin)	Antibiotic ointment
4 × 4 gauze	0.25% phenylephrine Neo-Synephrine)	Foley catheter or commercial balloon
		Rolled 4 × 4 gauze with silk suture

From Lucente F, Har-El G (eds): Essentials of Otolaryngology, 4th ed. New York, 1999; and Kucik CJ, Clenney T: Management of epistaxis. Am Fam Physician 7(12):305–311, 2005.

6. **How do I treat epistaxis?**
   Using the nasal speculum, suction, and with water-moistened cotton swabs, remove the existing clots until the bleeding site is seen. Alternatively you can ask the patient to blow the nose, which helps in the removal of clot. Insert a medicated pledget with topical anesthetic plus a vasoconstrictor (e.g., lidocaine 4% and Neo-Synephrine) for 5–10 minutes to allow vasoconstriction and anesthesia to occur. Remove the pledget and begin with simple methods.
   If the source is in Kiesselbach's plexus and is less than 1 cm^2, use silver nitrate or electrocautery. Alternatively, a small piece of absorbable gelatin sponge (Gelfoam), absorbable cellulose (Surgicel), or similar substance may be moistened with a vasoconstrictor and applied to the bleeding site.

If these methods are unsuccessful, an anterior nasal pack is used. In the past, stair-step application of ½-inch antibiotic-coated petrolatum gauze in an anterior-posterior direction was done with bayonet forceps until the entire nasal cavity was filled from the floor, superiorly. A better option includes a dry Merocel sponge or nasal tampon. Either can be used by coating the outside with antibiotic ointment and placing it into the nostril. Once in place, moisten this with saline or phenylephrine until it expands to fit the entire nasal cavity. If inspection of the posterior pharynx reveals no continued bleeding after the vasoconstrictor wears off (about 30 minutes), the patient may be discharged.

Shaw CB, Wax MK, Wetmore SJ: Epistaxis: A comparison of treatments. Otolaryngol Head Neck Surg 109:60–65, 1993.

7. **Any other pearls about treatment with silver nitrate?**
   - Silver nitrate is only helpful when the bleeding is slow or minimal. It won't work in the presence of active brisk bleed or in a pool of blood.
   - Only hold the silver nitrate to the septum for 5–10 seconds and only use electrocautery or chemical cauterization (silver nitrate) on *one* side of the septum. Cauterizing both sides can lead to perforation of the septum or permanent damage to the blood supply of the region.

8. **What are the important discharge instructions?**
   1. The pack (any type) should be left in place for 2–3 days.
   2. Treat each patient who has packing with prophylactic antistaphylococcal antibiotics to prevent sinusitis or toxic shock syndrome. Sinusitis may occur because the paranasal sinuses cannot drain properly with a pack in place. Cephalexin 500 mg four times a day is a good choice.
   3. If recurrences fail to respond to direct firm pressure for 10 minutes, the patient should seek medical attention.
   4. Regular application of petroleum jelly or antibiotic ointment and use of room humidifiers may prevent bleeding from desiccated nasal mucosa.

Rosen's Emergency Medicine: Concepts and Clinical Practice, 5th ed. St. Louis, Mosby, 2002.
Sparacino LL: Epistaxis management: What's new and what's noteworthy. Lippincotts Prim Care Pract 4:498–507, 2000.

KEY POINTS: INSTRUCTIONS FOR PATIENTS WITH AN ANTERIOR NASAL PACKING

1. The pack should be left in place for 2–3 days.

2. Treat each patient who has packing with prophylactic antistaphylococcal antibiotics.

3. If recurrences fail to respond to direct firm pressure for 10 minutes, the patient should seek medical attention.

4. Regular application of petroleum jelly or antibiotic ointment and use of room humidifiers may prevent bleeding from desiccated nasal mucosa.

9. **How do I diagnose posterior epistaxis?**
   If a properly placed anterior pack fails, the patient may have a posterior bleed, and more aggressive treatment is required. Posterior packs are accomplished with rolled 4 × 4 inch gauze, a Foley catheter (16 or 18 Fr), or other commercially available balloon products. Take a Foley and place in the nose until you can see it in the oropharynx. Fill the balloon with 10–15 mL of

saline and pull gently but firmly until the balloon is wedged in the far posterior nasal cavity. Clamp the Foley in this position with an umbilical clamp placed just outside the nose. Because the Foley will be stretched a bit, place gauze between the nose and clamp so as not to cause tissue necrosis of the nose.

10. **Do I discharge a patient to home with a posterior pack?**
No. All patients who require a posterior pack require an admission and an ear, nose, throat (ENT) consultation. Although the mechanism is unclear, posterior packs stimulate the "nasopulmonary reflex," which can lead to hypoxia and apnea. The patient should be on supplemental oxygen and continuous pulse oximetry. Also notable is that 10% of posterior bleeds are not controlled by the previously mentioned methods.

KEY POINTS: DIAGNOSIS AND MANAGEMENT OF POSTERIOR EPISTAXIS

1. When an anterior packing fails to control epistaxis, a posterior bleed originating from sphenopalatine artery must be suspected.

2. Treatment consists of an ENT consult for posterior nasal packing and hospital admission to monitor for hypoxia and apnea secondary to stimulation of the nasopulmonary reflex.

---

11. **When should I consult ENT?**

ENT referral is needed if you cannot control the anterior bleed with adequate **bilateral** nasal packing or with a posterior bleed. The patient may need endoscopic cauterization, ligation of the sphenopalatine artery, embolization, or septal surgery. An outpatient referral can be made for controlled anterior epistaxis that is recurrent.

Lucent F, Har-El G (eds): Essentials of Otolaryngology, 4th ed. New York, 1999.

12. **Didn't you forget to mention laboratory studies?**
No. Most patients don't need them. The exceptions are patients taking warfarin or with suspected coagulopathies and patients who are hemodynamically unstable or require admission.

FOREIGN BODIES

13. **How should I remove a foreign body from the ear?**
The following instruments can assist in extraction: alligator forceps, right-angle probe, tissue forceps, cyanoacrylate glue, Fraser tip suction, irrigation syringe, Adson forceps, Fogarty biliary catheter, ear curette, water-Pik, skin hook, and day hook.
If a live insect is in the external auditory canal (EAC), it should first be killed by instilling 2% lidocaine (which is quicker and less messy than mineral oil) before intact or segmental removal. If the tympanic membrane is intact and space exists between the EAC and the object, a stream of liquid can be directed behind the foreign body to force it out. A mixture of water and isopropyl alcohol as an irrigation solution tends to cause less swelling of organic matter and is evaporated more quickly. Direct instrumentation or suction removes most other objects. Occasionally, cyanoacrylate glue on the end of a suture or a small balloon-tipped catheter can do the trick.

14. **How do patients with nasal foreign bodies present?**
Unless the patient or witness reports the insertion of a foreign body, the chief complaint is that of unilateral, malodorous nasal discharge. The discharge may be thin and mucoid, serosanguinous, or, most often, purulent.

15. **Is there any special trick to removing foreign bodies from the nose?**

Prepare a 50/50 mixture of a topical vasoconstrictor and 4% topical lidocaine, and spray it into the involved nostril with an atomizer or spray bottle. Nebulized epinephrine has also been used with good results. This anesthetizes the sensitive nasal mucosa and reduces congestion to facilitate removal. When this is done, a simple measure, such as occluding the unaffected nostril and having the patient blow forcefully, can expel the object.

If the patient is unable or unwilling to attempt this maneuver, positive-pressure insufflation can be attempted. The unaffected nostril is occluded, and a quick breath is delivered through a facemask connected to an Ambu-bag. Alternatively, a parent or caregiver can do this in direct, mouth-to-mouth fashion. If insufflation maneuvers are unsuccessful, an attempt should be made to remove the foreign body with suction or instruments such as forceps. The techniques listed for ear foreign body removal can be applied to the nose. Because the nasal cavity is larger, a greater number and larger instruments can be used such as a Kelly clamp, bayonet forceps, or a Foley catheter. Consider antibiotics.

16. **"I think I've got something stuck in my throat." How is the patient with this complaint managed?**

The fact that the patient can talk is a good sign. Airway foreign body or compromise must be addressed and ruled out. The patient should be asked about the nature of the foreign body, duration of the sensation, the ability to swallow liquids or solids, and the perceived location of the object. Patient estimates of location are surprisingly accurate.

Direct visualization can identify sharp objects, such as fish bones, that may become impaled in the posterior pharynx or the base of the tongue. Indirect or fiberoptic laryngoscopy, in conjunction with local anesthesia (e.g., lidocaine nebulizer), can pinpoint objects stuck in the vallecula, epiglottis, or pyriform sinus.

It is important to note that the pain of myocardial ischemia can present as a "feeling of something stuck in my throat." If the history and physical are at all suspicious for acute coronary syndrome, get an electrocardiogram (ECG) and/or troponin measurement.

17. **If the physical examination does not reveal the foreign body, what should be done next?**

Soft tissue density lateral radiographs of the neck or chest radiographs should be obtained. Large and sharp, angulated objects tend to lodge in the esophagus. If these do not localize the foreign body, a water-soluble radiographic contrast agent like Gastrografin can be used as part of an esophagram done under fluoroscopy (by radiology). Barium should be avoided initially because it interferes with visualization during endoscopy. Esophagoscopy should be considered in patients with persistent symptoms or when the diagnosis is unclear.

18. **If I can see a foreign body, how do I remove it?**

After a topical spray anesthetic, such as topical benzocaine or nebulized 4% Xylocaine is administered, objects that can be seen can be removed with bayonet forceps or a Kelly clamp. Smooth objects such as coins in the esophagus can be removed by placing the patient in Trendelenburg position (head down), passing a Foley catheter beyond the object, expanding the balloon, and withdrawing the catheter. When the foreign body is more distal, this is often difficult to do and should usually be done only after gastrointestinal (GI) consultation.

It is more common to try pharmacologic treatments first. Sublingual nitroglycerin relaxes the lower esophageal sphincter and is often used to try to relieve a distal obstruction like a food bolus. Intravenous glucagon (0.5–2.0 mg) may relax the lower esophageal sphincter, allowing a distal obstruction to pass. Because glucagon commonly elicits vomiting, it can cause esophageal perforation if unsuccessful. *Never* use papain-containing agents; they dissolve meat and historically have been used but have a very high complication rate. Sharp objects should be removed endoscopically. Repeat esophagography should be done when the removal involves sharp or impaled objects or prolonged or aggressive manipulation or if perforation is a consideration.

KEY POINTS: ESOPHAGEAL FOREIGN BODIES

1. In the patient presenting with an esophageal foreign body sensation, esophagoscopy should be considered with persistent symptoms or an uncertain diagnosis.

2. Because glucagon commonly elicits vomiting, it can cause esophageal perforation if unsuccessful.

19. **Any other pearls?**
Eighty to 90% of esophageal foreign bodies pass through the GI tract without significant problems. The remainder require surgical removal. These latter objects tend to be sharp or long (>6.5 cm) and are among the 1% that cause perforation. A special case should be made for disk or button batteries. Because most are prone to leakage, every effort should be made to remove them if localized to the esophagus. Otherwise, their location in the GI system should be followed with serial x-rays until elimination is confirmed.

KEY POINTS: NATURAL HISTORY OF GI FOREIGN BODIES

1. Of foreign bodies, 80–90% pass through the gastrointestinal tract without significant problems.

2. The following often require surgical removal: sharp or long (>6.5 cm) objects, disk or button batteries, and those that have not migrated on serial radiographs.

SINUSITIS

20. **What is sinusitis? What are the common causes?**
Sinusitis is an inflammation of the paranasal sinuses, including the maxillary, ethmoid, frontal, and sphenoid sinuses. It is the consequence of ostia occlusion, most commonly caused by local mucosal swelling from a viral upper respiratory infection. Allergies, trauma, and mechanical obstruction from tumors, foreign bodies, or abnormal anatomy may also cause occlusion that leads to bacterial overgrowth and excess mucus production. Of all viral upper respiratory infections, 0.5–5% are complicated by bacterial rhinosinusitis. When symptoms last less than 3 weeks, the process is characterized as acute.

21. **How do I make the diagnosis?**
The four most helpful signs and symptoms when diagnosing bacterial rhinosinusitis are purulent nasal discharge, upper tooth or facial pain (especially unilateral), maxillary sinus tenderness (unilateral), and worsening of symptoms after initial improvement. The physical examination is often unrewarding. Anterior rhinoscopy with a headlamp and nasal speculum reveals the presence of pus, foreign bodies, masses, or anatomic abnormalities.

Scheid DC, Hamm RM. Acute bacterial rhinosinusitis in adults. Part 1: Evaluation. Am Fam Physician 70:1642–1645, 2004.

22. **Which other diagnostic studies should I pursue?**
Plain films and computed tomography (CT) are not recommended for initial diagnosis but may be used for recurrent or chronic conditions. A single Water's view is as sensitive as a full sinus series. Findings may include mucosal thickening (> 6 mm), air-fluid levels, and opacification. For uncomplicated sinusitis, CT is not specific because 40% of asymptomatic and 87% of patients with a recent upper respiratory infection have abnormal findings on CT scan. CT can be used to diagnose intrafacial or intracranial involvement. Nasal endoscopy is an excellent modality for identifying disease but is done only by an otolaryngologist and rarely on an emergent basis.

Fagnan LJ: Acute sinusitis: A cost-effective approach to diagnosis and treatment. Am Fam Physician 58:1795–1801, 1998.
Scheid, DC, Hamm RM: Acute bacterial rhinosinusitis in adults. Part 1: Evaluation. Am Fam Physician 70:1642–1645, 2004.

23. **How is sinusitis treated?**
Approximately 65% of cases of acute rhinosinusitis in adults and children will resolve spontaneously. Most patients with a viral upper respiratory infection improve within 7 days. Thus, antibiotics should be reserved for patients who meet the clinical criteria described previously and whose symptoms have persisted for more than 7 days. The most likely organisms are *Streptococcus pneumoniae,* nontypable *Haemophilus influenzae, Moraxella catarrhalis,* other *Streptococcus* species, and anaerobes.

Initial antibiotic therapy options include amoxicillin, trimethoprim-sulfamethoxazole, penicillin VK, amoxicillin-clavulanate, doxycycline, cefaclor, azithromycin, or clarithromycin. In children, use amoxicillin/clavulanate, high-dose amoxicillin, cefpodoxime, or cefuroxime. Duration of therapy is 10–21 days or 1 week past resolution of symptoms. The use of vasoconstrictor sprays such as phenylephrine (Neo-Synephrine) or oxymetazoline (Afrin) offer symptomatic relief but should not be used longer than 3–4 days because of the propensity for rebound edema. Antihistamines should not be used because they may worsen the course secondary to crusting and blockage of the ostia.

Lieser JD, Derkay CS: Pediatric sinusitis: When do we operate? Curr Opin Otolaryngol Head Neck Surg 13:60–66, 2005.
Poole MD: A focus on acute sinusitis in adults: Changes in disease management. Am J Med 106:38S–47S, 1999.
Scheid DC, Hamm RM: Acute bacterial rhinosinusitis in adults. Part 1: Evaluation. Am Fam Physician 70:1642–1645, 2004.

24. **Which patients need referral and admission? What are the complications?**
If there is no improvement after two complete courses of antibiotics, the patient should be referred to an otolaryngologist. Complications arising during therapy can be classified as local, orbital, and intracranial. Patients with sinusitis who show evidence of orbital or central nervous system involvement should be treated as medical emergencies.

Locally, mucoceles and osteomyelitis can develop. Orbital complications are the most frequent, especially in children, and range from cellulitis to abscess formation. Cavernous sinus thrombosis, resulting from the direct spread of infection through valveless veins, is imminently life threatening. It is heralded by a toxic appearance, high fever, cranial nerve palsies, retinal engorgement, and bilateral chemosis and proptosis. Other intracranial complications demanding aggressive intensive therapy include meningitis, subdural empyema, and brain abscess. The majority of these complications can be diagnosed by CT.

25. **Any other pearls?**
Yes. Check a fingerstick glucose in a sick patient with sinusitis. *Mucor* in diabetic patients and *Aspergillus* in immunocompromised patients can be life threatening. These patients require hospital admission and specialist consultation.

KEY POINTS: SINUSITIS

1. The four most helpful physical exam signs and symptoms when diagnosing bacterial rhinosinusitis are purulent nasal discharge, upper tooth or facial pain (especially unilateral), maxillary sinus tenderness (unilateral), and worsening of symptoms after initial improvement.

2. A single Water's view is as sensitive as a full sinus series. Findings may include mucosal thickening (> 6 mm), air-fluid levels, and opacification.

3. For uncomplicated sinusitis, CT is not specific because 40% of asymptomatic patients and 87% of patients with a recent upper respiratory infection have abnormal findings on CT scan.

4. Cavernous sinus thrombosis, resulting from the direct spread of infection through valveless veins, is imminently life threatening. It is heralded by a toxic appearance, high fever, cranial nerve palsies, retinal engorgement, and bilateral chemosis and proptosis.

5. *Mucor* in diabetic patients and *Aspergillus* in immunocompromised patients can be life threatening.

EPIGLOTTITIS

26. How did George Washington die?
George Washington is believed to have died from epiglottitis. It is recorded that on December 14, 1799, the morning of his death, he had a severe sore throat and later developed stridor and hoarseness and was unable to lie supine.

27. List the signs and symptoms of epiglottitis in adults.
Symptoms
- Sore throat (100%)
- Odynophagia/dysphagia (76%)
- Fever (88%)
- Shortness of breath (78%)
- Anterior neck tenderness
- Hoarseness or muffled ("hot potato") voice

Signs
- Lymphadenopathy
- Drooling
- Respiratory distress
- Extreme pain with palpation of the larynx

Carey MJ: Epiglottitis in adults. Am J Emerg Med 14:421–424, 1996.
Mayo-Smith MF, Spinale JW, Donsley CJ, et al: Acute epiglottitis: An 18-year experience in Rhode Island. Chest 108:1640–1648, 1995.

28. What is the thumbprint sign?
A finding on lateral neck radiographs caused by the presence of an edematous epiglottis. Lateral neck films are of limited use because they are only 38% sensitive and 76% specific.

29. Name the most common organisms identified in adult epiglottitis.
The two most common organisms found are *H. influenzae* and beta-hemolytic streptococci. In most cases, no organism is found, however, pointing to a viral cause. With the introduction of the Hib vaccine in children, the reservoir for *H. influenzae* has decreased dramatically so that epiglottitis is now seen more frequently in adults.

30. **How do I manage epiglottitis? What signs and symptoms indicate the need for airway intervention?**

Antibiotics should be started immediately. A second- or third-generation cephalosporin active against *H. influenzae* and beta-hemolytic streptococci is the drug of choice. Steroids are often used but remain controversial and have not been shown to provide any benefit. Patients with symptomatic respiratory distress, stridor, drooling, shorter duration of symptoms, and *H. influenzae* bacteremia are at increased risk for airway obstruction. Patients with a respiratory rate of less than 20 breaths/min and no respiratory distress should be observed closely in an intensive care unit (ICU). In patients with a respiratory rate greater than 30 breaths/min, moderate-to-severe respiratory distress, PCO_2 of greater than 45 mmHg, or cyanosis, consider immediate active airway intervention.

Shah RK, Roberson DW, Jones DT: Epiglottitis in the Haemophilus influenza type B vaccine era: Changing trends. Laryngoscope 114:557–560, 2004.

31. **How is the definitive diagnosis of epiglottitis made?**

The gold standard for definitive diagnosis of epiglottitis in **adults** is direct laryngoscopy and visualization of the inflamed or edematous epiglottis. In **children,** the appropriateness of direct visualization is more controversial. Some believe that any attempt at visualizing the inflamed epiglottis should take place in a controlled setting, such as the operating room. Others believe it is appropriate to use a tongue depressor or laryngoscope blade to depress the tongue and visualize the epiglottis of a small child sitting in his or her parent's lap. In either case, visualization should take place only by someone experienced in the management of pediatric airways.

OTITIS EXTERNA

32. **How does otitis externa present?**

The classic finding is pain with manipulation of the external ear. Cardinal symptoms are itching, pain, tenderness to palpation, and less commonly hearing loss and fullness. Common signs are erythema and edema of the auditory canal, with crusting, pus, or weeping secretions. Predisposing factors for otitis externa, also called swimmer's ear, are excessive moisture in the ear canal and trauma (typically from overzealous cleaning).

Bojrab DI, Bruderly T, Abdulrazzak Y: Otitis externa. Otolarynol Clin North Am 29:761–782, 1996.

33. **What bacteria are usually responsible?**

Pseudomonas aeruginosa, Staphylococcus aureus.

34. **How is it treated?**

The goals for treatment are twofold: to avoid precipitants and to eradicate infection. To treat infection, 2% acetic acid (for drying) combined with hydrocortisone (for inflammation) should be placed on a wick in the ear canal. Alternatively, topical antibiotic drops can be used. Cortisporin otic suspension works well as it has antibacterial, anti-inflammatory, and drying properties as well as a nontoxic pH.

Additionally, unlike cortisporin solution, **cortisporin suspension** can be used in the presence of a perforated tympanic membrane. If the external ear canal is extremely inflamed and narrowed, a wick can be placed to ensure drainage and instillation of medication. It otitis media coexists, be sure to add systemic antibiotics.

35. **What is malignant otitis externa?**

Malignant otitis externa is a potentially lethal extension of the external ear canal into the mastoid or temporal bone. It is caused most commonly by *P. aeruginosa* and occurs in patients with diabetes and immunocompromised states. The mortality rate can be greater than 50%. Malignant otitis externa should be considered when, despite adequate treatment, headache and otalgia persist or are greater than other clinical signs. CT or magnetic resonance imaging (MRI) confirms the diagnosis. Treatment includes admission, intravenous antipseudomonal antibiotics, and potentially surgical debridement.

PERITONSILLAR ABSCESS

36. **State the typical signs and symptoms seen with peritonsillar abscess.**
    - **Symptoms:** Fever, unilateral sore throat, odynophagia, trismus, and occasionally referred otalgia. Patients typically have had pharyngitis for some time with recent antibiotic treatment.
    - **Signs:** Limited opening of the mouth (usually cannot open more than 2.5 cm), drooling, speaking in a muffled "hot potato" voice, and rancid breath. Examining the oropharynx shows erythema with a deeper redness over the affected area. There is tense swelling of the anterior pillar and soft palate. Subsequently, the tonsil is pushed downward and toward the midline. The uvula may be in an abnormal position, either shifted away from or lying flat against the affected side.

37. **What are the treatment options for a peritonsillar abscess?**
    Needle aspiration followed by antibiotics is the treatment of choice, successful in 85–95% of patients. The patient should be seated with his or her head resting against the bed or dental chair headrest. Visualize the tonsils with the aid of a tongue depressor. Topical anesthetic should be applied using lidocaine or Cetacaine. A needle cover can be cut to provide a needle guard for an 18–20 G needle, exposing no more than 0.5 cm of the needle. The guarded needle is inserted at the most fluctuant portion of the abscess. The physician should not penetrate deeper than 1 cm and stay **medial** to avoid the more lateral positioned carotid artery. A positive aspiration is achieved if 1 mL or more of pus is obtained. If needle aspiration fails, referral to an ENT physician is necessary for surgical incision and drainage versus tonsillectomy.

38. **Describe the presentation of a retropharyngeal abscess.**
    Common presenting symptoms of retropharyngeal abscess include fever, odynophagia, and neck pain out of proportion to oropharyngeal findings. Patients are ill appearing and may hold the neck in slight extension and resist neck movement.

39. **Why is this diagnosis so concerning?**
    The retropharyngeal space of the neck involves three fascial layers between the paraspinal muscles and the pharynx. Infections and abscesses located here have the potential to cause airway compromise and offer a path of direct extension into the mediastinum.

Rosen's Emergency Medicine: Concepts and Clinical Practice, 5th ed. St. Louis, Mosby, 2002.

KEY POINTS: OTHER HEAD AND NECK SOFT TISSUE INFECTIONS

1. In the patient with respiratory compromise and suspected epiglottitis, evaluation is best performed in a controlled environment, with someone skilled at performing an emergent nonsurgical and surgical airway.

2. Malignant otitis externa is caused most commonly by *Pseudomonas aeruginosa* and occurs in patients with diabetes and immunocompromised states. The mortality rate can be greater than 50%.

3. Infections and abscesses in the retropharyngeal space can lead to airway compromise and direct extension into the mediastinum.

40. What organisms are found in retropharyngeal and peritonsillar abscesses?

Retropharyngeal and peritonsillar abscesses have similar microbial flora: anaerobes, group A streptococci (*Streptococcus pyogenes*), *S. aureus*, and *H. influenzae*.

Brook I: Microbiology and management of peritonsillar, retropharyngeal, and parapharyngeal abscesses. J Oral Maxillofac Surg 62:1545–1550, 2004.

41. How is a retropharyngeal abscess diagnosed and treated?

It is sometimes visible on a soft tissue lateral neck radiograph as an increase in soft tissue density best seen with the neck in slight extension. Definitive diagnosis is made by CT scan. Advanced airway management equipment should be at the bedside while an emergent consultation with an ENT physician is obtained. Intravenous antibiotics should be started, but as with pus formation anywhere in the body, definitive treatment is incision and drainage. The patient should be admitted to the ICU or taken directly to the operating room by the appropriate service. Mediastinal involvement mandates the involvement of a cardiothoracic surgeon.

Lee SS, Schwartz RH, Bahadori RS: Retropharyngeal abscess: Epiglottitis of the new millennium. J Pediatr 138:435–437, 2001.

CHAPTER 21

DENTAL AND ORAL SURGICAL EMERGENCIES

Richard D. Zallen, DDS, MD, and Gregory R. McGee, DMD

1. **When should an emergent dental/oral surgical consultation be obtained?**
    - Swelling associated with tooth pain
    - Avulsed tooth
    - Alveolar housing fractures
    - Refractory bleeding from tooth extraction
    - Facial fractures

2. **How are teeth numbered?**
    In adults, teeth are numbered starting from the upper right third molar (no. 1) and continuing around the teeth to the upper left third molar (no. 16). From here the numbering continues when you drop down to the lower left third molar (no. 17) and continues around to the lower right third molar (no. 32). (See Table 21-1.)

    In children, the 20 deciduous teeth (baby teeth) are lettered starting on the upper right second molar (A) and continuing around the teeth to the upper left second molar (J). From here the lettering continues on the lower left second molar (K) and continues around to the lower right second molar (T). (See Table 21-2.)

    Children between the ages of 6 and 13 are in a mixed dentition stage with some adult and some deciduous teeth. Their teeth are numbered and lettered as the previous descriptions.

3. **Describe the different types of tooth fractures. Which require treatment?**
    The two basic types are fractures of the crown and fractures of the root. Ellis classified tooth fractures for anterior teeth as I, II, III, and IV (Fig. 21-1). An Ellis class I fracture involves the enamel only and does not require emergent treatment. An Ellis class II fracture involves the enamel and dentin. An Ellis class III fracture involves the enamel, dentin, and pulp. Ellis class II and III fractures require placement of calcium hydroxide (Dycal). An Ellis class IV fracture involves the root of the tooth and may require extraction, root canal therapy, splinting with dental resin, ligature wire, or Erich arch bars depending on the level of fracture.

    www.iadt-dentaltrauma.org/
    www.dentsply.co.uk/products/restoratives/dycal.html

4. **How should an avulsed tooth be transported?**
    The best transport medium is the socket from which the tooth came if the tooth can be rinsed off and replaced. If this is not possible, Hank's balanced salt solution (EMT Tooth Saver) is the next best transport medium. If no transport solution is available, milk can be used or a wet handkerchief. The patient's (or caregiver) saliva or saline may also be used, but these can be damaging to the periodontal ligament that is adherent to the root surface.

TABLE 21-1. UNIVERSAL NUMBERING SYSTEM FOR PERMANENT TEETH

Maxillary right quadrant

1	2	3	4	5	6	7	8	9	10	11	12	13	14	15	16
Third molar	Second molar	First molar	Second premolar	First premolar	Cuspid	Lateral incisor	Central incisor	Central incisor	Lateral incisor	Cuspid	First premolar	Second premolar	First molar	Second molar	Third molar

Maxillary left quadrant

32	31	30	29	28	27	26	25	24	23	22	21	20	19	18	17
Third molar	Second molar	First molar	Second premolar	First premolar	Cuspid	Lateral incisor	Central incisor	Central incisor	Lateral incisor	Cuspid	First premolar	Second premolar	First molar	Second molar	Third molar

Mandibular right quadrant

Mandibular left quadrant

TABLE 21-2. UNIVERSAL LETTERING SYSTEM FOR PRIMARY TEETH

Maxillary right quadrant

										Maxillary left quadrant
A	B	C	D	E	F	G	H	I	J	
Second molar	First molar	Cuspid	Lateral incisor	Central incisor	Central incisor	Lateral incisor	Cuspid	First molar	Second molar	
T	S	R	Q	P	O	N	M	L	K	
Second molar	First molar	Cuspid	Lateral incisor	Central incisor	Central incisor	Lateral incisor	Cuspid	First molar	Second molar	

Mandibular right quadrant

Mandibular left quadrant

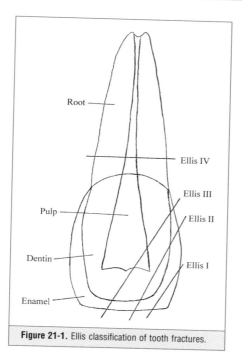

Figure 21-1. Ellis classification of tooth fractures.

KEY POINTS: PROCESS USED TO PREPARE AND APPLY CALCIUM HYDROXIDE PASTE (DYCAL)

1. Isolate and dry tooth with gauze.

2. Dispense equal volume of base and catalyst paste onto a mixing pad.

3. Stir immediately using an applicator (the wooden end of a cotton-tipped applicator will suffice) for 10 seconds until a uniform mixture occurs.

4. Quickly apply the mixed material onto the tooth and cover any exposed dentin or pulp.

5. Wait. The mixed material will set in about 2 minutes.

6. Remove excess paste with a sharp instrument. Be sure to check bite.

5. **When should an avulsed tooth be replanted? How is it stabilized?**
   An avulsed tooth should be replanted within 1 to 2 hours of injury. Teeth should not be replanted if more than 2 hours have passed since avulsion. Stabilization of replanted teeth is indicated provided that there is not extensive caries, periodontal disease, or large alveolar housing

fractures. Deciduous teeth should not be replanted. Teeth are stabilized by physiologic splinting with dental composite and ligature wire for 7–10 days.

6. **What are alveolar housing fractures? How are they treated?**
Fractures of the alveolar ridge encompassing the dentition of the maxilla or mandible. The usual treatment involves the manual reduction of the fracture and rigid splint fixation with an Erich arch bar for 4–6 weeks.

7. **Should antibiotics be prescribed for an alveolar housing fracture or reimplanted tooth?**
Yes. A 5-day course of penicillin is recommended. The oral dose of penicillin V is 500 mg four times a day for adults and 25–50 mg/kg/day in four divided doses for children. In penicillin-allergic patients, clindamycin is preferred. The oral dose of clindamycin is 300 mg four times a day for adults and 10–20 mg/kg/day in four divided doses for children.

8. **What are the concerns with electrical and thermal burns to the mouth?**
Electrical burns are deceptive. The ultimate extent of tissue damage is greater than is initially present on initial examination, and the full extent of the injury may not be appreciated for 4–7 days. Wound contracture may produce microstomia. Close observation is warranted due to the possibility of delayed arterial hemorrhage.

Thermal burns are typically treated with antibiotic ointment and topical steroids. Both electrical and thermal burn contractures may need to be treated with skin grafts and splinting.

9. **How should a tongue laceration with profuse bleeding be treated?**
Initially, packing with gauze and applying pressure should allow visualization of the source of bleeding. Securing the airway may be necessary with some tongue lacerations due to expanding hematoma and possible compromise of the airway. A silk traction suture placed into the tip of the tongue can aid in visualization of the laceration. Injection of a local anesthetic with 1:100,000 epinephrine aids with vasoconstriction. Clamping, ligating, or electrocautery helps to control the larger bleeders when the site can be identified clearly. If minor bleeding persists, the laceration should be closed in a layered fashion using resorbable sutures for deep approximation and Vicryl or Dexon for surface approximation.

10. **How should a through-and-through lip laceration be closed?**
Initial debridement of the wound may require surgical and saline debridement. Wound exploration and possible soft tissue radiographs to rule out foreign body (tooth fragments, metal, etc.) should be considered. Mucosal preparation with hexachlorophene (pHisoHex) is recommended. The mucosa is closed with 3–0 plain gut suture. Skin preparation with chlorhexidine following mucosal closure is recommended. A layered closure of the lip, using 4–0 Vicryl suture for deep tissue/muscle approximation and 5–0 or 6–0 nylon for skin, should be used. If the laceration involves the vermillion border, this should be approximated first, as any misalignment is extremely noticeable. Care should also be taken to align the orbicularis oris muscle to avoid any deformity. Prophylactic antibiotic coverage with penicillin for 5 days is recommended.

11. **How should human or animal bites of the mouth be treated?**
Human bites are managed best with copious irrigation, surgical debridement, and prophylactic antibiotics. The drug of choice is amoxicillin with clavulanic acid. Wounds should be closed primarily if possible, although delayed primary closure is an option in some cases. Animal bites are handled in a similar way. Antibiotics are recommended and may vary depending on species. Patients bitten by animals with suspected rabies must be treated aggressively, including irrigation with chlorhexidine solution followed by copious saline irrigation, rabies postexposure prophylaxis, and tetanus prophylaxis.

12. **When should antibiotics be used in management of dental infections?**

An acute dentoalveolar abscess usually requires antibiotic therapy, with penicillin being the drug of choice. Adjunctive therapy should include root canal treatment or extraction of the offending tooth with incision and drainage. The patient should be followed closely, usually within 24 hours.

Flynn TR, Halpern LR: Antibiotic selection in head and neck infections. Oral Maxillofac Surg Clin North Am 15:17-38, 2003.

13. **List some nonodontogenic sources of orofacial pain.**

- Temporomandibular joint
- Muscles of mastication
- Salivary glands
- Nose and paranasal sinuses
- Blood vessels (arteritis)
- Nerves
- Oral ulcers

14. **When should a patient with a dental abscess be admitted to the hospital?**

Admission criteria should be based on history and physical findings: size and location of swelling, rapidity of onset, dysphagia, dyspnea, fever, malaise, trismus, age, state of hydration, laboratory evaluation, and immune status of the patient. Urgent admission for airway concerns as well as intravenous (IV) antibiotics and fluid resuscitation may be necessary.

15. **Name the risks of dental local anesthesia.**

Local anesthetic toxicity including seizures, allergy, syncope, trismus, needle tract infection, intra-arterial or IV injection, paresthesia, hematoma, and transient Bell's palsy from accidental injection into the area of the parotid gland. Broken needles rarely occur.

16. **What is the best way to perform dental local anesthesia?**

Prior to all dental injections, the injection site should be cleansed with gauze and topical anesthetic applied if desired. The most predictable way to provide anesthesia to the maxilla is to infiltrate the buccal and palatal (painful injection) mucosa above the offending tooth with a 27G short or long needle.

For the mandible, an inferior alveolar nerve block is the best way to provide anesthesia for lower teeth on the affected side along with infiltration. To perform an inferior alveolar nerve block, a 25- or 27-G long needle with an aspirating syringe is needed. Using the nondominant hand, grasp the anterior mandible with your thumb intraorally near the ascending ramus at the level of the teeth. Aim the needle at the external auditory canal while inserting the needle in mucosa about 0.5–1 cm above the plane of teeth (bisecting your thumbnail) while approaching from the opposite mandibular premolars. The needle tip should enter the mucosa at the fold between the pharynx and buccal mucosa (pterygomandibular raphe). The needle tip should be advanced approximately 1.5–2 cm until the medial side of the mandible is felt, then the needle is withdrawn a few millimeters. After aspirating, approximately 1.8 mL of local anesthetic should have a therapeutic effect.

Malamed A: Handbook of Local Anesthesia. St. Louis, Mosby, 1996.

17. **What is anug? How is it treated?**

Acute necrotizing ulcerative gingivitis (ANUG) is an acute infection of the gingiva that can be precipitated by psychological stress, smoking, and poor oral hygiene. ANUG typically presents with blunted interdental papilla, which represents areas of necrosis, gingival bleeding, pain, fetor oris, gingival swelling, and lymphadenopathy. ANUG responds well to local debridement and irrigation. Oral rinses with chlorhexidine are necessary. Antibiotics should be used only in refractory cases, and penicillin is the drug of choice.

Marx R, Stern D (eds): Oral and Maxillofacial Pathology. Chicago, Quintessence Publishing, 2003, pp 53–54.

18. **Why is a lateral pharyngeal abscess of great concern?**
This infection is potentially life threatening because of airway obstruction and requires urgent incision and drainage. This abscess occurs between the pharyngeal mucosa and the superior constrictor muscle. Presenting symptoms usually include dysphagia, pain, trismus, and fever. Medial bulging of the lateral pharyngeal wall frequently occurs, causing displacement of the uvula to the opposite side. This complication is usually secondary to mandibular third molar extractions and/or needle tract infections.

   Topazian R, Goldberg M (eds): Oral and Maxillofacial Infections, 4th ed. Philadelphia, W.B. Saunders, 2002, pp 177-185.

19. **What is ludwig's angina?**
An infection of the submandibular, sublingual, and submental spaces bilaterally. A dental cause is present in 90% of cases. Treatment consists of maintaining the airway, removal of the offending tooth, incision and drainage, IV antibiotics, and hydration.

20. **How are apthous ulcers and herpetic lesions differentiated in the oral cavity?**
Recurrent aphthous ulcers, also known as *canker sores,* occur as a single circular ulcer and are usually less than 1 cm in diameter. The lesion has a central yellow area surrounded by a prominent band of erythema. Herpetic lesions usually present as clusters of small vesicles that eventually coalesce. Recurrent aphthous ulcers may occur anywhere in the oral cavity except the lips, hard palate, and attached gingiva. Recurrent herpes occurs exclusively in the lips, hard palate, and attached gingiva. Both of these types of lesions can be quite painful.

21. **How are oral cavity ulcers treated?**
Recurrent aphthous ulcers are treated many different ways, including topical corticosteroids, antibiotics, and anesthetic mouth rinses. An attapulgite (Kaopectate), diphenhydramine (Benadryl), and lidocaine (Xylocaine) **KBX** suspension has been shown to provide relief in cases of multiple recurrent aphthous ulcers. The treatment of herpes simplex virus is aimed at palliation of pain. Topical acyclovir, when used during the prodromal stage, has been shown to decrease size of lesions and duration of symptoms. Children may become dehydrated and require admission.

22. **How is postextraction hemorrhage evaluated and treated?**
The patient's past medical history and current medications should be thoroughly reviewed. Clinical inspection must include good lighting and suction to evaluate the alveolus for a bleeding source. Application of a gauze dressing maintained with firm digital pressure over the extraction site stops most bleeding episodes.

   Some hemostatic agents such as gelatin sponges (Gelfoam), absorbable knitted fabric (Surgicel), and topical thrombin may also be useful. Injecting the area with a local anesthetic containing a vasoconstrictor can also be effective. A carefully placed suture aids hemostasis. Refractory bleeding should be evaluated further with appropriate laboratory studies.

23. **What is the classification of mandibular fractures?**
The best clinical classification is by anatomic region: symphysis, parasymphysis, body, angle, ramus, condyle, and alveolar housing. These fractures may be further described by the specific type of fracture: simple, compound, comminuted, multiple, greenstick, or pathologic. (See Fig. 21-2.)

24. **List different ways to radiologically examine a patient for a mandible fracture.**
Panoramic, mandible series (Towne's, posteroanterior, lateral oblique right and left), dental periapical, computed tomography (CT) scan, and temporomandibular (rarely).

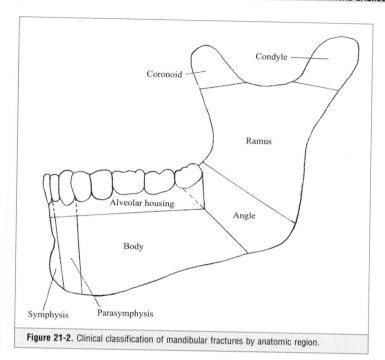

Figure 21-2. Clinical classification of mandibular fractures by anatomic region.

25. **How do you clinically examine a patient for a mandibular fracture?**
The main diagnostic criteria are a history of trauma, abnormal mandibular movements elicited by bimanual palpation, step deformities or changes in the occlusion, loose teeth, and soft tissue trauma including laceration or hematoma.

26. **Describe a lasso ligature.**
A 24-, 25-, or 26-G wire that is placed around one or two teeth adjacent to a fracture to approximate fragments of a mandible fracture. The wire is tightened as the patient's occlusion is maintained to bring the fracture into closer alignment. This helps to relieve pain, stop bleeding, and prevent the continued contamination of saliva into the fracture site.

27. **Are antibiotics indicated for a mandibular fracture?**
Antibiotics are indicated in all open mandibular fractures. All fractures involving teeth are considered open fractures. Fractures of the subcondylar/condylar region that do not communicate with the external auditory canal are closed and are not treated with antibiotics.

28. **List the immediate clinical problems associated with a fractured mandible.**
- Airway compromise
- Bleeding
- Pain
- Fracture displacement
- Displaced or aspirated teeth
- Lacerations

■ Trismus
■ Subcutaneous emphysema

29. What is a mandible contrecoup fracture?

A fracture distant from the site of trauma. A classic example is trauma to the symphysis or parasymphysis area with unilateral or bilateral subcondylar fractures.

30. Describe the treatment of dry socket (alveolar osteitis).

Dry socket is treated by gently irrigating the extraction site and placing a sedative dressing (BIPS and gauze or Alvogyl) into the socket. Local anesthetic may be necessary for pain relief during application of the dressing. Follow-up is needed to ensure pain relief and absence of infection. Multiple treatments are sometimes necessary.

KEY POINTS: COMMON CHARACTERISTICS OF DRY SOCKET (ALVEOLAR OSTEITIS)

1. Extraction 2–3 days prior to onset of pain

2. No purulence

3. No fever

4. No clot in extraction site (exposed bone)

5. No trismus

31. What oral complication is being seen with the use of bisphosphonates in the treatment of malignancy?

Osteonecrosis of the jaws with the clinical presentation of pain and denuded bone of the maxilla or mandible.

Mehrotra B, Rosenberg TJ, Engroff SL: J Oral Maxillofac Surg 62:527-534, 2004.

BIBLIOGRAPHY

1. Fonseca R, Walker R (eds): Oral and Maxillofacial Trauma, 3rd ed. St. Louis, Elsevier Saunders, 2005.

2. Kaban L, Pogrel M (eds): Complications in Oral and Maxillofacial Surgery. Philadelphia, W.B. Saunders, 1997.

3. Ghali GE, Larsen PE, Waite PD: Peterson's Principles of Oral and Maxillofacial Surgery, 2nd ed. London, BC Decker, 2004.

TRANSIENT ISCHEMIC ATTACK AND CEREBROVASCULAR ACCIDENT

Richard L. Hughes, MD, and Michael P. Earnest, MD

CHAPTER 22

1. What do you mean we're number 3?

Despite significant reductions in morbidity and mortality, stroke remains the third most common cause of death and the third most common diagnosis on admission to hospitals.

American Heart Association: 1991 Heart and Stroke Facts. Dallas, TX, American Heart Association, 1991.

2. What is the difference between a transient ischemic attack (TIA) and an ischemic stroke?

TIA and stroke refer to ischemia in the brain that results in neurologic deficits. If the **clinical deficit** resolves within 24 hours, the ischemia is referred to as a **TIA.** If the deficit is persistent at 24 hours, even if it resolves over a few days, it is called a **stroke.** The nomenclature becomes more complicated because 30–50% of patients with **clinically** defined TIA have a permanent abnormality on computed tomography (CT), magnetic resonance imaging (MRI), or in the brain at autopsy. TIAs can be the clinical expression of small areas of cell death in the brain, even though there is no permanent neurologic deficit.

3. Nothing can be done for most strokes, so what good is emergency therapy?

Although emergency resuscitation is possible and appropriate in only a few patients, complications of stroke and early stroke recurrence should be addressed in the emergency department (ED). This is philosophically similar to the approach taken with myocardial infarction (MI). The highest risk for a recurrent stroke is within the first few days and weeks after an initial stroke or TIA. It is crucial that patients have an appropriate evaluation to determine the cause of their stroke so that a second ischemic event can be prevented. Because the exact mechanism of stroke is usually not apparent in the ED, aspirin therapy or anticoagulation (heparin) therapy on a short-term basis should be initiated in the ED.

Adams H, Adams R, Del Zoppo G: Guidelines for the early management of patients with ischemic stroke. Stroke 36:916–923, 2005.

Coull BM, Goldstein LB, Johnston KC: Anticoagulants and antiplatelet agents in acute ischemic stroke. Stroke 33:1934–1942, 2002.

KEY POINTS: BEST WAYS TO EXACERBATE AN ISCHEMIC STROKE IN THE ED

1. Lower the blood pressure, compromising cerebral perfusion even more.

2. Neglect to rehydrate.

3. Wait until the patient is upstairs before giving an antithrombotic or anticoagulant.

4. Allow the patient to run a mild or moderate fever.

5. Let the glucose remain elevated.

4. **What is the role of thrombolytics for stroke?**

Tissue plasminogen activator (TPA) was approved in June 1996 for use in patients having ischemic stroke. In the paired studies resulting in Food and Drug Administration (FDA) approval, patients who were given TPA within 3 hours of stroke onset had better outcomes and showed no increase in death or severe disability. For patients who arrive in the ED early (i.e., within 2 hours), stroke is a medical emergency equal to major trauma because what you do in the first ED hour can greatly affect the eventual outcome.

5. **How can my hospital use thrombolytics safely in the treatment of stroke?**

First, basic support, such as CT scanning, laboratory testing, and an intensive care unit (ICU) level of care, must be available. Second, emergency physicians and neurologists must develop a rapid response protocol to stroke. Third, the basic indications and contraindications for thrombolytics based on the most current clinical guidelines must be followed. Fourth, a reasonable plan to deal with stroke complications, including hemorrhage, should be in place.

6. **How does the CT scan help me decide about using thrombolytics?**

The CT scan has become an important aspect of case selection for thrombolytic therapy. Although a completely normal scan is best, the presence of old strokes or early ischemic changes in small areas does not contraindicate administration of a thrombolytic. In 5–10% of cases, the deficit is caused by hemorrhage, tumor, trauma, or abscess. Because anticoagulant or antiplatelet therapy in these patients can be catastrophic, it is advisable to obtain a CT scan in all patients with strokes and TIAs before such therapies are instituted.

Kasner SE, Grotta JC: Emergency identification and treatment of ischemic stroke. Ann Emerg Med 30:642–653, 1997.

7. **Aren't thrombolytics dangerous to give?**

The safe use of TPA requires an understanding of the hemorrhage risks. Most notable is the use of intravenous (IV) TPA after the 3-hour limit. Although there are theoretically some patients who would benefit after the 3-hour window, this has not been well established. Many thrombolytic trials were done with a 6-hour limit from stroke onset and were uniformly negative. Thrombolytics are contraindicated if there is any hemorrhage, signs of significant recent trauma, or an area of obvious stroke that is sufficient to explain the patient's entire deficit—large (more than one third of the middle cerebral artery) area of obvious stroke.

Haley EC Jr, Lewandowski C, Tilley BC, for the NINDS rt-PA Stroke Study Group: Myths regarding the NINDS rtpPA trial: Setting the record straight. Ann Emerg Med 30:676–682, 1997.

Ingall TJ, O'Fallon WM, Asphind K, et al: Findings from the reanalysis of the NINDS tissue plasminogen activator for acute ischemic stroke treat trial. Stroke 35:2418–2424, 2004.

8. **What do I do if the patient is hypertensive?**

Blood pressure is often high in the first minutes after stroke but steadily falls over the first hour. An initial reading of 220/120 mmHg often drops to an acceptable level (185/110 mmHg) by the second or third hour. Some centers set fixed amounts that the blood pressure can be lowered (i.e., 15/7 mmHg) with medication to allow the use of thrombolytics. Severe or sustained hypertension that requires a continuous IV infusion of antihypertensive agents is another contraindication.

9. **What is the risk of intracerebral hemorrhage from TPA?**

The hemorrhage risk is higher in the largest strokes. This explains the lower death rate in the treated group because the patients suffering fatal or severe stroke have poor outcomes whether or not they receive TPA. Even in this subgroup, you are better off with treatment. An increased glucose level is a strong predictor of hemorrhage. This does not mean that patients with increased glucose should not be treated, but more caution should be exercised, and a greater risk should be expected. For all comers, the serious hemorrhage rate is about 6% for IV TPA compared with 0.6% without any treatment. In the PROACT study, the intra-arterial (IA) risks were 10% for lytic therapy and 2% for placebo as larger strokes were recruited. Factors that indicate higher risk of hemorrhage are size of stroke, elevated glucose, and delay to treatment.

10. Is there a role for selective IA thrombolytic infusion?

Enthusiasm has increased for the use of catheter-based thrombolytics or other devices to disrupt clot. The results of the PROCAT Trial have demonstrated the benefits for this approach and have made it clear that many patients can benefit after the 3-hour window. Further studies are being performed to better determine which patients should be selected for this approach to treatment. At large comprehensive stroke centers, the general approach is to use IV TPA for the small- to medium-size strokes and reserve intra-arterial treatment for patients with contraindications to IV TPA and those patients with very large strokes.

11. What if I treat something that turns out not to be a stroke?

After the CT scan excludes hemorrhages, the things that mimic stroke are not harmed by thrombolytics. Complicated migraine, psychogenic weakness, postictal weakness, and TIA are not likely to be affected.

Graham CD: Tissue plasminogen activator for acute ischemic stroke: A meta-analysis of safety data. Stroke 34:2847–2850, 2003.

12. Don't you need a detailed consent for TPA?

Obtaining informed consent can be difficult or impossible in patients with TPA-sized stroke; they are commonly aphasic (dominant hemisphere) or neglectful (nondominant hemisphere). Either condition makes obtaining meaningful consent questionable or impossible. Family members similarly can be so shocked that they balk at any decision making. Because IV TPA is approved by the FDA, a long and detailed consent is not needed. A general approach is to obtain whatever level of consent is possible from the patient and family. Failing that, approach the use of TPA as any other emergency procedure, with a thoughtful note that justifies treatment choice (either to treat or not to treat with TPA) in the individual circumstance.

Johnson JC: To use TPA or not? The legal implications. Neurology Today 5:4, 2005.

13. Is IA thrombolytic treatment better than IV TPA?

Until a clinical trial compares these methods of thrombolytic treatment, there can be no clear answer. Data from the PROACT trial of intra-arterial prourokinase showed better recanalization and better outcomes, even though they didn't begin treatment until 4–5 hours in most cases. It seems that IA techniques can achieve better recanalization, but it takes longer to initiate the treatment. Because "time is brain," this delay may counter any benefit.

IA treatments are favored in patients with systemic risk of hemorrhage because of the dosing changes. The dose of IV TPA in the 80-kg adult is 72 mg. When infusing TPA by IA catheter, the total dose is typically between 10 and 20 mg. The hemorrhage rate is thought to be about the same with either technique, but the systemic risks are much lower with the lower dose IA TPA. This is why patients who have a contraindication to IV TPA are typically candidates for IA TPA.

Furlan A, Higashada R, Wechsler L, et al: Intra-arterial prourokinase for acute ischemic stroke. The PROACT II Study: A randomized controlled trial. Prolyse in Acute Cerebral Thromboembolism. JAMA 282:2003–2011, 1999.

Kumpe DA, Hughes RL: Thrombolytic therapy for acute stroke. In Whittemore AD (ed): Advances in Vascular Surgery, vol. 4. Chicago, Mosby, 1996, pp 71–96.

KEY POINTS: INDICATIONS FOR CONSIDERING CONVENTIONAL ANGIOGRAPHY

1. To confirm the anatomic location and nature of aneurysms and arteriovenous malformations (AVMs)

2. When noninvasive imaging is equivocal

3. When an interventional procedure, such as angioplasty, stenting, or direct clot lysis, will be necessary

4. When noninvasive imaging protocol using CT, MRI, or ultrasound is not adequate

14. **What is the role of MRI in the stroke patient?**
   In general, MRI is indicated only when it can answer a specific question that CT cannot. Ischemic strokes usually do not show up on either CT or MRI within the first few hours. Smaller (i. e., milder) strokes may be viewed better with MRI, but specificity is a problem. MRI is the test of choice to image a stroke (or anything else) in the posterior fossa (brain stem and cerebellum), and MRI has the advantage of being better able to image small vessel infarctions (e.g., lacunar infarcts).

   As MRI and CT technology improves, we may be able to use either modality as a single test to look at the brain, intracranial vasculature, extracranial vasculature, and cerebral blood flow.

15. **When is computed tomography angiography (CTA) or magnetic resonance angiography (MRA) indicated? Should they be the initial studies?**
   The information provided by CTA or MRA can be helpful in theory, but unfortunately these tests take up too much time in practice (particularly the MRA). Some facilities perform the CTA with the CT routinely, adding only a few more minutes. This is useful if patients are being selected for IV or IA interventions. However, many other centers use the size of the stroke as well as IV TPA contraindications to select who needs an IA intervention.

16. **Should I give steroids to a patient with a stroke?**
   No. Despite the efficacy of steroids in cerebral edema associated with tumor and abscess, they do not work in ischemic stroke. The edema that is produced by stroke is more complicated than tumor edema. Because of anecdotal reports of success, steroids sometimes are used in large, life-threatening strokes as an act of desperation.

17. **Which patients should be monitored?**
   In general, patients without a known cause for TIA or stroke or patients with uncertain cardiac risks can benefit from short-term (i.e., 1-day) monitoring:
   Patients with a well-defined mechanism of stroke and a stable cardiac physiology do not usually require ICU or cardiac monitoring. Some institutions have dedicated stroke units, similar to step-down ICUs, to allow closer observation of stroke patients at less expense than a conventional ICU.

18. **What about hypothermia?**
   There is no doubt that hypothermia is effective in saving brain in the setting of cardiac arrest or the intraoperative settings of hypotension or circulatory arrest. Because it can be difficult to cool a person compared with a laboratory rat, clinical trials to demonstrate a benefit in ischemic stroke and to guide its use safely have not yet been completed. At this point, there

is a consensus that avoiding fevers in the first day or so after stroke is clearly of benefit. Thereafter, the determination of how much hypothermia and how early it must be instituted is not clear, and there is nothing more than theory to guide patient selection.

Adams H, Adams R, Del Zoppo G: Guidelines for the early management of patients with ischemic stroke. Stroke 36:916–923, 2005.

19. Do all stroke patients need a cardiac echocardiogram?

No, but all patients need to have the **mechanism** of their stroke defined. Cardiac ultrasound, either transthoracic or transesophageal, has shown a larger number of potential cardiac sources for emboli. This includes common sources, such as atrial fibrillation, prosthetic valves, endocarditis, and mural thrombi, and newer considerations, such as paradoxic emboli through a patent foramen ovale. Young stroke victims (< 45 years old) have a two to three times greater prevalence of patent foramen ovale than do normal age-matched controls, suggesting that these abnormalities have an important role in causing strokes.

20. How can I prevent strokes from occurring in my ED?

In the ED, three groups of patients are potentially identifiable before a stroke.
1. The first group includes patients with acute MI. Most emboli associated with MI occur soon after MI. Patients with anterior wall MIs are at highest risk. Appropriate intervention with anticoagulation or antiplatelet therapy in the ED may prevent a stroke a few hours later.
2. The second group includes patients with multiple traumatic injuries. These patients are notorious for having a stroke in the hospital after their "life has been saved." The highest risk of trauma-related stroke is in patients with direct trauma to the carotid or vertebral arteries. The vertebral artery is particularly prone to injury from rapid head motions. Facial fractures have been associated with a higher risk of carotid injury, leading to carotid occlusion, dissection, or artery-to-artery embolism. Recognition of high-risk patients and early angiography allow preventive measures, such as anticoagulation therapy, to be instituted if there are no contraindications.
3. The occasional patient will present with a stroke that occurred a few days earlier. Even if the stroke occurred a few days ago, the typical stroke patient is dehydrated and probably has some tendency toward a hypercoagulable state. Prompt rehydration and institution of antiplatelet agent are worthwhile in the ED and should not be deferred until the patient is admitted to the hospital floor.

21. Should stroke and TIA patients be allowed to eat?

Most stroke and TIA patients are able to swallow without difficulty. Patients with obviously garbled speech or reduced alertness or patients who have had very large strokes should be kept nil per os (NPO) until tested. Although feeding can be deferred until patients are admitted to a hospital bed, patients often need to take routine oral medications during their wait.

22. How much aspirin is enough to prevent stroke?

Although initially it was four per day, then later three per day, evidence has shown that one aspirin per day is as effective as the higher doses.

23. What good are these newer antiplatelet agents?

Looking at all studies in all ischemic areas, the **thienopyridines (clopidogrel** and **ticlopidine)** work better than aspirin. They are a great choice for aspirin-intolerant patients. Clopidogrel (Plavix) is a bit safer than ticlopidine (Ticlid) and requires no routine blood testing, so it is the popular choice.

Dipyridamole, a popular add-on to aspirin in the 1970s, was abandoned in the 1980s because studies failed to show it helped at all. Two more recent European trials (ESPS-1 and ESPS-2) have revived hope that the aspirin/dipyridamole combination may have some merit. Because these data are so inconsistent from trial to trial, the dipyridamole/aspirin combination benefit needs to be verified.

Overall, most will choose to use aspirin as the first-line antiplatelet agent because of the great cost benefit and the clear benefit for cardiac ischemia.

CAPRIE Steering Committee: A randomized, blinded trial of clopidogrel versus aspirin in patients at risk of ischemic events (CAPRIE). Lancet 348:1329–1338, 1996.

24. **What is the bottom-line risk/benefit analysis for TPA use in stroke?**
When used properly, thrombolytic therapy in ischemic stroke has an excellent overall benefit/ risk analysis for vascular interventions available in the modern hospital, on par with symptomatic carotid endarterectomy and coronary artery bypass grafting.

CONTROVERSIES

25. **What is the role for angioplasty or stenting in stroke?**
With smaller-caliber catheters and embolus protection devices that are placed distal to the stenosis, angioplasty with stenting is now the accepted approach for patients who have risks with general anesthesia and surgery. Further study is ongoing to see whether these approaches can be considered equivalent to carotid endarterectomy in the patients as described in the NASCET and ACAS trials.

26. **Is there any role for anticoagulation of stroke victims in the ED?**
Since this area has not been well studied, nonetheless, a choice must be made. Antiplatelet agents, unfractionated heparin, low-molecular-weight heparin, or no therapy (for patients with high bleeding risks) are all commonly used options based on the perceived risk of recurrence and mechanism of stroke. A brief conversation between the Emergency Medicine Physician and the Admitted Physician should be sufficient to choose an appropriate plan of care.

KEY POINTS: INDICATIONS FOR CONSIDERING ANTICOAGULATION

1. Atrial fibrillation

2. Mechanical heart valves

3. Hypercoagulable states

4. Recurrent embolization on antiplatelet therapy

5. Short-term protection from endothelial disruption such as dissection or endothelial catheter injury

BIBLIOGRAPHY

1. Adams H, Adams R, Del Zoppo G: Guidelines for the early management of patients with ischemic stroke. Stroke 36:916–923, 2005.

2. Alberts MJ, Latchaw RE, Selman WR: Recommendations for comprehensive stroke centers: A consensus statement from the Brain Attack Coalition. Stroke 36:1597–1618, 2005.

3. American Heart Association: 1991 Heart and Stroke Facts. Dallas, TX, American Heart Association, 1991.

4. Antiplatelet Trialists' Collaboration: Collaborative overview of randomized trials of antiplatelet therapy: I. Prevention of death, myocardial infarction, and stroke by prolonged antiplatelet therapy in various categories of patients. BMJ 308:87–106, 1994.

5. Atrial Fibrillation, Aspirin, Anticoagulation Study Group; Boston Area Anticoagulation Trial for Atrial Fibrillation Study Group; Canadian Atrial Fibrillation Anticoagulation Study Group; Veterans Affairs Stroke Prevention in Nonrheumatic Atrial Fibrillation Study Group: Risk factors for stroke and efficacy of antithrombotic therapy in atrial fibrillation. Arch Intern Med 154:1449–1457, 1994.

6. Burton TM: Stroke victims are often taken to wrong hospital, Wall Street Journal May 4, 2005.

7. Caplan LR: Diagnosis and treatment of ischemic stroke. JAMA 266:2413–2418, 1991.

8. CAPRIE Steering Committee: A randomised, blinded, trial of clopidogrel versus aspirin in patients at risk of ischemic events (CAPRIE). Lancet 348:1329–1338, 1996.

9. Coull BM, Goldstein LB, Johnston KC: Anticoagulants and antiplatelet agents in acute ischemic stroke. Stroke 33:1934–1942, 2002.

10. Executive Committee for the Asymptomatic Carotid Atherosclerosis Study: Endarterectomy for asymptomatic carotid stenosis. JAMA 273:1421–1428, 1995.

11. Furlan A, Higashada R, Wechsler L, et al: Intra-arterial prourokinase for acute ischemic stroke. The PROACT II Study: A randomized controlled trial. Prolyse in Acute Cerebral Thromboembolism. JAMA 282:2003–2011, 1999.

12. Graham CD: Tissue plasminogen activator for acute ischemic stroke: A meta-analysis of safety data. Stroke 34:2847–2850, 2003.

13. Haley EC Jr, Lewandowski C, Tilley BCfor the NINDS rt-PA Stroke Study Group: Myths regarding the NINDS rtpPA trial: Setting the record straight. Ann Emerg Med 30:676–682, 1997.

14. Hass WK, Easton JD, Adams HD, et al: A randomized trial comparing ticlopidine hydrochloride with aspirin for the prevention of stroke in high-risk patients. N Engl J Med 321:501–507, 1989.

15. Hughes RL: Carotid endarterectomy for the asymptomatic patient. J La State Med Soc 348:1329–1338, 1996.

16. Ingall TJ, O'Fallon WM, Asphind K, et al: Findings from the reanalysis of the NINDS tissue plasminogen activator for acute ischemic stroke treat trial. Stroke 35:2418–2424, 2004.

17. Johnson JC: To use TPA or not? The legal implications. Stroke 5:3, 2005.

18. Kasner SE, Grotta JC: Emergency identification and treatment of acute ischemic stroke. Ann Emerg Med 30:642–653, 1997.

19. Kidwell CS, Shepherd T, Lawyer TS: Establishment of primary stroke centers: A survey of physician attitudes and hospital resources. Neurology 60:1452–1456, 3003.

20. Kumpe DA, Hughes RL: Thrombolytic therapy for acute stroke. In Whittemore AD (ed): Advances in Vascular Surgery Vol 4. Chicago, Mosby-Year Book, 1996, pp 71–96.

21. Marler JR, Brott TG, Broderick JP: Early stroke treatment associated with better outcome. Neurology 55:1649–1655, 2000.

22. NASCET Collaborators: Beneficial effect of carotid endarterectomy in symptomatic patients with high-grade carotid stenosis. N Engl J Med 325:445–453, 1991.

23. Wyer PC, Osborn HH: Recombinant tissue plasminogen activator: In my community hospital ED, will early administration of rt-PA to patients with the initial diagnosis of acute ischemic stroke reduce mortality and disability? Ann Emerg Med 30:629–638, 1997.

CHAPTER 23

MENINGITIS

Maria E. Moreira, MD

1. **What is meningitis? Why is it important?**
   Meningitis is an inflammatory disease of the tissues surrounding the brain and spinal cord. Mortality from bacterial and fungal meningitis is 10–50%. This is an important issue because prompt recognition and treatment of bacterial meningitis can lessen morbidity and mortality.

2. **List the causes of meningitis.**
   Infectious
   - Bacteria
   - Viruses
   - Fungi
   - Parasites
   - Tuberculosis
   Noninfectious
   - Neoplastic
   - Collagen vascular

3. **Which organisms are most commonly involved in each age group?**
   See Table 23-1.

TABLE 23-1. ORGANISMS MOST COMMONLY INVOLVED BY PATIENT GROUP	
Age or Condition	**Most Commonly Encountered Organisms**
Newborns	Group B or D streptococci, non-group B streptococci, *Escherichia coli*
Infants and children	*Streptococcus pneumoniae, Neisseria meningitides, Haemophilus influenzae*
Adults	*S. pneumoniae, H. influenzae, N. meningitides,* staphylococci, streptococci, *Listeria* spp.
Patients with impaired cellular immunity	*Listeria monocytogenes,* gram-negative bacilli
Head trauma, neurosurgery, or CSF shunt	Staphylococci, gram-negative bacilli, *S. pneumoniae*
CSF = cerebrospinal fluid.	

4. **Who is at risk for meningitis?**
   Those older than 60 and younger than 5 are at highest risk. Medical conditions that put patients at risk include the following: diabetes, alcoholism, cirrhosis, sickle cell disease,

immunosuppressed states, history of splenectomy, thalassemia major, bacterial endocarditis, malignancy, history of ventriculoperitoneal shunt, and intravenous drug abuse. Other risks include recent exposure to others with meningitis, crowding, contiguous infection (e.g., sinusitis), and dural defect (e.g., traumatic, surgical, congenital).

5. **List the common presenting symptoms of meningitis.**
   - Fever
   - Change in mental status
   - Headache
   - Photophobia
   - Stiff neck
   - Lethargy
   - Irritability
   - Malaise
   - Confusion
   - Seizures

KEY POINTS: CLASSIC CLINICAL TRIAD FOR MENINGITIS

1. The classic clinical triad of fever, neck stiffness, and altered mental status is present in less than two thirds of patients with meningitis.

2. The absence of all three signs of the classic triad virtually eliminates a diagnosis of meningitis.

6. **What clinical signs are characteristic of meningeal irritation?**
   - Nuchal rigidity
   - Brudzinski sign: flexion of the neck results in flexion of the knees and hips
   - Kernig sign: pain or resistance of the hamstrings when the knees are extended with the hips flexed at 90 degrees

   These findings are often absent in the very young and older patients.

7. **What is jolt accentuation? What is its significance?**
   This is a physical finding that is found more reliably in meningitis than are the previously mentioned physical findings. Jolt accentuation is said to be present if the baseline headache increases when the patient is asked to turn the head horizontally two to three rotations per second.

   Attia J, Hatala R, Cook DJ, Wong JG: Does this adult patient have acute meningitis? JAMA 282:175–181, 1999.

   Edlow JA: Headache. In Wolfson AB (ed): Hardwood-Nuss' Clinical Practice of Emergency Medicine, 4th ed. Philadelphia, Lippincott Williams & Wilkins, 2005, pp 94–100.

8. **List the presenting signs of meningitis in infants.**
   - Bulging fontanelle (may not be present if patient is dehydrated)
   - Paradoxic irritability (quiet when stationary, cries when held)
   - High-pitched cry
   - Hypotonia
   - Skin or spine may have dimples, sinuses, nevi, or tufts of hair indicating a congenital anomaly communicating with the subarachnoid space.

9. **If the symptoms are not specific and physical findings are absent, what are the indications for lumbar puncture (LP)?**
LP should be done whenever meningitis is suspected because analyzing spinal fluid is the only way to diagnose meningitis.

10. **What tests should be done before doing an LP?**
A funduscopic exam should be performed checking for papilledema and spontaneous venous pulsations. A computed tomography (CT) scan should be done prior to LP if the following are present: papilledema, absence of spontaneous venous pulsations, altered mental status, focal neurologic exam, new-onset seizure, or clinical suspicion for recent trauma or subarachnoid bleed. If there is suspicion for a bleeding disorder, coagulation studies and platelet count should be checked prior to LP.

11. **What is the most common error in emergency department (ED) management of meningitis?**
Delaying administration of antibiotics until the LP is done. If there is a clinical suspicion of bacterial meningitis, antibiotics should be administered promptly. Intravenous antibiotics given 2 hours or less before the LP (and ideally after blood and urine cultures are obtained) will not affect the results of the cerebrospinal fluid (CSF) analysis.

12. **Discuss the risks of LP.**
Paralysis is highly unlikely because the needle is inserted below the level of the spinal cord at L2 or below in adults. However, patients can occasionally experience transient leg paresthesias during LP from irritation of nerve roots by the needle. There are rare reports of cauda equina syndrome from hematoma formation in patients with a coagulopathy. Headache is the most common sequela, occurring in 5–30% of patients. Tonsillar herniation is a potential complication after LP in a patient with increased intracranial pressure; however, the risk is eliminated if the patient has a normal head CT scan before the LP.

13. **What is the secret to performing LP successfully?**
Proper positioning of the patient is crucial. If the LP is done with the patient lying down, be sure the shoulders and hips are in a straight plane perpendicular to the floor. The patient should be in the tightest fetal position possible. If the LP is done with the patient sitting up, have the upper body rest on a bedside table and have the patient push his or her back toward you as if he or she is an angry cat.

14. **When is it essential to perform the LP with the patient lying down?**
This is important when you want to obtain an opening pressure. If you are unable to perform the LP with the patient lying down, you can place the needle with the patient sitting up and then have him or her lay down to obtain the opening pressure.

15. **What can cause a falsely elevated intracranial pressure?**
A tense patient, the head being elevated above the plane of the needle, marked obesity, or muscle contraction.

Euerle B: Spinal puncture and cerebrospinal fluid examination. In Roberts JR, Hedges JR (eds): Clinical Procedures in Emergency Medicine, 4th ed. Saunders, 2004, pp 1197–1222.

16. **Which laboratory studies should be ordered on the CSF?**
Four tubes are usually collected, each containing 1–1.5 mL. More CSF is needed if special tests are required.
- Tube 1: Cell count and differential
- Tube 2: Gram stain, culture, and sensitivities (Special tests that may be ordered include viral cultures, tuberculosis cultures and acid-fast stain, fungal antigen studies and India ink stain,

and serologic tests for neurosyphilis. Countercurrent immunoelectrophoresis is used occasionally to detect specific bacterial antigens in the CSF.)
- Tube 3: glucose and protein
- Tube 4: cell count and differential

In pediatric patients, three tubes are collected: tube 1 for microbiology, tube 2 for glucose and protein, and tube 3 for cell count and differential.

17. **What findings on LP are consistent with bacterial meningitis?**
See Table 23-2.

TABLE 23-2. FINDINGS CONSISTENT WITH BACTERIAL MENINGITIS

Parameter	Finding
Opening pressure	In range of 20–50 cmH$_2$O
Appearance	Cloudy
White blood cell count	1000–5000 cells/mm^3
Cells	Neutrophil predominance
Glucose	<40 mg/dL
Ratio of CSF to serum glucose	<0.4
CSF protein	Elevated (often >100 mg/dL)

CSF = cerebrospinal fluid.

KEY POINTS: CORRECTIONS FOR TRAUMATIC TAPS

1. CSF from a traumatic LP should contain 1 white blood cell (WBC) per 700 (red blood cells (RBCs).

2. When traumatic LP has occurred, correct CSF protein for the presence of blood by subtracting 1 mg/dL of protein for each 1000 RBCs.

3. A very high CSF protein level associated with a benign clinical presentation should suggest fungal disease.

18. **Which antibiotics should be prescribed when the causative organism is unknown?**
See Table 23-3.

Infectious Disease Society of America: www.idsociety.org.
Quagliarello VJ, Scheld WM: Treatment of bacterial meningitis. N Engl J Med 336:708–716, 1997.
  Talan DA: New concepts in antimicrobial therapy for emergency department infections. Ann Emerg Med 34:503–516, 1999.

19. **What about steroids?**
The rationale behind the use of steroids is that attenuation of the inflammatory response in bacterial meningitis may be effective in decreasing pathophysiologic consequences such as

TABLE 23-3. RECOMMENDATIONS FOR KNOWN ORGANISMS AND GENERALIZED RECOMMENDATIONS

Organism	Antibiotic Treatment
Neisseria meningitides	Penicillin G, 3–4 million IU IV every 4 hours, or ampicillin, 2 gm IV every 4 hours, or third-generation cephalosporin
Streptococcus pneumoniae	Vancomycin plus a third-generation cephalosporin
Haemophilus influenzae	Cefotaxime, 2 gm IV every 4 hours
Staphylococcus aureus	Nafcillin 2 gm IV every 4 hours
Escherichia coli and other gram-negative enterics except *Pseudomonas aeruginosa*	Cefotaxime, 2 gm IV every 4 hours
P. aeruginosa	Ceftazidime, 4 gm IV every 8 hours, plus gentamicin, 2 mg/kg IV at once, then 1.7 mg/kg IV every 8 hours (adjusted according to renal function) plus intrathecally every 12 hours if required
Listeria monocytogenes	Ampicillin, 2 gm IV every 4 hours, plus gentamicin (as for *P. aeruginosa*)
Group B streptococci	Ampicillin plus gentamicin
Generalized recommendations	
Age or condition	Antibiotic treatment
Age <3 months	Ampicillin + broad spectrum cephalosporin
Age 3 months to 50 yr	Vancomycin + broad-spectrum cephalosporin
Age >50 yr	Ampicillin + broad-spectrum cephalosporin + vancomycin
Impaired cellular immunity	Ampicillin + ceftazidime
Head trauma, neurosurgery, CSF shunt	Vancomycin + ceftazidime

CSF = cerebrospinal fluid, IV = intravenous.

cerebral edema, increased intracranial pressure, and altered cerebral blood flow. The current recommendations are listed here:

- The Infectious Disease Society of America includes dexamethasone in its algorithm for treatment of meningitis both in adults and in infants.
- Use dexamethasone (0.15 mg/kg) in adults with suspected or proven pneumococcal meningitis. Then only continue if CSF Gram stain shows gram-positive diplococci.
- Use dexamethasone (0.15 mg/kg) in children with suspected or proven *Haemophilus influenzae* meningitis.
- Do not give dexamethasone to adult patients who have already received antimicrobial therapy.

Infectious Disease Society of America: www.idsociety.org

Chaudhuri A: Adjunctive dexamethasone treatment in acute bacterial meningitis. Lancet Neurol 3:54–62, 2004.

20. **Do people exposed to a patient with meningitis need antibiotics?**
Individuals who have had close contact with someone who has, or is suspected to have, meningococcal meningitis should take rifampin, 600 mg twice a day for 2 days. Other accepted prophylaxis regimens for *Neisseria meningitides* include the following: ciprofloxacin, 500 mg single dose; ceftriaxone, 250 mg intramuscular (IM) (used in pregnancy); or a single oral dose of azithromycin, 500 mg. A 4-day course of rifampin is recommended for most individuals who have been in close contact with someone with *H. influenzae* type B meningitis. Individuals exposed to someone with another type of meningitis, especially viral, do not need prophylactic antibiotics.

BREATHING AND VENTILATION

David B. Richards, MD, and John L. Kendall, MD

CHAPTER 24

1. **How useful is the respiratory rate in the evaluation of a patient?**

   The respiratory rate is invaluable as a vital sign. Normal respiratory rate in children varies with age, whereas adults typically breathe 12–16 times per minute. As a testament to its usefulness, the respiratory rate can be helpful in the diagnosis of many conditions other than those with primary pulmonary pathology. For example, it is elevated in patients with anemia, arteriovenous fistula, pregnancy, cyanotic heart disease, metabolic acidosis, febrile illness, central nervous system pathology, anxiety, and those at high altitude. It is important that the respiratory rate be counted carefully for at least 30 seconds. The respiratory rate is often incorrectly estimated from a short period of observation.

2. **Which breathing patterns are associated with pathologic conditions?**

   - **Kussmaul** respirations are deep, rapid breaths that are associated with metabolic acidosis.
   - **Cheyne-Stokes** breathing comprises respirations that wax and wane cyclically so that periods of deep breathing alternate with periods of apnea. Causes include congestive heart failure (CHF), hypertensive crisis, hyponatremia, high altitude illness, and head injury.
   - **Ataxic** breathing is characterized by unpredictable irregularity. Breaths may be shallow or deep and may stop for short periods. Causes include respiratory depression and brain stem injury at the level of the medulla.

3. **Which pulmonary function tests are commonly used in the emergency department (ED)?**

   Other than the respiratory rate, the most useful pulmonary function test for ED patients is the peak expiratory flow rate. It is measured by having a patient exhale at a maximum rate through a peak flowmeter. Normal values range from 350 to 600 L/min in adults. Lower levels are characteristic of increased airway resistance as commonly seen in asthma and chronic obstructive pulmonary disease (COPD) exacerbations. Patients who present with values of 75–100 L/min have severe airflow obstruction. Comparing a patient's current peak expiratory flow rate to his or her personal best can provide good insight into the severity of respiratory distress and necessary treatment. Serial measurements are helpful for objectively quantifying response to treatment. A less commonly used test is the forced end-expiratory volume at 1 second, which helps quantify the severity of obstructive and restrictive lung disease.

4. **How does pulse oximetry work?**

   Pulse oximetry is based on a combination of spectrophotometry and plethysmography.

   - **Spectrophotometry** is based on the Beer-Lambert law, which holds that optical absorbance is proportional to the concentration of a substance and the thickness of the medium. Using this principle, the absorbance of light within a pulsatile vascular bed is used to distinguish between oxyhemoglobin (O_2Hb) and reduced hemoglobin (Hb).
   - **Plethysmography** measures the tissue displacement caused by an arterial pulse. This allows for assessment of the increase in light absorption caused by local arterial flow compared with the background of composite tissues and venous blood. Plethysmography also allows determination of the heart rate.

Pulse oximeters function by placing a pulsatile vascular bed between a light-emitting diode (LED) and a detector. Light is transmitted through the tissue at two wavelengths, 660 nm (primarily absorbed by O_2Hb) and 940 nm (primarily absorbed by Hb), allowing differentiation of O_2Hb from Hb. The detector compares the concentration of O_2Hb and Hb and displays the result as a percent saturation.

5. **How can pulse oximetry be useful? In which situations can it yield false readings?**
Pulse oximetry is useful when monitoring arterial O_2Hb saturation in cardiopulmonary disorders; monitoring oxygen saturation during conscious sedation, airway management, or in patients with a decreased level of consciousness; or quantifying the arterial O_2Hb saturation response to therapeutic interventions. Situations in which the usefulness of pulse oximetry is limited include vasoconstriction, excessive movement, low O_2Hb saturations ($< 83\%$), intravascular dyes, exposure of the measuring sensor to ambient light sources, and when nail polish is present. Oxygen saturation measurements may be falsely elevated in the presence of carboxyhemoglobin and falsely decreased in the presence of methemoglobin.

KEY POINTS: PULSE OXIMETRY

1. Pulse oximetry measures oxygenation not ventilation.

2. Poor peripheral perfusion is a frequent reason pulse oximeters provide unreliable readings.

6. **Why can a good pulse oximetry reading be falsely reassuring?**
Clinicians often rely on the pulse oximeter as part of monitoring a patient's respiratory status, particularly when using procedural sedation. The pulse oximeter only measures oxygenation and provides no information regarding CO_2 exchange and thus does not assess for adequate ventilation. A preoxygenated patient can be apneic for several minutes without an appreciable decrease in oxygen saturation, while significant hypercarbia is developing. Although the pulse oximeter has become indispensable, the clinician must always remember that it only assesses one part of a patient's respiratory status.

7. **What percentage of fraction of inspired oxygen (FiO_2) corresponds with the various types of oxygen delivery systems?**
The three primary means of oxygen delivery are nasal cannula, simple facemask, and facemask with an oxygen reservoir. A nasal cannula can be used to deliver oxygen at rates of 1–6 L/min. With a nasal cannula, every 1 L/min of flow increase increases the FiO_2 by 4%. As a result, a nasal cannula can deliver a FiO_2 between 25% and 45%. A simple facemask relies on an oxygen flow of 5–10 L/min with a resulting FiO_2 ranging from 35 to 50%. A facemask with an oxygen reservoir has a constant flow of oxygen so that higher concentrations of oxygen can be achieved. A properly fitted facemask with an oxygen reservoir with a 15 L/min flow rate can deliver up to 85% FiO_2.

8. **What is noninvasive ventilation?**
It is a means of delivering positive-pressure ventilation without placing a nasotracheal or endotracheal tube. As such, ventilatory assistance is possible without the risks of intubation and mechanical ventilation. Careful selection of patients can make noninvasive ventilation a useful tool to the emergency physician. Any patient who does not have an appropriate mental status, is unable to protect the airway, or unable to develop an adequate respiratory rate would not be a good candidate for noninvasive ventilation.

9. **What forms of noninvasive ventilation are available to emergency physicians?**
   The two most useful forms are mask continuous positive airway pressure ventilation and bilevel positive airway pressure. Each method involves placing a tight-fitting mask over the patient's face and delivering breaths by positive pressure.
   - **Continuous positive airway pressure (CPAP)** delivers a continuous amount of positive airway pressure during and after inspiration and expiration.
   - **Bilevel positive airway pressure (BiPAP)** not only provides a set positive pressure during exhalation but also delivers a set inspiratory pressure when the patient initiates a breath. The inspiratory pressure is always set higher than the expiratory pressure, can be sustained for various periods, and stops when the patient ceases to inhale or begins to exhale.

10. **In what circumstances would noninvasive ventilation be preferred over standard invasive ventilation?**
    Noninvasive ventilation has been shown to be useful in many conditions, including pulmonary edema, pneumonia, asthma, COPD, and nocturnal hypoventilation. In properly selected patients, CPAP is particularly useful in the treatment of pulmonary edema and BiPAP in respiratory distress due to COPD. Patients with COPD are notoriously difficult to wean from mechanical ventilators, and noninvasive ventilation can frequently be used to turn around COPD patients in moderate respiratory distress who would otherwise have required standard invasive ventilation. Lastly, some patients with advance directives forbidding mechanical ventilation can benefit from the respiratory support provided by noninvasive ventilation.

11. **How do I determine the initial ventilator settings in someone who has just been intubated?**
    Ventilator settings must take into account the patient's oxygenation status and his or her ventilation or acid-base status. The primary method for affecting the oxygenation of a patient is to alter the FiO_2 and positive end-expiratory pressure (PEEP). Initially, intubated patients should be given 100% oxygen or an FiO_2 of 1.00. Subsequently, if arterial blood gas analysis reveals that the PaO_2 is high, the FiO_2 and PEEP may be lowered incrementally.
    The main factors determining a patient's ventilatory status are tidal volume and respiratory rate. Changes in each are reflected by the carbon dioxide from arterial blood gas analysis. High respiratory rates and large tidal volumes decrease the carbon dioxide level, whereas the converse elevates the carbon dioxide level. Initially, the tidal volume can be estimated to be 8–10 mL/kg; for a 70-kg patient, that is 560–700 mL.
    The initial respiratory rate varies depending on the clinical situation. On average, the rate should be set between 10 and 16 breaths/min.

12. **Are ventilator settings always the same?**
    No. When you intubate a patient you must remember that you have now placed a bet that you can do a better job directing that patient's ventilation than his or her brain. Keep in mind that your patient's respiratory center has millions of years of evolution backing it up compared with your measly few years of experience. Imagining how your patient's respiratory center would respond to the clinical situation and where the failure has occurred will help you to determine the best ventilator settings for your patient. For example, a patient with an obstructive condition such as asthma does best with small tidal volumes, high respiratory rates, and low levels of PEEP. In contrast, a patient with a COPD exacerbation requires lower respiratory rates, higher tidal volumes, no PEEP, and a prolonged expiratory time. Following end-tidal CO_2 and pulse oximetry can provide real-time feedback of the adequacy of your settings. Other common ventilator settings for patients with closed head injury, CHF, metabolic acidosis, and sepsis are shown in Table 24-1.

13. **What are the different ventilator modes?**
    The main modes of ventilation are controlled mechanical ventilation (CMV), assist control (AC), intermittent mandatory ventilation (IMV), and synchronized intermittent mandatory ventilation

TABLE 24-1. VENTILATOR SETTINGS ACCORDING TO CONDITION

Condition	Tidal Volume (mL/kg)	Respiratory Rate (breaths/min)	FiO$_2$	PEEP (cm H$_2$O)
Asthma	5–10	10–16	100%	2.5–10
COPD	8–12	6–8	100%	None
Head injury	12–15	14–20	100%	None
CHF	8–12	8–12	100%	5–10
Metabolic acidosis	8–12	14–20	100%	2.5–5
SEPSIS	6	10–16	100%	2.5–5

CHF = congestive heart failure, COPD = chronic obstructive pulmonary disease, PEEP = positive end-expiratory pressure.

(SIMV). In the CMV mode, the ventilator delivers a certain volume or pressure at a preset rate, regardless of any ventilatory effort by the patient. AC is similar to CMV in that the tidal volume or inspiratory pressure and minimum respiratory rate are set. It differs from CMV by allowing patients to trigger the ventilator over a set minimum respiratory rate. IMV allows the patient to breathe spontaneously without having a preset tidal volume or pressure. A set rate similar to the CMV mode is in place. This allows the patient to breathe spontaneously, while ensuring a set respiratory rate and tidal volume. SIMV differs from IMV in that the ventilator senses the patient's spontaneous respirations and does not deliver a breath if the patient has already triggered the ventilator. This prevents stacking of respirations, which can be a component of the IMV mode.

14. **What is PEEP?**
Positive pressure applied during expiration. PEEP prevents collapse of alveoli at end-expiration leading to an increase in functional residual capacity. The end result is improved ventilation-perfusion matching in the pulmonary circulation, improving oxygenation. On the flip-side, PEEP can induce barotrauma, diminish venous return to the heart, and elevate intracranial pressure. PEEP is usually set at 2.5 or 5.0 cm H$_2$O.

KEY POINTS: VENTILATOR MANAGEMENT

1. Each clinical situation calls for a different approach to ventilator management.

2. Tidal volume and respiratory rate affect the patient's ventilation and pCO$_2$.

3. FiO$_2$ and PEEP affect the patient's oxygenation and pO$_2$.

4. Oxygenation and ventilation problems in patients on mechanical ventilators can be managed by removing them from the ventilator and following the DOPE mnemonic.

15. **What is auto-PEEP?**
Auto-PEEP develops when a positive-pressure breath is delivered before complete exhalation of the previous breath. As a result, air becomes trapped, and pressure within the lungs increases. This leads to increased airway pressures, diminished venous return to the right heart, and

consequently hypotension. The increased airway pressures can lead to barotrauma, pneumothorax, and inaccurate pulmonary artery catheter measurements. Auto-PEEP can be a particular problem in the mechanical ventilation of COPD and asthmatic patients. The immediate solution is to disconnect the ventilator circuit and allow a full exhalation followed by appropriate changes to the ventilator settings.

16. **What are the most common complications of mechanical ventilation?**
The most common direct complication seen in the ED is **barotrauma.** High pressure can lead to rupture of the alveolar wall, which can lead to pneumomediastinum, pneumothorax, tension pneumothorax, pneumoperitoneum, and subcutaneous emphysema. Pneumonia leads the list of ventilator complications overall, followed by sinusitis, tracheal necrosis, local trauma to the nares and mouth, increased intracranial pressure, renal failure, hyponatremia, and fluid retention.

17. **How do you approach a patient with acutely worsening oxygenation or ventilation already on a ventilator?**
A systematic approach to this situation will serve you well. The **DOPE** mnemonic taught in pediatric life support can be helpful in remembering the approach:
- First remove the patient from the ventilator and have an assistant hand ventilate the patient. Many problems involving a $30,000 ventilator can be solved with a $15 resuscitation bag.
- Confirm the endotracheal tube is in the proper place by using some combination of auscultation, CO_2 exchange, radiography, and direct visualization (**D**isplacement).
- Confirm that the endotracheal tube is patent by passing suction catheter. Sometimes an endotracheal tube can become kinked simply due to patient positioning (**O**bstruction).
- Confirm that there is no evidence of barotrauma, usually by a combination of physical exam and a chest radiograph (**P**neumothorax).
- Confirm that the ventilator circuit and ventilator itself are functioning properly (**E**quipment).

American Heart Association: Pediatric Advanced Life Support Provider Manual, Dallas, 2002, p 109.

18. **What is heliox therapy?**
Heliox is the mixture of oxygen and helium. A patient breathing ambient air inhales 21% oxygen and about 79% nitrogen. In heliox, helium replaces the nitrogen. The significance of this is that helium is seven times lighter than nitrogen, resulting in less turbulent flow and requiring less respiratory effort for ventilation. The standard mixture of heliox is 30% oxygen and 70% helium; thus, supplemental oxygen may be needed in the presence of significant hypoxia. As the concentration of oxygen goes up, the concentration of helium goes down, limiting the effectiveness of heliox to decrease the work of breathing.

McGee DL, Wald DA, Hinchliffe S: Helium-oxygen therapy in the emergency department. J Emerg Med 15:291–296, 1997.

19. **When should I use heliox?**
Heliox can be used in many respiratory conditions, including upper respiratory obstruction, severe COPD, and asthma exacerbation. An important point to stress is that heliox is not primary treatment for any of these conditions, but rather it is a temporizing measure while waiting for the primary treatment to take effect.

CHAPTER 25

ASTHMA, CHRONIC OBSTRUCTIVE PULMONARY DISEASE, AND PNEUMONIA

Rita K. Cydulka, MD, MS, and Jon Siff, MD, MBA

ASTHMA

1. **What is asthma and what are the presenting symptoms of asthma exacerbation?**
   Asthma is a chronic inflammatory disorder of the airways resulting in recurrent episodes of
   wheezing, breathlessness, chest tightness, and coughing. A key feature of asthma is airway
   hyper-responsiveness to a wide variety of stimuli.

2. **In addition to asthma, what should be included in the differential diagnosis of
   wheezing?**
   The following should also be included in the differential diagnosis of wheezing: chronic
   obstructive pulmonary disease (COPD), congestive heart failure (CHF), foreign body aspiration,
   anaphylaxis, epiglottitis, tracheobronchitis, reactive airway disease, viral respiratory infections,
   and vocal cord dysfunction.

3. **Which aspects of the asthmatic's history are important to the current
   exacerbation?**
   Ask questions regarding exposure to common precipitants, such as viral upper respiratory tract
   infections, allergens, cold, exercise, and possible aspirin or nonsteroidal anti-inflammatory drug
   use. Also important are duration and severity of symptoms, past history and frequency of
   sudden exacerbations, prior hospitalizations and intubations, number of recent emergency
   department (ED) visits, current medications, worsening of symptoms while on or if weaning off
   corticosteroids, and other comorbidities.

4. **Are there any helpful tests?**
   Tests of pulmonary function, such as forced expiratory volume in 1 second (FEV_1) or peak
   expiratory flow rate (PEFR) are helpful in determining the severity of airway obstruction. FEV_1 or
   PEFR $> 80\%$ of predicted (or personal best) indicates mild obstruction, FEV_1 or PEFR 50–80%
   of predicted (or personal best) indicates moderate obstruction, and FEV_1 or PEFR $< 50\%$ of
   predicted (or personal best) indicates severe obstruction. Most other tests, including arterial
   blood gases, complete blood counts, and electrocardiograms, are not useful in the management
   of asthma except in cases of active or impending respiratory failure. Chest films may be helpful if
   the patient does not respond to initial treatment or if a pulmonary complication, such as foreign
   body obstruction, pneumonia, pneumomediastinum, pneumothorax, or CHF, is suspected.

5. **What are the key objectives when treating an asthma exacerbation? How are
   they achieved?**
   The key objectives include correction of significant hypoxemia, rapid reversal of airflow
   obstruction, and reduction of the likelihood of recurrence of severe airflow obstruction
   First-line treatment includes β_2-agonists, corticosteroids, ipratropium if needed, and oxygen if
   needed. Relief of airflow obstruction (bronchoconstriction) is usually accomplished by
   administration of either intermittent or continuous doses of aerosolized β_2-agonists. Subcutaneous
   administration of terbutaline or epinephrine may be used in patients unable to tolerate aerosolized

medications. Early administration of systemic corticosteroids addresses the inflammatory component of acute asthma and has been demonstrated to prevent some hospitalization although beneficial effects of corticosteroids are often not noted until 4 hours after administration. High-dose inhaled corticosteroids may have some benefit in the acute setting and can be continued safely by patients already on inhaled steroids. Aerosolized ipratropium should be added if FEV_1 or PEFR is 80% of predicted as studies reveal that they increase pulmonary function modestly and decrease need for hospitalization in these patients. Hypoxemia is usually corrected by administration of supplemental oxygen with a goal of oxygen saturation of 90–95%. (See Table 25-1.)

National Institutes of Health, National Heart, Lung, and Blood Institute: Expert panel report 2: Guidelines for the diagnosis and management of asthma. NIH Pub No 97-4051. Bethesda, MD, NIH, 1997.

Rodrigo G, Rodrigo C: Corticosteroids in the emergency department therapy of acute adult asthma: An evidence-based evaluation. Chest 116:285–295, 1999.

Rodrigo G, Rodrigo C, Burschtin O: Ipratropium bromide in acute adult severe asthma: A metaanalysis of randomized control trials. Am J Med 107:363–370, 1999.

TABLE 25-1. MEDICATIONS USED TO TREAT ASTHMA AND COPD EXACERBATIONS	
Medications	**Dosage and Route**
Inhaled short-acting β_2-agonists	
Albuterol Nebulizer solution (5 mg/mL)	2.5–5 mg every 20 minutes for 3 doses, then 2.5–10 mg every 1–4 hours as needed, or 10–15 mg/hour continuously or 7.5 mg bolus
MDI (90 mcg/puff): *must be used with spacer device*	4–8 puffs every 20 minutes up to 4 hours, then every 1–4 hours as needed
Systemic (injected) β_2-agonists*	
Epinephrine 1:1000 (1 mg/mL)	0.3–0.5 mg every 20 minutes for 3 doses subcutaneously
Terbutaline (1 mg/mL)	0.25 mg every 20 minutes for 3 doses subcutaneously
Inhaled anticholinergics	
Ipratropium bromide nebulizer solution (0.25 mg/mL)	0.5 mg every 30 minutes for 3 doses then every 2–4 hours as needed
MDI (18 mcg/puff): *must be used with spacer device*	4–8 puffs as needed
Systemic corticosteroids	
Prednisone or prednisolone Methylprednisolone	40–60 mg by mouth or 125 mg IV

*Do not use in patients with known coronary artery disease

6. **How can I tell if my patients are improving?**
Ask them how they feel, re-examine them, and obtain objective measures of pulmonary function. Either FEV_1 or PEFR (the best of three attempts) should be obtained on presentation and after

treatment and compared with the patient's percent predicted (or personal best) FEV_1 or PEFR, if known, to determine the need for more aggressive therapy or hospitalization.

7. What measures are available if my patient isn't responding as expected?

Magnesium sulfate has been noted to help reverse bronchospasm in conjunction with standard therapy if PEFR is 25% or less of predicted but is not useful in patients with mild or moderate obstruction. Although widely discussed, the data for ketamine, heliox, and continuous positive pressure ventilation are less compelling.

There are no absolute indications for intubation except for respiratory arrest and coma. Possible indication for intubations include exhaustion, worsening respiratory distress, persistent or increasing hypercarbia, and changes in mental status. General anesthesia may be helpful for patients in status asthmaticus who continue to be refractory to treatment while intubated.

Ho Am LA, Karmakar MK, et al: Heliox vs air-oxygen mixtures for the treatment of patients with acute asthma: A systematic overview. Chest 123:882–890, 2003.

Silverman Ra, Osborn H, Runge J, et al: Magnesium sulfate in the treatment of acute severe asthma: A multicenter randomized controlled trial. Chest 122:489–497, 2002.

8. How should I decide whether a patient can be discharged or requires hospitalization?

This is the million dollar question. Relapse rates remain up to 25% because no sure-fire criteria for successful discharge and follow-up currently exist. Disposition of patients is usually determined by clinical response after the three doses of aerosolized β_2-agonist therapy, ipratropium (if used), and corticosteroids. If patients have clear breath sounds, are no longer are dyspneic or are back to baseline, and have an FEV_1 or PEFR 70% of predicted, they may be discharged home. Patients with an incomplete response to treatment, that is, FEV_1 between 50 and 70% of predicted and mild dyspnea, can be considered for discharge after assessing their individual circumstances. Patients with a poor response to bronchodilators, that is, $FEV_1 < 50\%$ of predicted, who have moderate to severe symptoms after treatment require hospitalization. If an ED observation capability exists, observation for 4–6 hours post steroid administration will decrease the number of inpatient admissions.

www.nhlbi.nih.gov/guidelines/asthma/asthgdln.htm

9. What should be considered at time of discharge?

Patients who received corticosteroids acutely should continue oral steroid therapy at home for up to 10 days. Dosing parameters are controversial, so choose a moderate regimen (about 40–50 mg prednisone per day); no tapering is required. Patients not already on controller medications who have mild persistent asthma should be started on low-dose inhaled corticosteroids or oral leukotriene modifiers, such as zafirlukast or montelukast. Long-acting β-agonists, such as salmeterol, should be added to the regimen of patients with moderate persistent asthma who are inadequately controlled on inhaled corticosteroids. All patients should be advised to use their short-acting β-agonists on a regularly scheduled basis for a few days and then as needed. Patient education should be provided at discharge, as well as an appointment for a follow-up visit within several days.

10. Does pregnancy change the management of acute asthma?

No. It is important to treat pregnant asthmatics aggressively to prevent maternal hypoxia and subsequent fetal morbidity and mortality. Patients should not be undertreated because of fear of teratogenicity; the risks from respiratory failure and severe acute asthma are greater than from therapy with standard medications.

Cydulka RK, Emerman CL, Schreiber DS: Acute asthma among pregnant women presenting to the emergency department. Am J Respir Crit Care Med 160:887–892, 1999.

CHRONIC OBSTRUCTIVE PULMONARY DISEASE

11. What is COPD? What are the presenting symptoms of COPD exacerbation?

COPD is a disease characterized by airflow limitation that is not fully reversible, is progressive, and is associated with an abnormal inflammatory response to noxious particles or gases. It includes emphysema and chronic bronchitis and can coexist with asthma. The characteristic symptoms of COPD are cough, sputum production, and dyspnea on exertion. Exacerbations are characterized by increased dyspnea, often accompanied by wheezing and chest tightness, increased cough and sputum, change in color or thickness of sputum, and fever. Smoking, exposure to occupational dusts and chemicals, and air pollution are the most common causes of COPD.

www.goldcopd.com/

KEY POINTS: EMERGENCY TREATMENT OF ASTHMA

1. Relieve significant hypoxemia: oxygen.

2. Reverse airflow obstruction: β-agonists + ipratropium.

3. Reduce of the likelihood of recurrence: corticosteroids.

4. Provide objective measure of improvement: PEFR or FEV_1.

5. Adequate discharge planning includes education, medications, and follow-up.

---

12. In addition to COPD, what should be included in the differential diagnosis of wheezing?

The differential diagnosis includes asthma, CHF, pneumonia, anaphylaxis, pulmonary embolism, tuberculosis (TB), and metabolic disturbances.

13. Which diagnostic tests are helpful in the management of COPD?

Pulse oximetry should be used in every patient with COPD. Oxygen saturation less than 90% indicates severe hypoxia. Arterial blood gas measurements often can identify patients with increased and continuing hypoxia, hypercarbia, and respiratory acidosis, especially if compared with the patient's baseline values. Check theophylline levels if indicated. Chest radiographs are appropriate in COPD exacerbations to help manage complications and concomitant disease. In patients with cor pulmonale, continuous cardiac monitoring may identify any associated arrhythmias. The use of B-type natriuretic peptide (BNP) does not substitute for clinical judgment when trying to differentiate COPD from CHF as a numeric cut-off value that differentiates between the two diseases remains elusive. In contrast to asthma, pulmonary function tests are less helpful because of the difficulty that sick patients with COPD have in performing these tests properly.

Cydulka RK, Dave M: Chronic obstructive pulmonary disease. In Tintinalli JE, Kelen GD, Stapczynski S (eds): Emergency Medicine: A Comprehensive Study Guide, 6th ed. New York, McGraw-Hill, 2004, pp 475–480.

McCullough PA, Hollander JE, Nowak RM: Uncovering heart failure in patients with a history of pulmonary disease: Rationale for the early use of B-type natriuretic peptide in the emergency department. Acad Emerg Med 10:198–204, 2003.

14. What are the key objectives when treating a COPD exacerbation? How are they achieved?

The key objectives are to relieve hypoxemia, alleviate reversible bronchospasm, and treat the underlying etiology of the exacerbation. First-line treatment includes $β_2$-agonists, corticosteroids, ipratropium if needed, and oxygen if needed. Relief of airflow obstruction (bronchoconstriction) is usually accomplished by administration of either intermittent doses of aerosolized β_2-agonists or anticholinergics, such as ipratropium. Systemic corticosteroids are indicated in severe exacerbations of COPD. Hypoxemia is usually corrected by administration of supplemental oxygen with a goal of oxygen saturation of 90% or greater. Excessive supplemental oxygen in this small subset of patients can cause respiratory arrest secondary to loss of their hypoxemia-induced ventilatory drive. Thus, oxygen administration should be carefully monitored by frequent clinical assessment, continuous pulse oximetry, and arterial blood gases, when needed.

Cydulka RK, Dave M: Chronic obstructive pulmonary disease. In Tintinalli JE, Kelen GD, Stapczynski S (eds): Emergency Medicine: A Comprehensive Study Guide, 6th ed. New York, McGraw-Hill, 2004, pp 475–480.

15. What about antibiotics?

Routine antibiotic coverage is controversial, but several guidelines recommend antibiotic therapy for patients with pneumonia, increased sputum production, fever, and worsening dyspnea. The antibiotic choices should reflect local antibiotic sensitivity to *Streptococcus pneumoniae, Haemophilus influenzae,* and *Moraxella catarrhalis.* Guidelines for treatment of pneumonia, if present, should be considered.

Saint S, Bent S, Vittinghoff E, Grady D: Antibiotics in chronic obstructive pulmonary disease exacerbations. A meta-analysis. JAMA 273:957–960, 1995.

16. How can I tell if my patient is improving?

Ask the patient how he or she feels, re-examine, and monitor the oxygen saturation. If the patient was able to perform objective measures of pulmonary function, compare FEV_1 or PEFR (the best of three attempts) obtained on presentation with that obtained after treatment.

17. When should a patient with COPD be intubated?

Noninvasive modalities such as continuous positive airway pressure (CPAP) and bi-level positive airway pressure often can obviate the need for intubation by improving gas exchange, decreasing hypoxia, and reducing work of breathing. Any patient with changes in mental status, increased respiratory distress with cyanosis, acute deterioration, or exhaustion should be intubated and mechanically ventilated immediately.

18. How should I decide whether a patient can be discharged or requires hospitalization?

This is the $2 million question. Relapse rates remain high because patients with COPD have less respiratory reserve and function that is not quickly reversible. These patients often take longer than an ED visit to recover and require hospitalization. Failure to improve while in the ED, failed outpatient management, and concerning pulmonary infections are reasons for hospitalization. Patients who return to near baseline with improvement from ED treatment and have good social support systems in place may be discharged home with close follow-up.

Kim S, Emerman CL, Cydulka RK, et. al: Prospective multicenter study of relapse following emergency department treatment of COPD exacerbation. Chest 125:473–481, 2004.

19. What should be considered at time of discharge?

Patients who received corticosteroids acutely should continue oral steroid therapy at home for up to 10 days. Dosing parameters are controversial, so choose a moderate regimen (about 40–50 mg of prednisone per day); no tapering is required. Patients should continue to use their short-acting rescue medications, that is, albuterol and/or ipratropium on a regular basis until the exacerbation resolves, in addition to their long-acting β-agonists and long-acting anticholinergics (i.e., tiotropium) The use of chronic inhaled corticosteroids is most beneficial for patients with an FEV_1 between 1 and 2 L. Antibiotics should be prescribed to patients deemed well enough for discharge who have experienced increase in sputum production, thickness, or change in sputum color. Patients with a $PaCO_2$ lower than 60 mmHg at baseline should be evaluated for home oxygen therapy. Patient education should be provided at discharge, as well as an appointment for a follow-up visit within several days.

Sin DD, Mcalister FA, Oaul Man SF, et al: Contemporary management of chronic obstructive pulmonary disease. JAMA 290:2301–2312, 2003.

20. **When is ipratropium bromide contraindicated in the management of patients with asthma or COPD?**
Ipratropium bromide contains derivatives of soya lecithin and related food products. Patients with soybean or peanut allergies may develop anaphylaxis if exposed to this medication in either metered dose inhaler (MDI) or nebulized forms.

KEY POINTS: EMERGENCY TREATMENT OF COPD

1. Relieve significant hypoxemia: oxygen.

2. Reverse airflow obstruction: β-agonists + ipratropium.

3. Consider antibiotics if there are changes in sputum production.

4. Patients with COPD have less respiratory reserve and require admission more frequently than patients with asthma.

5. Adequate discharge planning includes education, medications, and careful follow-up.

PNEUMONIA

21. **Why are the diagnosis and treatment of pneumonia important in the practice of emergency medicine?**
Pneumonia is the seventh leading cause of death overall and the leading cause of death from infectious disease in the United States. There are approximately 5 million identified cases of community-acquired pneumonia (CAP) each year, resulting in 1.3 million hospital admissions. The ED serves as the portal of entry for 75% of these admissions. When properly identified and treated as an outpatient, the mortality of CAP decreased from 30% to about 1%. The role of the emergency physician is to diagnose pneumonia accurately, initiate timely antibiotic therapy, and make an appropriate disposition.

Hoyert DL, Kung H-C, and Smith BL: Deaths: Preliminary Data for 2003; Vol. 53 no 15. Hyattsville, Maryland: National Center for Health Statistics. 2005.
www.cdc.gov/nchs/data/nvsr/nvsr53_15.pdf
www.cdc.gov/nchs/products/pubs/pubd/nvsr/nvsr.htm
www.emedicine.com/emerg/topic465.htm

22. **How does a pulmonary infection develop? What predisposes people to it?**
Pneumonia is an infection of the alveolar spaces of the lung. It commonly develops via inhalation of infectious particles or aspiration of oropharyngeal or gastric contents and less commonly through hematogenous spread of infection, direct invasion from contiguous structures, direct inoculation, and reactivation of prior disease. Table 25-2 lists predisposing factors.

www.clevelandclinicmeded.com\diseasemanagement\infectiousdisease\communitypneumonia.htm

23. **What are differences in presentation of ''typical'' pneumonia and ''atypical'' pneumonia?**
- **Typical** pneumonia presents with the abrupt onset of high fever, cough productive of purulent sputum, shortness of breath, and pleuritic chest pain. Infants may present with fever

TABLE 25-2. FACTORS PREDISPOSING TO DEVELOPMENT OF PNEUMONIA

Factor	Likely Populations
Impaired swallowing/airway protection	Patients with history of alcohol abuse, CVA, ET and NT intubation, head injury, impaired gag reflex, seizures
Extremes of age	Very young and very old
Underlying pulmonary disease	Pulmonary embolism, COPD, pulmonary foreign body or tumor, pulmonary contusion, atelectasis
Chest wall disorders Prevent good cough and clearing of secretions	Rib fracture, surgical wounds, myopathies affecting chest muscles
Impaired mucociliary clearance mechanisms	Smokers, smog, alcohol, underlying viral infection, chronic lung disease
Impaired immune function	HIV, cancer, chemotherapy, malnutrition, sickle-cell disease, chronic steroid use
Other predisposing risks—these may lead to more severe infections with more virulent organisms	Diabetes, alcoholism, recent antibiotic use, recent hospitalization

COPD = chronic obstructive lung disease, CVA = cerebrovascular accident, ET = endotracheal, HIV = human immunodeficiency virus, NT = nasotracheal.
Adapted from www.clevelandclinicmeded.com\diseasemanagement\infectiousdisease\ communitypneumonia.htm

associated with irritability, tachypnea, intercostal retractions, nasal flaring, and grunting. Cough may be absent in infants. Elderly or debilitated patients may present with nonspecific complaints and findings such as confusion or deterioration of baseline function, rather than classic symptoms.

- **Atypical** pneumonia has a more insidious onset and includes a prominent cough often with the absence of sputum production. Patients may have only a mild fever and are more likely to have extrapulmonary manifestations such as sore throat, dermatitis, headache, cardiac complications (pericarditis, myocarditis), hepatitis, and renal disease. There are no consistent clinical or radiographic criteria available to distinguish typical from atypical pneumonia.

24. **What are the most common causative agents in CAP and nosocomial pneumonia?**

The causative organism is unknown in 30–50% of patients with CAP. In those patients for whom the causative organism is known, *Streptococcus pneumoniae* is the most common agent (Table 25-3). During hospitalization, exposure to more virulent organisms changes the pattern of infection. Gram-negative bacilli, particularly *Klebsiella, Pseudomonas aeruginosa*, and *Escherichia coli*, are responsible for more than 50% of cases. *Staphylococcus aureus* accounts for another 10–20% of hospital-acquired pneumonias. The remainder of cases are usually due to

TABLE 25-3. IDENTIFIED PATHOGENS IN COMMUNITY-ACQUIRED PNEUMONIA

Pathogen	Percentage of Cases	Usual Pattern Caused
Streptococcus pneumoniae	20–60	Typical
Haemophilus influenzae	3–10	Typical
Mycoplasma pneumoniae	1–6	Atypical
Staphylococcus aureus	3–5	Typical
Viral (various incl. influenza)*	2–16	Atypical
Legionella species	2–8	Typical
Chlamydia pneumoniae	4–6	Atypical
Aspiration	6–10	Variable
Gram-negative bacilli (Klebsiella, Pseudomonas, etc.)	3–10	Typical
Others	3–5	Variable

*Percentage of viruses is highly variable and was as high as 36% in one study and may be higher in infants and young children than in adults.
Adapted from www.clevelandclinicmeded.com\diseasemanagement\infectiousdisease\communitypneumonia.htm

anaerobic oral flora, *S. pneumoniae, Legionella,* and *Moraxella catarrhalis* (each accounting for < 10% of cases). Patients who develop a hospital-acquired pneumonia have an attributable mortality of 27–50%.

McEachern R, Campbell GD Jr: Hospital-acquired pneumonia: Epidemiology, etiology, and treatment. Infect Dis Clin North Am 12:761–779, 1998.

Rello J, Paiva JA, Baraibar J, et al: International Conference for the Development of Consensus on the Diagnosis and Treatment of Ventilator-associated Pneumonia. Chest 120:955–970, 2001.

www.clevelandclinicmeded.com/diseasemanagement/pulmonary/hospital_pneumonia/hospital_pneumonia.htm

www.emedicine.com/emerg/topic465.htm

25. **Discuss the key aspects of the physical exam in assessing suspected pneumonia.**

Findings consistent with pneumonia include fever, tachypnea, tachycardia, and decreased oxygen saturation and abnormal breath sounds. With severe infection, patients may appear toxic, may be unable to communicate, and may have an altered mental status due to hypoxia. The presence or absence of any of these findings is not conclusive for pneumonia.

26. **What tests are useful in the evaluation of pneumonia?**

Although some providers will treat healthy, low-risk patients with suspected pneumonia empirically, others feel a chest x-ray is mandatory in every patient with a history and symptoms suggestive of pneumonia. The American Thoracic Society (ATS) and the Infectious Disease Society of America (IDSA) include radiographic findings as part of their definitions of pneumonia. The IDSA 2000 pneumonia guidelines state in their executive summary that "Chest radiography is considered critical for establishing the diagnosis of pneumonia."

An arterial blood gas may augment the information obtained through pulse oximetry to assess the need for respiratory support. In addition, the following laboratory tests are used to aid in risk stratification of patients: complete blood count and serum electrolytes. The use of sputum Gram stain and blood cultures is controversial.

Bartlett JG, Dowell SF, Mandell LA, et al: Practice guidelines for the management of community acquired pneumonia in adults. Clin Infect Dis 31:347–382, 2000.

27. **What radiographic findings are helpful in making a microbiologic differential diagnosis?**

Certain x-ray findings are suggestive of, but not diagnostic of, specific pathogens. In addition, dehydration and the radiographic manifestations of chronic diseases may obscure the infiltrates of pneumonia (Table 25-4).

TABLE 25-4. RADIOGRAPHIC APPEARANCES OF COMMUNITY-ACQUIRED PNEUMONIA*

Radiographic Pattern	Suggested Organisms
Lobar	*Streptococcus pneumoniae*, *Klebsiella* species, pneumonia due to bronchial obstruction
Diffuse patchy infiltrate involving multiple lobes	*Staphylococcus aureus*, *Haemophilus influenzae* or gram-negative organisms
Interstitial pattern	*Mycoplasma pneumoniae*, *Legionella*, viral, *Pneumocystis* (patients with HIV or HIV risks) *Chlamydia psittaci*
Cavitary lesions with air-fluid levels	*S. aureus*, *Klebsiella*, *Pseudomonas aeruginosa*, *Mycobacterium tuberculosis*[†]

*The development and resolution of x-ray findings may lag clinical findings by hours to days.
[†]Tuberculosis may take on almost any radiographic appearance with some predilection for the upper lobes.
HIV = human immunodeficiency virus.
Adapted from www.clevelandclinicmeded.com\diseasemanagement\infectiousdisease\communitypneumonia.htm

28. **How are patients with pneumonia risk stratified and how does that translate into a disposition decision?**

Once a diagnosis of pneumonia is strongly suspected by history, physical, and x-ray results, the next decision is whether the patient is appropriate for discharge or requires hospital admission. The Patient Outcome Research Team (PORT) studies have produced a pneumonia-specific severity of illness score (PSI). The PSI uses a combination of 20 parameters to evaluate patients, assign disease severity and mortality risk, and guide disposition. (See Tables 25-5 to 25-7.) Although there are no clear guidelines for intensive care unit (ICU) admission, several rules have been published. Patients requiring ventilatory assistance or pressors and those who have altered mental status, multilobar or bilateral infiltrates, and age > 65 are among the patients who should be considered for an ICU setting.

American College of Emergency Physicians: Clinical policy for the management and risk stratification of community-acquired pneumonia in adults in the emergency department. Ann Emerg Med 38:107–113, 2001.

Fine MJ, Auble TE, Yealy DM, et al: A prediction rule to identify low-risk patients with community acquired pneumonia. N Engl J Med 336:243–250, 1997.

Restrepo MI, Anzueto A: Antimicrobial treatment of community-acquired pneumonia. Clin Chest Med 26:65–73, 2005.

pda.ahrq.gov/clinic/psi/psi.htm.

TABLE 25-5. FACTORS IN PNEUMONIA DISPOSITION DECISION

PORT PSI Scoring

PORT Characteristics	Points given for presence of characteristic
Demographics	
Age—male patient	Age in years (one point per year)
Age—female patient	Age in years: 10
Lives in nursing home	+10
Coexisting illnesses	
Neoplastic disease	+30
Liver disease	+20
CHF	+10
Cerebrovascular disease (TIA or CVA)	+10
Renal disease	+10
Physical exam findings	
Acute disorientation, stupor or coma	+20
Respiratory rate 30/min	+20
Systolic blood pressure 90 mmHg	+20
Temperature < 35°C or 40°C	+15
Heart rate 125 bpm	+10
Laboratory and x-ray findings (if study performed)	
Arterial pH < 7.35	+30
Blood urea nitrogen 30 mg/dL	+20
Sodium < 130 mmol/L	+20
Glucose 250 mg/dL	+10
Hematocrit < 30%	+10
Partial pressure of arterial oxygen < 60 mmHg or oxygen saturation <90%	+10
Pleural effusion	+10
Total points = age + (−10 if female) + sum of above comorbidities, exam findings, and testing	

29. **What treatment should be started in the ED?**
Supportive care, including oxygen and ventilatory support, should be given as required. Rehydration, antipyretics, and pain control should also be started as indicated. Antibiotic therapy should begin, based on the most likely pathogens, as soon as the diagnosis of pneumonia is made or strongly suspected. Studies have shown a decreased mortality and length of stay in a group of patients admitted for CAP when antibiotics were administered within 4 hours of arrival. All patients being admitted for pneumonia from the ED should have their first dose begun prior to transfer to the floor or ICU.

TABLE 25-6. PSI CLASS BASED ON POINT TOTALS AND MORTALITY*

Points Calculated from PSI	Class	Mortality
< 51 points	I	0.1%
51–70	II	0.6%
71–90	III	0.9%
91–130	IV	9.5%
>130	V	26.7%

*Those patients who are under 50 years and without any comorbid illnesses or vital sign abnormalities fall into class I and may be safely treated as outpatients. Patients not falling into risk class I require additional laboratory testing so they may be assigned to risk classes II–V. Patients in classes II and III may be appropriate for outpatient management or a brief observation stay. Patients in class IV or V require hospital admission with a subset requiring ICU admission.

TABLE 25-7. OTHER FACTORS (NOT PART OF PORT PSI) THAT IMPACT DISPOSITION DECISION

- Patient's clinical appearance
- Patient's ability to tolerate oral intake
- Patient reliability
- Social factors such as home support
- Clinical judgment of the physician (most important)

PORT PSI = Patient Outcome Research Team pneumonia-specific severity of illness score.

American College of Emergency Physicians: Clinical policy for the management and risk stratification of community-acquired pneumonia in adults in the emergency department. Ann Emerg Med 38:107-113, 2001.
    Restrepo MI, Anzueto A: Antimicrobial treatment of community-acquired pneumonia. Clin Chest Med 26:65–73, 2005.

30. **Which antibiotic should I use?**
    The choice of which antibiotic to begin is based on the site of treatment and suspected pathogens. The suggestions in Table 25-8 should be used in consideration with the clinical picture, recent literature, local preference, and resistance patterns.

31. **Has the epidemiology of pneumonia changed in recent years?**
    The epidemiology of CAP continues to change due to a number of constantly changing factors such as the discovery of new pathogens, changing antibiotic resistance, an aging population, and new tools for fighting infection. Although *Pneumocystis carinii* pneumonia and TB continue to be significant pathogens, particularly in the developing world, a new pathogen has recently been discovered. The severe acute respiratory syndrome (SARS) was first described in 2002 in China and subsequently spread worldwide. SARS is now known to be caused by a previously undescribed coronavirus. Diagnostic and treatment guidelines are available on the CDC website at www.cdc.gov. Pneumonia due to *S. pneumoniae* continues to be a concern due to continually evolving resistance to a wider array of antibiotics.

TABLE 25-8. EMPIRICAL ANTIMICROBIAL THERAPY FOR COMMUNITY-ACQUIRED PNEUMONIA IN IMMUNOCOMPETENT ADULTS

Patient/Setting	Common Pathogens	IDSA Empiric Therapy	ATS Empiric Therapy
Outpatient <60 years old No comorbid diseases	S. pneumoniae M. pneumoniae C. pneumoniae H. influenzae Viruses	A macrolide or doxycycline	A macrolide or doxycyline
Outpatient > 65 years old or having comorbid disease or antibiotic therapy within last 3 months	S. pneumoniae (drug-resistant) M. pneumoniae C. pneumoniae H. influenzae Viruses Gram-negative bacilli*,† S. aureus*,†	A macrolide, doxycycline, or a fluoroquinolone*	A beta-lactam† and (macrolide or doxycycline) or a fluoroquinolone* alone
Inpatient Not severely ill	S. pneumoniae	A macrolide and cefotaxime or ceftriaxone or a beta-lactam/beta lactamase inhibitor‖; a fluoroquinolone‡ alone	Cardiopulmonary disease or risk factors: IV beta-lactam# and (IV or oral macrolide or doxycycline) or IV antipneumococcal fluoroquinolone* alone No cardiopulmonary disease or risk factors: intravenous azithromycin alone. If macrolide allergic: doxycycline and a beta-lactam# or an antipneumococcal fluoroquinolone alone.

Continued

TABLE 25-8. EMPIRICAL ANTIMICROBIAL THERAPY FOR COMMUNITY-ACQUIRED PNEUMONIA IN IMMUNOCOMPETENT ADULTS—CONT'D

Patient/Setting	Common Pathogens	IDSA Empiric Therapy	ATS Empiric Therapy
Inpatient Not severely ill	*H. influenzae* Polymicrobial Anaerobes *S. aureus* *C. pneumoniae* Viruses		
Inpatient Severely ill	*S. pneumoniae*[§] *Legionella* Gram-negative bacilli *M. pneumoniae* Viruses *S. aureus*	Erythromycin, azithromycin, or a fluoroquinolone[‡] and cefotaxime, ceftriaxone, or a beta lactam/beta lactamase inhibitor[ǁ]	*P. aeruginosa* unlikely: IV beta-lactam and (IV macrolide or fluoroquinolone). *P. aeruginosa* possible: (IV macrolide or fluoroquinolone and aminoglycoside IV) or (antipseudomonal quinolone) and antipseudomonal beta-lactam

*In the outpatient setting, many authorities prefer to reserve fluoroquinolones (levofloxacin, gatifloxacin, moxifloxacin, gemifloxacin) for patients with comorbid diseases/risk factors.
[†]In most cases, patients with pneumonias due to these organisms should be hospitalized.
[‡]Levofloxacin, gatifloxacin, moxifloxacin, or gemifloxacin
[§]Critically ill patients in areas with significant rates of high-level pneumococcal resistance and a suggestive sputum gram-stain should receive vancomycin or a newer quinolone pending microbiologic diagnosis.
[ǁ]Piperacillin-tazobactam or ampicillin-sulbactam
[¶]Cefpodoxime, cefuroxime, high-dose amoxicillin, amoxicillin/clavulanate; or parenteral ceftriaxone followed by oral cefpodoxime
[#]Cefotaxime, ceftriaxone, ampicillin/sulbactam, or high-dose ampicillin.

CONTROVERSY

32. What is the role of sputum Gram stain and culture?

The value of the Gram stain for expectorated sputum is controversial because it is uncertain how accurately expectorated sputum reflects lower respiratory tract secretions and pathology. Wide variability in the sensitivity and specificity of this test has been reported. Gram stain may be more useful in high-risk or hospitalized patients and should be considered in this group. The use of sputum with other stains (such as acid-fast for TB) and techniques such as direct fluorescent antibody staining have a continuing and developing role but are probably not helpful in ED management of these patients.

American College of Emergency Physicians: Clinical policy for the management and risk stratification of community-acquired pneumonia in adults in the emergency department. Ann Emerg Med 38:107–113, 2001.

33. Are routine blood cultures helpful in the management of community-acquired pneumomnia?

The utility of blood cultures to determine causative agent in unselected patients with CAP is only 6–11% and infrequently changes empirical management. However, in patients with severe symptoms and/or significant risk factors, blood cultures may demonstrate uncommon causative organisms or unexpected antibiotic resistance. In elderly patients, obtaining blood cultures within 24 hours of admission was associated with a decreased 30-day mortality. Currently, guidelines suggest that blood cultures be obtained in the ED prior to initiating antibiotics on all hospitalized patients, but future guidelines may be more selective.

American College of Emergency Physicians: Clinical policy for the management and risk stratification of community-acquired pneumonia in adults in the emergency department. Ann Emerg Med 38:107–113, 2001.
Meehan TP, Fine MJ, Krumholz HM, et al: Quality of care, process and outcomes in elderly patients with pneumonia. Chest 108:891–892, 1995.

KEY POINTS: EMERGENCY TREATMENT OF PNEUMONIA

1. Begin empiric treatment early based on suspected pathogens.

2. Calculation of the PORT score is a reliable predictor of mortality and a good tool to assist with disposition decisions.

3. Support oxygenation, ventilation, and circulation as indicated by the patient's condition.

4. Recently hospitalized and nursing home patients will be infected with different organisms and require additional antibiotic coverage.

5. Consider the presentation "typical" versus "atypical" when making therapy decisions.

CHAPTER 26

VENOUS THROMBOEMBOLISM

Stephen J. Wolf, MD

1. **What is virchow's triad of thromboembolism?**
   Venous stasis, vascular trauma, and hypercoagulable state.

2. **What two diseases represent the continuum of venous thromboembolism (VTE)?**
   Deep venous thrombosis (DVT) and pulmonary embolism (PE).

3. **What percentage of patients diagnosed with DVTs have concomitant PE when studied?**
   50%. Additionally, a similar percentage of patients with a diagnosed PE will have a concomitant DVT when studied.

KEY POINTS: MAJOR RISK FACTORS CARRYING A RELATIVE RISK OF 5–20 FOR VTE

1. Recent surgery ($\leq$ 4 weeks)

2. Immobilization (equivalent to bed rest $\geq$ 3 days)

3. Pregnancy (third > second > first trimester)

4. Postpartum (for up to 42 days)

5. Malignancy (treatment active, within 6 months, or palliative)

6. History of VTE

4. **List the minor risk factors for VTE**
   - Cardiovascular disease (heart failure, hypertension, congenital heart disease)
   - Indwelling vascular access
   - Estrogen use (hormone replacement or oral contraceptives)
   - Obesity
   - Neurologic disease (cerebrovascular accident [CVA], paresis)
   - Inflammatory bowel disease (Crohn's disease, ulcerative colitis)
   - Tobacco
   - Advanced age
   - Hypercoagulable states (factor V Leyden thrombophilia, prothrombin mutation, circulating lupus anticoagulant, antithrombin III deficiency, and protein C or S deficiency)

5. **What is the relative risk for VTE in a patient with a minor risk factor?**
   Two to four times that of a patient without a minor risk factor.

6. **Are there any signs or symptoms of PE that are diagnostic?**
    No. Although the common clinical signs and symptoms of shortness of breath, chest pain, tachypnea, and tachycardia occur in upwards of 97% of patients diagnosed with PE, they are nonspecific. Patient presentations can range from mild shortness of breath to cardiovascular collapse.

7. **Why is a clinician's pretest probability for VTE so important?**
    Because no diagnostic test available for the evaluation of VTE is absolute (with a perfect sensitivity and specificity), the results of any given test must be considered in combination with the pretest probability to yield a post-test likelihood of disease. Thus, the pretest probability should be used to determine when to initiate a patient work-up and how to interpret the results of any test.

8. **What are the Canadian Criteria for determining pretest probability for DVT?**
    - Malignancy (+1.0 point)
    - Paralysis/cast (+1.0 point)
    - Recent immobilization or surgery (+1.0 point)
    - Tenderness along deep veins (+1.0 point)
    - Swelling of entire leg (+1.0 point)
    - 3 cm difference in calf circumference (+1.0 point)
    - Pitting edema (+1.0 point)
    - Collateral superficial veins (+1.0 point)
    - Alternative diagnosis more likely than DVT (−2.0 points)

9. **Once you have calculated the total Canadian Criteria score for DVT, how do you interpret it?**
    The incidences of DVT based of off the Canadian Criteria for DVT are as follows:
    - Low pretest probability (<2 points): 3% incidence
    - Moderate pretest probability (2–6 points): 17% incidence
    - High pretest probability (>6 points): 75% incidence

10. **What are the Canadian Criteria for determining pretest probability for PE?**
    - Signs/symptoms of DVT (+3 points)
    - No alterative diagnosis more likely than PE (+3 points)
    - Heart rate >100 bpm (+1.5 points)
    - Recent immobilization or surgery (+1.5 points)
    - History of previous VTE (+1.5 points)
    - Hemoptysis (+1.0 point)
    - Malignancy (+1.0 point)

11. **Once you have calculated the total Canadian Criteria score for PE, how do you interpret it?**
    The incidences of PE based of off the Canadian Criteria for PE are as follows:
    - Low pretest probability (<2 points): 4% incidence
    - Moderate pretest probability (2–6 points): 21% incidence
    - High pretest probability (>6 points): 67% incidence

12. **What is a D-dimer test? How is it used?**
    D-Dimer, a degradation product of cross-linked fibronectin, is found in increased levels of the circulation of patients with acute VTE. The enzyme-linked immunosorbent assay (ELISA), rapid ELISA, turbidometric, and whole-blood agglutination D-dimer assay are useful to exclude thromboembolic disease. Traditional latex agglutination tests cannot be used in these algorithms

because of poor negative predictive values. Although useful in ruling out venothromboembolic disease in select populations, owing to a lack of specificity, D-dimer has not proved useful at ruling *in* the diagnosis.

13. **Which patients can have VTE excluded based off of a negative D-dimer?**
Low to low-moderate pretest probability patients only. You would miss the diagnosis anywhere from 5–20% (depending on the type of assay) of the time if you used a negative D-dimer to rule out VTE in a patient with a moderate to high pretest probability (>40%).

14. **What are some clinical situations that cause a false-positive D-dimer, lending to a decreased specificity?**
Sepsis, disseminated intravascular coagulation (DIC), aortic dissection, pregnancy, recent surgery, and severe trauma.

15. **What are some clinical situations that might cause a false-negative D-dimer?**
   - Subacute thrombosis (>7 days)
   - Recent anticoagulation

16. **What noninvasive imaging methods are available for the diagnosis of DVT?**
   - **Duplex ultrasound:** The sensitivity and specificity are operator dependent and related to patient symptomatology, but this test can detect more than 95% of acute symptomatic proximal DVTs. It should be noted that its specificity for acute thrombosis decreases in the settings of chronic or recurrent VTE.
   - **Radiofibrinogen leg scanning:** Good for detecting distal clots, including clots in the calf, popliteal ligament, and distal thigh vein, but relatively poor for more proximal clots.
   - **Impedance plethysmography:** The diagnostic sensitivity and specificity depend on the technical expertise of the person doing the study, but in many centers this test detects more than 95% of acute proximal lower extremity DVT.
   - **Spiral computed tomography (CT) venography:** Although rarely used and not extensively studied, reports show promise for this modality, with a sensitivity and specificity comparable to ultrasound.
   - **Magnetic resonance imaging (MRI) venography:** Can be useful, particularly for patients with inconclusive ultrasound studies or a contraindication to radiation or contrast dye (i.e., pregnant patients). It has proved accurate for both lower extremity and pelvic DVT.

17. **Are there classic chest x-ray (CXR) findings in patients with PE?**
No. The chest radiograph may be normal in up to 30%. Subtle abnormalities such as focal atelectasis, slight elevation of a hemidiaphragm, or focal hyperlucency of the lung parenchyma, may be present. Specifically, local oligemia of vascular markings (Westermark's sign) or a plural-based wedge-shaped infiltrate suggestive of pulmonary infarct (Hampton's hump) are relatively uncommon.

18. **Are there classic electrocardiogram (ECG) findings in patients with PE?**
No. Normal or near-normal ECGs with sinus tachycardia or nonspecific ST-T wave changes may be seen up to 30%. The findings classically associated with PE (S1, Q3, T3 pattern or a new right bundle-branch block) occur in less than 15% of patients and occur with the same frequency in patient work-up whether or not they are diagnosed with PE.

Chan TC, Vilke GM, Pollack M, et al: Electrocardiographic manifestations: Pulmonary embolism. J Emerg Med 21:263–270, 2001.

19. **What imaging studies can by used to evaluate PE?**
   - **Ventilation/perfusion (V/Q) scan.** Traditionally, a normal V/Q scan has been used to essentially rule out a diagnosis of PE with a post-test probability of disease of <4%. Likewise, a high-probability scan is considered to rule in the diagnosis. Unfortunately, upward of 60%

of V/Q scans are read as nondiagnostic (low or intermediate probability). This is frequently the case when the CXR is abnormal or the patient has underlying cardiopulmonary disease. A nondiagnostic scan should be followed up with further diagnostic work-up. Limitations of the V/Q scan include tech support, availability, and interpretation variability.

- **Computed tomography angiography (CTA) scan.** In the setting of an abnormal chest radiograph, CTA can be useful not only in diagnosing PE but also in defining other pathology. This modality is rapid and requires no additional technical support. However, it cannot be used in patients with a contraindication to contrast dye injection and requires radiologic expertise to interpret. Although shown to be highly sensitive in diagnosing central and segmental emboli, CTA is not as sensitive in ruling out subsegmental clots. However, outcomes data using new generation multirow detector CTAs of the chest are showing very high sensitivities, making this diagnostic modality the current standard of care.
- **Pulmonary angiogram.** This test has been the traditional gold standard for the diagnosis, even though its inter-rater agreement on interpretation has been reported to be as low as 65%. Limitations include contraindications to contrast dye injection, interventional radiology support, interpretation variability, and the need for expertise.
- **Magnetic resonance angiogram (MRA).** Limited studies have shown MRA has sensitivities and specificities comparable to standard pulmonary angiogram. Although often not immediately available, MRA is a useful modality when contraindications to conventional studies, such as contrast allergies or pregnancy, exist.

PIOPED Investigators: Value of the ventilation-perfusion scan in acute pulmonary embolism. JAMA 263:2753–5279, 1990.

Wolfe TR, Hartsell SC. Pulmonary embolism: Making sense of the diagnostic evaluation. Ann Emerg Med 37:504–514, 2001.

20. **What happens if the diagnosis of PE is missed?**
PE is listed as one of the most common causes of death in the United States, and yet only about 25% of cases are diagnosed. Of the undiagnosed 75%, a small number die within 1 hour of presentation, so it is unlikely that diagnosis and intervention could improve outcome in that group. In the rest, however, the mortality from untreated PE is approximately 30%.

21. **What is a massive PE?**
A massive PE can be either anatomically defined as the occlusion of greater than 50% of the pulmonary vasculature or physiologically defined as an embolus that is complicated by severe cardiopulmonary distress. These two definitions are not synonymous because a normal individual can lose 50% of pulmonary circulation without significant hemodynamic compromise, whereas a patient with significant underlying cardiopulmonary disease could suffer major hemodynamic compromise with a much smaller clot.

22. **What is the treatment for VTE?**
Anticoagulation should be started in the emergency department (ED). Studies suggest that patients with proximal DVTs and temporary risk factors can be anticoagulated with heparin (80 mg/kg loading dose followed by 18 mg/kg/hour infusion) followed by coumadin for 3 months, whereas patients with calf DVTs need to be treated for only 6 weeks. Patients with permanent risk factors potentially need lifelong treatment but should be anticoagulated for at least 6 months.

23. **What is the role of low-molecular-weight heparin (LMWH) in the treatment of VTE?**
LMWH is at least as effective as heparin for the treatment of DVT and probably should be considered the treatment of choice based on efficacy, low side effect profile, and cost-effectiveness. Outpatient management of DVT with LMWH is becoming commonplace and has

proved safe and effective. Subgroup analysis indicates that LMWH probably will be adopted for the treatment of PE as well, although further conclusive studies are needed.

24. **Under what conditions can an inferior vena caval filter be considered in the treatment of VTE?**
    - Contraindication to anticoagulation
    - Recurrent VTE despite adequate anticoagulation

    Hann CL, Streiff MB: The role of vena caval filters in the management of venous thromboembolism. Blood Rev 19:179–202, 2005.

BIBLIOGRAPHY

1. British Thoracic Society Standards of Care Committee Pulmonary Embolism Guideline Development Group: British Thoracic Society guidelines for the management of suspected acute pulmonary embolism. Thorax 58:470–484, 2003.
2. Craig F: Venous thrombosis and pulmonary embolism. In Marx JA, Hockberger RS, Walls RM (eds): Rosen's Emergency Medicine: Concepts and Clinical Practice, 5th ed. St. Louis, Mosby, 1998, pp 1770–1805.
3. Wells PS, Anderson DR, Bormanis J, et al: Value of assessment of pretest probability of deep-vein thrombosis in clinical management. Lancet 350:1795–1798, 1997.
4. Wells PS, Anderson DR, Rodger M, et al: Excluding pulmonary embolism at the bedside without diagnostic imaging: Management of patients with suspected pulmonary embolism presenting to the emergency department by using a simple clinical model and D-dimer. Ann Intern Med 135:98–107, 2001.

CONGESTIVE HEART FAILURE AND ACUTE PULMONARY EDEMA

Rodney W. Smith, MD, and Christopher R.H. Newton, MD

CHAPTER 27

1. What is congestive heart failure (CHF)?
Cardiac dysfunction that leads to an inability of the heart to work as a pump to meet the circulatory demands of the patient. As a result, pulmonary congestion occurs, and when the problem is severe enough, pulmonary edema results.

2. What causes CHF?
Myocardial disease, which may be primary (cardiomyopathies) or secondary (myocardial infarction secondary to coronary artery disease). Cardiac response to volume overload (as in mitral regurgitation) or pressure overload (as in hypertension or aortic stenosis) also can lead to CHF.

3. Describe the symptoms of CHF.
Common symptoms are **dyspnea** (the subjective feeling of difficulty with breathing) and **fatigue.** Early in the course of CHF, the patient reports exertional dyspnea; the heart is able to supply enough cardiac output for sedentary activities but does not have the reserve to increase cardiac output during exercise. As heart failure worsens, even minimal activity may be difficult. Patients also report orthopnea (dyspnea relieved by assuming an erect posture), paroxysmal nocturnal dyspnea (sudden onset of dyspnea at night), and nocturia.

KEY POINTS: CARDINAL SYMPTOMS OF CHF

1. Exertional dyspnea

2. Fatigue

3. Paroxysmal nocturnal dyspnea

4. Orthopnea

4. What causes these symptoms?
When the patient with CHF assumes the supine posture, fluid is redistributed from the abdomen and lower extremities to the pulmonary vasculature, causing increased pulmonary hydrostatic pressure and increased ventricular filling pressures. The patient has difficulty lying flat and sleeps with several pillows or sits in a chair to relieve these symptoms. Redistribution of fluid may lead to increased urine output and nocturia. In severe CHF, volume redistribution may be sufficient to lead to acute pulmonary edema.

5. Name the four main determinants of cardiac function in CHF.
- Preload
- Afterload

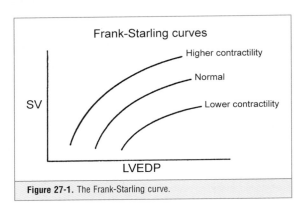

Figure 27-1. The Frank-Starling curve.

- Myocardial contractility
- Heart rate (HR)

6. **What is preload?**
Within limits, the amount of work cardiac muscle can do is related to the length of the muscle at the beginning of its contraction. This relationship is shown graphically by the **Frank-Starling curve,** in which left ventricular end-diastolic volume (LVEDV) represents muscle length, and the stroke volume (SV) represents cardiac work. (It is easier to measure pressure than volume, so we graph LVEDP versus SV.) Preload refers to LVEDP. As LVEDP increases, SV increases. At higher LVEDP, the increase in SV is less for a given increase in LVEDP. Note from Figure 27-1 that the heart can function on different Frank-Starling curves, depending on the contractility.

7. **What about afterload and HR?**
Afterload refers to the pressure work the ventricle must do. The important components here are ventricular wall tension and systemic vascular resistance. Ventricular wall tension is related directly to intraventricular pressure and ventricular radius and inversely related to ventricular wall thickness. Because cardiac output = SV × HR, **heart rate** is an important determinant of cardiac output. At high HRs, there may be insufficient time to fill the ventricle during diastole, leading to decreased LVEDP and SV, so that cardiac output may become compromised despite the tachycardia.

8. **How does this physiology relate to treatment?**
The goal of treatment of CHF is to improve cardiac output. This can be accomplished by modifying each of these parameters. Diuretics, dietary salt, and water restriction decrease preload and improve volume work. Inotropic agents such as Digoxin improve contractility. Vasodilators are helpful in reducing afterload and the pressure work required of the heart.

9. **Describe the role of natriuretic peptides in CHF.**
Natriuretic peptides are hormones produced by the heart in response to increased wall stress and are secreted into the circulation as a marker of failure. B-type natriuretic peptide (BNP) is an independent predictor of increased LVEDP, and levels correlate with symptoms and severity of disease. It has been suggested as a screening tool and for the diagnosis of CHF in the emergency department (ED). Natriuretic peptides also have been used to treat CHF and may affect mortality.

10. **How do I interpret BNP levels?**
    - < 100 pg/mL unlikely to be CHF
    - 100–500 pg/mL may be CHF

- 500 pg/mL most consistent with CHF (There is difficulty interpreting elevated BNP when patient has known severe CHF.)

McCullough PA, Nowak RM, McCord J, et al: B-type natriuretic peptide and clinical judgment in emergency diagnosis of heart failure: analysis from the Breathing Not Properly (BNP) Multinational Study. Circulation 106:416–422, 2002.

KEY POINTS: BNP LEVELS IN PATIENTS WITH UNDIFFERENTIATED DYSPNEA

1. < 100 pg/mL unlikely to be CHF

2. 100–500 pg/mL may be CHF

3. 500 pg/mL most consistent with CHF (There is difficulty interpreting elevated BNP when patient has known severe CHF.)

---

11. Discuss acute pulmonary edema.

The most dramatic presentation of CHF is acute pulmonary edema. To understand pulmonary edema, we must return to the physiologist Starling, who described the interaction of forces at the capillary membrane that lead to flow of fluid from capillaries to the interstitium. Simply put, there is a balance between hydrostatic pressure and osmotic pressure. Under normal circumstances, this leads to a small net movement of fluid from the capillaries into the lung interstitium. This fluid is carried away by lymphatics. In CHF, the capillary hydrostatic pressure increases to the point that the lymphatics no longer can handle the fluid. This then leads to interstitial edema, then subsequently to alveolar edema.

12. How do patients with acute pulmonary edema usually present?

Patients develop acute shortness of breath and generally are fighting for air. These patients sit upright to decrease venous return (preload); they cough up frothy, red-tinged sputum. Auscultation of the lungs reveals wet rales throughout and sometimes wheezes (owing to bronchospasm). This presentation is a true emergency and requires immediate aggressive therapy.

13. What is the treatment of acute pulmonary edema?

First, follow the ABCs (airway, breathing, circulation). In severe hypoxia, airway and breathing may be compromised, and the patient needs to be intubated. Intubation may be avoided with aggressive medical treatment. If you choose this route, however, constant attention to the patient is needed, and you need to set your decision point early. For example, you might decide, "I will intubate if the patient is not better in 15 minutes or worsens during that time." Administer oxygen to maintain sufficient oxygen saturation (> 90%), either by nasal cannula or nonrebreather mask. The use of continuous positive airway pressure has decreased the need for intubation of patients with pulmonary edema; however, this has not significantly affected in-hospital mortality. Continuously monitor oxygen saturation with pulse oximetry.

Pang D, Keenan SP, Cook DJ, et al: The effect of positive pressure airway support on mortality and the need for intubation in cardiogenic pulmonary edema. Chest 114:1185–1192, 1998.

Wigder HN: Pressure support noninvasive positive pressure ventilation treatment of acute cardiogenic pulmonary edema. Am J Emerg Med 19:179–181, 2001.

14. What about drug therapy?

Drug therapy is aimed at decreasing preload. Nitrates are first-line drugs and are useful in the form of sublingual nitroglycerin (NTG), topical NTG paste, or intravenous NTG drip. NTG is predominantly a venodilator, reducing preload, but also dilates coronary arteries, so it may be especially helpful in the setting of coronary artery disease. Furosemide is given as a 40-mg intravenous bolus (larger amounts if the patient is on diuretics). Within 5 to 15 minutes of the injection, venodilation occurs and accounts for the rapid response to this drug. This action is followed within 30 minutes by diuresis. In addition to furosemide, morphine is given, 5–10 mg intravenously, to decrease anxiety and the work of breathing. It also is a venodilator, decreasing preload. With decreased anxiety, there is decreased sympathetic response and decreased afterload.

Carson P: Beta-blocker therapy in heart failure. Cardiol Clin 19:267–278, 2001.

15. Are there other drugs that are useful in the treatment of acute pulmonary edema?

Yes. For the patient who is hypertensive, it is often helpful to lower the blood pressure (afterload). Hypertension and tachycardia generally result from reflex mechanisms because of the acute decompensation and often correct themselves with the initial treatment outlined previously. With severe hypertension, nitroprusside is the treatment of choice. It is a venodilator and arterial dilator, reducing preload and afterload. Start the infusion at 10 mg/min and titrate upward every 5 minutes. It is important to monitor the blood pressure closely. If the patient becomes hypotensive, stopping the infusion causes a prompt increase in blood pressure because nitroprusside has such a short half-life. Generally, doses of 0.5–2 mg/kg/min are sufficient.

Carson P: Beta-blocker therapy in heart failure. Cardiol Clin 19:267–278, 2001.
Gomberg-Maitland M, Baran DA, Fuster V: Treatment of congestive heart failure: Guidelines for the primary care physician and the heart failure specialist. Arch Intern Med 161:342–352, 2001.

16. What about giving positive inotropic drugs?

Digoxin, which is used in the treatment of chronic CHF, has little role in the treatment of acute pulmonary edema. Inotropic agents that are helpful include dobutamine, dopamine, and milrinone. Dobutamine and dopamine are positive inotropic agents. Dopamine has more alpha effect, especially at higher doses, and should be reserved for hypotensive patients. In cardiogenic shock that is refractory to these agents, milrinone infusion may be given. The ideal situation for administering these agents is in an intensive care unit (ICU) with pulmonary artery monitoring to measure filling pressures, cardiac output, and other hemodynamic parameters.

17. When the initial treatment has begun, what else needs to be done?

After the patient is stabilized, routine tests are done, the most important being chest radiograph and electrocardiogram (ECG). Cardiac monitoring is begun; pulse oximetry is monitored continuously, and vital signs are recorded frequently. It is generally necessary to insert a Foley catheter for close monitoring of urine output. The search is on to try to discover the underlying reason for acute decompensation.

18. Do all patients with CHF need to be admitted to the hospital?

Patients with a new diagnosis of CHF need an in-patient work-up that includes serial cardiac enzymes and an assessment of the global function of the heart. Patients with known CHF who have mild symptoms or signs may be managed on an outpatient basis, assuming that they are compliant with medications, have an appropriate social network, and follow up with their primary care physician.

Graff L, Orledge J, Radford MJ, et al: Correlation of the Agency for Health Care Policy and Research congestive heart failure admission guideline with mortality: Peer Review Organisation Voluntary Hospital Association Initiative to Decrease Events (PROVIDE) for congestive heart failure. Ann Emerg Med 34:429–437, 1999.

19. **What are the usual precipitating causes of acute pulmonary edema?**
The most common cause is undermedication, either as a result of patient noncompliance with medication orders or dietary salt restrictions or as a result of a change in medication under a physician's supervision. Other causes include pulmonary embolism, acute myocardial infarction, infection, anemia, arrhythmias, and severe hypertension. When precipitating factors are identified, specific therapy should be initiated.

20. **What is the outpatient treatment of CHF?**
Angiotensin-converting enzyme (ACE) inhibitors are the mainstay of long-term treatment of CHF, leading to a decrease in mortality and an increase in functional capacity. Other drugs that act on the renin-angiotensin system (angiotensin receptor antagonists and spironolactone) also are effective. Beta-blockers are useful in that they block the cardiac effects of long-term adrenergic stimulation. Diuretics also are beneficial, especially in patients with volume overload. Digoxin causes an improvement in symptoms but no overall decrease in mortality. Combined therapy with hydralazine and isosorbide dinitrate has shown a decrease in mortality and is particularly useful in patients who have contraindications to other classes of drugs.

   Digitalis Investigation Group: The effect of digoxin on mortality and morbidity in patients with heart failure. N Engl J Med 336:525–533, 1997.

   Miller AB, Srivastava P: Angiotensin receptor blockers and aldosterone antagonists in chronic heart failure. Cardiol Clin 19:195–202, 2001.

21. **How do ACE inhibitors work in CHF?**
In response to cardiac decompensation, the renin-angiotensin system is activated. Angiotensin is a potent vasoconstrictor, leading to increased afterload. Stimulation of aldosterone leads to sodium retention and extracellular fluid volume expansion and increased preload. ACE inhibitors help to decrease afterload by decreasing angiotensin II-mediated vasoconstriction and decrease preload by blocking sodium retention and volume expansion.

22. **What is the long-term prognosis for patients with CHF?**
Prognosis depends on the cause and severity of the heart failure. The prognosis is good when the underlying cause can be corrected, as in valvular heart disease. Patients with mild disease that can be controlled with ACE inhibitors with or without low doses of diuretics generally do well. Overall, however, patients with CHF have a 10–20% yearly death rate, and fewer than half survive 5 years.

BIBLIOGRAPHY

1. Carson P: Beta-blocker therapy in heart failure. Cardiol Clin 19:267–278, 2001.
2. Dao Q, Krishnaswamy P, Kazanegra R, et al: Utility of B-type natriuretic peptide in the diagnosis of congestive heart failure in an urgent-care setting. J Am Coll Cardiol 37:379–385, 2001.
3. DeNofrio D: Natriuretic peptides for the treatment of congestive heart failure. Am Heart J 138:597–598, 1999.
4. Digitalis Investigation Group: The effect of digoxin on mortality and morbidity in patients with heart failure. N Engl J Med 336:525–533, 1997.
5. Gomberg-Maitland M, Baran DA, Fuster V: Treatment of congestive heart failure: Guidelines for the primary care physician and the heart failure specialist. Arch Intern Med 161:342–352, 2001.
6. Graff L, Orledge J, Radford MJ, et al: Correlation of the Agency for Health Care Policy and Research congestive heart failure admission guideline with mortality: Peer Review Organisation Voluntary Hospital Association Initiative to Decrease Events (PROVIDE) for congestive heart failure. Ann Emerg Med 34:429–437, 1999.
7. McCullough PA, Nowak RM, McCord J, et al: B-type natriuretic peptide and clinical judgment in emergency diagnosis of heart failure: analysis from the Breathing Not Properly (BNP) Multinational Study. Circulation 106:416–422, 2002.

8. Miller AB, Srivastava P: Angiotensin receptor blockers and aldosterone antagonists in chronic heart failure. Cardiol Clin 19:195–202, 2001.

9. Pang D, Keenan SP, Cook DJ, et al: The effect of positive pressure airway support on mortality and the need for intubation in cardiogenic pulmonary edema. Chest 114:1185–1192, 1998.

10. Wigder HN: Pressure support noninvasive positive pressure ventilation treatment of acute cardiogenic pulmonary edema. Am J Emerg Med 19:179–181, 2001.

CHAPTER 28

ISCHEMIC HEART DISEASE

Edward P. Havranek, MD

1. **How is acute ischemic heart disease classified?**
   1. Chronic stable ischemic heart disease
      - Asymptomatic
      - With angina
      - Post myocardial infarction (MI), with or without angina
   2. Acute coronary syndromes
      - Unstable angina
      - Acute non-ST segment elevation myocardial infarction (NSTEMI)
      - Acute ST segment elevation MI (STEMI)

2. **How do patients with acute ischemic heart disease present?**
   The most common presenting symptom is **central chest discomfort.** The discomfort also may be felt (in descending order of frequency) in the right or left chest, the right or left shoulder or arm, the throat or jaw, the epigastrium, and, rarely, the ear. Less commonly, patients may present with episodic dyspnea. Some patients may have ischemia and even acute MI with no symptoms.

3. **To define the discomfort better, what information should be obtained?**
   - Chronology
   - Frequency
   - Location
   - Precipitating factors
   - Radiation
   - Alleviating factors
   - Duration
   - Quality
   - Intensity
   - Associated symptoms

4. **Describe the typical features of the chest discomfort in ischemic heart disease.**
   Typically, patients with **stable angina** have discomfort during exertion relieved within minutes by rest. The degree of exertion bringing on the discomfort can vary from day to day. The discomfort is often vague, is described most often as a tightness or heaviness, and is substernal in location, with radiation to the jaw, shoulder, or upper extremity common.

   Patients with **unstable angina** usually have similar pain, but it occurs at rest or with progressively less exertion (crescendo angina). Patients with unstable angina who have pain at rest also should have pain with exertion. **Prinzmetal's angina,** which is caused by coronary artery spasm, is an exception to this rule. Patients with Prinzmetal's angina typically have pain at rest, usually in the early morning hours, and often do not have exertional discomfort. True vasospastic angina is uncommon.

   Patients with **acute MI** typically have pain that is more severe than any preceding angina. It may be described as crushing but usually not ripping or tearing.

5. **What other symptoms are associated with the chest discomfort of ischemic heart disease?**
Shortness of breath commonly accompanies angina. Many conditions other than angina that cause chest discomfort, such as pulmonary disease and anxiety disorder, also are accompanied by shortness of breath. Diaphoresis occurs less frequently with angina but should raise one's level of suspicion of angina because it does not occur often with other disorders that cause chest pain. Nausea and vomiting can occur with acute MI—the larger the infarction, the more common are nausea and vomiting. Thus, patients with anterior MI are more likely to have nausea and vomiting than are patients with inferior MI.

KEY POINTS: TYPICAL FEATURES OF ANGINA

1. Substernal location

2. Radiation to the arm, neck, or jaw

3. Precipitation by exertion, relief with rest

4. Sensation of tightness or heaviness

5. Accompanied by shortness of breath

6. **Is there anything different about evaluating elderly patients?**
The symptoms associated with ischemic heart disease in patients older than 75 years are more likely to be atypical. The older the patient, the more atypical the symptoms become.

7. **What about diabetics?**
Although it is often taught that patients with diabetes are more likely to present with atypical symptoms or no symptoms at all, the literature suggests that diabetic patients present just like everyone else except perhaps for being a little more likely to have shortness of breath.

Funk M, Naum JB, Milner KA, Chyun D: Presentation and symptom predictors of coronary heart disease in patients with and without diabetes. Am J Emerg Med 19:482–487, 2001.

Kentsch M, Rodemerk U, Gitt AK, et al: Angina intensity is not different in diabetic and non-diabetic patients with acute myocardial infarction. Z Kardiol 92:817–824, 2003.

8. **Should demographic features and the presence or absence of coronary risk factors change your mind about the diagnosis?**
They are not particularly useful for making a diagnosis except in patients who have objective evidence of prior ischemic heart disease in whom the likelihood of another ischemic event occurring is rather high. A young woman with no risk factors but with typical symptoms and electrocardiogram (ECG) changes should be suspected of having ischemic disease. Conversely, a middle-aged man with diabetes and hypertension whose chest pain has no typical features should still be treated as if he may have the disease.

9. **List the key elements of the initial evaluation of a patient with a suspected acute coronary syndrome**
   - The patient should be placed on O_2 and a cardiac monitor and have intravenous (IV) access established.
   - The patient should have an **ECG** within 5–10 minutes of arrival.
   - **Vital signs** are vital. The presence of hypertension, hypotension, or tachycardia must be dealt with early.

- A **history** directed at the key elements described previously and a **cardiovascular examination** come next; the examination is useful for ruling out other diagnoses, such as pericarditis and aortic dissection.
- Administer aspirin (325 mg).

10. **What is the significance of abnormal ST segment changes on an ECG?**
    Abnormal ST segment changes may or may not represent ischemic cardiac injury. The *current of injury* that accompanies ST segment elevation MI is typically a convex-downward elevation of the ST segment. It may be confused with pericarditis or early repolarization. Other causes of ST elevation are as follows:
    - Left ventricular hypertrophy
    - Acute pericarditis
    - Acute cor pulmonale
    - Hyperkalemia
    - Hypercalcemia
    - Hypothermia
    - Left ventriculare aneurysm

    ST depression may be caused not only by cardiac ischemia but also by such things as ventricular hypertrophy, drugs (e.g., digoxin), atrioventricular junctional rhythm with a retrograde P wave, or electrolyte abnormalities.

11. **What is the typical time course of ECG changes in ischemic cardiac injury?**
    The initial changes are T-wave prolongation and increased T-wave magnitude, either upright or inverted. Next, the ST segment displays elevation or depression. A Q wave may be seen in the initial ECG or may not develop for hours to days. As the ST segment returns to baseline, symmetrically inverted T waves evolve. This classic evolution is documented in approximately 65% of patients with acute MI.

12. **Can the ECG be normal while a patient is having cardiac ischemia or an acute MI?**
    Although serial ECGs showing evolving changes are diagnostic for acute MI in greater than 90% of patients, 20–50% of initial ECGs are normal or show only nonspecific abnormalities. The initial ECG may be diagnostic for acute MI in only half of patients. Therefore, an early repeat ECG may be helpful.

13. **Are cardiac markers useful in the emergency department (ED)?**
    Maybe. Troponin I, the most commonly used cardiac marker, doesn't begin to rise until 4–6 hours after the onset of ischemia, so single determinations are generally not sufficiently specific to make a diagnosis. Myoglobin levels begin to rise within 1–2 hours after the onset of pain, but elevations of this protein are nonspecific. Creatine phosphokinase (CPK) levels also don't begin to rise until 4–6 hours after onset. Conversely, patients may have unstable angina, necessitating ICU admission but still have normal levels of cardiac markers.

14. **How can echocardiography be useful in ED patients with suspected acute coronary syndrome?**
    It may be useful when the ECG is nondiagnostic, such as when there is a left bundle-branch block or minimal ST elevation. The presence of a wall motion abnormality is evidence that supports the diagnosis of ischemia, although it may be the result of an old rather than acute infarction. Echocardiography also may provide information about complications, such as mitral regurgitation and pericardial effusion.

    A negative echocardiogram in the setting of a typical history and ECG *does not* rule out the diagnosis of an acute coronary syndrome.

15. **What other diagnoses should be considered in a patient with chest pain?**
    The patient's history is paramount:
    - A life-threatening condition, **dissecting aortic aneurysm,** also may cause sustained chest pain or typical angina.
    - Pleuritic chest pain may be caused by pleuritis, pericarditis, pneumothorax, or pulmonary embolism.
    - Nonanginal pain may be found with the onset of herpes zoster or with cervical or thoracic nerve root compression.
    - Esophagitis, esophageal spasm, and esophageal rupture may mimic pain of cardiac origin.
    - Patients with anxiety or depression syndromes often complain of chest pain.

16. **What are the indications for reperfusion therapy in acute MI?**
    - ST elevation greater than 1 mm in two leads
    - Pain not immediately responsive to nitroglycerin
    - Pain lasting less than 6 hours (In many patients, reperfusion therapy still may be of benefit 12 hours after the onset of pain.)

17. **What is the preferred method of reperfusion therapy in acute MI, thrombolytic therapy or primary angioplasty?**
    Angioplasty (usually with coronary stenting) in the setting of acute MI if done within approximately 90 minutes of arrival reduces mortality to a greater degree than does thrombolytic therapy. Primary coronary intervention has the added advantages of lower rates of reocclusion in the subsequent few days and lower risks of intracranial bleeding. The problem is that studies from community settings show that optimally delivered angioplasty is not often accomplished. Unless a skilled catheterization laboratory team can do an angioplasty in less than 90 minutes after presentation, thrombolytic therapy is probably preferable.

18. **How do you choose which thrombolytic agent to use?**
    Streptokinase (and its modified form, anistreplase) is currently the least popular agent in acute MI because it is thought to be slightly less effective than the other available agents. Reteplase and tenecteplase have become more popular than alteplase because they can be administered in bolus form rather than an infusion with a varying dose schedule.

19. **What is the preferred therapy for cardiogenic shock?**
    The only therapy shown to decrease the historically high mortality associated with this syndrome is primary coronary intervention. This should be performed without delay. An exception to this is cardiogenic shock caused by **right ventricular infarction.** This problem should be suspected whenever shock accompanies an acute inferior MI. The presence of jugular venous distention is an important clue to the diagnosis of this syndrome, and volume expansion usually reverses the hypotension.

20. **List the contraindications to thrombolytic therapy.**
    Absolute contraindications
    - Active bleeding
    - Major surgery or trauma in the past 3 weeks
    - Neurosurgery or stroke in the past 3 months
    - Prolonged (>10 minutes) or traumatic cardiopulmonary resuscitation (CPR)
    - Hypertension (systolic >180 mmHg, diastolic >110 mmHg)

    Relative contraindications
    - Major trauma or surgery more than 3 weeks ago
    - Neurosurgery or stroke more than 3 months ago
    - Active peptic ulcer
    - Hemorrhagic ophthalmic condition, especially diabetic retinopathy

Patients with a known allergy to streptokinase or anistreplase (also known as APSAC [anisoylated plasminogen-streptokinase activator complex]) should be treated with another agent. Exposure to streptokinase or anistreplase in the previous 6 months or streptococcal infection in the previous 6 months are reasons to use another agent.

21. **What other diagnoses should be considered before giving thrombolytic therapy?**

    Aortic dissection and **acute pericarditis** can mimic acute MI. Both have had fatal outcomes when thrombolytics were given. Dissection can be excluded with a careful history, examination of peripheral pulses, and chest radiograph or chest CT scan. Pericarditis can be excluded by carefully listening for a rub and examining the ECG for widespread, concave-upward ST elevation.

22. **What is the risk for fatal complications of thrombolytic therapy for acute MI?**

    Mortality, which almost invariably results from intracranial hemorrhage, occurs in about 0.5% of treated patients.

23. **What are reperfusion arrhythmias?**

    Approximately 45 minutes after initiation of a thrombolytic agent, blood flow is restored in most patients. This event may be accompanied by arrhythmias, especially ventricular tachycardia or accelerated idioventricular rhythm. In patients with inferior MI, sinus bradycardia or heart block may occur. These arrhythmias are transient (generally lasting <30 seconds). Reperfusion may be accompanied by a brief increase in pain.

24. **What other medications are useful adjuvants to thrombolytic therapy?**

    - **Morphine.** MI can cause excruciating pain and severe fear and anxiety. IV morphine sulfate should be administered in increments of 2–4 mg to alleviate these symptoms.
    - **Aspirin.** Unless the patient has had an aspirin, it should be given immediately because it reduces mortality independent of thrombolytic therapy.
    - **Beta-blockers.** Given intravenously during thrombolytic therapy, metoprolol, atenolol, or esmolol reduce mortality and infarct size further. They are better tolerated than one may think and are underused. Contraindications include heart failure, bradycardia (heart rate <55 bpm), and bronchospasm.
    - **Heparin.** With tissue plasminogen activator (t-PA), initiation of heparin is imperative at least 1 hour before the completion of the thrombolytic infusion. With streptokinase or APSAC, administration of heparin should be delayed 4–6 hours. There is currently controversy over whether low-molecular-weight heparin is superior to unfractionated heparin for reducing recurrent events.
    - **Nitroglycerin.** If control of blood pressure is an issue, nitroglycerin is the preferred agent.

KEY POINTS: MOST IMPORTANT MEDICATIONS FOR ALL PATIENTS WITH AN MI IN THE ED

1. Aspirin

2. Intravenous beta-blockers

25. **What other arrhythmias occur with acute MI?**

    Ventricular irritability, with frequent premature ventricular contractions, nonsustained ventricular tachycardia, and ventricular fibrillation, may occur and should be treated with lidocaine or amiodarone. Sustained ventricular tachycardia (lasting >30 seconds) is uncommon in acute MI. Accelerated idioventricular rhythm (heart rate, 60–100 bpm) should not be treated.

Bradyarrhythmias also may occur. Second-degree or third-degree heart block that accompanies inferior MI is usually transient, and a temporary pacemaker generally is not required. When heart block accompanies an anterior MI, a temporary pacer *is* required. A prophylactic temporary pacer should be considered when severe conductive system disease (bifascicular block or left bundle-branch block plus first-degree block) accompanies an anterior acute MI.

26. **Which patients with unstable angina are at highest risk for MI and benefit from more aggressive treatment?**
    - ECG changes: Transient or fixed ST segment depression or T-wave inversion, especially when these changes are in leads V_1 through V_3
    - Elevated troponin levels
    - Age greater than 65
    - Known coronary artery disease
    - Presence of three or more coronary risk factors (smoking, hypertension, diabetes, elevated cholesterol, family history)
    - Severe angina within the prior 24 hours

    These patients are thought to benefit more from more aggressive medical treatment (see question 24) and early catheterization.

    Antman EM, Cohen M, Bernink PJ, et al: The TIMI risk score for unstable angina/non-ST elevation MI: A method for prognostication and therapeutic decision making. JAMA 284:835–842, 2000.

27. **How should unstable angina be managed in the ED?**
    - Always administer **aspirin.** Evidence suggests that addition of clopidogrel to aspirin may reduce risk of death and MI better than aspirin alone.
    - Virtually all patients with unstable angina should be treated with **beta-blockers.** It may be desirable to start this therapy in the ED.
    - For patients with ongoing pain, always treat with **nitroglycerin.** Start with the sublingual route of administration, and move to IV nitroglycerin if that does not work. Nitroglycerin is the preferred agent when the patient has concurrent hypertension.
    - **Heparin** should be started. For low-risk or intermediate-risk patients, heparin may be reserved for patients refractory to aspirin, nitrates, and beta-blockers. It is currently unclear if low-molecular-weight heparin reduces subsequent risk of MI or death more than unfractionated heparin does. Some low-molecular-weight heparin preparations may reduce these endpoints better than others.
    - High-risk patients (*see* question 26) benefit from use of the IV antiplatelet agents **tirofiban** or **eptifibatide.** The other agent in this class of antiplatelet drugs (glycoprotein IIB/IIIA inhibitors), abciximab, is not effective in acute coronary syndromes (although it is an effective adjuvant during percutaneous coronary interventions).
    - Add **calcium channel blockers** when symptoms recur despite aspirin, nitrates, and beta-blockers. *Never* use short-acting dihydropyridines, such as nifedipine, without beta-blockers. In the setting of unstable angina, use of calcium channel blockers without concurrent beta-blockade increases the risk of MI.

28. **Which is better, low-molecular-weight heparin or unfractionated heparin?**
    There is no consensus about which type of heparin is clinically more effective, so practical considerations are important. The advantage of low-molecular-weight heparin is that it can be given in the ED as a single bolus and doesn't require an infusion pump. The major disadvantage of low-molecular-weight heparin is that it may be difficult to communicate to other providers

that the patient has received it (as a result some patients have gotten double doses) and that the effects last longer, making invasive procedures more problematic.

BIBLIOGRAPHY

1. ACC/AHA 2002 Guideline update for management of patients with chronic stable angina. J Am Coll Cardiol 41:159–168, 2003 (www.acc.org/clinical/guidelines/stable/stable_clean.pdf).
2. ACC/AHA Guidelines for the Management of Patients With ST-Elevation Myocardial Infarction (www.acc.org/clinical/guidelines/stemi/Guideline1/index.htm).
3. ACC/AHA 2002 Guideline update for management of patients with unstable angina and non-ST-segment elevation myocardial infarction. J Am Coll Cardiol 40:366–374, 2002 (www.acc.org/clinical/guidelines/unstable/incorporated/index.htm).

CHAPTER 29

CARDIAC DYSRHYTHMIAS, PACEMAKERS, AND IMPLANTABLE DEFIBRILLATORS

Christopher B. Colwell, MD

1. **What is a sinus beat?**
   At the end of each heartbeat, all myocardial cells are depolarized and experience a refractory period. At this point, certain cardiac cells (sinoatrial and atrioventricular [AV] nodes and some ventricular cells) float back up through phase IV depolarization toward *threshold potential*. It is like a race, and typically the sinoatrial node cells win this race, achieve threshold, fire, and assume the pacemaker *sinus beat* function of the heart.

2. **What is the AV node?**
   The AV node is not simply a passive connection between the atria and ventricles. It is "smart." Normally, all atrial impulses are conducted to the ventricles. When the ventricular rate becomes sufficiently rapid that cardiac output is compromised, conduction velocity begins to slow in the AV node. This progressive slowing filters the rapid atrial impulses so that serial atrial impulses are not conducted at all (otherwise known as **Wenckebach block**). This progressive AV nodal conduction block is a protective mechanism to prevent dysfunctionally rapid ventricular rate.

3. **Is it necessary to identify a dysrhythmia before treating it?**
   No.

4. **How do I know whether a patient's dysrhythmia is causing hemodynamic compromise?**
   Typically, if a patient's ventricular rate is between 60 and 100 bpm, any hemodynamic instability is caused by something else. It is unusual, although not impossible, for a tachydysrhythmia with a rate of less than 150 bpm to be the primary cause of hemodynamic instability. It is unusual that a heart rate of less than 150 bpm requires electrical cardioversion.

   Harken AH, Honigman B, Van Way C: Cardiac dysrhythmias in the acute setting: Recognition and treatment (or) anyone can treat cardiac dysrhythmias. J Emerg Med 5:129–134, 1987.

5. **How do I treat bradyarrhythmias?**
   Do not treat a bradycardia if the patient is hemodynamically stable and asymptomatic. Always treat the patient not a number. If the patient has a heart rate less than 60 bpm and is hemodynamically unstable:
   1. Give 0.5 mg (0.01 mg/kg in a child) intravenous atropine (may repeat as needed).
   2. Initiate pacemaker (do not forget the external pacemaker). The transvenous pacemaker (especially without fluoroscopy) always takes much longer than you think it will.

6. **Define premature ventricular contraction.**
   A premature ventricular contraction occurs when a ventricular site wins the "race" among myocardial cells and ventricular depolarization originates from an ectopic ventricular site.

7. **What is a narrow-complex tachycardia?**
   The AV node attaches directly to the Purkinje system, which courses over the endocardial surface of the ventricles. An electrical impulse travels over the Purkinje fibers fast: 2–3 m/sec. If an impulse enters the ventricles from the AV node, it can activate electrically the entire

ventricular muscle mass rapidly—in 0.12 sec, 120 msec, or three little boxes on electrocardiogram (ECG) paper. *Narrow complex* refers to the width of the QRS complex. A narrow-complex tachycardia must originate above the AV node and is a supraventricular tachycardia (SVT).

8. **Is there a limit above which tachycardia no longer increases cardiac output?**
   A reasonable rule of thumb is that you can increase cardiac output by increasing the heart rate up to 200 bpm minus the age of the patient.

9. **Do I need to distinguish the multiple varieties of narrow-complex tachycardia (i.e., rapid atrial fibrillation [AF], SVT, atrial flutter) to treat effectively?**
   No, as long as it is unstable. You do not want to convert stable AF or atrial flutter if there is any chance it has been going on for more than 48 hours because of the risk of embolizing clot. Electrical conversion is always the treatment if the tachycardia is unstable.

10. **How do I treat narrow-complex tachycardia in a hemodynamically stable patient?**
    A narrow-complex tachycardia must be supraventricular, originating above the AV node (*see* question 9). To control the ventricular rate, you need to block the AV node pharmacologically. Verapamil, 5–10 mg, or diltiazem, 20 mg, intravenously over 1–2 minutes, terminates or controls the ventricular response rate in 80–90% of cases. Alternatively, adenosine, 6 mg intravenous rapid bolus followed by 12 mg (which may be repeated), has a response rate of 85–90%. Although more expensive than verapamil, adenosine has no serious side effects. Adenosine exhibits little effect on infranodal conduction, which has led some authors to recommend its use as a diagnostic agent in wide-complex tachycardias.

11. **What is a wide-complex tachycardia?**
    When an impulse originates from a typically damaged or ischemic bit of ventricular muscle, it takes awhile to access the Purkinje superhighways, permitting electrical activation of the entire ventricular mass. The QRS is measured from its initial deflection (at the ectopic site) to the completion of all ventricular activity. When the major conduction pathways are not used primarily, it takes a long time (>0.12 second, 120 msec, or three little boxes on the ECG paper) to inscribe the QRS complex. This ectopic, ventricular origin complex is referred to as *wide*.

12. **What is the most common cause of wide-complex tachycardia?**
    Ventricular tachycardia (VT). Of patients presenting to the emergency department (ED) with a wide-complex tachycardia, 80–90% have VT, and only 10–20% have SVT with aberrancy. VT is even more likely if the patient has a history of a prior myocardial infarction or congestive heart failure.

13. **How do I treat wide-complex tachycardia?**
    See Table 29-1.

14. **What is synchronized cardioversion?**
    Synchronization of delivered energy to match the QRS complex. This reduces the chance that a shock will induce ventricular fibrillation, which can occur when electrical energy impinges on the relative refractory portion of the cardiac electrical activity (downslope of the T wave).

15. **How do I perform synchronized cardioversion?**
    Select a lead on the monitor that clearly reveals an R wave of greater amplitude than the T wave. Turn on the defibrillator. Engage the synchronization mode by pressing the sync control button, and look for markers on the R waves indicating the sync mode is functioning and capturing the QRS complex and not the T wave. You may need to adjust the R wave gain until the sync markers occur with each QRS complex. Then select the appropriate energy level; position the

TABLE 29-1.   TREATMENT OF WIDE-COMPLEX TACHYCARDIA

Clinical Situation	Treatment
Unstable patient	**Cardioversion**
Wide-complex tachycardia of unknown type with preserved cardiac function (no clinical congestive heart failure)	**Procainamide** (17 mg/kg IV at a rate of 20 mg/min, to be stopped if the dysrhythmia is suppressed, hypotension occurs, or the QRS complex widens by 50% of its original width) or **amiodarone** (0.75 mg/kg IV given over 10–15 minutes)
Wide-complex tachycardia of unknown type in a patient with clinical evidence of congestive heart failure	**Amiodarone**
Rhythm known to be ventricular in origin	**Amiodarone, procainamide,** or **lidocaine** (1.0 to 1.5 mg/kg IV, repeated every 5 minutes to a maximum of 3 mg/kg

IV = intravenous.
Adapted from Shah CP, Thakur RK, Xie B, Hoon VK: Clinical approach to wide QRS complex tachycardias. Emerg Med Clin North Am 16:331–360, 1998.

paddles appropriately; apply 25 lb of pressure on both paddles, and press the discharge buttons simultaneously. Always remember to use adequate sedation in any awake patient.

16. **What is a supraventricular rhythm with aberrancy?**
Usually a supraventricular rhythm traverses the AV node and courses through the large endoventricular conduction fibers, activating the ventricles rapidly and resulting in a narrow QRS complex (<0.12 sec). A wide-complex tachycardia typically represents a tachycardia of ventricular origin. Although less frequent, a supraventricular origin impulse that travels through the ventricle in an aberrant fashion also can be wide and is called supraventricular rhythm with aberrancy.

17. **How do I treat tachyarrhythmias?**
Any unstable patient with a tachyarrhythmia that either is or may be the cause of the instability requires cardioversion. An unstable patient is any patient with hypotension (systolic blood pressure <90 mmHg) plus altered level of consciousness or complaining of chest pain or shortness of breath. SVT and atrial flutter often respond to low voltages (50 J), whereas most other tachyarrhythmias typically require at least 100 J to convert to a sinus rhythm. One may consider vagal maneuvers or pharmacotherapy before cardioversion in stable patients.

18. **Does it make sense to cardiovert asystole?**
Strictly speaking, no. Theoretically, electrical cardioversion synchronously depolarizes all myocardial cells simultaneously. All cells then should repolarize synchronously and spontaneously reinitiate sinus rhythm. With asystole, there is nothing to depolarize and nothing to cardiovert. Clinicians in favor of attempting to cardiovert apparent asystole point out, however, that you have nothing to lose. Conceivably, the major QRS vector is perpendicular to the axis of the ECG lead, making ventricular fibrillation appear as asystole. In this instance, cardioversion of apparent asystole could help.

19. **How do I make the diagnosis of AF when the ventricular rate is fast?**
Rapid AF may be impossible to differentiate from SVT on a cardiac rhythm strip. The diagnosis of AF is made by palpating a peripheral pulse and simultaneously auscultating the heart or visualizing the cardiac rhythm. AF is the only arrhythmia that results in a pulse deficit (fewer beats palpable than observed or auscultated) and that has an irregular pulse with varying intensity of the pulse. When rapid AF is present on ECG or monitor, it is difficult to differentiate it from paroxysmal atrial tachycardia or atrial flutter because it appears regular.

20. **What drug is contraindicated in the treatment of any wide-complex tachycardia?**
Verapamil. Because all wide-complex tachycardias must be considered to be of ventricular origin, verapamil is likely to cause hypotension and may cause degeneration of the rhythm to ventricular fibrillation or asystole. Procainamide may induce hypotension, particularly in patients with impaired left ventricular function.

21. **Is VT always hemodynamically unstable?**
No. Hemodynamic status should not be used to determine the nature of a wide QRS tachycardia: Do not assume a wide-complex tachycardia is not VT if the patient is hemodynamically stable.

22. **Differentiate VT from SVT with aberrancy based on findings on the 12-lead ECG.**
In general, assume VT and treat accordingly whenever there is any question. Findings on the 12-lead such as AV dissociation, fusion or capture beats, left or right axis deviation, a QRS width of greater than 140 msec, concordance of QRS complexes, monophasic or biphasic QRS in lead V1, or an RS or QS in lead V6 all strongly suggest VT. A history of coronary artery disease or congestive heart failure, or evidence of AV dissociation on physical exam (Cannon A waves) also suggests VT. Heart rate is *not* an accurate way to differentiate VT from SVT with aberrancy. Again, if there is any doubt, assume VT. Treating SVT with aberrancy as if it were VT is less problematic than treating VT as if it were SVT with aberrancy.

23. **When is it necessary to anticoagulate a patient with AF?**
In a stable patient who presents to the ED in AF, rate control is the primary goal. Beta-blockers (metoprolol, 5–10 mg over 2 minutes) and calcium channel blockers (diltiazem, 20 mg over 2 minutes) are effective AV nodal blocking agents and can achieve adequate rate control in most patients with AF. Anticoagulation in patients who have AF for less than 48 hours is unnecessary because the risk of thromboembolism is lower. If the duration of AF has been greater than 48 hours and the patient is stable, cardioversion should be delayed until the patient is fully anticoagulated.

Weigner MJ, Caulfiel TA, Danias PG, et al: Risk for clinical thromboembolism associated with conversion to sinus rhythm in patients with AF lasting less than 48 hours. Ann Intern Med 126:615–620, 1997.

24. **What does amiodarone do? Should we be using it in the ED?**
Amiodarone (Cordarone) is a class III antiarrhythmic that prolongs the action potential duration and refractory period, slows automaticity in pacemaker cells, and slows conduction in the AV node. It is approved for the treatment of ventricular and supraventricular arrhythmias, including AF, atrial flutter, and accessory pathway syndromes. Amiodarone is a good option to consider in a hemodynamically stable patient with known VT or a wide-complex tachycardia of unknown mechanism, particularly in patients in whom lidocaine and procainamide have been ineffective. Primary side effects are hypotension, bradycardia, and heart failure. The loading dose is 0.75 mg/kg given over 10–15 minutes. Amiodarone exhibits a slow onset of action and an even slower clearance. Current advanced cardiac life support (ACLS) guidelines suggest amiodarone can be used instead of lidocaine for monomorphic VT, but its use as a primary agent probably

should wait until the results of direct comparative trials with long-term survival outcomes measured become available.

Connolly SJ: Evidence-based analysis of amiodarone efficacy and safety. Circulation 100:2025–2034, 1999.

25. **Should we be using monophasic or biphasic waveform defibrillation in the ED?**
Theoretical advantages to biphasic waveforms include less energy required to achieve effective defibrillation and less postshock myocardial damage and dysfunction at equivalent energy levels. Studies have shown some promise for biphasic waveform defibrillation, but there are no data at this point that show a benefit in terms of long-term survival when biphasic waveforms are used. Biphasic defibrillation may or may not be beneficial and cost-effective for patients; the jury is still out at this point. Although it may be prudent to go with biphasic defibrillators if buying new equipment, it is unnecessary to replace well-functioning monophasic defibrillators with new expensive biphasic defibrillators.

Martens PR, Russell JK, Wolcke B, et al: Optimal Response to Cardiac Arrest Study: Defibrillation waveform effect. Resuscitation 49:233–243, 2001.

26. **What is a pacemaker?**
An external source of energy used to stimulate the heart. It consists of a pulse generator (i.e., power source), an output circuit, a sensing circuit, a timing circuit, and pacing leads. The battery most commonly used in permanent pacers is a lithium-iodide type and has a life span of 5–8 years. Temporary pacemakers use an external generator with transvenous, transcutaneous, or transthoracic leads. Temporary transvenous pacers use a household 9-volt battery.

27. **What are the indications for temporary pacemakers?**
Temporary emergency pacing is indicated for therapy of significant and hemodynamically unstable bradyarrhythmias and prevention of bradycardia-dependent malignant arrhythmias. Pacemakers also can be used for overdrive pacing in an attempt to terminate VT by placing a ventricular extrasystole during the vulnerable period of the cardiac cycle. Prophylactic temporary pacing is indicated for insertion of a pulmonary artery catheter in a patient with an underlying left bundle-branch block or use of medications that may cause or exacerbate hemodynamically significant bradycardia. It is also indicated in the setting of an acute myocardial infarction (AMI) with symptomatic sinus node dysfunction, Mobitz II second-degree AV block, complete heart block, or newly acquired left bundle-branch block (LBBB) or bifascicular block.

28. **Pacemakers are indicated for what specific arrhythmias?**
Sinus node dysfunction
- Symptomatic sinus bradycardia
- Sinus pauses >3 seconds
AV nodal block
- Symptomatic second-degree AV block (Mobitz I)
- Symptomatic complete heart block
Infranodal block
- New bifascicular block associated with AMI
- Alternating bundle-branch block with changing PR interval
- Second-degree AV block (Mobitz II)
- Complete heart block

Glikson M, Hayes DL: Cardiac pacing: A review. Med Clin North Am 85:369–421, 2001.

29. **Where are external/transcutaneous pacemakers placed? How are they operated?**
Pacing pads and monitor leads are placed preferably in the midanterior chest and just below the left scapula. The desired heart rate is chosen, and the current is set to 0 mA.

The external pacemaker is turned on, and the current is increased as tolerated until capture is achieved.

30. State the limiting factors in the use of external pacemakers.
Skeletal muscle contraction can be uncomfortable and often limits use of external pacemakers. Placing electrodes over areas of least skeletal muscle may minimize the discomfort. The physician should use the lowest effective current. Sedation should be considered if these measures are inadequate.

31. What are the complications of long-term external cardiac pacing?
Continued patient discomfort is the only significant problem because no enzymatic, electrocardiographic, or microscopic evidence of myocardial damage has been found after pacing for 60 minutes.

Cardall TY, Chan TC, Brady WJ, et al: Permanent cardiac pacemakers: Issues relevant to the emergency physician: Part I. J Emerg Med 17:479–489, 1999.

32. Can an external pacemaker be used if a permanent pacemaker malfunctions?
Yes, but be careful to place the external pacer on a *pace only* (fixed-rate) mode and not the sensing mode; otherwise, it may sense spikes from the permanent pacemaker and not fire.

33. What are the advantages of transvenous versus transcutaneous pacemakers?
Transcutaneous leads are the easiest to use for rapid initiation of temporary pacing. Transvenous leads are the more reliable and more comfortable because external pacing requires 30–100 times the current needed for internal transvenous pacing.

Bocka JJ: External transcutaneous pacemakers. Ann Emerg Med 18:1280–1286, 1989.

34. How are transvenous and transthoracic pacemakers placed?
Semifloating or flexible balloon-tipped catheters can be placed with central venous access into the subclavian or internal jugular veins. In the ED, using ECG guidance, an alligator clip is connected to a precordial lead such as V_1 with another clip attached to the pacing wire. When a current of injury (ST elevation) is seen on the monitor, the wire should be withdrawn slightly, leaving it in pacing position. If available, fluoroscopy is preferred to ensure proper placement. Transthoracic catheters are inserted directly into the right ventricle through a left parasternal or subxiphoid approach and can be used in a cardiac arrest situation. This procedure, generally reserved for cardiac arrest, has many complications and rarely produces effective mechanical cardiac contraction.

35. Can cardiopulmonary resuscitation (CPR) be performed with a pacemaker?
CPR can be performed safely with the external pacing pads in place. Turning the external pacemaker off during CPR is advisable, in particular when defibrillating or cardioverting a patient. Defibrillator paddles should be placed at least 2–3 cm away from pacing pads to prevent arching of current.

36. List the indications for a permanent pacemaker.
Absolute indications
- Sick sinus syndrome
- Symptomatic sinus bradycardia
- Tachycardia-bradycardia syndrome
- AF with a slow ventricular response
- Complete heart block
- Chronotropic incompetence (inability to increase the heart rate to match a level of exercise)
- Long QT syndrome

Relative indications
- Cardiomyopathies (hypertrophic or dilated)
- Severe refractory neurocardiogenic syncope
- Paroxysmal AF

Hayes DL: Evolving indications for permanent pacing. Am J Cardiol 83:161D–165D, 1999.

37. **Describe the complications of permanent pacemaker implantation.**
Routine placement of a pacemaker generator into a subcutaneous or submuscular pocket carries the risk of pocket hematoma, which if large enough to palpate often needs surgical drainage. Pocket infection, manifest as local inflammation, fluctuance, and abscess formation or local cellulitis, is common. Rarely, the pocket itself may erode with extrusion of the generator, secondary to infection, trauma, or local tissue ischemia. Infection usually is caused by *Staphylococcus aureus* acutely and *Staphylococcus epidermidis* in chronic infections. Treatment is empirical antibiotics and ultimately removal of the device and reimplantation at a remote site. Wound dehiscence may require admission for debridement and reapproximation of wound edges.

Cardall TY, Brady WJ, Chan TC, et al: Permanent cardiac pacemakers: Issues relevant to the emergency physician: Part II. J Emerg Med 17:697–709, 1999.

38. **What are the complications of lead placement?**
Placement of transvenous leads can lead to pneumothorax or hemothorax, venous thrombosis, or lead infection. Thrombosis may occur at the lead implant, the tricuspid valve, or the subclavian vein and may cause superior vena cava syndrome.

39. **What does a pacer setting of *DDD* mean?**
The letters represent a pacing code. The code consists of three to five letters that describe the different types of pacer function (Table 29-2). The first letter indicates the chamber paced; the second indicates the chamber in which electrical activity is sensed, and the third indicates the response to a sensed event. A fourth and fifth letter may be added to describe whether the pacemaker is programmable and whether special functions to protect against tachycardia are available. A DDD pacer is able to pace and sense atria and ventricles ([D]ual chambers) and has a (D)ual response to the sensed ventricular and atrial activity (i.e., can pace either the atrium or the ventricle). Spontaneous atrial and ventricular activity inhibits atrial and ventricular pacing; atrial activity without ventricular activity triggers only ventricular pacing.

TABLE 29-2. PACING CODE		
First Letter: Chamber Paced to a Sensed Event	**Second Letter: Chamber Sensed**	**Third Letter: Response**
A (atrial)	A (atrial)	O (no response)
V (ventricle)	V (ventricle)	I (inhibition)
D (dual chamber)	D (dual chamber)	T (triggering)
		D (dual response)

40. **How can the type of permanent pacemaker be identified in the ED?**
Patients should carry a card with them providing information about their particular model. Most pacemaker generators have an x-ray code that can be seen on a standard chest radiograph. The markings, along with the shape of the generator, may assist with determining the manufacturer of the generator and pacemaker battery.

41. What are the complications of permanent pacemakers?
See Table 29-3.

TABLE 29-3. COMPLICATIONS OF PERMANENT PACEMAKERS

Complication	Description
Oversensing	Occurs when a pacer incorrectly senses electrical activity and is inhibited from correctly pacing. This may be due to muscular activity, electromagnetic interference, or lead insulation breakage.
Undersensing	Occurs when a pacer incorrectly misses intrinsic depolarization and paces despite intrinsic activity. This can be due to poor lead positioning, lead dislodgement, magnet application, low battery states, or myocardial infarction.
Operative failures	This includes malfunction resulting from mechanical factors (such as a pneumothorax, pericarditis, infection, hematoma, lead dislodgement, or venous thrombosis).
Failure to capture	Occurs when a pacing spike is not followed by either an atrial or ventricular complex. This may be due to lead fracture, lead dislodgement, a break in lead insulation, an elevated pacing threshold, myocardial infarction at the lead tip, drugs, metabolic abnormalities, cardiac perforation, poor lead connection, and improper amplitude or pulse width settings.

42. What is the most common cause of permanent pacemaker malfunction?
Today, most pacemaker failures are the result of problems with the electrodes or the wires, not the battery or the pulse generator. Because of greater technologic sophistication, patients with pacemaker problems present to the ED much less commonly now than in the past.

McComb JM, Gribbin GM: Effect of pacing mode on morbidity and mortality: Update of clinical pacing trials. Am J Cardiol 83:211D–213D, 1999.

43. What is pacemaker syndrome?
A clinical spectrum of lightheadedness, fatigue, palpitations, syncope, dyspnea on exertion, and hypotension that usually is attributed to asynchronous AV contraction and loss of atrial functional support.

44. Name the most common reason for early pacemaker malfunction.
Lead dislodgement.

45. How do I assess a patient with potential pacemaker malfunction?
1. Take a focused history on symptoms related to pacemaker malfunction, including palpitations, weakness, fatigue, shortness of breath, hiccups, syncope, or pain or erythema at the generator site.
2. The physician examination should focus on vital signs, mental status, cardiovascular system, and inspection of the generator site.
3. An ECG should be obtained to evaluate pacemaker function, and anteroposterior and lateral chest radiographs should be obtained to check pacemaker lead placement and lead and connector integrity.

Sarko JA, Tiffany BR: Cardiac pacemakers: Evaluation and management of malfunctions. Am J Emerg Med 18:435–440, 2000.

46. What is twiddler's syndrome?
The most common cause of late lead dislodgement. It results from the twisting or *twiddling* of a pulse generator in its pouch to the point of twisting leads around the generator box, shortening and dislodging them from their proper position. The pulse generator may erode through the skin.

47. What is pacemaker-mediated tachycardia?
A normally functioning pacemaker may initiate a tachyarrhythmia. Retrograde conduction of a ventricular beat may cause the atrium to trigger a second ventricular contraction that falls during the pacemaker's refractory period. Because this contraction is not sensed by the pacemaker, the pulse generator fires, initiating a reentrant tachycardia.

48. How is pacemaker-mediated tachycardia treated?
Treatment consists of lengthening the AV time by any of the following methods:
- Programming an increase in the atrial refractory time
- Administering adenosine or verapamil
- Increasing atrial sensory threshold
- Applying a magnet to stop atrial sensing by the pacemaker

49. What is a runaway pacemaker?
Malfunction of the pacemaker that is manifested by tachycardias secondary to rapid ventricular pacing. The problem is recognized when rates are greater than the upper rate limit settings of the pacemaker and may require drastic measures, such as cutting the pacer leads.

50. What happens as pacemakers lose battery power?
Pacemakers usually show a decline in the rate of magnet-mediated pacing, usually to a predetermined manufacturer's rate. Pacer response varies with manufacturer; some models may change pacer mode also (e.g., DDD to VVI).

KEY POINTS: CARDIAC DYSRHYTHMIAS

1. An unstable patient with any tachydysrhythmia, regardless of the mechanism, requires cardioversion.

2. When trying to decide if the rhythm your patient is in is VT or SVT with aberrancy, assume VT and treat accordingly.

3. The common reason for early pacemaker malfunction is lead dislodgement. The most common cause of late lead dislodgement is Twiddler's syndrome.

4. Pacemakers should be used for hemodynamically unstable bradycardias as well as for overdrive pacing in an attempt to terminate VT.

5. Calcium channel blockers should *not* be used to treat wide-complex tachycardias.

51. What is the most reliable indicator of pacer malfunction?
Rates that are usually inappropriate for paced hearts. A nonpaced ventricular rate less than 60 bpm or a paced rate greater than 100 bpm is probably secondary to pacemaker malfunction.

52. What does a magnet do?
Placing a pacemaker magnet over the pulse generator stops the pacemaker from sensing or responding to a sensed event. The pacemaker reverts to one of three fixed rate modes: the AOO (atrium paced), the VOO (ventricle paced), or the DOO (atrium and ventricle paced) mode. The

purpose is to check the pacing rate, which should be done quickly because the pulse generator no longer is prevented from firing during the T wave or from inhibiting serious arrhythmias. Magnets can also be used to turn off some automatic implantable cardioverter defibrillators (AICDs).

53. **Can a patient with a permanent pacemaker be defibrillated?**
Yes, but it is important to place the paddles away from the pulse generator, preferably in the anteroposterior position.

54. **Can defibrillation damage the pulse generator when current passes through?**
Yes. Temporary and even permanent loss of ventricular or atrial capture may occur secondary to elevation of the capture threshold of the pacer leads.

55. **What is an AICD?**
An **automatic implantable cardioverter defibrillator (AICD)** is a specialized device designed to treat a cardiac tachyarrhythmia. If the device senses a ventricular rate that exceeds the programmed cutoff rate of the implantable cardioverter defibrillator, the device performs cardioversion/defibrillation. Alternatively, the device may attempt to pace rapidly for a number of pulses, usually around 10, to attempt pace termination of the VT. Newer AICDs are a combination of implantable cardioverter defibrillator and pacemaker in one unit.

Gillis AM: The current status of the implantable cardioverter defibrillator. Annu Rev Med 47:85–93, 1996.

56. **Discuss complications associated with an AICD.**
See Table 29-4.

TABLE 29-4. COMPLICATIONS ASSOCIATED WITH AN AICD

Complication	Description
Operative failure	Similar to operative failures in pacemakers
Sensing failure	Oversensing and undersensing occur, for similar reasons as with pacemakers
Inappropriate cardioversion	May occur if a patient presents in atrial fibrillation or has received multiple shocks in rapid succession
Ineffective cardioversion	Can be seen because of T wave oversensing, lead fracture, lead insulation breakage, electrocautery, MRI, or electromagnetic interference. Can also be caused by inadequate energy output, a rise in the defibrillation threshold because of antidysrhythmic medications, myocardial infarction at the lead site, lead fracture, insulation breakage, or dislodgement of the leads of the cardioversion patches
Failure to deliver cardioversion	Can be caused by failure to sense, lead fracture, electromagnetic interference, and inadvertent AICD deactivation

AICD = automatic implantable cardioverter defibrillator, MRI = magnetic resonance imaging.
Adapted from Higgins GL III: The automatic implantable cardioverter-defibrillator: Management issues relevant to the emergency care provider. Am J Emerg Med 8:342–347,1990.

57. **Name the most frequent complication associated with AICDs.**
Inappropriate cardioversion.

58. **What will a magnet do when placed over an AICD?**
Use of a magnet over the AICD inhibits further shocks, but it does not inhibit bradycardiac pacing should the patient require it. In older devices, application of a magnet produces a beep for each QRS complex. If the magnet is left on for 30 seconds, the AICD is disabled, and a continuous tone is produced. To reactivate the device, the magnet is removed and replaced. After 30 seconds, a beep returns for every QRS complex.

HYPERTENSION, HYPERTENSIVE CRISIS, AORTIC ANEURYSMS, AND AORTIC DISSECTION

Neide Fehrenbacher, MD

CHAPTER 30

1. **Describe the blood pressure (BP) classification system used by the latest Joint National Committee (JNC 7) report.**
   Normal BP is <120/80 mmHg, and abnormal is considered >140/90 mmHg. Stage 1 is <160/100 mmHg, and Stage 2 is >160/100 mmHg. Note that a patient must have at least three elevated BP readings documented at three separate office visits to be labeled as having hypertension (HTN).

2. **Define hypertensive emergency/crisis and list some examples.**
   It is defined as acute end-organ damage in the presence of severely elevated BP. Examples include hypertensive encephalopathy, ischemic and hemorrhagic stroke (CVA), acute myocardial infarction (AMI), congestive heart failure (CHF), aortic dissection, acute renal failure (ARF), and preeclampsia/eclampsia. Except for those patients with cerebrovascular involvement, rapid lowering of BP should occur within 1 hour of presentation.

3. **How does hypertensive emergency differ from hypertensive urgency?**
   With hypertensive urgency, a patient has very high BP but no evidence of acute end-organ damage. There may be a history of chronic HTN and chronic end-organ damage, but if there is no acute worsening, it is classified as an urgency. There is no evidence to support acutely decreasing BP in the emergency department (ED) prior to discharge, but it is very important to refer these patients back to their primary care physician for follow-up within 1–2 days.

   Nguyen TT, Rohrback SM, Lenamond C: Distinguishing and managing hypertensive emergencies and urgencies. Emerg Med Pract 7(7):1–20, 2005.

4. **What symptoms might be present in a patient with hypertensive emergency?**
   Central nervous system involvement may cause headache, lethargy, dizziness, confusion, focal weakness, paresthesias, or vision changes. Chest pain, back pain, shortness of breath, and lower extremity swelling may reveal cardiopulmonary compromise. Decreased urine output, nausea, and generalized malaise and weakness may suggest ARF.

5. **What signs support the diagnosis of hypertensive crisis?**
   Confusion, altered level of consciousness, and focal neurologic findings, along with arteriovenous (AV) nicking, copper-wiring, flame-shaped hemorrhages, exudates, and papilledema on funduscopy exam. Crackles, hepatomegaly, and lower extremity edema may be present as well as a gallop, jugular venous distension, and a displaced point of maximal impulse.

6. **What studies should be considered in a patient with a hypertensive emergency?**
   If neurologic symptoms or signs are present, order a computed tomography (CT) of the head to evaluate for hemorrhagic or ischemic stroke or hypertensive encephalopathy. Obtain an electrocardiogram (ECG) to screen for hypertrophy, ischemia, or infarction and a chest x-ray (CXR) to look for CHF and aortic dissection. A troponin should be sent in a patient with chest pain, back pain, and/or shortness of breath, and, if there is concern for dissection, a stat CT angiogram is necessary. A chemistry panel will screen for renal failure, and a urine sample can be obtained to check for protein, blood, and glucose.

7. **Is ED testing necessary in a patient with elevated BP and no symptoms?**
No testing is necessary, because these patients should receive urgent follow-up with a primary care physician who can confirm the diagnosis and perform diagnostic studies such as a serum creatine to evaluate renal function.

Nguyen TT, Rohrback SM, Lenamond C: Distinguishing and managing hypertensive emergencies and urgencies. Emerg Med Pract 7(7):1–20, 2005.

8. **What is the difference between primary and secondary HTN?**
Essential or primary HTN accounts for more than 90% of patients with true HTN and the cause is unknown. Its etiology is likely multifactorial, a combination of both genetics and environment.
Secondary HTN has an identifiable cause. It can result from a primary neurologic (increased intracranial pressure), renal (glomerulonephritis, polycystic kidney disease, chronic pyelonephritis), vascular (coarctation of the aorta, renal artery stenosis), or endocrine (Cushing's syndrome—increased cortisol, Conn syndrome—increased aldosterone, pheochromocytoma—increased catecholamines, thyrotoxicosis) disorders and from pregnancy-induced HTN, that is, preeclampsia and eclampsia.

9. **List other causes of transient HTN.**
Anxiety, pain, illicit drug use (cocaine, amphetamines, phencyclidine [PCP], lysergic acid diethylamide [LSD]), over-the-counter medications containing sympathomimetics, certain toxidromes, and alcohol withdrawal.

10. **Describe the pathophysiology of hypertensive encephalopathy.**
With abrupt, severe elevations in BP, cerebral autoregulation fails. When this occurs, blood flow to the brain is no longer controlled, causing overperfusion, vasodilation, and increased vascular permeability. This leads to cerebral edema and elevated intracranial pressure (ICP).

11. **How do I diagnose hypertensive encephalopathy?**
The classic triad associated with hypertensive encephalopathy is altered mental status (AMS), HTN, and papilledema. Acute onset of headache, vomiting, drowsiness, confusion, seizures, vision changes, focal neurologic findings, and decreased level of consciousness may occur. Symptoms are reversible with appropriate BP reduction, but if left untreated coma and death occur within hours.

12. **What is the characteristic head CT finding in hypertensive encephalopathy?**
Posterior leukoencephalopathy, most prominent in the occipital-parietal areas.

Shayne PH, Pitts SR: Severely increased blood pressure in the emergency department. Ann Emerg Med 41:513–529, 2003.

13. **Why is it important to understand cerebral autoregulation?**
Cerebral autoregulation works only within a certain range of mean arterial pressure (MAP), and overtreatment of cerebrovascular hypertensive emergencies can be just as damaging as no treatment at all. Cerebral blood flow (CBF) depends on cerebral perfusion pressure (CPP), which is the difference between MAP and ICP. MAP = diastolic blood pressure (DBP) + {1/3} [systolic blood pressure (SBP) − DBP]. To maintain CBF and CPP at relatively constant levels, cerebral arteries vasoconstrict when MAP increases and vasodilate when MAP decreases. In normotensive individuals, cerebral autoregulation maintains constant CBF between a MAP of 60 and 120 mmHg.

14. **What happens to CBF in patients with chronic HTN?**
In patients with chronic HTN, this lower limit for autoregulation is reset to a higher level. Attempts to reach a "normal BP" with treatment will likely lead to inadequate CBF and subsequent ischemia and infarction. This is because autoregulation fails when MAP is >160 mmHg or <60 mmHg.

15. **In a patient with a cerebrovascular hypertensive emergency, how much should I decrease the BP?**

When treating cerebrovascular hypertensive emergencies, it is recommended that MAP not be lowered by more than 20–25% or that the DBP not be lowered to less than 110 mmHg over 30 minutes to 1 hour. Careful monitoring of therapy is essential to avoid precipitous drops in BP.

Shayne PH, Pitts SR: Severely increased blood pressure in the emergency department. Ann Emerg Med 41:513–529, 2003.

16. **How do I treat a patient with hypertensive encephalopathy?**

One of several medications may be chosen. They work by different mechanisms but should have three important properties in common: (1) an intravenous (IV) drip enabling easy titration, (2) rapid onset, and (3) short duration of action. Traditionally, the drug of choice has been nitroprusside, a powerful vasodilator. Note that it can cause elevated ICP and has cyanide as an intermediate metabolite, limiting its use in patients with liver or kidney disease. For equally effective treatment with potentially fewer limitations, consider labetalol, esmolol, or fenoldopam mesylate.

17. **What other neurologic syndromes are associated with HTN?**

Patients with ischemic and hemorrhagic strokes may have elevated BP due to an adaptive response by the brain to try to maintain CPP. **Lowering or *normalizing* BP is potentially dangerous in patients with ischemic stroke and is not recommended.** The Stroke Council for the American Heart Association recommends cautious lowering of BP in stroke *only* when BP is >220/120 mmHg or MAP is >130 mmHg, or if BP >185/110 mmHg in an otherwise possible thrombolytic candidate. Decision making regarding BP management should be done in close consultation with a neurologist or neurosurgeon.

Nguyen TT, Rohrback SM, Lenamond C: Distinguishing and managing hypertensive emergencies and urgencies. Emerg Med Pract 7(7):1–20, 2005.

18. **How do I treat a patient with severe HTN and evidence of pulmonary edema?**

Start with standard treatment for pulmonary edema: oxygen, diuretics, and afterload reduction with nitrites.

19. **How do I treat a patient with severe HTN and chest pain due to ischemia?**

Acute ischemia of the left ventricle is often accompanied by severe HTN. Reduction of BP is crucial to decrease the work of the myocardium and prevent ongoing ischemia. First-line treatment is IV nitroglycerin combined with beta-blocker and morphine. If this fails to control BP, nicardipine or fenoldopam can be added. Avoid nitroprusside as it can cause a coronary-steal phenomenon in patients with coronary artery disease, causing increased mortality in the presence of an AMI.

20. **Is ischemia the only cause of chest pain to worry about in a hypertensive patient?**

No. Always think about the possibility of acute aortic dissection because this can be a rapidly fatal cause of chest pain, and HTN is the most common risk factor. Other risk factors include congenital heart disease, Ehlers-Danlos, Marfan syndrome, intra-aortic balloon pump use, or major trauma (due to deceleration injury—not to be discussed here).

Ankel F: Aortic dissection. Rosen's Emergency Medicine, 5th ed. St. Louis, Mosby, 2002, pp 1171–1176.

21. **What symptoms/signs may be present in a patient with thoracic aortic dissection?**

Classic symptoms include sudden onset, severe chest pain, and/or back pain, often described as sharp, ripping, or tearing. Proximal dissections may cause aortic regurgitation (31%) and tamponade. Occlusion of aortic branches may cause AMI (coronary artery involvement), stroke (carotid involvement), or paresthesias and arm pain (subclavian artery involvement), which may be suggested by unequal bilateral arm pressures and unequal pulses. Extension into the abdomen may cause abdominal pain or leg ischemia. Spinal artery occlusion will cause neurologic compromise, and hoarseness may result from recurrent laryngeal nerve compression.

www.surgical-tutor.org.uk/system/vascular/dissection.htm

22. **What diagnostic studies should be done when thoracic aortic dissection is suspected?**
Order a CXR followed by a CT, magnetic resonance imaging (MRI), or transesophageal echocardiography (TEE), because a CXR may be normal in up to 20% of patients. Spiral CT is the most practical modality in the ED as it is quick, accurate, and most readily available. MRI is very sensitive and specific, but scan times are long, and access to the patient during the study is limited. TEE is great for determining involvement of the aortic valve and coronary arteries and can detect the presence of pericardial effusion or tamponade, but emergent access to this study is likely limited. Aortography, once considered the gold standard, is rarely used any longer as the initial diagnostic study.

23. **What findings on a CXR suggest thoracic aortic dissection?**
Widened mediastinum, loss of the aortic knob, left pleural effusion, deviation of the trachea or nasogastric tube to the right, apical pleural capping, and the "calcium sign" (displacement of the intimal calcium layer in the aorta).

24. **Describe the difference between type A and type B thoracic aortic dissections.**
Type A dissections (60%) involve the proximal/ascending aorta and require emergent surgical repair, whereas type B dissections (40%) affect the descending aorta (distal to the great vessels) and are managed medically.

Bettmann MA, Dake MD, Hopkins LN, et al: Atherosclerotic vascular disease conference. Circulation 109:2643–2650, 2004.

25. **How do I treat a patient with suspected aortic dissection?**
Start IV antihypertensive BP medications immediately if hypertensive and call a cardiothoracic surgeon before the patient heads for the scanner. ED therapy for both types of dissections aims to lessen the pulsatile load and shear forces on the aorta. Rapid reduction of SBP to a range of 100–110 mmHg is indicated. Traditional therapy includes IV nitroprusside and an IV beta-blocker such as esmolol, which should be started first. This prevents the reflex tachycardia associated with nitroprusside and subsequent propagation of the dissection. Alternative treatment regimens include IV labetalol used as a single agent and IV nicardipine or fenoldopam in place of nitroprusside.

26. **What are the agents of choice in a patient with severe HTN and ARF?**
IV fenoldopam is a dopamine–1-receptor agonist, which is short acting and has advantages over traditional nitroprusside therapy. It increases renal blood flow, creatinine clearance, sodium excretion, and diuresis, and there is no issue with potential cyanide toxicity. It is as effective as nitroprusside with no reported adverse effects. It is, however, more costly. Other reasonable alternatives include nicardipine and labetalol. Angiotensin-converting enzyme (ACE) inhibitors should be avoided if bilateral renal artery stenosis has not yet been ruled out.

Shayne PH, Pitts SR: Severely increased blood pressure in the emergency department. Ann Emerg Med 41:513–529, 2003.

27. **What should you always think about in a pregnant or postpartum woman with HTN?**
Preeclampsia! If she is between 20 weeks' gestation and 2-weeks postpartum with HTN, edema, and proteinuria, start magnesium for seizure prophylaxis and to prevent progression to eclampsia. (See Chapter 82.)

28. **What are the two types of antihypertensive medications that if stopped abruptly can cause rebound HTN?**
Short-acting sympathetic blockers, such as clonidine, and beta-blockers.

29. **What antihypertensive medications are contraindicated in a catecholamine-induced hypertensive emergency?**
Beta-blockers. Beta-receptor-induced vasodilation results in unopposed alpha-adrenergic vasoconstriction and elevates BP further. In patients with concomitant cocaine ingestions, beta-blockers enhance coronary artery vasoconstriction, increase BP, fail to decrease heart rate, decrease the seizure threshold, and increase mortality. Labetalol, an alpha- and beta-blocker, theoretically avoids the problem of unopposed alpha, but some sources say it may still cause harm in patients with cocaine ingestion or pheochromocytoma. Antihypertensive agents that can be used for treatment of a catecholamine-induced hypertensive emergency include nicardipine, fenoldopam, phentolamine, and nitroprusside. However, most cocaine or amphetamine-induced HTN responds to appropriate doses of benzodiazepines.

KEY POINTS: SPECIAL CONSIDERATIONS WITH HYPERTENSIVE EMERGENCIES

1. Avoid precipitous or excessive drop in BP with cerebrovascular emergencies.

2. Start esmolol before nitroprusside with aortic dissections.

3. Do not give pure beta-blockers for catecholamine-induced hypertensive emergencies.

30. **What about using oral agents to treat hypertensive emergencies?**
Oral agents are acceptable for use in patients with hypertensive urgencies but not hypertensive emergencies because they yield unpredictable responses, cannot be titrated, and cannot be discontinued immediately if the patient's BP drops to unsafe levels.

31. **Are there any new medications out on the horizon that look promising for treating hypertensive emergencies?**
Yes. Urapidil is an alpha–1 adrenergic antagonist and a serotonin 5-HT1A receptor antagonist. It causes vasodilation without concomitant reflex tachycardia. It appears to be safe and as effective as nitroprusside, but it has not yet received Food and Drug Administration (FDA) approval. It is currently being used in many other countries.

Shayne PH, Pitts SR: Severely increased blood pressure in the emergency department. Ann Emerg Med 41:513–529, 2003.

32. **Summarize the common parenteral antihypertensive medications and their indications and contraindications.**
See Table 30-1.

33. **Describe the two different types of aortic aneurysms.**
A true aneurysm, as seen with most abdominal aortic aneurysms (AAAs), involves dilation of all three layers of the arterial wall: the intima, media, and adventitia. In a **pseudoaneurysm,** blood communicates with the arterial lumen but is contained solely within the adventitia or surrounding soft tissue. This is much less common.

TABLE 30-1. PARENTERAL ANTIHYPERTENSIVE MEDICATIONS

Drug	Dose	Onset	Duration	Indications	Contraindications
Nitroprusside	0.3–10 mcg/kg/min IV	1–2 min	1–2 min	CHF, aortic dissection, catecholamine excess, hypertensive encephalopathy	Pregnancy, AMI, hepatic or renal insufficiency, caution with increased ICP
Nitroglycerin	10–100 mcg/min IV	2–5 min	3–5 min	AMI, CHF	CVA, ARF
Nicardipine	5–15 mg/hr IV	15 min	6 hr	AMI, ARF, eclampsia, hypertensive encephalopathy, catecholamine excess	CHF, 2nd or 3rd degree AVB
Fenoldopam	0.1–1.7 mcg/kg/min IV	5–15 min	1–4 hr	AMI, CHF, ARF, aortic dissection, hypertensive encephalopathy, catecholamine excess	Glaucoma (can cause increased IOP)
Hydralazine	10–20 mg IV bolus; repeat q4–6h prn, (max 40 mg)	10–20 min	3–8 h	Eclampsia	AMI, CVA, aortic dissection
Esmolol	500 mcg/kg IV bolus over 1 min, then 50–300 mcg/kg/min	1–2 min	10–20 min	CAD, aortic dissection	CHF, 2nd or 3rd degree AVB
Labetolol	20 mg IV bolus, then 40–80 mg q10 min up to 300 mg or 2 mg/min IV	2–10 min	2–4 h	CAD, aortic dissection, hypertensive encephalopathy, eclampsia	CHF, 2nd or 3rd degree AVB, asthma
Phentolamine	5 mg IV, repeat prn (max 20 mg)	1–2 min	10–30 min	Catecholamine excess	AMI

34. **Are aortic dissections and aortic aneurysms somehow related?**
No. These two disease processes are totally unrelated, have different symptoms, require different work-ups, and are managed differently. Aortic dissection is caused by a weakness/tear of the intima leading to the formation of a false lumen within the media. Blood enters here and dissects proximally, distally or both.

Bessen HA: Abdominal aortic aneurysm. Rosen's Emergency Medicine, 5th edition. St. Louis, Mosby, 2002, pp 1171–1176.

35. **What risk factors are associated with aortic aneurysms?**
Aneurysms result from a degenerative process that affects the aortic wall. Its prevalence is higher with advanced age, male sex, and family history of AAA in a first-degree relative and in patients with atherosclerosis, diabetes, hyperlipidemia, smoking, and HTN. Other rare causes include infection, such as tertiary syphilis (which leads to aneurysmal dilation in the aortic root/ascending aorta), after blunt chest trauma (usually resulting in pseudoaneurysms), patients with connective tissue diseases (such as Marfan syndrome and Ehlers-Danlos), and in arteritis. Although aneurysms can develop anywhere along the aorta, 75% are AAAs.

36. **What are common presenting signs and symptoms of AAA?**
Most patients with AAAs are asymptomatic, and their aneurysm is found incidentally on physical exam or on diagnostic studies done for other reasons. Approximately 75% of aneurysms >5 cm can be palpated, but only 5–10% of patients with an AAA have an abdominal bruit. A patient with an acutely expanding or ruptured aneurysm will likely complain of constant **abdominal pain,** often localizing to the left side with radiation to the back/flank area. It could be described as dull, throbbing, or colicky. Hypotension, syncope, or low hematocrit may signify significant blood loss.

Bessen HA: Abdominal aortic aneurysm. Rosen's Emergency Medicine, 5th ed. St. Louis, Mosby, 2002, pp 1171–1176.

37. **What should I do when I suspect a ruptured AAA?**
Place two large bore IVs, type and cross for at least two units of packed red blood cells, and call a vascular surgeon. The goal should be to get the patient to the operating room (OR) as soon as possible, and transport should not be delayed for definitive studies or to attempt full resuscitation in the ED. A bedside ultrasound can be done quickly to screen for an AAA, but it cannot reliably rule out rupture as it can miss retroperitoneal blood. Ultrasound may be limited by obesity or bowel gas and is user dependent. CT, on the other hand, will pick up 100% of AAAs and is much more sensitive in picking up retroperitoneal blood.

Lederle FA: Ultrasonographic screening for abdominal aortic aneurysms. Ann Intern Med 522:516–522, 2003.

KEY POINTS: ABDOMINAL AORTIC ANEURYSMS

1. The triad is abdominal pain, pulsatile mass, hypotension.

2. Do not wait for a definitive study before calling surgery.

3. Bedside ultrasound is an excellent screening tool for AAA.

4. CT is the gold standard for making the diagnosis of a ruptured AAA.

38. **Discuss the dilemmas behind aggressive fluid resuscitation in a hypertensive patient with ruptured AAA.**

Unfortunately, no prospective studies exist to guide optimal fluid resuscitation, and the appropriate amount of volume to give is controversial. Allowing some degree of hypotension may slow bleeding, allow some clot formation and temporarily tamponade the bleeding. Too much fluid may have the opposite effect and may also cause a dilutional coagulopathy, further increasing bleeding. On the other hand, these patients likely have other comorbid conditions that could be potentially fatal in the presence of prolonged hypotension. The goal should be to maintain adequate perfusion to the vital organs using warm saline/blood without intentionally raising the BP above 90–100 mmHg systolic.

Bessen HA: Abdominal aortic aneurysm. Rosen's Emergency Medicine, 5th ed. St. Louis, Mosby, 2002, pp 1171–1176.

39. **How do I treat a patient with HTN and a ruptured AAA?**

Morphine is a good choice as it helps with pain, BP, and shear forces. Esmolol is the best antihypertensive medication because it decreases shear forces, is easily titratable, and has a short half-life.

40. **What common diseases may mimic ruptured AAA?**

Renal colic, pancreatitis, perforated peptic ulcer, AMI, gallbladder pathology, musculoskeletal back pain, and intestinal ischemia. Thus, always consider this diagnosis in middle-aged or elderly patients with any one of the symptoms in the classic triad: pain, hypotension, and pulsatile mass.

www.emedicine.com/EMERG/topic27.htm

41. **List some atypical symptoms that may be related to the presence of an AAA.**

Gastrointestinal bleeding in a patient with previous aortic repair may signify fistula formation between the wall of the aorta and the small or large bowel. A large aneurysm may cause mass effect on surrounding structures causing a bowel or ureteral obstruction. Radicular pain may occur if the bleeding is retroperitoneal. Leg ischemia may occur due to peripheral embolization of mural plaques.

42. **When do you need to worry about an AAA?**

The risk of rupture is minimal for an AAA measuring <4 cm, but the risk increases dramatically if it's >6 cm to 25% per year. Rapid expansion is the greatest predictor of impending rupture and routine screening with known AAAs is important as it significantly affects mortality. The mortality for elective repair of an AAA is approximately 5% as opposed to 50% if it has already ruptured.

www.surgical-tutor.org.uk/system/vascular/aaa.htm

43. **How are AAAs surgically repaired?**

Traditional repair involves laparotomy and cross-clamping the aorta. A newer, less invasive approach involves placement of a self-expanding stent graft via the femoral artery under fluoroscopic guidance.

Sakalihasan NS, Limet R, Defawe OD: Abdominal aortic aneurysm. Lancet 365:1577–1589, 2005.

CHAPTER 31

PERICARDITIS AND MYOCARDITIS

John L. Kendall, MD, and Christopher B. Colwell, MD

PERICARDITIS

1. **Describe a normal pericardium.**
   The pericardium is 1–2 mm thick and envelops the heart. It has two layers. Between the two layers is the pericardial space, which normally contains 25–50 mL of fluid.

2. **What is pericarditis?**
   Inflammation of the pericardium.

3. **What causes pericarditis?**
   Infectious agents, such as viruses and bacteria, can cause pericarditis as a result of direct spread of infection to the pericardium. Pericarditis also may be caused by the antibody-mediated autoimmune reaction that occurs 2–4 weeks after a viral illness (Table 31-1). This postviral pericarditis, termed *idiopathic* because a viral source has not been isolated, is probably the most common form of pericarditis. An autoimmune reaction to cardiac antigens may occur after cardiac instrumentation or acute myocardial infarction (MI). The likelihood of postinfarction pericarditis is reduced by half (from approximately 12% to 6%) when a thrombolytic agent is used.

TABLE 31-1. CAUSES OF PERICARDITIS		
Infection	**Immunologically Mediated Diseases**	**Trauma**
Viral	Postinfectious	Blunt
Coxsackie B	Postcardiac injury syndrome	Penetrating
		Drugs
Cytomegalovirus	Postpericardiotomy	Procainamide
Echovirus	Postinfarction (Dressler's syndrome)	Cromolyn sodium
HIV	Autoimmune disorders	Hydralazine
Bacterial	Acute rheumatic fever	Uremia
Tuberculosis	Rheumatoid arthritis	Radiation
Staphylococcus	Connective tissue diseases	Neoplasm
Fungal	Lupus erythematosus	
Parasitic		

HIV = human immunodeficiency virus.

4. **Who is most susceptible to infectious pericarditis?**

Viral and idiopathic pericarditis occur most commonly in healthy persons between 20 to 40 years old. Bacterial pericarditis occurs in patients with a bacterial infection of the lungs, endocardium, or blood. Patients with human immunodeficiency virus (HIV) are susceptible to pericarditis caused by opportunistic infections.

5. **Describe the clinical presentation of pericarditis.**

The most common symptom is chest pain, described as midline and sharp. The pain is worse with movement and breathing, and relief is obtained from sitting up and leaning forward. It may radiate to the neck, back, or left shoulder. Dyspnea, malaise, and fever may occur. The pathognomonic clinical finding is a friction rub, which is a scratchy noise, similar to creaking leather. The optimal patient position for a rub to be auscultated is sitting up, leaning forward, and in full expiration. The diaphragm of the stethoscope should be pressed firmly to the chest at the lower left sternal border. A little luck is needed to detect a rub because it occurs intermittently.

6. **How does the electrocardiogram (ECG) appear in pericarditis?**

The ECG typically evolves through four stages:
- **In stage 1,** The first hours to days of illness may show ST segment elevation and PR segment depression in all leads except aVR and V_1, in which reciprocal changes occur.
- **In stage 2,** the ST and PR segments normalize, and the T waves flatten.
- **In stage 3,** deep T-wave inversion occurs.
- **In stage 4,** the ECG reverts to normal. Occasionally, stage 4 does not occur, which results in permanent generalized or focal T-wave inversions and flattenings. The ST segment displacement seen in stage 1 is attributed to the associated subepicardial myocarditis, whereas the PR segment depression is attributed to subepicardial atrial injury.

Chan TC, Brady WJ, Pollack M: Electrocardiographic manifestations: Acute myopericarditis. J Emerg Med 17:865, 1999.

7. **How can acute pericarditis be distinguished from acute MI?**

ST segment elevations in stage 1 of acute pericarditis tend to be upwardly concave rather than convex, and simultaneous T-wave inversions are not typically seen. The progression to T-wave inversions in stage 2 tends to occur after the ST segments have returned to baseline, whereas in acute MI, the T-wave inversion is more likely to accompany ST segment elevation. The ST segment elevations in acute pericarditis typically are diffuse as opposed to an anatomic distribution, which typically is seen in acute MI.

Clinically, patients with acute pericarditis are more likely to be younger, to be otherwise healthy, and to have a history of a preceding viral illness and pleuritic-type chest pain. Patients with acute MI are more likely to be older with risk factors for coronary disease. Ventricular arrhythmias are not associated with isolated pericardial disease and suggest the presence of underlying cardiac disease.

8. **How can acute pericarditis be distinguished from musculoskeletal chest pain?**

Musculoskeletal chest pain generally is not relieved by sitting up, and the characteristic friction rub and ECG abnormalities of pericarditis are not present.

9. **Is pericardial effusion a concern in patients with pericarditis?**

Yes. Pericardial effusion occurs most commonly in patients with acute viral or idiopathic, neoplastic, postradiation, or posttraumatic pericarditis. Its effects range from insignificant to life threatening if tamponade occurs.

10. **How much pericardial effusion is significant?**

The answer depends entirely on the clinical situation. A patient with a stab wound to the heart may be able to accommodate only 80–200 mL of pericardial fluid before tamponade develops.

Patients with longstanding pericardial fluid collections may tolerate 2000 mL without hemodynamic compromise.

11. How can a pericardial effusion be diagnosed?

The physical examination is unreliable in detecting or excluding a pericardial effusion. Similarly, the cardiac silhouette is not enlarged on chest radiograph until at least 250 mL of fluid has accumulated. **Echocardiography** has excellent sensitivity and specificity; it can detect as little as 15 mL of pericardial fluid.

12. What is cardiac tamponade?

Cardiac tamponade exists when accumulating pericardial fluid leads to increased pericardial pressure to the point that it prevents the atria and ventricles from filling adequately during diastole, decreasing the volume of blood available to be pumped during systole and causing hemodynamic compromise. Although any form of pericarditis may lead to cardiac tamponade, acute tamponade usually is caused by trauma. Subacute tamponade occurs most commonly in neoplastic pericarditis.

Spodick DH. Pathophysiology of cardiac tamponade. Chest 113:1372–1378, 1998.

13. How is cardiac tamponade diagnosed?

The first step is to confirm the presence of a pericardial effusion by echocardiography. Absence of a pericardial effusion rules out cardiac tamponade. If an effusion is present, a combination of physical examination and echocardiographic findings can confirm of the diagnosis of tamponade. Physical examination findings suggestive of tamponade include tachycardia, hypotension, cyanosis, dyspnea, jugular venous distention, pulsus paradoxus, and elevated central venous pressure (>15 mmHg). Echocardiographic findings are more specific and develop sequentially as pericardial pressure increases: right atrial collapse, right ventricular collapse, and bowing of the interventricular septum. Another helpful finding is to perform the *sniff test*. Instruct the patient to inhale quickly through the nose while the ultrasonographer visualizes the inferior vena cava. Incomplete collapse of the inferior vena cava correlates well with elevated central venous pressure measurements.

14. What is pulsus paradoxus?

An abnormally large (>10 mmHg) drop in the systolic blood pressure with inspiration. Kussmaul termed this phenomenon *paradoxical* because of the disappearance of the pulse during inspiration when the heart was obviously beating. Pulsus paradoxus is a pulse, not a pressure, change and is an exaggeration of the normal inspiratory fall in arterial flow and systolic pressure. Inspiration favors right-sided heart filling by decreasing pericardial pressure, whereas expiration favors left-sided heart filling. Pulsus paradoxus usually signals large reductions in ventricular volumes and equilibration of mean pericardial and all cardiac diastolic pressures. The detection of pulsus paradoxus on physical examination suggests (and may be one of the earliest clues to) the existence of cardiac tamponade.

15. What is the appropriate emergency department (ED) management of pericarditis?

Antiinflammatory agents, such as indomethacin (Indocin), 25–75 mg four times a day; aspirin, 650 mg every 3–4 hours; or ibuprofen, 600 mg four times a day, should be administered. The use of corticosteroids is controversial. Although corticosteroids are effective anti-inflammatory agents, 10–20% of patients develop recurrent pericarditis as tapering occurs. Echocardiography is indicated to rule out pericardial effusion. If cardiac tamponade is present, percutaneous pericardiocentesis must be done to relieve intracardiac pressure. Intravenous fluids should be infused rapidly to increase arterial pressure and cardiac output.

16. **What is the prognosis for patients with pericarditis?**
Most patients recover fully, although 15–20% have a recurrence, probably because of an autoimmune mechanism. Nonsteroidal anti-inflammatory drugs are used for recurrences. If these agents are ineffective, corticosteroid therapy is initiated. Colchicine holds promise as an adjunctive therapy in recurrent pericarditis. If medical interventions fail, pericardiectomy usually is done.

17. **Is pericarditis seen in pediatric patients?**
Yes, but the frequency is unknown, and there does not appear to be any age or gender predilection. Viral etiologies (Coxsackie, echovirus, influenza) seem to be the most common in children. Signs and symptoms, as well as physical findings, are very similar to those seen in adults.

MYOCARDITIS

18. **What is myocarditis?**
An inflammation of the myocardium in the absence of ischemia.

19. **What causes myocarditis?**
In the **United States,** myocarditis is caused most commonly by viruses. Enteroviruses, especially the Coxsackie B virus, predominate as causative agents. Infectious agents cause myocardial damage by three basic mechanisms: (1) the direct invasion of the myocardium, (2) production of a myocardial toxin (e.g., diphtheria), or (3) immunologically mediated myocardial damage. The immunologically mediated destruction of cardiac tissue from infiltration of host cellular immune components is probably the more common mechanism in adults, whereas in neonates, damage from direct viral invasion is more likely.
   Worldwide, Chagas' disease is the leading cause of myocarditis. Other organisms that are known to infiltrate the myocardium include influenza A and B, adenovirus, hepatitis A and B, tuberculosis, *Chlamydia pneumoniae, Borrelia burgdorferi* (Lyme disease), *Legionella pneumophila,* cytomegalovirus, *Toxoplasma gondii, Trichinella spiralis,* and *Corynebacterium diphtheriae.*

   Wynne J, Braunwald E: The cardiomyopathies and myocarditides. In Braunwald E, Zipes DP, Libby P (eds): Heart Disease: A Textbook of Cardiovascular Medicine, 6(th) ed. Philadelphia. W.B. Saunders, 2001, pp 1783–1806.

20. **When should a diagnosis of myocarditis be considered in the ED?**
Diagnosing myocarditis in the ED can be a challenge, and because the presenting symptoms and signs are typically nonspecific, this is often a diagnosis of exclusion. Nonspecific symptoms include fatigue, myalgias, dyspnea, palpitations, and precordial discomfort. Chest pain often reflects associated pericarditis. Patients may present with dilated cardiomyopathy without evidence of ischemia or valvular disease. Myocarditis probably should be considered in any previously healthy person who develops dyspnea, orthopnea, decreased exercise tolerance, palpitations, or syncope when no other obvious cause is found. Patients should be asked about concomitant or recent upper respiratory or gastrointestinal illness.

21. **What clinical findings may be present?**
Flulike complaints, such as fatigue, myalgias, nausea, vomiting, diarrhea, and fever, are usually the earliest symptoms and signs of myocarditis. Tachycardia is common and can be disproportionate to the temperature or apparent toxicity. This may be the only clue that something more serious than a simple viral illness exists. Clinical evidence of congestive heart failure occurs only in more severe cases. Typical findings in patients with congestive heart failure include tachypnea, rales, and pedal edema. A pericardial friction rub may be auscultated if myopericarditis is present. Complications of myocarditis include ventricular arrhythmias and left ventricular aneurysms.

22. **Are there any chest radiograph or ECG abnormalities?**
    - The **chest radiograph** may be normal or abnormal, depending on the extent of disease. The cardiac silhouette may be enlarged, which can be due to a dilated cardiomyopathy or a pericardial effusion.
    - The **ECG** commonly shows a sinus tachycardia and low electrical activity. Nonspecific ST segment and T-wave abnormalities, a prolonged corrected QT interval, atrioventricular block, or acute MI pattern also may occur. Atrial arrhythmias have been described.

KEY POINTS: PERICARDITIS AND MYOCARDITIS

1. The physical exam or chest radiography is neither sensitive or specific for pericardial effusion; echocardiography is the gold standard.

2. Myocarditis should be considered in patients with significant tachycardia that cannot otherwise be explained.

3. Viruses are the most common causes of pericarditis and myocarditis, and a history of preceding or concurrent viral illness is quite common.

4. Myocarditis is very common in AIDS patients, with rates at autopsy as high as 52%.

23. **How is myocarditis diagnosed?**
    Making the diagnosis clinically can be difficult. Endocardial biopsy currently is considered the gold standard, although it has highly variable sensitivity and specificity. In contrast to patients with pericarditis, cardiac enzymes frequently are elevated in patients with myocarditis. White blood cell count and erythrocyte sedimentation rate may be elevated but are nonspecific. Indium–111 antimyosin antibodies show myocardial necrosis by binding to exposed myosin in damaged myocardial cells. When myocarditis is suspected clinically, indium–111 antimyosin imaging may be helpful. Viral titers have been suggested but have a low yield. Echocardiography often shows global dysfunction that does not correspond to a specific coronary artery distribution.

    Brady WJ, Ferguson JD, Ullman EA, et al: Myocarditis: eEmergency department recognition and management. Emerg Med Clin North Am 22:4865–885, 2004.

24. **How can acute myocarditis be distinguished from acute MI?**
    Myocarditis occurs primarily in young healthy patients without significant cardiac history or risk factors for coronary artery disease. Chest pain, dyspnea, ECG abnormalities, and cardiac enzyme elevation may occur in both conditions. In the ED, it may be impossible to distinguish between these two entities, in which case treatment for acute MI should be initiated.

25. **Is myocarditis a concern in acquired immunodeficiency syndrome (AIDS)?**
    Yes. The incidence of myocarditis found at autopsy of AIDS patients has been reported as high as 52%, compared with almost 10% in the population as a whole. The increased risk of myocarditis in patients with AIDS may be due to an abnormal autoimmune reaction, opportunistic infections, or HIV itself.

26. **In what other clinical situations should myocarditis be considered?**
    Myocarditis and dilated cardiomyopathy have been associated with cocaine use. Myocarditis is a common autopsy finding in patients who have died from cocaine abuse.

27. **Describe the appropriate ED management of a patient with myocarditis.**
    The current recommended treatment consists of supportive therapy. The only uniformly accepted beneficial therapy is bed rest. All patients with suspected myocarditis should be

admitted to a monitored bed in the hospital. Antibiotics are appropriate when a bacterial cause is suspected. Dilated cardiomyopathy is treated with diuresis, afterload reduction, and digoxin. In severe cases, temporary pacing and external circulatory support may be needed. Patients with a fulminant clinical course may require cardiac transplantation. Immunosuppressive therapy has been studied, but controlled studies have not established efficacy. High-dose gamma globulin has been studied and may be associated with improved left ventricular function and better survival during the first year after initial presentation.

Jouriles NJ: Pericardial and myocardial disease. In Marx JA (ed): Rosen's Emergency Medicine: Concepts and Clinical Practice, 5(th) ed. St. Louis, Mosby, 2002, pp 1130–1149.

28. What is the prognosis for patients with acute myocarditis?

Mortality for patients with myocarditis has been reported to be 20% at 1 year and 56% at 4 years, although many patients do recover completely.

McCarthy RE III, Bochmer JP, Hruban RH, et al : Long-term outcome of fulminant myocarditis as compared with acute (non-fulminant) myocarditis. N Engl J Med 342:690–695, 2000.

ESOPHAGUS AND STOMACH DISORDERS

Philip L. Henneman, MD

CHAPTER 32

1. **How are gastrointestinal (GI) problems differentiated from acute myocardial infarction?**

   Esophageal or gastric pain can present with visceral-type chest pain (e.g., ache, pressure) or upper abdominal pain and nausea that are difficult to differentiate from pain and nausea related to myocardial ischemia or infarction. Description of the pain, determination of cardiac risk factors, and appropriate use of an electrocardiogram (ECG) in adult patients with visceral-type pain or cardiac risk factors will minimize clinical errors. Nitroglycerin, antacids, and GI cocktails are therapeutic interventions not diagnostic tests. Patients with esophageal spasm may respond to nitroglycerin and antacids, or GI cocktails may provide a placebo-like benefit to patients with cardiac ischemia.

2. **What is a GI cocktail?**

   The two most commonly used GI cocktails contain antacids (30 mL), viscous lidocaine (10 mL), and either Donnatal (10 mL) or dicyclomine (Bentyl) (20 mg). These cocktails may provide temporary symptomatic relief of minor esophageal and gastric irritation. Recent studies show that antacids alone are as effective in temporary relief of symptoms as these cocktails.

3. **What is heartburn?**

   Retrosternal burning discomfort that may radiate to the sides of the chest, neck, or jaw. The description of the pain may be similar to the pain of cardiac ischemia. Heartburn is characteristic of reflux esophagitis and often is made worse by bending forward or lying recumbent after meals. It may be relieved by upright posture, liquids (including saliva or water), or, more reliably, antacids. Heartburn is probably due to heightened mucosal sensitivity and can be reproduced by infusion of dilute hydrochloric acid into the esophagus (Bernstein test).

4. **How is reflux esophagitis treated?**

   In addition to antacids, general measures include elevation of the head of the bed (e.g., 4 inches), weight reduction, and elimination of factors that increase abdominal pressure. Patients should avoid alcohol, chocolate, coffee, fatty foods, mint, orange juice, smoking, ingestion of large quantities of food and drink, and certain medications (e.g., anticholinergics or calcium channel blockers). Antacids after meals, H_2-blockers (e.g., cimetidine) before bedtime or daily proton pump inhibitors (omeprazole) are often helpful. Treatment is usually for 1–2 months, and the disease may recur.

5. **What are the esophageal causes of odynophagia?**

   Odynophagia, or painful swallowing, is a characteristic of nonreflux esophagitis. Infectious esophagitis is a common cause and usually occurs in immunocompromised patients, and it can be due to fungal (e.g., monilial), viral (e.g., herpes, cytomegalovirus), bacterial (e.g., *Lactobacillus,* β-hemolytic streptococci), or parasitic organisms. Other types of nonreflux esophagitis include radiation, corrosive, pill-induced, and certain systemic diseases (e.g., Behçet's, Crohn's, pemphigus vulgaris, Stevens-Johnson syndrome). Odynophagia is unusual in reflux esophagitis but may occur with a peptic ulcer of the esophagus (Barrett's ulcer).

6. **How does esophageal obstruction present?**

   Except in infants, there is usually a history of eating or swallowing something that is followed by the onset of chest pain, odynophagia, or inability to swallow. Foreign bodies usually lodge at one of four locations: cervical esophagus, upper esophageal sphincter, aortic arch, and lower esophageal sphincter. Obstruction by food may occur wherever there is narrowing of the lumen because of stricture, carcinoma, or a lower esophageal ring. Round, blunt objects may be removed using a Foley catheter that is inserted beyond the object; the balloon is inflated, then the catheter is withdrawn gently with the patient in a steep head-down position. This procedure most often is done under fluoroscopy. Foreign bodies, especially those that are sharp (e.g., needle); impacted food; or objects that cannot be removed with the Foley method are best removed endoscopically. Meat tenderizer should not be used to facilitate passage of obstructed meat. Glucagon (0.5–2 mg intravenously) may relieve distal esophageal food obstruction in a minority of patients.

7. **What is Mallory-Weiss syndrome?**
   A mucosal tear that usually involves the gastric mucosa near the squamocolumnar mucosal junction; it also may involve the esophageal mucosa. It usually is caused by vomiting and retching. Patients may present with upper GI bleeding.

8. **What causes esophageal perforation, and how is it diagnosed and treated?**
   Esophageal perforation, a true emergency, can be caused by iatrogenic damage during instrumentation, trauma (most often penetrating), increased intraesophageal pressure associated with forceful vomiting (Boerhaave's syndrome), or diseases of the esophagus (e.g., corrosive esophagitis, ulceration, neoplasm). Esophageal perforation causes chest pain that is often severe and may be worsened by swallowing and breathing. Chest radiograph may reveal air within the mediastinum, pericardium, pleural space (pneumothorax), or subcutaneous tissue. Esophageal perforation may lead to leakage of gastric contents into the mediastinum and secondary infection (i.e., mediastinitis). The diagnosis is confirmed by swallow and leakage of radiopaque contrast material. Treatment includes broad-spectrum antibiotics, gastric suction, and surgical repair and drainage as soon as possible.

9. **What are causes of abdominal pain that are gastric or duodenal in origin?**
   An estimated 10% of cases of abdominal pain seen in the emergency department (ED) are due to gastric or duodenal disease. Gastritis and peptic ulcer disease (PUD) (i.e., ulcer of the stomach or duodenum owing to gastric acid) account for most patients with abdominal pain secondary to gastric or duodenal disease. Perforated PUD and gastric volvulus are the two most serious conditions requiring immediate diagnosis and treatment.

10. **What are the common causes of gastritis and PUD?**
    Gastritis is associated with alcohol, salicylates, nonsteroidal anti-inflammatory drugs (NSAIDs), and hiatal hernia. PUD is related to family history, associated diseases (e.g., chronic obstructive pulmonary disease [COPD], cirrhosis, chronic renal failure), male gender, advanced age, and smoking. The use of certain drugs, such as aspirin or NSAIDs, and the psychological profile may be related to PUD, but diet (e.g., caffeine and spicy foods) and alcohol are not. *Helicobacter pylori* has been shown to be the frequent cause of duodenal ulcers. These patients should be treated with antibiotics (amoxicillin or clarithromycin) and proton pump inhibitors (omeprazole).

11. **How does perforated PUD present?**
    Perforated PUD (and gastric volvulus) presents with sudden onset of abdominal pain that may or may not be related to eating. The pain is usually steady and refractory to antacids; it often radiates to the back but also may radiate to the chest or upper abdomen. Vomiting is present in approximately 50%.
    On **physical examination,** patients appear in acute distress and often have tachycardia. Blood pressure may be elevated secondary to pain or decreased secondary to extensive fluid loss from generalized peritonitis. Patients usually lie still and avoid movement. Involuntary guarding, rebound tenderness, and abdominal rigidity are common. Bowel sounds are usually absent or significantly decreased.

Laboratory work may reveal nonspecific leukocytosis (40% have a white blood cell count greater than 14,000 per mm³). If vomiting has been protracted, hypochloremic, hypokalemic, metabolic alkalosis may be seen. A small percentage of patients have mild elevation in amylase or lipase. Free air is present on upright chest radiograph or abdominal left lateral decubitus view in more than 70% of patients.

12. **How should a patient suspected of having a perforated ulcer be managed?**
Patients with severe abdominal pain should be undressed, placed on cardiac and SaO_2 monitors, and have a large-bore intravenous catheter placed for fluid resuscitation with crystalloid (e.g., normal saline). Patients with oxygen saturation <93% should be given supplemental oxygen. A prompt but thorough physical examination should be done, including pelvic and rectal examinations. Blood should be drawn for complete blood count, electrolytes, blood urea nitrogen (BUN), creatinine, lipase, and type and screen. An ECG should be obtained on patients older than 40 years. A Foley catheter should be placed and urinalysis and urine pregnancy done as appropriate. A portable upright chest radiograph or abdominal left lateral decubitus view often helps to show free intraperitoneal air. A nasogastric (NG) tube should be placed after anesthetizing the nasopharynx and prompt surgical consultation obtained. Broad-spectrum antibiotics should be given and the patient prepared for emergency laparotomy. Finally, intravenous analgesics (opiates) should be given for patient comfort.

13. **What differentiates upper from lower GI hemorrhage?**
Upper GI hemorrhage is bleeding that is proximal to the ligament of Treitz, and lower GI bleeding is distal. In the ED, this is evaluated by placement of an NG or orogastric tube and aspiration of gastric and proximal duodenal contents. Physical appearance of the aspirate (coffee grounds, red-tinged fluid, or fresh blood) is the best way of determining the presence of significant upper GI bleeding; testing of gastric content for blood with various cards (e.g., Hemoccult) is not reliable.

14. **List the causes of upper GI bleeding.**
    - PUD (45%)
    - Gastric erosions (23%)
    - Varices (10%)
    - Mallory-Weiss tear (7%)
    - Esophagitis (6%)
    - Duodenitis (6%)

    Henneman PL: Gastrointestinal bleeding. In Rosen P, Barkin RM (eds): Emergency Medicine and Clinical Practice, 5th ed. St. Louis, Mosby, 2002, pp 194–200.

15. **Discuss the emergency management of upper GI bleeding.**
Management begins with a rapid assessment and management of the patient's airway, breathing, and cardiovascular status. Patients should be undressed, placed on cardiac and SaO_2 monitors, and given supplemental oxygen (i.e., SaO_2 <93%). The history of GI bleeding (i.e., vomiting blood or passing black or bloody stool) is sufficient to lead to the placement of a large-bore, peripheral intravenous catheter with infusion of normal saline. A focused physical examination should be done, checking for signs of shock (e.g., altered mental status, tachycardia, hypotension, cool extremities, delayed capillary fill). Patients who have abnormal vital signs or signs of shock should have two or more intravenous lines placed and be given rapid infusion of crystalloid (20–40 mL/kg). The evaluation should include testing of stool for blood. During the initial examination and resuscitation, a history should be obtained. Patients with stable vital signs should be cautiously evaluated for postural changes in blood pressure or pulse. Blood should be drawn for type and crossmatching, hematocrit, platelet count, prothrombin time, electrolytes, BUN, and creatinine. Elderly patients, patients with a history of cardiovascular disease or chest pain, and patients who are severely anemic should have an ECG

to evaluate for signs of cardiac ischemia (i.e., ST depression). Obtain a chest radiograph (upright) to rule out subdiaphragmatic air or aspiration. An NG (or orogastric) tube should be placed to determine the presence of blood in the stomach, then removed.

16. What happens to these patients with GI hemorrhage?

GI bleeding usually stops spontaneously, and no further ED management is necessary other than admission and perhaps transfusion if there is significant anemia (i.e., hematocrit <25%). In 20% or less of patients, continued GI hemorrhage requires prompt management and treatment.

17. How do I facilitate the placement of an NG tube?

Applying an anesthetic spray to the nose and posterior pharynx or having the patient breathe nebulized 4% lidocaine decreases the discomfort of placing the NG tube.

18. How should a patient with continued GI hemorrhage be managed?

Blood replacement should begin in patients who continue to show signs of shock or cardiovascular instability. Patients who do not respond promptly (i.e., remain hypotensive) to a 30 mL/kg infusion of crystalloid should be given O-negative blood if type-specific blood is not yet available. Crossmatched blood takes approximately 45–60 minutes to become available. If patients continue to show signs of shock or require more than 3 or 4 U of blood, surgery and gastroenterology consultation should be initiated promptly. Upper GI bleeding may be stopped through the endoscope, but emergency operative repair often is required in patients with persistent GI bleeding.

19. Is placement of an NG or orogastric tube contraindicated in someone with esophageal varices?

There is no evidence that a properly placed NG or orogastric tube results in a significantly increased risk of tearing varices or increased size of a Mallory-Weiss tear. NG or orogastric tubes can perforate the esophagus or posterior pharynx if they are placed too aggressively. Diagnostic NG or orogastric tubes are unnecessary if the patient vomits gastric contents in the ED because this may be inspected for the presence of blood.

20. Does iced saline lavage decrease gastric bleeding?

No. The use of iced fluid to lavage patients with upper GI hemorrhage no longer is recommended because it may result in hypothermia.

KEY POINTS: ESOPHAGUS AND STOMACH DISORDERS

1. Epigastric pain may be due to myocardial ischemia, so an ECG should be obtained in all elderly patients with epigastric discomfort.

2. Antacids often provide symptomatic relief of abdominal discomfort related to gastroesophageal disease.

3. *H. pylori* is a common, treatable cause of peptic ulcer disease.

4. Upper gastrointestinal bleeding in most patients stops spontaneously.

5. All patients with gastrointestinal bleeding should be risk stratified for proper management and disposition.

21. When should gastric lavage be used in patients with upper GI bleeding?
Gastric lavage is necessary only in patients who have no aspirate after the tube is placed. Lavage fluid need not be saline or sterile; regular tap water is fine. The only other indication for gastric lavage in patients with upper GI bleeding is immediately before endoscopy to improve visualization.

22. Should all patients with upper GI bleeding undergo endoscopy?
Endoscopy is the most accurate diagnostic tool available in the evaluation of patients with upper GI bleeding, identifying a lesion in 78–95% of patients if it is done within 12–24 hours of hemorrhage. Accurate identification of the bleeding site allows risk stratification with respect to predicting rebleeding and mortality. Risk stratification facilitates a proper disposition decision.

23. How does one risk-stratify patients with GI bleeding?
See Tables 32-1 and 32-2.

24. What are the low-risk criteria that allow a patient who is complaining of GI bleeding to be sent home?
- No comorbid diseases
- Normal vital signs
- Normal or trace positive stool guaiac
- Negative gastric aspirate, if done
- Normal or near-normal hemoglobin and hematocrit
- Good home support
- Proper understanding of signs and symptoms of significant bleeding
- Immediate access to emergent care if needed
- Follow-up arranged within 24 hours

TABLE 32-1. INITIAL ED RISK STRATIFICATION FOR PATIENTS WITH GI BLEEDING		
Low Risk	**Moderate Risk**	**High Risk**
Age <60 years	Age >60 years	
Initial SBP ≥100 mmHg	Initial SBP <100 mmHg	Persistent SBP <100 mmHg
Normal vitals for 1 h	Mild ongoing tachycardia for 1 h	Persistent moderate-to-severe tachycardia
No transfusion requirement	Transfusion required ≤4 U	Transfusion required >4 U
No active major comorbid diseases	Stable major comorbid diseases	Unstable major comorbid diseases
No liver disease	Mild liver disease—PT normal or near normal	Decompensated liver disease—coagulopathy, ascites, encephalopathy
No moderate or high-risk clinical features	No high-risk clinical features	

ED = emergency department, GI = gastrointestinal, SBP = systolic blood pressure, PT = prothrombin time.
Adapted from Terdiman PK, Lindenauer: Acute gastrointestinal bleeding. In Wachter RM, Goldman L, Hollander H (eds): Hospital Medicine. 2nd ed. Philadelphia, Lippincott Williams & Wilkins, 2005, pp 767–779.

TABLE 32-2. FINAL RISK STRATIFICATION FOR PATIENTS WITH UPPER GI BLEEDING AFTER ENDOSCOPY

	Clinical Risk Stratification		
Endoscopy	Low Risk	Moderate Risk	High Risk
Low risk	Immediate discharge*	24-h inpatient stay (floor)†	Close monitoring for 24 h‡; ≥ 48-h hospitalization
Moderate risk	24-h patient stay†	24–48 h inpatient stay (floor)†	Close monitoring for 24 h; ≥ 48-h hospitalization
High risk	Close monitoring for 24 h; 48–72 h hospitalization	Close monitoring for 24 h; 48–72 h hospitalization	Close monitoring ≥ 72-h hospitalization

GI = gastrointestinal.

*Patients with low-risk clinical and endoscopic findings can be discharged home with appropriate treatment based on diagnosis, scheduled follow-up evaluation within 24 h, and proper patient education to ensure immediate return if signs of rebleeding.

†Patients may be discharged after 24–48 h of in-hospital observation if there is no evidence of rebleeding, vital signs are normal, there is no need for further transfusion, and the hemoglobin or hematocrit has remained stable. They should be provided with appropriate treatment based on diagnosis, scheduled follow-up evaluation within 24 h, and proper patient education to ensure immediate return if signs of rebleeding.

‡Patients with high-risk clinical or endoscopic findings should be admitted and closely monitored for evidence of rebleeding.

Adapted from Terdiman PK, Lindenauer: Acute gastrointestinal bleeding. In Wachter RM, Goldman L, Hollander H (eds): Hospital Medicine. 2nd ed. Philadelphia, Lippincott Williams & Wilkins, 2005, pp 767–779.

BIBLIOGRAPHY

1. Henneman PL: Gastrointestinal bleeding. In Marx JA, Hockberger RS, Walls RM (eds): Rosen's Emergency Medicine Concepts and Clinical Practice, 6th ed. St. Louis, Mosby, 2006, pp 220–227.

2. Lowell MJ: Esophagus, stomach, and duodenum. In Marx JA, Hockberger RS, Walls RM (eds): Rosen's Emergency Medicine Concepts and Clinical Practice, 6th ed. St. Louis, Mosby, 2006, pp 1382–1401.

CHAPTER 33

BOWEL DISORDERS

James S. Eadie, MD, and Vikhyat S. Bebarta, MD

1. **When do you consider evaluating a patient for appendicitis?**
   Consider appendicitis in anyone presenting with abdominal pain. It can occur at any age, but is most prevalent in the teens and 20s. With the high prevalence of appendicitis in the population, atypical presentations are common. Appendicitis is one of the most commonly missed diagnoses in the emergency department (ED), and it is the most common nonobstetrical emergency during pregnancy.

   e-medicine.com: www.emedicine.com/emerg/topic41.htm

2. **What are the cause and pathogenesis of acute appendicitis?**
   The appendix lumen becomes obstructed, most commonly by a fecalith, leading to bacterial overgrowth and dilation of the appendix. Early on, the distended lumen causes dull, diffuse abdominal pain. As the inflammation progresses, a localized peritonitis develops, producing the classic right lower quadrant (RLQ) pain with involuntary guarding and rebound on physical examination.

3. **How does appendicitis clinically present?**
   The classic presentation is nonspecific, umbilical abdominal pain that migrates over several hours to the RLQ of the abdomen. Associated symptoms include nausea, anorexia, and fever. However, variation of the appendix location leads to varied clinical presentations. For example, a retrocecal appendix may cause back or flank pain that can be mistakenly diagnosed as pyelonephritis or symptomatic nephrolithiasis. An extra long appendix with an inflamed tip may produce left lower quadrant pain. In pregnancy, the appendix is displaced into the right upper quadrant and, when inflamed, may be mistaken for symptomatic gallbladder disease. Other diagnoses of RLQ pain should be also be considered (Table 33-1).

TABLE 33-1. DIFFERENTIAL DIAGNOSIS FOR RIGHT LOWER QUADRANT ABDOMINAL PAIN

Acute ileitis	Inflammatory bowel disease
Diverticulitis	Acute cholecystitis
Perforated gastric or duodenal ulcer	Volvulus
Intussusception	Small bowel obstruction
Inflammation of Meckel's diverticulum	Uterine or tubo-ovarian pathology (e.g., tubo-ovarian abscess, ovarian torsion, ovarian cysts)
Incarcerated inguinal hernia	Ectopic pregnancy
Testicular torsion or epididymitis	Mittelschmerz
Mesenteric adenitis	Pyelonephritis, symptomatic nephrolithiasis

4. **Is the physical exam reliable in appendicitis?**

   Unfortunately, the classic physical exam findings of appendicitis—RLQ guarding and rebound, and positive psoas, obturator, or Rovsing's signs—are neither specific nor sensitive enough to accurately diagnose appendicitis. Standard laboratory test results may raise or lower your clinical suspicion, but only an abdominal computed tomogram (CT) scan or direct visualization with surgery can reliably diagnose an inflamed appendix. Frequently, nonspecific RLQ pain and tenderness are the only clinical findings of appendicitis.

   Rao PM, Rhea JT, Rattner DW, et al: Introduction of appendiceal CT: impact on negative appendectomy and appendiceal perforation rates. Ann Surg 229:344–349, 1999.

5. **What laboratory tests are helpful in evaluating RLQ pain?**

   Although no laboratory test is diagnostic of appendicitis, tests can aid in the evaluation of the patient and exclude other diagnoses:
   - **White blood cell count:** >10,000 per mm^3 in approximately 90% of cases
   - **Urinalysis:** To exclude urinary tract infection (However, mild pyuria or hematuria may be present when an inflamed appendix lies near the bladder or ureter.)
   - **Beta-human chorionic gonadotropin:** To exclude ectopic pregnancy

6. **What radiologic study is best at imaging the appendix?**

   The **abdominal CT** is the imaging modality of choice for appendicitis. The scan is routinely done with intravenous and oral or rectal contrast enhancement. It has a reported accuracy of 93–98% in ruling in or out the diagnosis of appendicitis and is more sensitive and specific than any combination of physical exam and laboratory findings. The CT is cost effective because it reduces negative laparotomy rates. Additionally, the CT scan may show other diseases responsible for the patient's symptoms.

   Rao PM, Rhea JT, Novelline RA, et al: Effect of computed tomography of the appendix on treatment of patients and use of hospital resources. N Engl J Med 338:141–146, 1998.

7. **What is the treatment for appendicitis?**

   Appendectomy is the definitive treatment. Once appendicitis has been diagnosed, or is highly suspected, a surgical consult should be obtained. Fluid resuscitation, pain control, and broad-spectrum antibiotics should be started while waiting for surgery. A delay in diagnosis and treatment increase the risk of perforation.

8. **What is mesenteric ischemia?**

   Mesenteric ischemia is caused by insufficient blood supply to the intestines leading to tissue ischemia and infarction. The most common causes are arterial emboli (most common) or thrombus, venous thrombosis, or nonocclusive hypoperfusion states. Patients should be assessed for risk factors of mesenteric ischemia (Table 33-2).

TABLE 33-2.   RISK FACTORS FOR MESENTERIC ISCHEMIA

Age greater than 50 years	Recent myocardial infarction
Valvular or atherosclerotic heart disease	Arrhythmias (e.g., atrial fibrillation)
Peripheral vascular disease	Critical illness with hypotension or sepsis
Congestive heart failure	Diuretics or vasoconstrictive drugs

9. **How do patients with mesenteric ischemia present?**

   Patients complain of a diffusely painful abdomen. In the early state, patients complain of severe pain but have minimal physical findings—the characteristic "pain out of proportion to the examination." As the infarction develops, peritoneal signs develop. Vomiting, hematochezia, hematemesis, abdominal distention, fever, and shock are late signs that often indicate infarcted bowel.

10. How do I diagnose mesenteric ischemia?

Diagnosing mesenteric ischemia can be difficult. The combination of clinical suspicion, radiographic imaging, and laboratory findings can help lead to the correct diagnosis. Direct surgical visualization of the bowel remains the gold standard. The abdominal CT with intravenous and oral contrast can show the location of the vascular occlusion and secondary findings consistent with ischemia, such as air within the bowel wall, intestinal wall thickening, and local inflammation. Laboratory findings may include leukocytosis; hemoconcentration; metabolic acidosis; and elevated phosphate, lactate, or lactate dehydrogenase. These lab findings may indicate ischemic bowel but lack sensitivity and specificity.

Segatto E, Mortele KJ, Ji H, et al: Acute small bowel ischemia: CT imaging findings. Semin Ultrasound CT MR. 24:364–376, 2003.

11. How is mesenteric ischemia treated?

Initial treatment includes vigorous resuscitation, parenteral antibiotics, correction of predisposing factors, and early surgical consultation. Definitive management involves selective vasodilator infusion, anticoagulation in venous occlusion, or embolectomy. Laparotomy is necessary for resection of necrotic bowel.

12. What is intussusception?

Intussusception occurs when an intestinal segment invaginates and telescopes into an adjacent segment. This is a disease predominately seen in children, but it can occur in adults (*see* Chapter 62). Typical pathologic lesions include tumors, Meckel's diverticulum, and inflammatory lesions. The high frequency of mass lesions in adults mandates surgical exploration.

13. What is IBD?

Inflammatory bowel disease (IBD) is an idiopathic, chronic inflammatory disease of the intestine. It encompasses two main groups: **Crohn's disease (CD)** and **ulcerative colitis (UC)**. CD is also known as *regional enteritis* or *granulomatous ileocolitis*. CD and UC are rising in incidence. Common clinical features are summarized in Table 33-3.

TABLE 33-3. COMMON FEATURES FOR INFLAMMATORY BOWEL DISEASE		
	Crohn's Disease	**Ulcerative colitis**
Clinical feature		
Weight loss	Common	Fairly common
Fever	Common	Fairly common
Diarrhea	Fairly common	Very common
Rectal bleeding	Fairly common	Very common
Perianal disease	Common	None
Site		
Colon	{2/3} of patients	Exclusively
Ileum	{2/3} of patients	None
Jejunum, stomach, or esophagus	Uncommon	None

Continued

TABLE 33-3. COMMON FEATURES FOR INFLAMMATORY BOWEL DISEASE—CONT'D

	Crohn's Disease	Ulcerative colitis
Intestinal complications		
Stricture	Common	Unknown
Fistulas	Fairly common	None
Toxic megacolon	None	Unknown
Perforation	Uncommon	Unknown
Cancer	Fairly common	Common
Endoscopic findings		
Friability	Fairly common	Very common
Aphthous and linear ulcers	Common	None
Cobblestone appearance	Common	None
Rectal involvement	Fairly common	Very common
Radiologic findings		
Distribution	Discontinuous, segmental	Continuous
Ulceration	Deep	Superficial
Fissures	Common	None
Strictures for fistulas	Common	Rare
Ileal involvement	Narrowed, nodular	Dilated

Adapted from Podolsky DK: Inflammatory bowel disease. N Engl J Med 347:417–429, 2002.

14. **How do CD and UC present?**
    Although they are pathologically distinct diseases, CD and UC can present in a similar fashion
    and affect all age groups (*see* Table 33–3). Both diseases may present with diarrhea, abdominal
    pain, fever, anorexia, weight loss, and bloody diarrhea; however, UC is more likely to present
    with bloody diarrhea. In nonfulminating colitis, the diagnosis can be confirmed by endoscopy or
    barium enema.

15. **What is the ED management for IBD?**
    Patients with mild disease and no signs of life-threatening complications can be treated as
    outpatients with close follow-up. Treatment usually consists of sulfasalazine, steroids (oral or
    rectal), steroid-sparing agents such as 6-mercaptopurine, antidiarrheal agents (e.g., loperamide,
    Lomotil, and cholestyramine), and analgesia. Antidiarrheal agents should be used with caution
    because they can predispose to toxic megacolon. Metronidazole may help treat the chronic
    perirectal complications of CD. Patients should be admitted if they have severe disease or any life-
    threatening complications. Extraintestinal manifestations of IBD can also occur (Table 33-4).

    Podolsky DK: Inflammatory bowel disease. N Engl J Med 347:417–429, 2002.

16. **Describe what happens during intestinal obstruction.**
    When the large and small bowels become obstructed, loss of the normal forward flow of
    digested food and secretions occurs. Proximal to the obstruction, a build up of bowel gas,
    gastric secretions, and food develops. The bowel then becomes distended, causing pain,
    vomiting, and decreased oral intake. The cause of the obstruction can be mechanical or

TABLE 33-4. COMMON EXTRAINTESTINAL MANIFESTATIONS OF INFLAMMATORY BOWEL DISEASE

Clinical Category	Disorder
Ocular	Uveitis, episcleritis
Dermatologic	Erythema nodosum, pyoderma gangrenosum
Musculoskeletal	Ankylosing spondylitis, peripheral arthritis, sacroiliitis
Hepatobiliary	Cholelithiasis, pericholangitis, hepatitis, fatty liver, primary sclerosing cholangitis, cholangiocarcinoma, pancreatitis
Hematologic	Thromboembolic disease, chronic anemia
Renal	Nephrolithiasis, amyloidosis leading to renal failure

adynamic. Mechanical obstruction from adhesions or tumors frequently requires surgical intervention, whereas an adynamic ileus usually resolves spontaneously within a few days.

17. **What are the common causes of small bowel obstruction (SBO)?**
Overall, adhesions, hernias, and cancer account for more than 90% of SBO cases. **Postoperative adhesions** are the most common cause of a SBO (56%), followed by **incarcerated hernia** (25%) and **cancer** (10%). Other less common causes include IBD, gallstones, volvulus, intussusception, radiation enteritis, abscesses, congenital lesions, and bezoars.

18. **What are the clinical features of SBO?**
Patients present with diffuse abdominal pain, distention, and occasionally, vomiting. Early on, the pain is mild, crampy, and colicky in nature. An SBO in its early state can be difficult to diagnose. The patient complains of pain but continues to have flatus and passage of some stool. As the obstruction progresses, the intestinal contents build up proximally, leading to nausea and vomiting. The intestine distal to the obstruction empties of stool and has decreased peristaltic motion leading to obstipation (inability to pass feces or flatus). Auscultation may reveal high-pitched, hyperactive *tinkling* or *rushing* sounds. Rectal examination may reveal impacted stool.

19. **Describe the radiographic findings in SBO.**
The classic finding on abdominal plain films is multiple air-fluid levels and distended loops of small bowel. When the obstructed intestine contains more fluid than gas, small round pockets of air may line up to form the *string of pearls* sign. A paucity of stool and gas is noted distal to the obstruction. Plain films have sensitivity of 41–86% and a specificity of 25–88%; therefore, an early SBO may be missed by using only radiographs to diagnose the obstruction. Abdominal CT scan has a higher sensitivity (100%) and specificity (83%). Additionally, CT scan can show the location of the obstruction and help identify the cause (e.g., mass, or infection such as appendicitis or diverticulitis).

20. **What is the treatment for SBO?**
The initial emergency management includes cardiopulmonary support, electrolyte replacement, decompression with a nasogastric tube, and intravenous fluids. Patients lose a large amount of fluid into the obstructed bowel and can be significantly intravascularly depleted. SBOs can often be managed nonoperatively with observation, intravenous fluid resuscitation, and bowel rest. However, some complete or mechanical obstructions require surgery. A surgical consultation is indicated during the ED visit.

21. **What are the characteristics of an ileus?**

    The terms *ileus* and *adynamic ileus* are synonymous for a paralyzed intestine. The bowel is unable to perform peristalsis. This is the most common cause of SBO. Causes of an ileus include infection (e.g., peritonitis), drugs (e.g., narcotics, anticholinergics), electrolyte imbalance (e.g., hypokalemia), spinal cord injuries, and recent bowel surgery. Patients present with abdominal distention, nausea and vomiting, and obstipation. Abdominal examination reveals hypoactive bowel sounds, mild tenderness, and absence of peritoneal signs. Radiographs usually show minimally distended bowel throughout the entire gastrointestinal (GI) tract, with diffuse air-fluid levels in the small bowel.

22. **How is an ileus treated?**

    Management is similar to SBO. Limit oral intake, resuscitate with intravenous fluids, and correct electrolyte abnormalities, particularly hypokalemia. If abdominal distention is present, place a nasogastric or orogastric tube to decompress the stomach. Identify and limit the patient's medications, such as opioids, that slow intestinal motility. If the ileus is prolonged ($> 3–5$ days), obtain additional imaging to search for an underlying cause.

23. **What are the causes of large bowel obstruction (LBO)?**

    LBO is caused most commonly by colon cancer (60%), volvulus (20%), and diverticular disease (10%). Primary adenocarcinoma accounts for most cancerous lesions. Other less likely causes include metastatic carcinoma, gynecologic tumors, IBD, intussusception, and fecal impaction. In infants, consider congenital disorders, such as Hirschsprung's disease or an imperforate anus. Hernias and adhesions are uncommon causes of LBO.

24. **What are diverticula and what are common complications?**

    Diverticula are saclike outpouchings of the colon that occur through weakened areas of the muscularis of the colon wall. They commonly occur in persons of industrialized nations and increase in frequency with age. It is estimated that one third of the U.S. population will develop diverticula by age 50, and two thirds by 85 years. Complications from diverticula include bleeding and diverticulitis, a localized infection. Diverticulitis is caused by obstruction of the opening of a diverticula, usually by stool, leading to infection from the proliferation of colonic bacteria and build-up of bowel secretions within the diverticula.

25. **How does diverticulitis clinically present?**

    The most common symptom of diverticulitis is abdominal pain. The pain usually evolves over 1–2 days from dull, diffuse abdominal pain to more intense, localized left lower quadrant pain. Patients may complain of fevers, nausea, vomiting, and decreased appetite. Diverticulitis occurs most frequently in the descending and sigmoid regions of the colon but can occur throughout the colon. The abdominal CT scan is the diagnostic procedure of choice and can show evidence for abscesses, bowel perforation, and severity of disease.

26. **How do you manage diverticulitis?**

    Management consists of intravenous fluids, electrolyte replacement, parenteral analgesics, bowel rest, and broad-spectrum antibiotics. Patients with mild symptoms who are able to eat and have close follow-up can be managed as outpatients with oral antibiotics and close follow-up. Patients who have systemic or severe symptoms, older age, comorbidities, abscess, or bowel perforations require hospitalization, intravenous antibiotics, and serial examinations. Surgery may be required for repeat episodes or for bowel perforation. Abscess requires surgical or interventional radiology catheter drainage.

Ferzoco LB, Raptopoulos V, Silen W: Current concepts: Acute diverticulitis. N Engl J Med 338:1521–1526, 1998.

KEY POINTS: BOWEL DISORDERS

1. Appendicitis is common, and unusual presentations are frequent; therefore, always consider appendicitis in a patient with abdominal pain.

2. A patient with atrial fibrillation and abdominal pain has mesenteric ischemia until proven otherwise.

3. Surgical adhesions are the most frequent cause of a small bowel obstruction.

4. Patients with a small bowel obstruction should be aggressively resuscitated with intravenous fluids in the ED due to the extensive depletion of intravascular fluid.

5. Although diverticulitis is most commonly seen in the older patient population, younger patients (20–40 years) also develop it.

6. Inflammatory bowel disease can cause complicated rectal abscesses or fissures that require surgical consultation.

27. What are common causes of lower GI bleeding?

Patients frequently present to the ED with complaints of rectal bleeding. Lower GI bleeds occur from many causes, and a thorough history and exam are vital to diagnose the bleeding source. Investigating anatomically from the rectum proximally, evaluate for hemorrhoids and rectal fissures, then, based on history and exam, consider diverticulosis, polyps, cancer, arteriovenous (AV) malformation, IBD, ischemic colitis, infectious diarrhea, and finally an upper GI source.

28. How do you perform anoscopy?

Anoscopy can provide a direct view of the anus and distal rectum. A lubricated anoscope with the obturator in place is advanced gently through the anal orifice. The obturator is removed to view the distal rectal mucosa; a light source is shined into the barrel of the anoscope, and the anoscope is withdrawn slowly while searching for internal hemorrhoids, fissures, abscess, masses, or bleeding proximal to the rectum.

29. What are hemorrhoids?

Hemorrhoids are engorged vascular cushions comprised of internal or external hemorrhoidal veins and present most often with bleeding, pain, or rectal itching. They are associated with prolonged increase in resting pressure in the anal canal most often from constipation but also seen in pregnancy, excessive straining, and in certain occupations (e.g., truck driver).

30. How do internal and external hemorrhoids differ?

- **Internal hemorrhoids** arise above the dentate line, are covered by mucosa, and are not usually palpable or painful. They are seen during anoscopy and typically present as bright red blood in the toilet bowl or on toilet paper.
- **External hemorrhoids** are covered by skin and are easily visible and palpable at the anal orifice. A common complication of external hemorrhoids is thrombosis, which is very painful and requires excision of the thrombus.

31. How are hemorrhoids treated?

Treat mildly symptomatic hemorrhoids with irrigation during the shower or bath, stool softeners, high-fiber diet, bulk laxatives (e.g., psyllium or methycellulose), increased fluid consumption, proper anal hygiene, and analgesics if necessary. Nonthrombosed prolapsed hemorrhoids should be gently reduced. Thrombosed hemorrhoids should be excised. Patients with intractable symptoms need surgical referral.

32. **What is an anal fissure?**

An anal fissure is a linear crack or ulcer in the epithelium in the distal anal canal. Anal fissures are the most common cause of rectal pain. Most are idiopathic, but any anal canal trauma can cause a fissure. Most benign anal fissures occur in the posterior midline, followed by the anterior midline. Fissures in other locations are associated with CD, infection, malignancy, or immunodeficiency.

33. **How do I treat an anal fissure?**

Most anal fissures can be managed conservatively with sitz baths, stool softeners, high-fiber diet, bulk laxatives (e.g., psyllium or methycellulose), additional fluid consumption, proper anal hygiene, and analgesics. Recent studies have shown good success with the use of topical 0.2% nitroglycerin ointment applied twice daily for 6 weeks or a single botulinum injection. Fissures that do not improve with conservative therapies should be referred to a surgeon for consideration of a lateral internal sphincterotomy.

Brisinda G, Maria G, Bentivoglio AR, et al: A comparison of injections of botulinum toxin and topical nitroglycerin ointment for the treatment of chronic anal fissure. N Engl J Med 341:65–69, 1999.

34. **Can I drain anorectal abscesses in the ED?**

Small isolated perianal abscesses can be drained successfully in the ED. These abscesses can be very painful, requiring both local anesthetic and oral or parenteral sedation. For complicated or deep rectal abscesses, consult surgery for operative drainage.

CHAPTER 34

LIVER AND BILIARY TRACT DISEASE

Kaushal Shah, MD, and Larry Nathanson, MD

1. **What are the common manifestations of biliary disease?**

   Cholelithiasis is the presence of gallstones in the gallbladder without evidence of infection. Among adults, 8% of men and 17% of women have gallstones, and the incidence increases with age.

   - **Biliary colic** is right upper quadrant or epigastric pain sometimes radiating to the right shoulder or scapula. It usually lasts less than 6 hours, occurs after a fatty meal, and is thought to be due to transient obstruction of the cystic duct by a gallstone.
   - Of patients with colic, 30% progress to **cholecystitis,** a bacterial overgrowth and infection of the gallbladder caused by obstruction of the cystic duct.
   - **Choledocholithiasis** occurs when the gallstone lodges in the common bile duct and can cause cholecystitis or pancreatitis (if the ampulla of Vater is obstructed) or both.
   - **Cholangitis** is a severe infection of the biliary tract that presents as right upper quadrant pain, fever and chills, and jaundice (Charcot's triad) and may include shock and mental status changes (Reynold's pentad).
   - **Emphysematous cholecystitis** is caused by gas-forming bacteria and is seen with vascular insufficiency. It is more frequent in men and diabetic patients and often is accompanied by sepsis.

   Feldman M (ed): Sleisenger and Fordtran's Gastrointestinal and Liver Disease, 7th ed. Philadelphia, W.B. Saunders, 2002, pp 1065–1090.

   Lum DF, Leung JW: Bacterial cholangitis. Curr Treat Opt Gastroenterol 4:139–146, 2001.

   See rad.usuhs.mil/medpix/medpix.html?mode=tsearch2&srchstr=cholecystitis for excellent imaging and pathology images of these conditions.

2. **Do all gallstones produce pain? Does a lack of stones preclude cholecystitis?**

   Of patients with gallstones, 80% are asymptomatic. Fifteen to 30% of asymptomatic patients develop symptoms within 15 years. Although 90–95% of cholecystitis cases are in the setting of gallstones, 5–10% are not secondary to cholelithiasis and are termed *acalculous cholecystitis*. This can be a challenging diagnosis because these patients often have concomitant medical conditions, such as diabetes, burns, multisystem trauma, acquired immunodeficiency syndrome (AIDS), or sepsis.

   Yusoff IF, Barkun JS, Barkun AN: Diagnosis and management of cholecystitis and cholangitis. Gastroenterol Clin North Am 32:1152–1153, 2003.

3. **What is Murphy's sign?**

   The sign is named after a prominent Chicago surgeon, John B. Murphy (1857–1916). The patient is asked to take a deep breath while the examiner applies pressure over the area of the gallbladder. If the gallbladder is inflamed, the descending diaphragm forces it against the examiner's fingertips, causing pain and often a sudden halt to the inspiration. A sonographic Murphy's sign uses the ultrasound probe instead of the examiner's fingers and is positive when the site of maximal tenderness localizes to the gallbladder.

4. **Can a plain radiograph of the abdomen aid diagnosis?**

   Maybe. Only 10–15% of gallstones contain sufficient calcium to be radiopaque. Air can be seen in the biliary tree or the gallbladder wall when infection is due to gas-forming bacteria or there is a biliary-intestinal fistula. In cases in which the cause of upper abdominal pain is unclear, a flat plate may help by showing free air, pancreatic calcifications, ileus, obstruction, pneumatosis, or lower lobe lung consolidation.

5. **What is the gold standard for diagnosing cholecystitis?**
   Although ultrasound is the test of choice in the emergency department (ED), a **hepatobiliary iminodiacetic acid (HIDA) scan** is 95% accurate if the gallbladder does not fill with radioisotope within 4 hours after injection.

6. **Is an elevated temperature or white blood cell count necessary for diagnosis?**
   No, they are not helpful for diagnosis, as is seen in one study in which 71% of patients with acute nongangrenous cholecystitis were afebrile, and 32% had normal white blood cell count.

   Gruber PJ, Silverman RA, Gottesfeld S, et al: Presence of fever and leukocytosis in acute cholecystis. Ann Emerg Med 28:273–277, 1996.

7. **Describe the ultrasound findings in cholecystitis.**
   Gallstones can be detected directly, or sometimes their presence can be inferred by interference with transmission of ultrasound waves (*acoustic shadowing*) (Fig. 34-1). Other helpful findings include a thickened gallbladder wall (>3 mm), fluid collections around the gallbladder (*pericholecystic fluid*), and common ductal dilation (>6 mm).

   Shah K, Wolfe R: Hepatobiliary ultrasound. Emerg Med Clin North Am 22:661–673, 2004.

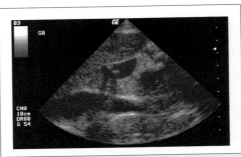

Figure 34-1. Gallstones can be detected directly, or sometimes their presence can be inferred by interference with transmission of ultrasound waves (*acoustic shadowing*).

KEY POINTS: ULTRASOUND FINDINGS OF CHOLECYSTITIS

1. Presence of gallstones

2. Gallbladder wall thickening >3 mm

3. Pericholecystic fluid

4. Common bile duct dilatation >6 mm

8. **When should elective surgery be considered in patients with asymptomatic cholelithiasis?**
   Cholecystectomy should be considered in diabetics, patients with a porcelain gallbladder, and patients with a history of biliary pancreatitis.
   - Diabetics have increased morbidity and mortality when urgent cholecystectomy is done in the setting of cholecystitis.

- Calcified or porcelain gallbladders have a 22% association with carcinoma.
- The risks of pancreatitis may outweigh the risks of elective cholecystectomy.

9. **What are Courvoisier's law, Klatskin's tumor, and Fitz-Hugh-Curtis syndrome?**
   - **Courvoisier's law** states that a palpable gallbladder in the setting of painless jaundice is likely to represent obstruction of the common bile duct by a malignancy, usually carcinoma of the pancreatic head.
   - **Klatskin's tumor** is a malignant tumor located where the hepatic ducts form the common duct.
   - **Fitz-Hugh-Curtis syndrome** is caused by pelvic inflammatory disease extending up the right paracolic gutter, causing inflammation of the capsule of the liver (perihepatitis), and can lead to adhesions between the liver and abdominal wall.

10. **What is a porcelain gallbladder?**
    A gallbladder with calcified walls. This is an important finding because 22% are associated with carcinoma, and it is an indication for cholecystectomy in asymptomatic patients. There is a higher incidence in women and Native Americans, especially members of the Pima tribe.

    Sheth S, Bedford A, Chopra S: Primary gallbladder cancer: Recognition of risk factors and the role of prophylactic cholecystectomy. Am J Gastroenterol 95:1402–1410, 2000.

11. **Are all gallstones created equal?**
    No. Cholesterol stones usually are found in the stereotypical, **female, fat, forty, fertile** patient. Asian patients and patients with parasitic infections, chronic liver/biliary disease, or chronic hemolysis states (i.e., sickle cell, spherocytosis) are more likely to have pigment stones.

12. **What is ERCP? What is the most common complication that presents to the ED after an ERCP procedure?**
    Endoscopic retrograde cholangiopancreatography (ERCP) is a procedure that examines the pancreatic and bile ducts for disease or irregularities with the ability of removing lodged stones and opening narrowed ducts with stents. The most common serious complication is pancreatitis, which occurs in approximately 1% of cases.

13. **What are liver function tests?**
    Elevated blood levels of the intracellular enzymes aspartate aminotransferase (AST) and alanine aminotransferase (ALT), correlate with liver injury not function. Liver function is analyzed best by measuring factors affected by hepatic protein synthesis. Acute liver failure results in a decrease in vitamin K–dependent coagulation factors (except factor VIII), leading to a prolonged prothrombin time. The liver also synthesizes albumin, although its longer half-life makes it a better marker of subacute or chronic liver disease.

14. **What is the difference between conjugated and unconjugated bilirubinemia?**
    Bilirubin is a breakdown product of hemoglobin and related proteins. In its **unconjugated,** hydrophobic form, it is unable to be excreted into bile, although it can traverse the blood–brain barrier and placenta. Bilirubin is **conjugated** in the liver with glucuronic acid, making it more water soluble for excretion into the bile. A predominance of unconjugated bilirubin occurs when there is overproduction (due to hemolysis) or decreased conjugation (due to inborn metabolism syndromes of medications). A primarily conjugated bilirubinemia results from reflux into the plasma from impaired excretion, secondary to biliary obstruction from cholestasis, gallstones, tumors, or strictures.

15. **State the major causes of acute hepatitis.**
    Viruses such as hepatitis A through E viruses, Epstein-Barr virus, and cytomegalovirus. It also can result from exposure to toxins such as ethanol, *Amanita phalloides* mushrooms, carbon tetrachloride, acetaminophen, halothane, and chlorpromazine.

16. **What are the risk factors for viral hepatitis? Which can result in a carrier state?**
    Hepatitis B and C are transmitted via blood and body fluid exposures: sexual intercourse, intravenous drug abuse, blood transfusions, tattoos or body piercings, hemodialysis, and needle sticks. Hepatitis A and E are transmitted via fecal/oral exposure (i.e., foreign travel, raw seafood ingestion, poor hygiene or sewage management, and close contact with a person infected with hepatitis). Hepatitis A and E are often self-limited, whereas hepatitis B and C can result in a carrier state and progress to chronic hepatitis.

    Hepatitis B: www.hepb.org/
    Hepatitis C: hepatitis-central.com/

17. **What is the most common form of liver disease in the United States?**
    Alcoholic hepatitis. It is most often diagnosed by history, but the following are highly suggestive associated findings: spider angiomas, gynecomastia, palmar erythema, ascites, and an elevated AST and ALT in a ratio of greater than 2:1.

18. **Which patients with hepatitis should be admitted?**
    Patients who are coagulopathic (international normalized ratio >3), actively bleeding, encephalopathic, and unable to tolerate oral fluids and whose social situation (including drug and alcohol abuse) would make proper care and follow-up difficult or impossible.

19. **What is the initial treatment of hepatic encephalopathy? What is asterixis?**
    In addition to supportive care, lactulose, neomycin, and a low-protein diet are the mainstays of treatment. Lactulose reduces ammonia absorption by increasing gastrointestinal (GI) motility and by trapping ammonia as ammonium in the stool via fecal acidification in the form of lactic acid; neomycin is an aminoglycoside that reduces the bacteria that produces ammonia.

    Asterixis is a clinical manifestation of moderate hepatic encephalopathy in which the hands "flap" (low-amplitude alternating flexion and extension) when the wrists are held in extension.

    Guss DA. Liver and biliary tract. In Marx J, Hockenberger R, Walls R (eds): Rosen's Emergency Medicine: Concepts and Clinical Practice, 5th ed. St. Louis, Mosby, 2002, pp 1258–1260.

KEY POINTS: TREATMENT OF HEPATIC ENCEPHALOPATHY

1. Supportive care
2. Lactulose, 15–30 mL PO every 6–8 hours
3. Neomycin, 0.5 gm PO every 4–6 hours
4. Low-protein diet

20. **What are complications of chronic liver disease to watch for in the ED?**
    The most common complication of cirrhotic ascites is **spontaneous bacterial peritonitis,** which can present with fever, abdominal pain, or mental status changes. Paracentesis is diagnostic if it shows white blood cell count greater than 1000 cells/mm^3, neutrophils greater than 250 cells/mm^3, or a positive Gram stain or culture. Portal hypertension causes the development of **esophageal varices,** which can lead to massive GI bleeding. Management should focus on resuscitation, local control (balloon tamponade or endoscopic ligation/sclerotherapy), and reduction of portal pressure (vasopressin plus nitroglycerin, somatostatin,

octreotide, and, if necessary, emergent transjugular intrahepatic portosystemic shunt). Patients with chronic liver disease are at greatly **increased risk of bleeding** because of deficits of the coagulation cascade proteins, platelet abnormalities, and increased fibrinolysis. Renal failure in cirrhotic patients with structurally normal kidneys represents the **hepatorenal syndrome.** One study showed 38% 1-year survival in patients with the hepatorenal syndrome.

KEY POINTS: PERITONEAL FLUID CRITERIA FOR SPONTANEOUS BACTERIAL PERITONITIS

1. White blood cell count >1000 cells/mm^3

2. Neutrophil count >250 cells/mm^3

3. Positive Gram stain

4. Positive culture result (gold standard)

21. **Are there any special issues to watch for in the post-liver-transplant patient?**
    Transplant rejection is common and manifests as fever, pain, and elevated transaminases and bilirubin. This can be treated with high-dose steroids and increased immunosuppressive medication. Other causes of transplant dysfunction include biliary strictures, recurrence of viral hepatitis, and vascular thrombosis. Immunosuppressive therapy can cause nephrotoxicity, neurotoxicity, and hypertension. As with other immunosuppressed patients, opportunistic infections, such as cytomegalovirus, Epstein-Barr virus, mycobacteria, and *Pneumocystis* and fungal infection should be considered.

RENAL COLIC AND SCROTAL PAIN

Christopher M.B. Fernandes, MD, and Ayad Al-Dharrab, MD

CHAPTER 35

1. What are the most common forms of renal stones?

Calcium stones account for 80% of all renal stones: Two-thirds are calcium oxalate, and the remainder are calcium phosphate. Struvite (magnesium ammonium phosphate), uric acid, and cystine account for 20% of renal stones.

Manthey DE, Teichman J: Nephrolithiasis. Emerg Med Clin North Am 19:633–654, 2001.

2. List factors that predispose to stone formation.

Calcium stones

- Chronic dehydration
- Antacid use
- Hypercalciuria
- Hyperoxaluria
- Acid urine
- Ingestion of vitamins A, C, and D

Struvite stones: chronic infection by urea-splitting organisms

Cystine stones: cystinuria

Wasserstein AG: Nephrolithiasis. Am J Kidney Dis 45:422–428, 2005.

3. Name the lethal conditions that often are misdiagnosed as renal colic.

Aortic and iliac aneurysms. A careful search for bruits and pulsatile masses is mandatory when renal colic is suspected.

Rogers RL: Aortic disasters. Emerg Med Clin North Am 22:887–908, 2004.

4. What clinical features help distinguish renal colic from other causes of abdominal pain?

Renal colic usually begins abruptly, causing terrible pain in the flank, costovertebral angle, lateral abdomen, and genitals. Patients often are profoundly distressed, more so than patients with other abdominal pathologies. Pallor, diaphoresis, restlessness, and nausea are prominent. Renal colic causes flank tenderness, but in contrast to other causes of lateralized abdominal pain (e.g., appendicitis, diverticulitis, cholelithiasis, and ectopic pregnancy), it produces little or no abdominal tenderness.

Portis AJ: Diagnosis and initial management of kidney stones. Am Fam Physician 63:1329–1338, 2001.

5. In which patients would imaging be absolutely indicated to confirm the diagnosis of renal colic?

- Patients with a first episode of renal colic
- Patients in whom the diagnosis is unclear
- Patients in whom a proximal urinary tract infection, in addition to a calculus, is suspected
- Elderly patients

Manthey DE, Teichman J: Nephrolithiasis. Emerg Med Clin North Am 19:633–654, 2001.

6. What is the role of the abdominal flat plate in diagnosing renal colic?

The abdominal flat plate, or *kidneys-ureter-bladder (KUB),* is less sensitive and less specific than the clinical examination and, by itself, has no role in the work-up of suspected renal colic. If a stone is diagnosed on ultrasound, it may be appropriate to view the stone on a plain film. Subsequent radiographs may be helpful to document stone progression.

Eray O: The efficacy of urinalysis, plain films, and spiral CT in ED patients with suspected renal colic. Am J Emerg Med 21:152–154, 2003.

7. **Has helical computed tomography (CT) supplanted the intravenous pyelogram (IVP) as the diagnostic test of choice? Why or why not?**
Helical noncontrast CT has replaced IVP as the preferred diagnostic test. The IVP pinpoints stone size and location, clarifies the degree of obstruction, and shows ongoing renal function. Helical CT has been shown to be 97% sensitive and 96% specific in diagnosing renal stones. Used for this purpose, helical CT does not require intravenous contrast material and is faster than IVP—requiring only 1–2 minutes of scanner time to complete a study. Even though helical CT provides no information about renal function, this can be ascertained by a urinalysis and serum creatinine. The marginal cost is less, and it can identify other important causes of flank pain.

Worster A, Preyra I, Weaver B, et al: The accuracy of noncontrast helical computed tomography versus intravenous pyelography in the diagnosis of suspected acute urolithiasis: A meta-analysis. Ann Emerg Med 40:280–286, 2002.

8. **Is pregnancy a contraindication to IVP?**
Ultrasound is the investigation of choice in pregnant patients, but if ultrasound is nondiagnostic, a limited IVP (scout film and 20-minutes postinjection film, preferably coned to the area of concern) is appropriate because the risk of radiation from CT KUB is greater than the limited exposure of plain film radiography with this limited IVP.

Manthey DE, Teichman J: Nephrolithiasis. Emerg Med Clin North Am 19:633–654, 2001.

9. **What IVP findings suggest a renal stone?**
Typical findings include a delayed, intense, and often prolonged nephrogram on the involved side, delayed filling and dilation of the affected collecting system (hydroureter and hydronephrosis), and an uninterrupted column of dye extending from the kidney to the calculus. An unobstructed ureter, because it is peristaltic, does not normally appear opacified with contrast in its entirety.

10. **Why is the postvoid film important? What other special views are helpful?**
Contrast in the bladder obscures the distal ureter. The postvoid film provides optimal visualization of the distal ureter and the ureterovesical junction. The postvoid film also shows whether the bladder is emptying completely. Oblique views help to confirm that a visualized stone is in, rather than overlying, the ureter. Prone films often provide a better view of the ureter than do standard supine films.

KEY POINTS: MOST COMMON FORMS OF RENAL STONES

1. Calcium stones (80%)

   - Calcium oxalate: two thirds

   - Calcium phosphate: one third

2. Struvite, uric acid, and cystine (20%)

11. **What if the ureter is not visualized on the standard IVP?**

In high-grade ureteral obstruction, contrast material may not reach the distal ureter for many hours. If the ureter cannot be visualized at 1 hour, take a 2-hour film. If this fails, take a 4-hour film. The interval between films should be doubled until adequate visualization is achieved. It is important not to abandon the IVP until contrast material reaches the calculus.

Koelliker SL, Cronan JJ: Acute urinary tract obstruction: Imaging update. Urol Clin North Am 24:571–582, 1997.

12. **Name the most common sites of stone impaction.**

The ureteropelvic junction, the pelvic brim (where the ureter crosses the iliac vessels), and the ureterovesical junction (the most narrow point in the ureter).

Engineer R, Peacock IV WR: Renal and ureteral stones. In Tintinalli JE, Kelen GD, Stapczynski JS (eds): Emergency Medicine A Comprehensive Study Guide, 6th ed. New York, McGraw-Hill, 2004, pp 620-625.

13. **Can the likelihood of spontaneous passage be predicted based on the size and location of the stone?**

Stones reaching the distal ureter are more likely to pass than those impacting proximally. Stones 2–4 mm pass 95% of the time; stones 4–6 mm pass 50% of the time, and stones greater than 6 mm pass 10% of the time. When estimating stone size, remember that the x-ray image is magnified; the actual size is 80% of what is measured on the films.

Miller OF, Kane CJ: Time to stone passage for observed ureteral calculi: A guide for patient education. J Urol 162:688–690, 1999.

Morse RM, Resnick MI: Ureteral calculi: Natural history and treatment in the era of advanced technology. J Urol 145:263–265, 1991.

14. **What if the imaging study is normal, but the patient still appears to have renal colic?**

Reexamine the patient carefully to ensure that you have not missed another cause of abdominal pain and that the patient is not developing a condition requiring surgery. If the physical examination is still compatible with renal colic, treat the patient, not the test result. Occasional false-negative results occur with all tests, and imaging modalities may miss small stones, but this may not be clinically relevant because small stones are unlikely to require specific therapy. Persistent severe flank pain can be caused by a leaking abdominal aortic aneurysm (AAA).

Manthey DE, Teichman J: Nephrolithiasis. Emerg Med Clin North Am 19:633–654, 2001.

15. **Isn't an ultrasound just as accurate as helical CT or an IVP?**

Ultrasound is safe and noninvasive but is more prone to false-negative results than the other studies. Ultrasound is sensitive for stones in the bladder and renal pelvis but often fails to visualize those in the mid and distal ureter—the most common sites for stone impaction. When ultrasound fails to identify a stone, however, it may show dilation of the renal collecting system, providing evidence of ureteral obstruction.

Noble VE: Renal ultrasound. Emerg Med Clin North Am 22:641–659, 2004.

16. **List secondary signs of ureteral obstruction shown on helical CT.**
   - Unilateral obstruction
   - Stranding of perinephric fat
   - Hydronephrosis
   - Nephromegaly

Smith RC, Verga M, Dalrymple NC, et al: Acute ureteral obstruction: Value of secondary signs on helical unenhanced CT. AJR 167:1109–1113, 1996.

17. **What is the soft tissue rim sign on helical CT? How is it useful?**
This sign shows soft tissue attenuation around a ureteral calculus and helps differentiate a calculus from a phlebolith.

Spencer BA, Wood BJ, Dretler SP: Helical CT and ureteral colic. Urol Clin North Am 27:231–241, 2000.

18. **What other tests are useful in the emergency department (ED)?**
Urine dipsticks are sensitive for microscopic hematuria, which is present in 80% of patients with renal colic. Urinalysis is recommended to rule out pyuria and bacteriuria. Urine culture is indicated if symptoms, signs, or urinalysis findings suggest infection. Determination of blood urea nitrogen (BUN), creatinine, and electrolyte levels is helpful if the patient has been vomiting or if presence of an underlying renal disease is suspected. There is usually no need for a more extensive metabolic work-up in the ED.

Bove P, Kaplan D, Dalrymple N, et al: Reexamining the value of hematuria testing in patients with acute flank pain. J Urol 162:685–687, 1999.

19. **Why is coexistent infection a major problem?**
Bacteria in an obstructed collecting system can cause abscess formation, renal destruction, and bacteremia quickly. The presence of infection in an obstructed ureter mandates immediate consultation with a urologist and high-dose intravenous antibiotics.

Manthey DE, Teichman J: Nephrolithiasis. Emerg Med Clin North Am 19:633–654, 2001.

20. **Has lithotripsy supplanted percutaneous and open surgical methods of stone removal?**
Not always. Optimal therapy depends on the size, type, and location of the stone. Ureteroscopic techniques probably are still preferable for lower ureteral stones. Extracorporeal shock wave lithotripsy (ESWL) is optimal for stones 2 cm in size, particularly those in the renal pelvis. Percutaneous stone removal techniques are indicated for larger stones, when there is obstructive uropathy, and when less invasive techniques have failed. For some stones, a combination of ESWL followed by percutaneous instrumentation is optimal. Some large stones still require open surgery. The method of removal is best determined by a urologist.

Gravenstein D: Extracorporeal shock wave lithotripsy and percutaneous nephrolithotomy. Anesthesiol Clin North Am 18:953–971, 2000.

21. **What are the basics of ED treatment of renal colic?**
Hydration, analgesia, and antiemetics. Patients who have clinical dehydration secondary to vomiting and decreased oral intake should receive intravenous fluid hydration, as well as if radiocontrast media study is planned. Various analgesics and antiemetics are available for rapid control of symptoms (Table 35-1). Intravenous pain control is the mainstay ED treatment. Analgesic treatment should not be delayed waiting for test results. Opiate analgesics have long been the standard medication. Rectal or intravenous nonsteroidal anti-inflammatory drugs (NSAIDs), which inhibit renal prostaglandin synthesis, are effective and may be given concurrently with opioids. A recent systematic review suggested that for the management of acute renal colic, NSAIDs achieve slightly better pain relief, reduce need for rescue analgesia, and produce much less vomiting than do opioids. Optimal ED pain control involves the combined administration of NSAIDs and opioids (balanced analgesia).

Holdgate A, Pollock T: Systematic review of the relative efficacy of non-steroidal anti-inflammatory drugs and opioids in the treatment of acute renal colic. BMJ 328:1401–1406, 2004.

22. **Who requires hospitalization? Urology consultation?**
Patients with high-grade obstruction, intractable pain or vomiting, associated urinary tract infection, a solitary or transplanted kidney, and in whom the diagnosis is uncertain. Obtain urologic consultation for patients with stones larger than 5 mm in diameter, urinary extravasation, and renal insufficiency regardless of symptoms.

Manthey DE, Teichman J: Nephrolithiasis. Emerg Med Clin North Am 19:633–654, 2001.

TABLE 35-1. ANALGESICS AND ANTIEMETICS FOR RENAL COLIC

Opioid analgesics

Meperidine (Demerol)	IV 25–50 mg	q 5–10 min	prn
Hydromorphone	IV 1–2 mg	q 2–4 h	
	IM 1–2 mg/kg	q 2 h	prn*
Morphine sulphate	IV 3–5 mg	q 5–10 min	prn
	IM 0.1–0.2 mg/kg	q 3 h	prn*
Oxycodone and acetylsalicylic acid (Percodan)	PO 2 tabs	q 4 h	prn
Oxycodone and acetaminophen (Percocet)	PO 2 tabs	q 4 h	prn
Anileridine (Leritine)	PO 50 mg	q 4 h	prn
Antiemetics			
Metoclopramide (Reglan)	IV 10–20 mg	q 15 min prn	
Perphenazine (Trilafon)	IM 5 mg	q 6 h	prn*
	PO 4 mg	q 6 h	prn
Prochlorperazine (Compazine)	IV 5–10 mg	q 4 h	prn
	IM 5–10 mg	q 6 h	prn*
	PO 5–10 mg	q 4 h	prn
Nonsteroidal analgesics			
Ketorolac (Toradol)	IV 30 mg	q 6 h†	
	IM 30 mg	q 6 h†	
Indomethacin	50- or 100-mg suppositories, 200 mg/day		
Diclofenac (Voltaren)	50- or 100-mg suppositories, 150 mg/day		

IM = intramuscular, IV = intravenous, PO = per os, prn = as needed.
*IM route not recommended for emergency department (ED) management of acute, severe pain.

23. What advice should I give to patients being discharged from the ED?
Patients should be advised to drink plenty of fluids, strain their urine, and return to the ED if they develop symptoms of infection or recurrent severe pain. Follow-up with a urologist within a week should be recommended.

Singal RK, Denstedt JD: Contemporary management of ureteral stone. Urol Clin North Am 24:59–70, 1997.

24. Which analgesics are recommended for outpatient pain control?
Gastrointestinal irritation limits the usefulness of oral NSAIDs in patients with renal colic; however, rectal NSAIDs (diclofenac, indomethacin) may provide adequate analgesia. If necessary, oral opioids can be combined with NSAIDs in patients with documented ureteral calculi.

Manthey DE, Teichman J: Nephrolithiasis. Emerg Med Clin North Am 19:633–654, 2001.

KEY POINTS: INDICATIONS FOR HOSPITALIZATION

1. Patients with high-grade obstruction

2. Intractable pain or vomiting

3. Associated urinary tract infection

4. Solitary or transplanted kidney

5. Patients in whom the diagnosis is uncertain

6. Stones larger than 5 mm in diameter

7. Urinary extravasation

8. Renal insufficiency regardless of symptoms

25. **Why should patients be given a urine strainer on discharge?**
If the stone can be analyzed, the patient can then receive follow-up counseling on dietary modification or medications that may reduce the risk of recurrence.

    Borghi L: Medical treatment of nephrolithiasis. Endocrinol Metab Clin North Am 31:1051–1064, 2002.

26. **When should patients return to the ED?**
Patients should be instructed to seek medical care immediately if they have continued or increasing pain, nausea and vomiting, fever or chills, or any other new symptoms.

27. **What is the differential diagnosis in a patient presenting with an acutely painful scrotum?**
The differential diagnosis of acute scrotal pain includes testicular torsion, torsion of the testicular or epididymal appendages, epididymitis, orchitis, scrotal hernia, testicular tumor, renal colic, Henoch-Schönlein purpura, and Fournier's gangrene. Although not life threatening, testicular torsion is a significant cause of morbidity and sterility in the male. Thus, any case of an acute scrotum should be considered testicular torsion until proven otherwise.

    Marcozzi D, Suner S: The nontraumatic, acute scrotum. Emerg Med Clin North Am 19:547–568, 2001.

28. **What is testicular torsion?**
Testicular torsion results from maldevelopment of the normal fixation that occurs between the enveloping tunica vaginalis and the posterior scrotal wall. This maldevelopment then allows the testis and the epididymis to hang freely in the scrotum (the so-called bell-clapper deformity), allowing the testis to rotate on the spermatic cord. The degree of testicular ischemia is dependent on the number of rotations of the cord.

    Rosenstein D, McAninch J: Urologic emergencies. Med Clin North Am 88:495–518, 2004.

29. **When is testicular torsion most likely to occur?**
The annual incidence of testicular torsion is estimated to be 1 in 400 for males under the age of 25. Testicular torsion has a bimodal distribution, with peak incidence in the neonate within the first few days of life and preadolescence.

    Hawtrey CE: Assessment of acute scrotal symptoms and findings. A clinician's dilemma. Urol Clin North Am 25:715–723, 1998.

KEY POINTS: SIX DIFFERENTIAL DIAGNOSES OF ACUTE SCROTUM

1. Testicular torsion

2. Torsion of the testicular or epididymal appendages

3. Epididymo-orchitis

4. Scrotal hernia

5. Testicular tumor

6. Fournier's gangrene

30. **What history is suggestive of testicular torsion?**

Usually, there is a history of trauma or strenuous event before the onset of scrotal pain in testicular torsion. One study reported sudden onset of scrotal pain to be present in 90% of patients with testicular torsion, compared with 58% of patient with epididymitis and 78% of patients with normal scrotum. Fever was present in 10% of patients with testicular torsion compared with 32% of patients with epididymitis.

Van Glabeke E, Khairouni A, Larroquet M, et al : Acute scrotal pain in children: Results of 543 surgical explorations. Pediatr Surg Int 15:353–357, 1999.

31. **What clinical features are suggestive of testicular torsion?**

In testicular torsion, the affected testis usually is firm, tender, and aligned in a horizontal rather than a vertical axis. The presence of cremasteric reflex appears to be one of the most helpful signs in ruling out testicular torsion with 96% negative predictive value. It is elicited by gently stroking the inner aspect of the involved thigh and observing more than 0.5 cm of elevation in the affected testis.

Van Glabeke E, Khairouni A, Larroquet M, et al. Acute scrotal pain in children: Results of 543 surgical explorations. Pediatr Surg Int 15:353–357, 1999.

32. **What is the proper management of testicular torsion?**

The proper management of a suspected testicular torsion is immediate urologic consultation and surgical exploration. If surgical consultation is not immediately available, manual detorsion should be attempted.

Marcozzi D, Suner S: The nontraumatic, acute scrotum. Emerg Med Clin North Am 19:547–568, 2001.

KEY POINTS: PROPER MANAGEMENT OF TESTICULAR TORSION

1. Emergent urologic consultation

2. Attempt at manual detorsion

33. **How is manual detorsion performed?**
This procedure is best done by standing at the foot or right side of the patient's bed.
The torsed testis is detorsed in fashion similar to opening a book. The patient's right testis
is rotated counterclockwise, and the left testis is rotated clockwise. A testis viability rate of
100%, 70%, and 20% for 6, 6–12, and 12–24 hours of symptoms respectively has been
reported.

Patriquin HB, Yazbeck S, Trinh B, et al: Testicular torsion in infants and children: Diagnosis with Doppler
sonography. Radiology 188:781–785, 1993.
Schneider R: Male genital problems. In Tintinalli JE, Kelen GD, Stapczynski JS (eds): Emergency Medicine:
A Comprehensive Study Guide, 6th ed. New York, McGraw-Hill, 2004, pp 613–620.

34. **Is imaging testing helpful to confirm the diagnosis of testicular torsion?**
Testicular torsion is mainly a clinical diagnosis. If it is suspected, immediate urologic
evaluation is mandatory and should precede any further testing as time is critical. However,
imaging tests could be helpful adjuncts to the work-up of the acute scrotum when the diagnosis
is unclear.

Marcozzi D, Suner S: The nontraumatic, acute scrotum. Emerg Med Clin North Am 19:547–568, 2001.

35. **What are the diagnostic imaging tests that can be used to evaluate the acute
scrotum?**
Doppler ultrasound and radionucleotide scintigraphy are the two imaging tests that can be used
to evaluate the acute scrotum. Both measure the blood flow to the testis, with Doppler
ultrasound curries a sensitivity of 86% and 97% accuracy, whereas radionucleotide scintigraphy
has 80% sensitivity and 97% specificity.

Dorga V, Bhatt S: Acute painful scrotum. Radiol Clin North Am 42:49–63, 2004.
Lewis A, Bukowski P: Evaluation of acute scrotum and the emergency department. J Pediatr Surg
30:277–282, 1995.

36. **How is testicular torsion treated surgically?**
The involved testis must be detorsed then checked for viability. If it is viable, it is fixed
(orchidopexy). Because approximately 40% of patients have a bell-clapper deformity of the
contralateral testis, the unaffected tested should be fixed to prevent recurrence.

McCollough M, Sharieff G: Abdominal surgical emergencies in infants and young children. Emerg Med Clin
North Am 21:909–935, 2003.

37. **What are testis and epididymal appendix?**
The appendix testis is a müllerian duct remnant that is attached to the superior pole of the
testicle and rests in the groove between the testis and epididymis. The appendix epididymis is a
wolffian duct remnant that is attached to the head of the epididymis.

Wan J: Genitourinary problems in adolescent males. Adolesc Med 14:717–731, 2003.

38. **What are clinical features of torsion of testis and epididymal appendix?**
Both torsion of testis and epididymal appendix result in unilateral pain. The pain of epididymal
appendix torsion typically is more gradual in onset and is usually not quite as severe as that
associated with true testicular torsion. The most important aspect of the physical examination is
pain and tenderness localized to the involved appendix. However, late in its course, generalized
scrotal swelling and tenderness may be encountered, making it difficult to differentiate from
testicular torsion. The classic blue dot sign (visualization of the ischemic or necrotic appendix
testis through the scrotal wall on the superior aspect of the testicle) is pathognomonic for
appendix testis torsion, but it is also relatively uncommon.

Jayanthi VR: Adolescent urology. Adolesc Med Clin 15:521–534, 2004.

39. **How is torsion of testis or epididymal appendix treated?**

Torsion of epididymal and testicular appendix are self-resolving, benign processes. Rest, scrotal elevation, and analgesia are the mainstays of treatment. Resolution of the swelling and pain should be expected within 1 week.

Marcozzi D, Suner S: The nontraumatic, acute scrotum. Emerg Med Clin North Am 19:547–568, 2001.

40. **What is epididymitis?**

Epididymitis arises from swelling and pain of the epididymis. It usually arises secondary to infection or inflammation from the urethra or bladder. Patients with epididymitis present with increasing, dull, unilateral scrotal pain during a period of hours to days. Possible associated symptoms include fever, urethral discharge, hydrocele, erythema of the scrotum, and palpable swelling of the epididymis. Involvement of the ipsilateral testis is common, producing epididymitis-orchitis.

Kodner C: Sexually transmitted infections in men. Prim Care 30:173–191, 2003.

41. **List the most common causes of epididymitis.**

The most common causes of epididymitis in males older than 35 years are gram-negative organisms such as *Escherichia coli*, *Klebsiella*, and *Pseudomonas* species. Among sexually active men younger than 35 years, epididymitis is often caused by *Chlamydia trachomatis* or *Neisseria gonorrhoeae*. *E. coli* infection also may occur in men who are insertive partners during anal intercourse.

Kodner C: Sexually transmitted infections in men. Prim Care 30:173–191, 2003.

42. **What is the treatment for epididymitis?**

Admission should be considered for any febrile, toxic-appearing patient with epididymitis or when testicular or epididymal abscess should be excluded. In-patient therapy includes bed rest, analgesia, scrotal elevation, nonsteroidal anti-inflammatory drugs, and parenteral antibiotics based on presumed etiology.

When sexually transmitted disease is suspected to be the cause for epididymitis, or in males younger than 35 years, urethral culture should be taken for *Chlamydia* and gonorrhea, followed by empirical treatment with ceftriaxone 250 mg intramuscularly once, plus doxycycline 100 mg orally twice a day for 10 days OR ofloxacin 300 mg orally twice a day for 10 days. When gram-negative bacilli are suspected to be the cause for epididymitis, or in males older than 35 years, treatment includes ciprofloxacin 500 mg orally twice a day or levofloxacin 750 mg once a day for 10–14 days.

Treatment in all patients should also include bed rest, analgesia, and scrotal elevation. Follow up with an urologist within 5–7 days is recommended.

Gilbert DN, Moellering RC, Eliopoulos GM, Sande MA: The Sanford Guide to Antimicrobial Therapy. Antimicrobial Therapy Inc, Sperryville, VA, 2004.

43. **What is Fournier's gangrene?**

Fournier's gangrene is a life-threatening disease characterized by necrotizing fasciitis of the perineal and genital region. It is generally the result of a polymicrobial infection from bacteria that are normally present in the perianal area. The diagnosis and treatment of Fournier's gangrene are similar to those of necrotizing fasciitis. Diabetes mellitus, alcohol abuse, and local trauma are known risk factors. Empirical broad-spectrum antibiotics with early aggressive surgical debridement are the mainstays of therapy. Reexploration commonly is needed, and some patients require diverting colostomies or orchiectomies.

Schneider JI: Rapid infectious killers. Emerg Med Clin North Am 22:1099–1115, 2004.

CHAPTER 36

ACUTE URINARY RETENTION

John P. Marshall, MD, and Samuel J. Killian, MD

1. **What is acute urinary retention (AUR)?**
   A painful inability to urinate. AUR is most commonly the result of bladder outlet obstruction, but it also may result from neurogenic, pharmacologic, or other causes of detrusor muscle dysfunction. Urine is produced normally but is retained in the bladder, which then becomes distended and uncomfortable.

2. **Is there chronic urinary retention?**
   Yes. It generally represents prolonged retention. The hallmarks of chronic urinary retention are the absence of pain and overflow incontinence. It most frequently occurs in mentally debilitated or neurologically compromised patients.

3. **What is the most common cause of AUR? Who gets it?**
   Obstruction of the lower urinary tract (bladder and urethra) is the most common cause encountered in the emergency department (ED). The usual site of obstruction is the prostate gland, but lesions of the urethra or penis also may cause retention. In general, AUR is a disease of older men, although it occasionally is encountered in women. Patients with indwelling catheters (suprapubic or Foley) are at risk for episodes of retention because of obstruction or dysfunction of these drainage systems.

4. **How does benign prostatic hypertrophy (BPH) cause AUR?**
   BPH with bladder neck obstruction is the most common cause of AUR. Of men older than age 60, 50% have histologic evidence of BPH. As the prostate hypertrophies, urine outflow is obstructed by enlargement of the median lobe of the gland impinging on the internal urethral lumen. The typical patient with BPH gives a progressive history suggestive of urinary outlet obstruction. Symptoms such as hesitancy, diminished stream quality, dribbling, nocturia, and the sensation of incomplete bladder emptying may precede the episode of acute retention. New medications or increased fluid loads may precipitate an acute episode of retention in these patients.

5. **List the other causes of AUR.**
   1. **Obstructive:** BPH, prostate carcinoma, prostatitis, urethral stricture, posterior urethral valves, phimosis, paraphimosis, balanitis, meatal stenosis, calculi, blood clots, circumcision, urethral foreign body, constricting penile ring, clogged or crimped Foley catheter
   2. **Neurogenic:** Spinal cord injuries, herniated lumbosacral disks (cauda equina syndrome), central nervous system (CNS) tumors, stroke, diabetes, multiple sclerosis, encephalitis, tabes dorsalis, syringomyelia, herpes simplex, herpes zoster, alcohol withdrawal
   3. **Pharmacologic:** Anticholinergics, antihistamines, antidepressants, antispasmodics, narcotics, sympathomimetics, antipsychotics, antiparkinsonian agents (see question 14)
   4. **Psychogenic:** Diagnosis of exclusion

6. **What are the important features in the history and physical examination?**
   When taking the history, any previous prostate or urethral conditions should be elicited. Patients often have a history of chronic voiding hesitancy, a decreased force to the urinary stream, a

feeling of incomplete bladder emptying, or nocturia. Information about neurologic symptoms, trauma, previous instrumentation, back pain, and current medication is essential. On physical examination, the distended bladder often is palpable above the pubic rim and indicates at least 150 mL of urine in the bladder. The penis and particularly the urethra should be examined carefully for any signs of stricture, which may be evident on palpation. A rectal examination is essential and often provides clues to the diagnosis of BPH, prostate carcinoma, or prostatitis. A careful neurologic examination, including rectal tone and perineal sensation, is vital in any patient suspected of having a neurologic lesion.

7. **Are there any red flags in the history and physical examination that might indicate a more serious, potentially surgical, cause?**
Yes. New urinary symptoms, particularly obstruction, in patients with a history of trauma or back pain should alert the examiner to the possibility of spinal cord compression resulting from disk herniation, fracture, epidural hematoma, epidural abscess, or tumor. Be especially suspicious if there is no prior history of bladder, prostate, or urethral disorders.

8. **How do I treat AUR?**
Catheterization and bladder decompression using a Foley catheter.

9. **What if I can't pass a Foley catheter?**
Occasionally, simple passage of a 16- or 18-Fr Foley catheter cannot be accomplished. One trick that often helps is to fill a 30-mL syringe with lidocaine (Xylocaine) jelly and inject it into the urethral meatus. Still no luck? Try an 18 or 20 Fr coudé catheter. The coudé-tipped catheter has a gentle upward curve in the distal 3 cm that may be helpful in pointing the catheter up and over the enlarged prostatic lobe. Never force a catheter through an area of significant resistance because this can cause urethral perforation, false lumens, and subsequent stricture formation.

10. **Is bigger better?**
A loaded question. If you are unable to pass a 16-Fr (standard adult) catheter, it is generally recommended to move up in size to a 18- or 20-Fr Foley catheter. Usually, the stiffness and larger bulk of the bigger catheter are more successful in passing through the bladder neck than a smaller, more flexible catheter. Remember, never force a catheter through significant resistance.

11. **What if nothing is working?**
If you still cannot pass a catheter, the obstruction may be more severe than anticipated, or a stricture may be present. One clue to the presence of a stricture is that the obstruction occurs less than 16 cm from the external meatus. If this is the case, an attempt may be made using a pediatric-sized urinary catheter. If this fails, more sophisticated instrumentation may be required, such as filiforms and followers or catheter guides. These techniques should be done only by a urologist or practitioner with extensive training in their use. If AUR cannot be relieved by transurethral bladder catheterization, placement of a suprapubic catheter may be necessary.

12. **What is suprapubic catheterization? How is it done?**
A procedure used to pass a urinary catheter directly into the bladder through the lower anterior abdominal wall (Fig. 36-1). It is indicated when bladder drainage is necessary and other methods have failed or when urethral damage from trauma is suspected. The procedure is done under sterile conditions with local anesthesia. The presence of a distended bladder is confirmed by ultrasound or percussion. A small midline incision is made 2 cm above the symphysis pubis. Depending on the technique, either a needle or a trocar is used to penetrate the bladder through the incision. When urine is aspirated, a catheter is advanced over the cannula.

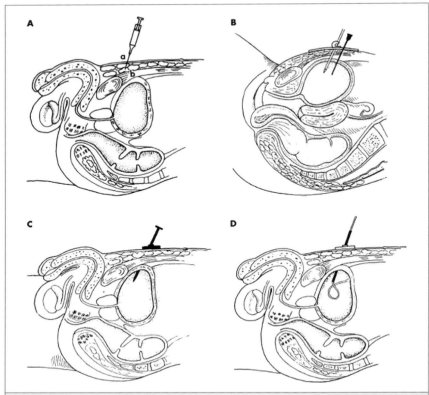

Figure 36-1. Suprapubic catheterization. (From Roberts J, Hedges J: Clinical Procedures in Emergency Medicine. Philadelphia, W.B. Saunders, 2000.)

KEY POINTS: TREATMENT OPTIONS FOR AUR

1. Foley catheter placement

2. Coudé catheter placement

3. Filiforms and followers

4. Suprapubic catheterization

13. **What diagnostic studies are useful in the evaluation of AUR?**
    Bedside ultrasonography can be helpful during the initial evaluation, and, if needed, suprapubic aspiration can be done. Always check a urinalysis with microscopic examination and urine culture. It is generally recommended to check blood urea nitrogen and creatinine levels to evaluate renal function, especially in cases of suspected chronic retention.

14. Which medications may cause AUR?

Table 36-1 presents the broad categories as well as some specific medications that can cause AUR.

TABLE 36-1. MEDICATIONS THAT CAN CAUSE ACUTE URINARY RETENTION

Sympathomimetics (Alpha-Adrenergic)	**Antipsychotics**
Ephedrine	Haloperidol
Pseudoephedrine (Sudafed, Actifed)	Chlorpromazine (Thorazine)
Phenylephrine hydrochloride (Neo-Synephrine)	Prochlorperazine (Compazine)
Phenylpropanolamine hydrochloride (Contac)	Risperidone (Risperdal)
Amphetamine	Clozapine (Clozaril)
Cocaine	Quetiapine (Seroquel)
Sympathomimetics (Beta-Adrenergic)	**Antihypertensives**
Isoproterenol	Nifedipine (Procardia)
Terbutaline	Hydralazine
Antidepressants	Nicardipine
Tricyclics	**Muscle Relaxants**
Fluoxetine (Prozac)	Diazepam (Valium)
Antiarrhythmics	Cyclobenzaprine (Flexeril)
Quinidine	**Narcotics**
Disopyramide (Norpace)	Morphine sulfate
Procainamide	Codeine
Anticholinergics	Meperidine (Demerol)
Antihistamines	Hydromorphone hydrochloride (Dilaudid)
Antiparkinsonian Agents	**Miscellaneous**
Benztropine (Cogentin)	Indomethacin
Amantadine (Symmetrel)	Metoclopramide (Reglan)
Levodopa (Sinemet)	Carbamazepine (Tegretol)
Trihexyphenidyl (Artane)	Mercurial diuretics
Hormonal Agents	Dopamine
Progesterone	Vincristine
Estrogen	MDMA
Testosterone	Cannabis

MDMA = 3,4-methylenedioxymethamphetamine.

15. Summarize the different neurogenic causes of AUR.

1. **Upper motor neuron lesions:** Lesions located in the spinal cord above the sacral micturition center (L2 vertebral level, S2–4 spinal segments) result in a spastic or reflex bladder. Common causes are spinal cord trauma, tumor, and multiple sclerosis. Lesions of the cerebral cortex (e.g., acute stroke, bleed) usually cause chronic loss of bladder control and incontinence, except in the acute phase, when the lesions typically produce AUR.
2. **Lower motor neuron lesions:** Lesions at the micturition center in the cauda equina interrupt the sacral reflex arc and produce vesical dysfunction. There is loss of sensation of bladder

fullness leading to overstretch, muscle atony, and poor contraction. Large residuals are common. The most common causes include spinal trauma, tumor, herniated intervertebral disks, and multiple sclerosis.

3. **Bladder afferent and efferent nerve dysfunction:** Dysfunction in this pathway disrupts the micturition reflex arc that is necessary for proper urination, causing AUR. Common causes include diabetes mellitus, herpes simplex infection, and the postoperative state.

16. **Name the most common complications of AUR.**
Infection, hemorrhage, and postobstruction diuresis. All three are more common in patients with chronic urinary retention.

17. **What is autonomic dysreflexia/hyperreflexia, and what does it have to due with AUR?**
An abnormality of the autonomic nervous system seen in patients with longstanding cervical or high thoracic spinal cord lesions (i.e., quadriplegics and high paraplegics). It is caused primarily by unchecked reflex sympathetic discharge secondary to visceral or somatic stimuli below the level of the spinal injury. This potentially life-threatening syndrome includes severe paroxysmal hypertension, diaphoresis, tachycardia or bradycardia, anxiety, headache, flushing, seizures, and coma. Morbidity has resulted from cerebrovascular accident, subarachnoid hemorrhage, and respiratory arrest. One of the most common precipitating stimuli is overdistention of the bladder (AUR) owing to a plugged or kinked catheter. Therefore, it is always important to evaluate these types of patients for potential Foley catheter problems.

Givre S, Freed HA: Autonomic dysreflexia: A potentially fatal complication of somatic stress in quadraplegics. J Emerg Med 7:461–463, 1989.

18. **What is postobstruction diuresis? How is it managed?**
The inappropriate excretion of salt and water after relief of urinary obstruction. Patients with abnormal renal function or chronic urinary retention are most susceptible. A physiologic diuresis is normal because the kidneys excrete the overload of solute and volume retained while obstructed. If urine output persists at high levels, significant fluid and electrolyte abnormalities may develop. Any patient who exhibits a continuous diuresis after clinical euvolemia is reached requires hospitalization for hemodynamic monitoring and fluid and electrolyte repletion.

19. **Whom can I send home? Who needs admission? Can I remove that catheter?**
Most patients with AUR caused by an obstruction require Foley catheterization with continuous drainage. Reliable patients in good health and without signs of serious systemic infection are candidates for careful outpatient management with a leg bag and timely urologic follow-up. The use of prophylactic antibiotics in these patients is controversial. Patients with new neurogenic causes, severe infection, systemic toxicity, or any lesion that may need surgical intervention require hospital admission. Some younger patients with pharmacologic urinary retention may have the catheter removed after decompression. The causative medication should be discontinued, and the patient should be discharged with instructions to return if symptoms recur. If the catheter is removed, it is prudent to be sure that patients can void on their own prior to discharge from the emergency department (ED).

Hastie KJ, Dickinson AJ, Ahmad R, Maoisey CU: Acute retention of urine: Is trial without catheter justified? J R Coll Edinb 35:225–227, 1990.

CONTROVERSY

20. **I have heard that gradual emptying of the distended bladder best helps to prevent complications. Is this true?**
Traditionally, the medical literature has recommended gradual emptying of the obstructed, distended bladder to decrease the risk of hematuria, hypotension, and postobstructive diuresis.

The validity of this practice has long been questioned and inadequately studied. Recently, however, one study reviewed all of the available literature for each of these complications and compared quick, complete decompression with gradual emptying. Their review revealed that, although hematuria, transient hypotension, and postobstructive diuresis occasionally do occur after rapid emptying of the bladder, they are rarely of any clinical significance and do not require any treatment. The recommendation is that gradual, incremental bladder decompression is unnecessary.

Nyman MA, Schwenk NM, Silverstein MD: Management of urinary retention: Rapid vs. gradual decompression and risk of complications. Mayo Clin Proc 72:951–956, 1997.

BIBLIOGRAPHY

1. Dawson C, Whitfield H: ABC of urology: Urologic emergencies in general practice (education and debate). BMJ 312:838–840, 1996.
2. Emberton M, Anson K: Acute urinary retention in men: An age old problem. BMJ 319:1004–1005, 1999.
3. eMedicine: Urinary Obstruction:www.emedicine.com.
4. Escobar JI, Eastman ER, Harwood-Nuss AL: Selected urologic problems. In Marx J, Hockenberger R, Walls R (eds): Rosen's Emergency Medicine: Concepts and Clinical Practice, 5th ed. St. Louis, Mosby, 2002, pp 1400–1433.
5. Fontanarosa PB, Roush WR: Acute urinary retention. Emerg Med Clin North Am 6:419–437, 1988.
6. Higgins PM, French ME, Chadalavada VS: Management of acute retention of urine: A reappraisal. Br J Urol 67:365–368, 1991.
7. Jones DA, George NJR: Interactive obstructive uropathy in man. Br J Urol 69:337–345, 1992.
8. Samm BJ, Domchowski RR: Urologic emergencies: Conditions affecting the kidney, bladder, prostate, and ureters. Postgrad Med 100:177–180, 183–184, 1996.
9. Wolf SJ: Urinary incontinence and retention. In Wolfson A, Linden C, Luten RC, et al (eds): Harwood-Nuss' Clinical Practice of Emergency Medicine, 4th ed. Philadelphia, Lippincott-Raven, 2005, pp 443–448.

CHAPTER 37

URINARY TRACT INFECTION: CYSTITIS, PYELONEPHRITIS, AND PROSTATITIS

Nicola E.E. Schiebel, MD, and Gayle Braunholtz, MD

1. **Define the terms relevant to the spectrum of urinary tract infection (UTI).**
   - **Bacteriuria:** The presence of bacteria anywhere in the urinary tract
   - **Cystitis:** Significant bacteriuria with bladder mucosal invasion, clinically characterized by dysuria, urgency, frequency, and sometimes suprapubic discomfort
   - **Pyelonephritis:** An infection of the renal parenchyma and collecting system, characterized by flank pain, fever, costovertebral angle tenderness, and significant bacteriuria
   - **Urethritis** or **acute urethral syndrome:** The clinical syndrome of dysuria, frequency, and urgency in the absence of significant bacteriuria
   - **Prostatitis:** A chronic or acute syndrome of prostatic inflammation that presents with a wide range of symptoms

KEY POINTS: CHARACTERISTICS OF URETHRITIS

1. Dysuria

2. Frequency

3. Urgency

4. Absence of significant bacteriuria

2. **What are the most common causes of UTI?**
   Escherichia coli is the most common pathogen. *Staphylococcus saprophyticus* is the second most common. In immunocompromised or chronically ill patients and in complicated UTI, *Pseudomonas* and many members of the Enterobacteriaceae family, such as *Klebsiella, Proteus,* and *Enterobacter,* are commonly involved. *Proteus* and *Klebsiella* predispose to stone formation and grow more frequently in patients with calculi. Remember these organisms by the mnemonic SEEK PP.

3. **What is asymptomatic bacteriuria?**
   The presence of greater than or equal to 10^5 uropathogens/mL on voided midstream urine from an asymptomatic patient. When two consecutive specimens contain the same organism at this concentration, the probability of true bacteriuria rises from 80–95%.

   Patterson TF, Andriole VT: Detection, significance, and therapy of bacteriuria in pregnancy. Infect Dis Clin North Am 11:593–608, 1997.
   www.idsociety.org

4. **When should asymptomatic bacteriuria be treated?**
   During pregnancy because it is associated with a 20–40% risk of developing symptomatic UTI, including pyelonephritis. Pyelonephritis during pregnancy is associated with increased risk of prematurity and low birth weight. Also, treating asymptomatic bacteriuria before urologic surgery decreases the risk of postoperative complications, including bacteremia. There is no evidence to support the treatment of asymptomatic bacteriuria in catheterized patients or in the elderly.

Nicolle L, Bradley S: Infectious Diseases Society of America guidelines for the diagnosis and treatment of asymptomatic bacteriuria in adults. Clin Infect Dis 40: 643–654 2005.

5. **List the differential diagnoses of dysuria.**
   - **Infectious:** Cystitis, urethritis, pyelonephritis, epididymitis, prostatitis, vulvovaginitis
   - **Structural:** Calculi, occasionally neoplastic lesions
   - **Traumatic:** Blunt trauma, sexual intercourse, sexual assault, chemical irritants, allergy

6. **When should a pelvic examination be done in a female patient with dysuria?**
   Whenever there is a suspicion that the cause is not a classic UTI. Clinical situations include external dysuria suggestive of vulvovaginitis, low abdominal pain or bilateral flank pain to rule out pelvic inflammatory disease, any history of trauma or chemical irritant, and any patient at high risk for a sexually transmitted disease or sexual abuse. Any patient who fails to respond to empirical antibiotic therapy for cystitis or who has a negative urinalysis or cultures with a suspected UTI should have a pelvic examination.

   Winkens RAG, Leffers P, Trienekens TAM: The validity of urinary examination for urinary tract infections in daily practice. Fam Pract 12:290–293, 1995.

7. **What is a routine urinalysis?**
   There is no standardization of what constitutes a *routine urinalysis* in the literature. The definition of *significant bacteriuria* depends on the relatively costly and slow results of urine culture. Many screening tests have been evaluated to try to detect UTI earlier and to predict negative cultures, reducing the number of full urine cultures ordered. These screening tests include the following:
   - **Pyuria:** This involves the measurement of white blood cells (WBCs) in the urine. The most commonly used technique is to examine microscopically the centrifuged urine sediment and to quantitate the number of WBCs per high-power field (HPF) ($>$5 WBCs/HPF is abnormal). This technique, however, is hampered by a lack of standardization. The most accurate method to measure pyuria is with a hemocytometer on unspun urine (10 leukocytes/mm^3 is considered abnormal). This test is not widely available.
   - **Microscopic evaluation for bacteria:** Variable techniques include examination of unstained and Gram-stained specimens of centrifuged and uncentrifuged urine. Standardization of this technique is poor, and it is an insensitive test because pathogens in quantities less than 10^4 colony-forming units (CFUs)/mL are difficult to find by this technique.
   - **Epithelial cells:** Estimates of epithelial cells per HPF are used mainly to estimate perineal contamination of midstream specimens. Although epithelial cells can be derived from anywhere in the urinary tract, their presence on urinalysis is usually from vaginal epithelial cells and suggests contamination.
   - **Leukocyte esterase:** This test depends on the ability of any leukocytes present to convert indoxyl carboxylic acid to an indoxyl moiety. When positive, it is suggestive of but not confirmatory for pyuria.
   - **Nitrite:** This test depends on the ability of most urinary pathogens to reduce urine nitrates to nitrite. To be positive, the bacteria must act on the urine for 6 hours, making a first-voided morning specimen necessary for optimal testing. Methods used to detect leukocyte esterase and nitrite include urine dipsticks and automated urine analyzers in the laboratory.

   Sheets C, Lyman JL: Urinalysis. Emerg Med Clin North Am 4:263–280, 1986.
   Stamm WE: Measurement of pyuria and its relation to bacteriuria. Am J Med 75:53–58, 1983.

8. **What is the role of urinalysis and urine dipsticks in the diagnosis of UTI?**
   The reported sensitivities, specificities, and likelihood ratios for the previously mentioned screening tests vary widely in the literature. Given that the clinical presentation of most UTIs is

classic, the utility of any of the screening tests becomes questionable. The pretest probability of cystitis in a population of patients presenting with any symptoms of dysuria, frequency, or urgency has been estimated to be approximately 70%. Estimates of screening test sensitivities and specificities vary so much that the predictive value of a positive test ranges from 75–99%, and the predictive value of a negative test ranges from 40–99%. Evidence suggests that urinalysis and dipstick testing done under practice conditions are not as reliable as when done under research protocol conditions. The role of urine screening tests is unclear. As a result, it may be sensible to continue to develop clinical guidelines involving the empirical treatment of uncomplicated UTI, limiting the use of screening tests to only patients with low-to-moderate pretest probability estimates.

Sultana RV, Zalstein S, Cameron P, Campbell D: Dipstick urinalysis and the accuracy of the clinical diagnosis of urinary tract infection. J Emerg Med 1:13–19, 2001.

9. **When should I order a urine culture?**
A urine culture generally is not required to treat presumptively uncomplicated cystitis in women. Most clinicians recommend a culture with sensitivities in suspected pyelonephritis because of the potential for serious sequelae if an inappropriate antibiotic is used. All cases of potentially complicated UTI should also have a urine culture done.

10. **What is the difference between complicated and uncomplicated UTI?**
A complicated infection is associated with a clinical condition that increases the risk for acquiring infection, patients who have failed initial therapy, and patients who have increased morbidity. Factors that predispose to a complicated UTI include structural abnormalities (e.g., calculi, urinary catheters, stents, prostatic infection, and urinary diversion procedures), metabolic or hormonal abnormalities (e.g., diabetes or pregnancy), immunocompromise, recent urinary tract instrumentation, male gender, extremes of age (the elderly, young children), unusual pathogens, recent antibiotic use or failed treatment for UTI, and presence of symptoms for longer than 7 days. It can be argued that true uncomplicated UTIs occur only in nonpregnant, healthy women with no neurologic or structural dysfunction; 80% of UTIs fall into this group.

KEY POINTS: CHARACTERISTICS OF COMPLICATED UTIS

1. Structural abnormality

2. Immunocompromised host

3. Recent instrumentation

4. Failed treatment

5. Male gender or extremes of age

11. **How should acute, uncomplicated cystitis be treated?**
The causative agents are quite predictable. The Infectious Diseases Society of America (IDSA) has recommended that a 3-day regimen of trimethoprim-sulfamethoxazole (TMP-SMX) be standard therapy for acute uncomplicated cystitis. Fluoroquinolones, such as ofloxacin, norfloxacin, or ciprofloxacin, for 3 days are considered to have similar effectiveness as TMP-SMX but are considerably more expensive. Also, in an effort to postpone emergence of resistance to these drugs, the IDSA dose not recommend them as initial empirical therapy except in regions with known resistance to TMP-SMX of greater than 10–20% among

uropathogens. Nitrofurantoin for 7 days or a single dose of fosfomycin may become more useful as resistance to TMP-SMX increases.

Gupta K, Scholes D, Stamm WE: Increasing prevalence of antimicrobial resistance among uropathogens causing acute uncomplicated cystitis in women. JAMA 281: 736–738, 1999.

Warren JW, Abrutyn E, Hebel JR, et al: Guidelines for antimicrobial treatment of uncomplicated acute bacterial cystitis and acute pyelonephritis in women. Clin Infect Dis 29: 745–758, 1999

KEY POINTS: CHARACTERISTICS OF CYSTITIS

1. Dysuria

2. Frequency

3. Urgency

4. Suprapubic discomfort

5. Significant bacteriuria

12. How should acute, uncomplicated pyelonephritis be treated?

The IDSA recommends 14 days of antimicrobial therapy for young, nonpregnant women with normal urinary tracts. In mild cases, oral fluoroquinolones are considered the first choice for outpatient treatment of pyelonephritis (e.g., ciprofloxacin, 500 mg every 12 hours; levofloxacin, 250 mg daily; or ofloxacin, 200–300 mg every 12 hours). TMP-SMX for 14 days is an inexpensive option, but because of increasing antibiotic resistance to this agent in pyelonephritic strains, the IDSA recommends it be used only if the organism is known to be susceptible. In patients with a contraindication to fluoroquinolones, alternatives include cefixime, 400 mg daily, and cefpodoxime proxetil, 200 mg every 12 hours, for 14 days. A single-dose parenteral antibiotic (gentamicin or ceftriaxone) followed by any of the aforementioned regimens is an acceptable alternative.

www.idsociety.org

KEY POINTS: CHARACTERISTICS OF PYELONEPHRITIS

1. Fever

2. Flank pain

3. Costovertebral angle tenderness

4. Significant bacteriuria

13. Which patients with pyelonephritis should be admitted?

Admission should be strongly considered for patients who are unable to maintain oral hydration or to take oral medications and patients with uncertain social support or concern about compliance. Other indications include uncertain diagnosis or severe illness with extreme pain or marked debility. Any patients with evidence of complicated UTI also should be considered for admission. There is increasing evidence that some subsets of complicated pyelonephritis can be treated successfully on an outpatient basis. Pregnant patients at less than 24 weeks' gestation who are hemodynamically stable have been treated safely as outpatients if they can be reached easily by phone and are likely to be compliant with medication and follow-up. Further study is needed to define what other subsets of complicated pyelonephritis may be managed safely outside of the hospital.

14. **When should emergency imaging of the urinary tract be obtained in acute pyelonephritis?**
If the patient remains febrile for more than 72 hours on appropriate antibiotic therapy, computed tomography (CT) or ultrasound should be considered to rule out obstruction and renal or perinephric abscess.

KEY POINTS: FACTORS THAT MAY REQUIRE ADMISSION FOR PATIENTS WITH PYELONEPHRITIS

1. Pregnancy

2. Severe illness

3. Inability to maintain oral hydration

4. Uncertain social support/compliance

5. Complicated UTIs

15. **What are the signs and symptoms of acute bacterial prostatitis?**
The presentation can be dramatic and usually includes frequency, urgency, dysuria, and some obstructive voiding symptoms in greater than 80% of patients. Other common complaints include fever (60%), rigors, myalgias, and perineal discomfort (38%). Some patients also complain of low back pain or rectal pain. The prostate is warm, swollen, and extremely tender.
    Lummus WE, Thompson I: Prostatitis. Emerg Med Clin North Am 19:691–707, 2001.

16. **How is acute prostatitis managed?**
The pathogen usually can be isolated from voided urine. Prostatic massage and urethral catheterization should be avoided because they are painful and may precipitate bacteremia. Severely ill patients should be admitted and treated with intravenous antibiotics. An aminoglycoside-penicillin derivative combination is often used. Less severely ill patients respond well to oral fluoroquinolones or TMP-SMX. In one study, more than 95% of cultured organisms were sensitive to aminoglycosides, cephalosporins, ciprofloxacin, and imipenem as opposed to 83% sensitivity to TMP-SMX. The duration of therapy should be at least 30 days to prevent chronic bacterial prostatitis. Supportive measures include hydration, nonsteroidal anti-inflammatory drugs, sitz baths, and stool softeners. If urinary retention is a problem, suprapubic aspiration or suprapubic catheter placement is recommended.
    Lummus WE, Thompson I: Prostatitis. Emerg Med Clin North Am 19:691–707, 2001.

17. **Name the most common cause of recurrent UTI in men.**
Chronic bacterial prostatitis.

KEY POINTS: DURATION OF ANTIBIOTIC TREATMENT FOR UNCOMPLICATED DISEASE

1. Cystitis: 3–7 days

2. Pyelonephritis: 14 days

3. Prostatitis: At least 30 days

18. **What are the signs and symptoms of chronic bacterial prostatitis?**
    This is a syndrome of relapsing subacute illness characterized by mild symptoms of frequency, urgency, and dysuria. Other symptoms may include back pain, scrotal or perineal pain, voiding dysfunction, hematospermia, and painful ejaculation. Fever and rigors should not occur. Symptoms must be present for more than 3 months. Examination is highly variable and may be normal. A premassage and postmassage of the prostate urinalysis generally should be done and show repeated postmassage bacteriuria with the same organism.

19. **How is chronic bacterial prostatitis treated?**
    Treatment is difficult with poor cure rates and frequent relapse. Prolonged treatment (2–3 months) with fluoroquinolones is the mainstay of therapy. Recalcitrant infection may require long-term, low-dose therapy or resection of the prostate. Referral to a urologist generally is recommended, if possible, before treatment with antibiotics. α_1-Blocking agents show some promise for relief of symptoms and prevention of recurrence.

    e-Medicine.com/emerg/topic488.htm

CHAPTER 38

CHRONIC RENAL FAILURE AND DIALYSIS

Allan B. Wolfson, MD

1. **Isn't renal failure just another genitourinary disorder?**

   No. **End-stage renal disease (ESRD)** is a complex multisystem disorder. The absence of renal function has obvious consequences for the regulation of total body fluid and electrolyte balance, limiting the ability to handle fluid and electrolyte loads. Chronic renal failure results in subtle metabolic abnormalities, such as glucose intolerance and lipid disturbances. Renal failure is associated with numerous end-organ effects, ranging from pericarditis to renal osteodystrophy, that compromise comfort and normal function.

   Wolfson AB: Renal failure. In Marx JA, Hockberger RS, Walls RM, et al (eds): Rosen's Emergency Medicine: Concepts and Clinical Practice, 6th ed. Philadelphia, Mosby, 2006, pp 1524–1556.

   Wolfson AB: Chronic renal failure and dialysis-related emergencies. In Wolfson AB, Hendey GW, Hendry PL, et al (eds): Harwood-Nuss's Clinical Practice of Emergency Medicine, 4th ed. Philadelphia: Lippincott Williams & Wilkins, 2005, pp 457–463.

2. **What are the special concerns in patients with renal failure?**

   Iatrogenic illness is one important consideration, whether through overadministration of fluids or drug toxicity. Because the effects of renal failure on drug metabolism and disposition are often complex, it is always advisable to check recommended dosage adjustments for patients with ESRD before administering or prescribing medications. Even apparently innocuous drugs, such as antacids and cathartics, may cause morbidity and mortality if used improperly. Patients with ESRD have complications both from the underlying disease that caused renal failure and from complications of dialysis therapy. They have a limited capacity to respond to infection, trauma, or other intercurrent illnesses.

   Aronoff GR, Berns JS, Brier ME, et al: Drug Prescribing in Renal Failure: Dosing Guidelines for Adults. Philadelphia: American College of Physicians, 2002.

3. **How is hemodialysis performed?**

   In hemodialysis, the patient's blood is brought into contact with a semipermeable artificial membrane, on the other side of which is a chemically balanced aqueous dialysis solution. Metabolic waste and electrolytes flow from the patient's blood into the dialysate, and other substances (e.g., calcium) may flow from the dialysate into the blood, acting to normalize blood chemistries. To achieve adequate total body clearances over the time available for hemodialysis, a high blood-flow rate is necessary. This requires the cannulation of large vessels or, for long-term dialysis, the creation of an artificial vascular access that can be used repeatedly. Hemodialysis typically is performed for 4–5 hours, three times per week.

4. **How is peritoneal dialysis performed?**

   The patient's peritoneal membrane serves as the semipermeable barrier between the blood (in the peritoneal capillaries) and a balanced dialysate solution. The latter is introduced into the patient's peritoneal cavity and allowed to dwell for a period of hours before being drained and replaced. An osmotic gradient is created by using a dialysate with high concentrations of glucose that, through osmosis, pulls water from the intravascular space into the dialysate, acting to correct volume overload. For patients with ESRD on **chronic ambulatory peritoneal dialysis (CAPD),** about 2 L of dialysate dwells continuously within the peritoneal cavity. It is exchanged for fresh dialysate in a sterile fashion by the patient four times a day. Special peritoneal access is required in the form of a surgically implanted Teflon catheter (Tenckhoff catheter), through which dialysate is infused and drained.

5. **What is the most common problem relating to the vascular access device in the emergency department (ED)?**
Thrombosis should be suspected when patients report loss of a pulse or thrill in the vascular device. More often, they present to the ED when there has been a problem establishing adequate flow during a hemodialysis session. The only intervention necessary is a prompt call to a vascular surgeon. An angiogram defines the nature and extent of the obstruction and delineates anatomic lesions, allowing the surgeon to revise or replace the access.

KEY POINTS: PROBLEMS WITH VASCULAR ACCESS DEVICES

1. Thrombosis

2. Hemorrhage

3. Infection (often inapparent)

6. **How do I diagnose and treat a vascular access infection?**
Infection is obvious when the patient presents with signs of inflammation localized to the access area. The difficulty is that many patients present only with fever and without specific localizing signs. A useful rule of thumb in such instances is to assume that an endovascular access infection is present and to treat accordingly. After blood cultures are obtained, patients typically can be sent home after one dose of an appropriate antibiotic, provided that they look well and are reliable for follow-up. A single dose of vancomycin, 1 g intravenously, is the treatment of choice because most infections are staphylococcal and the drug's duration of action is 5–7 days in ESRD. Vancomycin is not hemodialyzable, and its major toxicity is to the kidneys. If gram-negative infection is suspected, a third-generation cephalosporin, aztreonam, or an aminoglycoside should be added to the regimen. Careful follow-up should be arranged with the patient's dialysis nurse or physician.

7. **When can the vascular access device be used for giving intravenous (IV) infusions or for drawing blood?**
Hemodialysis patients are instructed never to allow their blood pressure to be taken in the arm with the vascular access or to allow their blood to be drawn or IV fluids to be infused through the vascular access. This is to protect the access device, which is truly the patient's lifeline. Occasionally, there is no reasonable alternative but to use the access device for blood drawing or IV lines. In these situations, cautious use of the vascular access device is permissible, provided that certain guidelines are followed.
When using the access to draw blood, a tourniquet should not be used. At most, one finger can be used to tourniquet the vein lightly. The presence of a thrill should be documented before and after the procedure. The area should be cleaned thoroughly with povidone-iodine or another antiseptic, and sterile technique should be observed. Care should be taken not to puncture the back wall of the vessel, and after the puncture, firm but nonocclusive pressure should be applied to the site for several minutes to ensure that extravasation does not occur. Obvious aneurysms should not be punctured.

When using the vascular access for an IV line, similar precautions should be observed. Because the vessel is under arterial pressure, a pressure bag or, preferably, an automated infusion device is an absolute requirement (certainly when infusing medications).

8. How is CAPD-associated peritonitis diagnosed?

Peritonitis associated with CAPD occurs about once per year in even the most fastidious and well-motivated patients. In contrast to other types of peritonitis, it tends to be mild clinically, and most patients can be managed without hospital admission. CAPD-associated peritonitis is caused most commonly by gram-positive organisms, which are thought to be introduced during the exchange procedure. The diagnosis is suspected by the patient on the basis of the new appearance of cloudiness of the dialysis effluent. Patients are instructed to seek medical attention promptly when this occurs, and for this reason most episodes of peritonitis are relatively mild. If the patient delays seeking attention, however, the symptoms tend to become progressively more severe. Most patients have abdominal pain and tenderness, but only a few have fever, nausea, vomiting, or even (at least early on) an elevated peripheral white blood cell count. Localized peritoneal findings are suggestive of an acute surgical abdomen rather than CAPD-associated peritonitis.

9. How is CAPD-associated peritonitis treated?

When fluid has been obtained from the effluent bag and laboratory studies have confirmed the presence of a significant number of white cells (>100 cells/mm^3 with $>50\%$ polymorphonuclear leukocytes) or a positive Gram stain, antibiotic treatment is initiated. Commonly, vancomycin (30 mg/kg) is given intraperitoneally and may be repeated weekly. Gram-negative coverage, with a third-generation cephalosporin, aztreonam, or an aminoglycoside, can be added if thought appropriate. These may be given intraperitoneally as well and should be followed by daily intraperitoneal maintenance doses as an outpatient. Usually, each center has its own protocols for treatment, so the patient's nephrologist or dialysis nurse should be consulted. Follow-up should be in 48 hours, at which time cultures and clinical findings are rechecked and therapy adjusted as necessary. Admission criteria include severe pain, nausea and vomiting, a toxic appearance, or the inability of the patient to comply with outpatient therapy and follow-up.

Keane WF, Bailie GR, Boeschoten E, et al: Adult peritoneal dialysis-related peritonitis treatment recommendations: 2000 update. www.ispd.org/guidelines/articles/update (Accessed June 24, 2005).

KEY POINTS: CAPD-ASSOCIATED PERITONITIS

1. Diagnosis: Cloudy dialysate effluent, abdominal pain, fever

2. Treatment: Typically with intraperitoneal antibiotics

10. What are the indications for emergency dialysis?

Acute pulmonary edema, life-threatening hyperkalemia, or life-threatening intoxication or overdose secondary to dialyzable toxins that ordinarily are excreted by the kidneys.

11. What is unique about a dialysis patient with cardiac arrest?

Two potentially reversible entities always should be considered in an ESRD patient with cardiac arrest:

1. **Severe hyperkalemia** may cause severe rhythm disturbances and ultimately cardiac arrest without any other warning or clinical signs. When a patient suffers an arrest from whatever cause, respiratory and metabolic acidosis and the efflux of potassium from cells can be

expected to produce hyperkalemia secondarily. In the patient who already may have a tendency toward hyperkalemia, this further increase could cause the patient to be refractory to standard advanced cardiac life support (ACLS) interventions. ESRD patients in cardiac arrest always should be given IV calcium if they do not respond immediately to the first round of ACLS measures.

2. **Acute pericardial tamponade** may result from accumulation of pericardial fluid or spontaneous bleeding into the pericardial sac. Patients with tamponade tend to display refractory hypotension or pulseless electrical activity or both. Although less likely than other entities to be the cause of refractoriness to resuscitation measures, the possibility of pericardial tamponade always should be considered in patients in whom other measures have failed. Emergency pericardiocentesis may be life saving.

KEY POINTS: INDICATIONS FOR EMERGENCY DIALYSIS

1. Acute pulmonary edema

2. Life-threatening hyperkalemia

3. Life-threatening intoxication or overdose with agents normally excreted by the kidneys

12. **What are the treatment options for acute pulmonary edema in patients with ESRD?**

ESRD patients with pulmonary edema do not have the ability to rid themselves of excess fluid through the kidneys and ultimately require dialysis to correct volume overload. Interventions that are useful in patients with functioning kidneys also are useful in patients with ESRD while awaiting the initiation of acute dialysis. The patient should be given oxygen and placed in a sitting position. Nitrates administered sublingually or intravenously are the mainstay of temporizing therapy. Sublingual nitroglycerin can be given every 3 minutes to decrease preload and afterload as blood pressure permits. IV nitroglycerin is a useful alternative. IV morphine, although less popular, also may be helpful in decreasing pulmonary venous hypertension, although patients may be more likely to require intubation and mechanical ventilation because of its sedative action. IV furosemide, although it cannot act as a diuretic, has some action in decreasing pulmonary venous pressure.

Dialysis is the definitive therapy and should be instituted as early as possible. The CAPD patient with acute pulmonary edema presents a slightly different problem because intensified dialysis, even with 4.25% glucose solution, is a slow means of removing fluid and because the presence of 2 L of dialysate in the peritoneal cavity tends to have an adverse effect on diaphragmatic excursion and pulmonary mechanics. Intubation and mechanical ventilation may be necessary while continuing hourly exchanges of high-concentration dialysate.

13. **How should I treat hyperkalemia in a dialysis patient?**

The approach is similar to that taken with nondialysis patients. IV calcium gluconate (10 mL of a 10% solution) acts rapidly to antagonize the cardiotoxic effects of hyperkalemia (without affecting the serum potassium level), but its effects last for only a few minutes. It should be used only as a temporizing measure in patients with cardiovascular compromise or a widened QRS complex on the electrocardiogram (ECG).

Nebulized albuterol (10–20 mg by inhalation) acts within a few minutes to shift potassium into cells. It is easy to administer, generally has minimal side effects, and is effective for a few hours. The dose can be repeated as necessary.

Glucose and insulin (typically 50 g and 0.1 units/kg, respectively, as a slow IV infusion) also moves potassium into cells but requires close serial monitoring of blood glucose levels.

IV sodium bicarbonate (50 mEq over 5 minutes) has a similar action but can exacerbate volume overload and can acutely decrease the ionized calcium.

If dialysis is not immediately available to remove potassium from the body, sodium polystyrene sulfonate (Kayexalate), a sodium-potassium exchange resin typically given orally wih sorbitol to enhance passage through the gut, can remove significant amounts of potassium from the body. It is slow acting, however, and should be reserved for situations in which the patient is stable but requires continuing control of the serum potassium over hours, until dialysis can be performed.

In all cases of acute hyperkalemia, the serum potassium level should be checked frequently, and continuous ECG monitoring is mandatory until definitive treatment with dialysis can be initiated.

KEY POINTS: TREATMENT OF HYPERKALEMIA

1. IV calcium

2. Inhaled albuterol

3. IV glucose and insulin

4. IV sodium bicarbonate

5. Oral or rectal Kayexalate

6. Dialysis

14. **What about air embolism?**

Air embolism is an uncommon complication of hemodialysis. Although air embolism has become rare with the advent of sophisticated monitoring and alarm systems on hemodialysis machines, when it does occur it is often a devastating event and one for which the patient almost surely will be brought to the nearest ED.

Air embolism should be suspected when a patient experiences a sudden acute decompensation during the course of hemodialysis treatment. Several immediate measures are thought to be helpful. Any IV lines should be clamped. The patient should be given 100% oxygen and laid on the left side with the head down, in an attempt to cause the air to collect at the apex of the right ventricle. At this point, if the patient is reasonably stable, an interventional radiologist or cardiologist can be consulted for consideration of passage of a central venous catheter into the right ventricular apex, through which the air can be aspirated directly out of the heart. For patients who are in close proximity to a hyperbaric chamber, treatment with 100% oxygen at several atmospheres can shrink the size of the bubbles and enhance resorption of the gas. One should be certain before embarking on this course, however, that the patient's symptoms are due to air embolism rather than, for example, a sudden spontaneous pneumothorax.

15. **How should a patient with acute shortness of breath be evaluated?**

The rule of thumb is to dialyze ESRD patients who are short of breath, because volume overload is the most common cause. It is sometimes difficult to make the diagnosis of volume overload. The patient's weight may be the best guide. Physical examination is not always helpful, and chest radiographs may be misleading.

16. **What are the main differential diagnostic considerations for chest pain in ESRD?**

Always think first of either angina or pericarditis. Some patients with ESRD, particularly those who are anemic, may have angina and cardiac ischemia even if a previous cardiac catheterization has shown a *noncritical* coronary obstruction. This is due to increased cardiac oxygen demands and decreased oxygen delivery to the heart. Although cardiac enzyme levels may be altered in ESRD, renal failure does not obscure the usual ECG and enzyme changes of acute myocardial infarction.

17. **What is the differential diagnosis of hypotension in a patient with ESRD?**
The most common entities are hypovolemia after dialysis, sepsis, hemorrhage, and acute pericardial tamponade.

KEY POINTS: MOST COMMON CAUSES OF HYPOTENSION IN DIALYSIS PATIENTS

1. Hypovolemia after dialysis

2. Sepsis

3. Hemorrhage

4. Pericardial tamponade

18. **What are the major causes of altered mental status in patients with ESRD?**
Dysequilibrium syndrome, caused by rapid solute shifts during hemodialysis, is a consideration, but a major pitfall is to attribute every change in mental status to this entity. Drug effects are a major cause, as is spontaneous intracranial hemorrhage. Any patient with localizing signs should have a computed tomography (CT) scan of the head; patients without localizing signs should also undergo CT scanning, however, because subdural hematoma may not cause focal findings.

HEMOSTASIS AND COAGULOPATHIES

Thomas B. Barry, MD

CHAPTER 39

1. What is meant by hemostasis?

Hemostasis is a balance between excessive bleeding and thrombosis. It is the active process of clot formation and degradation in response to injury of a blood vessel. This response normally occurs through the coordinated efforts of the blood vessel endothelium, platelets, the clotting factor cascade, and fibrinolysis.

KEY POINTS: THREE PHASES OF HEMOSTASIS

1. Platelet plug formation

2. Propagation of the coagulation cascade and fibrin clot formation

3. Balanced fibrinolysis

2. Is hemophilia the main cause of hemostatic abnormality?

Most hemostatic abnormalities result from drugs such as heparin, warfarin, and aspirin or from associated disease such as liver or kidney failure. The hemophilias are important but less common.

3. Do I really need to know the whole clotting cascade to manage patients?

A working knowledge should include the basics of the three phases of hemostasis, some key clotting factors, and familiarity with basic testing and therapeutics.

In **primary hemostasis,** after injury, platelets and von Willebrand factor (vWF) from the endothelium interact to form a plug (platelet adhesion). Platelet activation and aggregation occur along with vessel constriction. Disorders include problems with platelet quantity and function as well as vWF problems and vascular abnormalities such as hereditary telangiectasia. Platelet count and bleeding time are used to assess this phase of hemostasis.

In **secondary hemostasis,** the platelet plug is reinforced with cross-linked fibrin from the coagulation cascade (factor XIII causes covalent cross-links). Effective functioning of the cascade may be impaired by deficiencies of coagulation factor activity (hemophilia A and B) or by inadequate factor production such as with warfarin use.

In **tertiary hemostasis,** the fibrin clot is enzymatically broken down by plasmin. Endothelial cells release plasminogen activator, which converts plasminogen to plasmin. The plasmin breaks down fibrin and fibrinogen into fibrin split products and D-dimers. Excessive fibrinolytic activity or deficiencies of fibrinolytic inhibitors can increase bleeding. Because protein C and protein S are involved in the regulation of blood clotting, deficiencies can result in excessive intravascular clotting.

Hamilton GC, Janz TG: Disorders of hemostasis. In Rosen P, Barkin RM (eds): Emergency Medicine: Concepts and Clinical Practice, 5th ed. St. Louis, Mosby, 2002, pp 1688–1700.

4. **What are the intrinsic and extrinsic coagulation pathways? How can I tell the difference?**

   Prothrombin time (PT) is affected by the extrinsic (and common) pathways of the cascade and partial thromboplastin time (PTT) by defects in the intrinsic (and common) paths. The extrinsic pathway is activated by tissue factor exposed at the site of injury. The intrinsic pathway is initiated by blood exposure to a negatively charged surface. A patient with a prolonged PTT and a normal PT is considered to have a defect in the intrinsic coagulation pathway. The name indicates that all of the components of the PTT test (except kaolin) are "intrinsic" to the plasma. On the other hand, a patient with a prolonged PT and a normal PTT has a defect in the "extrinsic" coagulation pathway (tissue factor being extrinsic to the plasma). Prolongation of both the PT and the PTT implies that the defect is in a common pathway. Both pathways converge to activate factor X, which activates prothrombin to thrombin.

5. **What parts of the history and physical can help me assess a suspected bleeding abnormality?**

   It is important to ask about medications, previous medical history (especially liver, kidney, and malignant disease), previous problems with bleeding (such as with dental work and surgeries), and family history of bleeding disorders. In patients with known bleeding disorders, ask about the nature of their disease and previous therapies. They are frequently very knowledgeable about their individual disease. Platelet disorders frequently result in petechia, purpura, epistaxis, and gum and other mucosal bleeding. They are common in women and usually acquired as opposed to congenital. Problems with coagulation are more commonly congenital, found more often in men, and are likely to present as deep muscle or joint bleeding. Postsurgical bleeding from coagulopathy usually occurs after a delay of up to 3 days. Coagulopathy is rarely the cause of epistaxis, menorrhagia, or gastrointestinal (GI) bleed.

6. **How do I interpret PT, PTT, and international normalized ratio (INR)?**

   PT tests the factors of the extrinsic and common pathways. It is prolonged by deficiencies of prothrombin, fibrinogen, and factors V, VII, and X. A PT 2 seconds more than the control is significant. PTT tests all the intrinsic and common pathways, including all factors except VII and XIII. INR reduces interlaboratory variation by indexing thromboplastin test lot activity to an international standard. Liver disease, warfarin use, and other abnormalities of the vitamin K sensitive factors (II, VII, IX, X) affect the PT and INR. INR of 1 is normal. An INR between 2–3 indicates a therapeutic level of warfarin.

7. **What are the causes of thrombocytopenia?**
   - Decreased production: Marrow disease, chemotherapy, alcohol or thiazide effect
   - Immune destruction: Idiopathic thrombocytopenic purpura (ITP), systemic lupus erythematosus (SLE), lymphoma, quinine, quinidine, postinfectious disease
   - Toxic destruction: Disseminated intravascular coagulation (DIC), thrombotic thrombocytopenic purpura (TTP), hemolytic uremic syndrome (HUS), hemolysis with elevated liver enzymes and low platelets (HELLP) syndrome
   - Splenic sequestration (hypersplenism; rare): Hematologic malignancy, portal hypertension, autoimmune hemolytic anemia, hereditary spherocytosis
   - Dilution: Massive transfusion
   - Lab error: It happens. "I'm shocked, shocked..." (Claude Rains, *Casablanca,* Warner Brothers, 1942)

8. **What are the differences between idiopathic and chronic thrombocytopenic purpura?**
   - **ITP** should be a diagnosis of exclusion after considering SLE, antiphospholipid syndrome, human immunodeficiency virus (HIV), and lymphoproliferative disorders. It is associated with

antiplatelet antibody IgG. The acute form is seen in children 4–6 years old several weeks after a viral prodrome. It is self-limited with a 90% rate of spontaneous remission. Morbidity and mortality rates are low, and steroid therapy does not seem to alter the course.

- **Chronic ITP** is found in adults. It is three times more common in women than men. Severity waxes and wanes with only a 1% mortality, but spontaneous remission is rare. It may respond to therapy with glucocorticoids, intravenous (IV) immunoglobulin, and splenectomy if recurrent. Other treatments include plasmapheresis, androgen therapy with danazol, cyclophosphamide, azathioprine, vincristine, thrombopoietin, antiCD40 ligand, rituximab, and anti-D immunoglobulin (WinRho) in Rh-positive presplenectomy patients. Platelet transfusion is reserved for life-threatening bleeds because it may increase antiplatelet antibodies.

9. **What are the five clinical signs of TTP?**
   Only 40% of patients have all five:
   - Fluctuating change in mental status
   - Thrombocytopenia
   - Fever (in 90% of patients)
   - Microangiopathic hemolytic anemia
   - Renal impairment

10. **What causes TTP? Is it worse than ITP?**
    TTP results from subendothelial and intraluminal deposits of fibrin and platelet aggregation in capillaries and arterioles. Prostacyclin and abnormal platelet aggregation are thought to contribute to its origins. It may affect patients of any age or gender although most are 10–40 years old and 60% are female. When untreated, there is 80% mortality at 3 months as a result of microthrombi in the heart, brain, and kidneys. Recently plasmapheresis has reduced this to 17%. Other therapies include steroids, splenectomy, gamma-globulin, vincristine, and antiplatelet agents such as aspirin and dipyridamole (Persantine). Platelet transfusions may cause additional microcirculatory thrombi and should be avoided unless bleeding is life threatening.

11. **What is HUS?**
    HUS is similar to TTP. HUS causes less change in mental status and more kidney damage. Patients with HUS tend to be younger, and onset is often associated with a bacterial gastroenteritis such as *Escherichia coli* 0157:H7 and *Shigella* sp.

12. **Should I worry about thrombocytopenia during large-volume blood transfusion?**
    Stored banked blood is platelet poor because platelets have a life span of only 9 days. Follow platelet counts after 10 units of blood. Transfuse platelets when count is down to 50,000/mL.

13. **How does aspirin increase bleeding?**
    Aspirin blocks cyclooxygenase, which decreases thromboxane formation leading to decreased platelet aggregation and less vasoconstriction. Aspirin poisons this reaction for the life of the platelet. Nonsteroidal anti-inflammatory drugs such as indomethacin have this effect only while in the circulation. Uremia has a similar reversible effect.

14. **When do I need to transfuse platelets?**
    As previously noted, platelet transfusion should be delayed in ITP and TTP to avoid disease-specific complications and alloimmunization. It is more commonly indicated for primary bone marrow problems. In a patient with a platelet count greater than 50,000/mL, hemorrhage due to the deficiency is unlikely. From 10,000–50,000/mL there is variable risk with trauma, ulcer, and invasive procedures. The less mature platelets of peripheral consumption and sequestration are

less likely to allow spontaneous hemorrhage. Choosing when to transfuse at these levels is not an exact science. Platelet transfusion is indicated with counts less than 10,000/mL because there is a significant risk of spontaneous hemorrhage. Each bag of random donor platelets may be expected to raise the platelet count 5000/mL. They are usually ordered six at a time. One single-donor apheresis unit results in the same 30,000/mL increase.

15. **What is the most common inherited bleeding disorder?**
It is von Willebrand's disease (5–10 cases per million population). It is usually autosomal dominant. There is a deficiency or dysfunction of vWF and a mild factor VIII defect. Treatment is with desmopressin in the mild, most common, type I form of the disease.

In more severe types, therapy is with cryoprecipitate based on the factor VIII level. Usual dose is 1–2 bags/10 kg. In vonWillebrand's this is found to stimulate factor VIII activity and less is needed in redosing.

16. **Do people with hemophilia A have low levels of factor VIII?**
It is the activity of factor VIII that is impaired, technically not its level. Seventy percent of cases are transmitted by sex-linked recessive (X chromosome) inheritance; 30% of cases are due to spontaneous mutation. Severe disease has less than 1% activity, and spontaneous bleeding (joints, deep muscles, urinary tract, and central nervous system [CNS]) is a problem. Between 1% and 5% activity is classified as moderate disease with problems mostly after trauma and surgery. Above 5% is mild disease, but some trauma and surgical risk persist PTT is only prolonged with less than 35% activity.
Pearl: 1 unit of factor VIII per kilogram increases the activity level by 2%. (Unless adversely affected by anti-factor VIII antibodies (IgG), which develop in 7–20% of patients.) Recombinant DNA factor VIII is the replacement of choice and lacks the hepatitis B, C, and HIV risks of fresh frozen plasma (FFP) and cryoprecipitate.

17. **How is factor VIII dosed in hemophilia A?**
Twenty-five units per kilogram for moderate bleeding, 50 units/kg for severe hemorrhage or life-threatening bleeding site (GI, neck, sublingual, retroperitoneal, intra-abdominal, head injury, CNS bleed, and necessary surgical procedures). Because the half-life is 8–12 hours, redose with half the loading dose after 8–12 hours. Recombinant factor VIII unit concentration is noted on the label. Cryoprecipitate (of FFP) is assumed to be 80–100 units of factor VIII per bag.

18. **What is Christmas disease?**
Hemophilia B, which involves decreased factor IX activity. The clinical presentation is the same as hemophilia A. The genetic pattern is the same, although less prevalent in the population with only {1/5} the number of cases. Treatment is with factor IX, 50 U/kg or FFP.
Pearl: There is no factor IX in cryoprecipitate.

19. **What does desmopressin (DDAVP) do?**
Desmopressin is a synthetic analog of antidiuretic hormone. It works by causing release of vWF from endothelial storage sites and increases levels of factor VIII in hemophilia A and some cases of von Willebrand's. The dose is 0.3 μg/kg IV; it lasts 4–6 hours and is most effective in mild to moderately deficient patients.

20. **What factors are affected by vitamin K deficiency? Warfarin? Liver disease? Banked blood?**
- Vitamin K deficiency affects II, VII, IX, and X, the same ones affected by warfarin.
- Hepatic insufficiency affects all factors except VIII.
- Stored blood is low in V, VIII, and platelets.

KEY POINTS: HEMOSTATIC DEFICIENCIES

1. With hemophilia A and B, the bleeding time is normal (as is the PT and the PTT in mild and moderate cases).

2. Bleeding time is increased with von Willebrand's disease.

3. PT reflects extrinsic pathway abnormality through factor VII deficient activity.

4. Factor VII has the shortest half-life of the factors (3–5 hours) and causes the first manifestations of production deficiency.

5. An INR of 2–3 is recommended with most warfarin therapy.

6. Deficiency of factors VIII, IX, and XI account for 99% of inherited bleeding disorders. If congenital bleeding disorder is suspected, FFP at 15 mL/kg will support hemostasis while a definitive diagnosis is being made.

---

21. What happens in DIC?

Platelets and clotting factors (especially V, VIII, and XIII) are consumed. Thrombin formation overwhelms fibrinolysis and activates fibrinogen. Fibrin is deposited in small vessels of multiple organ systems. Fibrin degradation products are released, and platelet function as well as fibrin polymerization are decreased.

Treatment is with platelets and FFP. Heparin may be used if fibrin deposition and thrombosis dominate the clinical picture.

22. What are HIT and HITT?

Heparin-induced thrombocytopenia (HIT) is caused by antibodies to heparin/platelet factor 4 complex. It results in platelet activation and clot formation. It usually occurs 5–10 days after exposure to heparin but may occur after as little as 10 hours. It occurs in 2% of patients on unfractionated heparin anticoagulation therapy and is even less common with low-molecular-weight heparin (LMWH). Platelet counts drop to 50,000–100,000/mL. HITT (HIT with thrombosis) develops in 50% of the patients with HIT. HIT and HITT require discontinuation of heparin (including heparin flushes). A direct thrombin inhibitor is indicated in patients with thrombosis (Hirudin or Argatroban). Doppler ultrasound of the legs is indicated in HIT, because recent studies have found subclinical deep venous thrombosis (DVT) in up to 50% of HIT patients. DVT requires anticoagulation for 3–6 months.

Hassel K: The management of patients with heparin-induced thrombocytopenia who require anticoagulant therapy. Chest 127:1s–8s, 2005.

23. Need help with HELLP?

HELLP criteria:

- Microangiopathic hemolytic anemia
- Serum aspartate transaminase levels greater than 70 U/L
- Platelets less than 100,000/mL

The HELLP syndrome is a form of preeclampsia. Gestational thrombocytopenia (100,000–150,000/mL) is found in 5–10% of third trimester pregnancies. It is even more common in pregnancies complicated by preeclampsia (15–20%) and eclampsia (40–50%). Fetal and maternal mortality are increased. Treatment is primarily supportive although platelet transfusion may be required prior to cesarean section. DIC may develop.

24. **How do heparin and LMWH work?**

Heparin catalyzes the inactivation of thrombin and factor X by antithrombin. It also has some effect on II, IX, and XI. Factor VII is not affected. At usual doses, it will prolong the PTT (and thrombin time [TT]) but not the PT. Occult GI bleeding is a relative contraindication to its use, and clearance is prolonged in hepatic and renal dysfunction.

25. **How do I treat hemorrhage secondary to heparin therapy?**

With major bleeding episodes, heparin can be 100% reversed with protamine sulfate at a dose of 1 mg/100 U of circulating heparin to a maximum dose of 250 mg. It is given slowly, IV, over 10 minutes. Rapid infusion increases the risk of anaphylaxis. (Protamine is only 60% effective in reversing LMWH, resulting in unfractionated heparin being the choice when surgery or invasive procedures may become necessary.) LMWH is derived from smaller pieces of the heparin molecule. Weight-based subcutaneous dosing of LMWH without anticoagulation monitoring has proven safe and effective in clinical trials. (This is fortunate, because LMWH inactivates factor X more than it does thrombin, so PTT is not significantly affected and cannot be used to monitor clinical effect and therapeutic plasma concentrations.) Weight-based pharmacokinetic predictions for LMWH are not reliable in patients weighing more than 100 kg, pregnant patients, and those with decreased creatinine clearance. If LMWH is used in these patients, anti-X activity must be monitored. (Unfractionated heparin usually becomes the drug of choice in these patients.)

KEY POINTS: DIAGNOSIS AND TREATMENT OF COAGULOPATHIES

1. Thrombocytopenia: Increased bleeding time, epistaxis, purpura, petechia, mucosal bleeding (6 bags random donor platelets yields 30,000/mL increase)

2. PT and INR: Extrinsic and common paths—warfarin (II, VII, IX, X)

3. PTT: Intrinsic and common paths (all factors *except* VII and XIII)—heparin

4. For severe bleeding with hemophilia A, 50 U/kg factor VIII

5. FFP, 15 mL/kg (will support hemostasis until definitive diagnosis)

26. **How does warfarin work? How do I deal with elevated INR?**

Warfarin (an oral anticoagulant therapy [OAT]) inhibits the reduction of vitamin K to its active form causing depletion of factors II, VII, IX, and X. Starting dose is 5 mg/day, with 4–5 days required for full anticoagulant effect. (Heparin or LMWH is continued in the interim.) Target is usually an INR of 2–3. Significant bleeding occurs in 3% of patients on chronic OAT. Drug interactions are common, and INR must be monitored. Head computed tomography (CT) evaluation should be considered even in minor head trauma with therapeutic dosing. Minor bleeding with elevated INR less than 5 can be treated by withholding doses until INR returns to the desired range. The underlying need for anticoagulation should be considered. Asymptomatic patients with INR of 5–9 may receive vitamin K 1–2.5 mg per os (PO) without significantly altering the ability to control anticoagulation. Give 3–5 mg PO for INR greater than 9 in asymptomatic patients. Serious bleeding is treated with FFP (10–15 mL/kg) and 10 mg IV vitamin K, given slowly (FFP for immediate effect; vitamin K effect takes several hours).

27. **What's new in antithrombotics?**

Activated protein C. Sepsis causes a cascade of inflammation and coagulation with impaired fibrinolysis. Microvascular hypoperfusion and organ dysfunction contribute to mortality. Among its effects, activated protein C inactivates factors V and VIII inhibiting thrombosis and promoting fibrinolysis. Treatment with activated drotrecogin alfa (Xigris), a recombinant human activated protein C, has shown a reduction in 30-day mortality in adult sepsis patients with acute organ dysfunction who are at a high risk of death.

Shapiro NI, Howell M, Talmor D: A blueprint for a sepsis protocol. Acad Emerg Med 12:352–359, 2005.

28. **What's new in prothrombotics?**

Recent studies are investigating the use of recombinant activated factor VII (NovoSeven) to promote hemostasis in a number of hemorrhagic conditions including transfusion-resistant hemorrhage, acute intracranial hemorrhage, and battlefield injury.

Mayer SA, Brun NC, Begtrup K, et al: Recombinant Activated factor VII for acute intracerebral hemorrhage. N Engl J Med 352:777–785, 2005.

29. **Is it true they are close to developing safe and effective fake blood?**

Development of a blood substitute has been a major goal of transfusion research groups for many years. Advantages could include improved storage requirements and shelf-life, and decreased antigen reactions and viral and bacterial contamination.

Hemoglobin-based oxygen carriers (HBOCs) had been developed in the 1980s and seem to have taken the lead over perfluorocarbon blood substitutes. Initial renal toxicity was eliminated and clinical trials started. Two trials with diaspirin cross-linked hemoglobin (DCLHb) showed worse outcomes in the treatment groups than the controls. Hemopure, a bovine hemoglobin solution, did reduce the need for standard transfusions but appeared to cause massive vasoconstriction. Hemolink, an oligomeric human HBOC, also reduced transfusion requirements, but a phase IIb study was suspended when an increase in adverse cardiac events was detected. Polyheme, a human polymeric HBOC, has reduced transfusion requirements without causing vasoconstriction. It is currently undergoing phase 4 clinical trials. Despite more than a decade of significant advances, much remains to be done.

Bone HG, Westfall M: The prospect of hemoglobin-based blood substitutes: Still a long stony road to go. Crit Care Med 33:694–695, 2005.

CHAPTER 40

SICKLE CELL DISEASE

Kurt Whitaker, MD

1. **What is sickle cell disease (SCD)?**
   SCD (also known as sickle cell anemia) is an autosomal recessive disease that results from a single amino acid substitution—valine for glutamine—at the sixth position on the β-globulin chain of the hemoglobin molecule. This substitution affects hemoglobin solubility. When sickle hemoglobin (hemoglobin S [HgS]) is deoxygenated, the abnormal hemoglobin polymerizes. This results in abnormal, sickle-shaped, nondeformable red blood cells, which cannot pass through capillaries. These sickle cells are responsible for the vaso-occlusive phenomena that are the hallmark of the disease.

2. **What is sickle cell trait?**
   A patient with sickle cell trait has one copy of the sickle cell gene (SCD patients have two). These patients have a normal life span and are generally asymptomatic.

3. **What are hemoglobin C and β-thalassemia?**
   Both are abnormal hemoglobins that create hemolytic anemias of their own. Hemoglobin C (HbC) is an inherited abnormal beta chain, which when combined with the sickle cell gene produces a less severe form of SCD known as HbSC. β-Thalassemia is also an inherited abnormal beta chain. When combined with a copy of the sickle cell gene, the clinical presentation of the disease can range from a mild to severe form of SCD. Table 40-1 summarizes the spectrum of SCD.

TABLE 40-1. THE SPECTRUM OF SICKLE CELL DISEASE (SCD)		
Disease	**Genetics**	**Clinical Severity**
Sickle cell disease	Two copies of sickle cell gene	Most severe
Sickle cell trait	One copy of sickle cell gene, other Hb gene is normal	Usually asymptomatic with a normal life span
HbSC disease	One copy of sickle cell gene, one of Hb C gene	Less severe symptoms, life span ≈ 20 years longer than in SCD
Sickle cell-β-thalassemia	One copy of sickle cell gene, one of β-thalassemia gene	20% have symptoms as severe as those with SCD; 80% have less severe symptoms.

4. **What causes red blood cells to sickle?**
   The rate and extent of polymer formation in a circulating SS red cell depend primarily on three independent variables: the cell's degree of deoxygenation, the intracellular hemoglobin concentration, and the presence or absence of hemoglobin F (fetal hemoglobin). Any factors that promote global or local hypoxia, such as circulatory stasis, cardiovascular disease, pulmonary

disease, and high altitude, can cause sickling. Low temperature promotes sickling through vasoconstriction. Acidosis also promotes sickling, as does radiographic contrast dye. The presence of hemoglobin F in a red blood cell prevents sickling.

Bunn HF: Mechanisms of disease: Pathogenesis and treatment of sickle cell disease. N Engl J Med 337:762–769, 1997.

5. Is sickling reversible?

Yes. Cells sickle and unsickle as they are exposed to different conditions in the microcirculation and central bloodstream. After repeated episodes of sickling, permanently deformed sickle cells may be formed.

6. How common is SCD?

In the United States, 1 of every 650 (about 0.15%) people of African descent is born with SCD. Approximately 8% are heterozygous for the sickle cell gene. The prevalence is increasing in the United States, due to both population growth and improved longevity of patients with SCD. Mortality rates for children with SCD have declined with the advent of newborn screening programs, education initiatives for parents, antibiotic prophylaxis, and *Haemophilus influenzae* and *Streptococcus pneumoniae* vaccination. Despite these improvements in the care provided, the median age at death is 42 years for men and 48 years for women.

Minter KR, Gladwin MT: Pulmonary complications of sickle cell anemia. Am J Respir Crit Care Med 164:2016–2019, 2001.

7. What are the treatments for SCD?

Currently no therapies are widely available to provide long-term cure. In the acute care setting, the goal is to stop the cycle of deoxygenated sickling and microvascular sludging. Therapies include rest, hydration, oxygenation, and analgesia. Transfusion and antibiotic therapy for infection are also indicated in some cases. Hydroxyurea, which increases fetal hemoglobin levels, may be used as an adjunct for chronic therapy. Fetal hemoglobin alters the dynamics of hemoglobin S polymerization, thereby decreasing the rates of vaso-occlusive crisis, acute chest syndrome (ACS), and transfusion. Advances have been made in gene therapy. Bone marrow transplantation for SCD may be curative.

8. What are the typical baseline laboratory findings in patients with SCD?

Because sickle cells have a shorter half-life than normal red blood cells, most patients will have a mild to moderate anemia with a hematocrit from 20–30% and a reactive reticulocytosis of 3–15%. In an analysis of laboratory values collected on more than 2700 patients in the Cooperative Study of Sickle Cell Disease, the white blood cell count, platelet count, and alkaline phosphatase levels were elevated. Mean bilirubin levels and lactate dehydrogenase levels were also elevated secondary to early red cell death. Creatinine and electrolyte levels were generally normal.

West MS, Wethers D, Smith J, Steinberg M: Laboratory profile of sickle cell disease: A cross-sectional analysis. The Cooperative Study of Sickle Cell Disease. J Clin Epidemiol 45:893–909, 1992.

9. What are the four different types of sickle cell crises?

- **Vaso-occlusive (pain) crisis** is caused by ischemic injury, which can lead to tissue infarction. The pain may affect any organ, but common sites include digits, joints, back, bone, abdomen, and chest. The patient will be able to tell you if the presentation is typical for his or her acute painful crises. If the presentation is atypical for the patient, a more extensive evaluation must be performed to identify the underlying cause. Children often present with "hand-foot syndrome" with pain in their digits.
- **Hemolytic crisis** usually occurs in response to infection or drugs, resulting in a more rapid rate of hemolysis. A rapidly falling hematocrit, an elevated reticulocyte count, pallor, and

jaundice are observed. Patients with glucose 6-phosphate dehydrogenase (G6PD) deficiency are even more prone to hemolysis and hypoxia. It can be precipitated by certain foods (fava beans) and medications (aspirin and sulfonamides).

- **Aplastic crisis** is frequently a response to infection, with parvovirus B19 being a known precipitant. It is characterized by decreased hematocrit, depressed reticulocyte count, fatigue, dyspnea, and pallor.
- **Sequestration crisis** occurs when large numbers of red blood cells pool in the spleen due to their abnormal shape and stiffness. Patients present with splenic enlargement, abdominal pain, a falling hematocrit, pallor, tachycardia, and dyspnea. Massive sequestration can lead to hypovolemic shock and death. This usually occurs between the ages of 5 months and 2 years, because the spleen is typically autoinfarcted by the age of two due to multiple vaso-occlusive events. It is the most dangerous crisis for young children, with a mortality of 10–15%.

Embury SH, Vichinsky EP: Overview of the clinical manifestations of sickle cell disease. UpToDate, version 13.1, December, 2004. Available at http://www.utdol.com/utd/content/topic.do?topicKey=red_cell/24936&type=A&selectedTitle=2~102

10. How should vaso-occlusive (pain) crisis be managed?

Vaso-occlusive crises are managed with oral (in mild cases) or intravenous rehydration, oxygen, and analgesics. A fingerstick spun hematocrit and urine dipstick to screen for worsened anemia and urinary tract infections should be obtained. Overtesting in this population can lead to elimination of valuable future venous access sites. If pain is refractory to treatment, the patient should be admitted.

11. How should aplastic crisis be managed?

These patients are generally admitted. They need to be monitored for possible transfusion needs.

12. How should sequestration crisis be managed?

This is a life-threatening emergency. A complete blood count and reticulocyte count are necessary. Other intra-abdominal pathology must be considered and ruled out. The patient should be admitted and serial exams and laboratories performed.

13. What is abdominal crisis?

Abdominal pain is common in SCD with vaso-occlusive crises. It can be very challenging to distinguish the abdominal pain of a vaso-occlusive crisis from a true abdominal emergency such as appendicitis, pyelonephritis, or cholecystitis. Because SCD patients are functionally asplenic, rapid diagnosis of abdominal pathology is important.

14. How is abdominal pathology distinguished from abdominal crisis?

Patients with vaso-occlusive crises should be afebrile and should not have any rebound or guarding on abdominal exam. A complete blood count and urinalysis should be ordered if any suspicion exists. An abdominal computed tomography (CT) or ultrasound is useful, depending on the location and nature of complaint. Of note, biliary disease is common because pigment-related cholelithiasis is seen in 30–70% of patients with SCD. These patients do not require admission if:

- Thorough work-up is negative.
- Pain can be managed with oral medications.
- They can return for re-evaluation in the emergency department (ED) or at their primary care doctor's office in 12–24 hours.
- They can follow and comply with precautions and instructions for immediate return if their condition worsens.

15. Do cerebrovascular accidents (CVAs) occur in SCD?

Yes. Children with SCD carry a 300-fold increased risk for stroke, making it the most common cause of childhood stroke. By age 20, 10–20% of patients with SCD will have experienced a clinical stroke syndrome, and a further 17–22% will have subclinical evidence of cerebral infarction on brain magnetic resonance imaging (MRI). The mean age of onset of CVA is 10 years. Of patients with CVA, 67% will suffer another, usually within 36 months.

Hoppe C: Defining stroke risk in children with sickle cell anaemia. Br J Haematol 128:751–766, 2005.

KEY POINTS: INDICATIONS FOR ADMISSION OF PATIENTS WITH SCD

1. Pain not controlled with oral medications

2. Unable to hydrate orally

3. Neurologic findings

4. Pulmonary findings (e.g., hypoxia, infiltrate on chest x-ray, new rales)

5. Sequestration crisis

6. Aplastic crisis

7. Fever

16. Is there a role for blood transfusion in SCD?

Simple transfusion is appropriate for single transfusions to restore oxygen carrying capacity or blood volume. Partial exchange transfusions are required in emergencies and in the setting of chronic transfusions.

KEY POINTS: INDICATIONS FOR CONSIDERATION OF TRANSFUSION IN PATIENTS WITH SCD

1. Aplastic crisis

2. Sequestration crisis

3. Priapism

4. Cerebrovascular accident

5. Prior to major surgery

6. Severe acute chest syndrome

7. Pregnancy

17. **What is ACS?**

    Acute chest syndrome (ACS) is defined as a new pulmonary infiltrate on chest radiograph accompanied by fever, chest pain, and a variety of respiratory symptoms including coughing, wheezing, and tachypnea. ACS often develops after a vaso-occlusive crisis and is the leading cause of death in SCD.

18. **What causes ACS?**

    Infection, vaso-occlusion, fat embolism, reactive airway disease, fluid overload, and atelectasis due to splinting can cause ACS. Regardless of the root cause, the final common pathway in the pathogenesis of ACS is small-vessel vaso-occlusion, infarction, and inflammation with alveolar wall necrosis. In a vicious cycle, these factors lead to regional hypoxemia and acidosis, which in turn causes increased sickling and sludging.

    Vichinsky EP, Neumayr LD, Earles A, et al: Causes and outcomes of the acute chest syndrome in sickle cell disease. N Engl J Med 342:1855–1865, 2000.

19. **How should ACS be managed?**

    If ACS is suspected after a thorough history and physical, a complete blood count, reticulocyte count, blood cultures, and chest x-ray should be ordered. Sputum cultures may also be of use in this population. If ACS is diagnosed, the patient should be admitted and treated with intravenous hydration, antibiotics, oxygen, and analgesics. Early treatment with broad-spectrum antibiotics (cefuroxime and erythromycin or azithromycin) is recommended until culture results are available. In many cases, exchange transfusion is indicated to lower the concentration of HbS. Those who present with severe anemia, thrombocytopenia, or multilobar pneumonia should receive a transfusion before respiratory distress develops. Early aggressive ventilatory support is mandatory.

20. **Is there a role for heparin prophylaxis in ACS?**

    There are no clear data supporting its use. Given the increased risk of bleeding, heparin should be reserved for patients with proven evidence of deep vein thrombosis or pulmonary embolism.

    Lakkireddy DR, Patel R, Basarakodu K, Vacek J: Fatal pulmonary artery embolism in a sickle cell patient: Case report and literature review. J Thromb Thrombol 14:79–83, 2002.

21. **How should a patient with SCD be managed when he or she presents with fever?**

    Patients with SCD are functionally asplenic, so they are at increased risk for serious bacterial infection. Children require a thorough search for the source, blood cultures, and empiric antibiotics. The clinician should also have a low threshold for admitting adults and/or administering empiric antibiotics. One approach is to divide patients into two categories:
    - **High risk:** Patients with SCD or sickle cell-β-thalassemia who appear toxic, have temperature $>40°$C, or are not receiving prophylactic penicillin. Admit for intravenous ceftriaxone.
    - **Low risk:** Patients with SCD or sickle cell-β-thalassemia who appear to be well, have temperature $<40°$C, and are taking prophylactic penicillin; OR patients with HbSC who have temperatures $>38.5°$C. Obtain blood cultures, observe for several hours in the ED, administer ceftriaxone, and arrange follow-up within 24 hours.

    Embury SH, Vichinsky EP: Overview of the management of sickle cell disease. UpToDate, version 13.1, December, 2004. Available at http://www.utdol.com/utd/content/topic.do?topicKey=red_cell/22897& type=A&selectedTitle=3~102

22. **How is bone infarction differentiated from osteomyelitis in SCD?**

    It is extremely challenging. Both entities cause bone pain and fever. In attempting to make the diagnosis, fever greater than 38.4°C may indicate osteomyelitis, although this cutoff is imperfect. A presentation of multifocal, rather than unifocal, bone pain is more consistent with bone infarction. The absence of leukocytosis or elevated erythrocyte sedimentation rate (ESR) may also suggest infarction. Although positive cultures of bone can diagnose osteomyelitis, a period of at least 48 hours is required to process them, and sensitivity is not 100%. The leading cause of osteomyelitis is *Salmonella,* followed by *Staphylococcus aureus.* Plain radiographs, contrast-enhanced CT, MRI, and radionucleotide bone scans have all had disappointing results. Therefore, antibiotics are recommended for all patients with fever and bone pain until osteomyelitis can be ruled out.

Wong AL, Sakamoto KM, Johnson EE: Differentiating osteomyelitis from bone infarction in sickle cell disease. Pediatr Emerg Care. 17:60–63, 2004.

CHAPTER 41

ONCOLOGIC EMERGENCIES

Nicholas J. Jouriles, MD

1. **What is an oncologic emergency?**
   An oncologic emergency is a life- or limb-threatening problem in a patient with an underlying neoplastic disease. These problems may be caused by the cancer or its systemic effects or by therapeutic interventions against the cancer.

2. **Is this important?**
   Yes. Cancer is the second leading cause of death in the United States. It is also second only to trauma in years of potential life loss.

3. **Name several oncologic emergencies.**
   See Table 41-1.

TABLE 41-1. EMERGENCIES IN PATIENTS WITH UNDERLYING NEOPLASTIC DISEASES (PARTIAL LIST)	
Airway compromise	Graft vs. host disease
Head and neck mass	Hemorrhagic cystitis
Tracheal compression	Chemotherapy-induced
Adrenal crisis	Radiotherapy-induced
Primary tumor	Hyperviscosity syndrome
Metastatic lesion	Infection
Anemia	With neutropenia
Bone marrow replacement with tumor	Postobstructive pneumonia
Chemotherapy effects	Intestinal obstruction
Bleeding	Intestinal perforation
Primary mass	Malignant pericardial effusion
Low platelet count	With tamponade
Abnormal clotting factors secondary to liver metastases	Metabolic abnormalities
Carcinoid syndrome	Hypercalcemia
Complications of chemotherapy	Acute tumor lysis syndrome
Bone marrow suppression	Hyponatremia/SIADH
Cardiac toxicity	Hyperuricemia
GI toxicity	Hypoglycemia
Pulmonary toxicity	Obstructive jaundice
Renal toxicity	Obstructive uropathy
	Pain

TABLE 41-1. EMERGENCIES IN PATIENTS WITH UNDERLYING NEOPLASTIC DISEASES (PARTIAL LIST)—CONT'D

Complications of radiotherapy	Peptic ulcer disease
Dermatitis	Seizures
GI toxicity	Spinal cord compression
Emotional stress	Motor/sensory loss
Death and dying	Incontinence
DNR orders	Back pain
Family issues	Superior vena cava syndrome
	Tinnitus

DNR = do not resuscitate; SIADH = syndrome of inappropriate secretion of antidiuretic hormone.

4. **Which on this list are life- or limb-threatening?**
   The life-threatening diseases are those that can lead to shock or death. They can be divided into the standard categories of shock: volume loss (bleeding) or impaired vascular return (superior vena cava syndrome), pump impairment (cardiac tamponade), and derangement of systemic vascular resistance or afterload (infection or sepsis). In addition to life-threatening problems, there are diseases that can cause serious metabolic derangements (hypercalcemia) and those that can lead to neurologic impairment including paralysis (spinal cord compression [SCC]).

5. **Tell me about these.**
   - **Superior vena cava syndrome:** Caused by obstruction of the superior vena cava. Although it may be caused by mediastinitis or aortic aneurysms, today 85% of all cases are caused by a neoplastic process. Lung cancer is the most common cause, usually the small cell or squamous types. Adenocarcinoma of the breast, lymphoma, and thymus neoplasms are also common. Superior vena cava syndrome may also occur secondary to metastatic lesions from distant primary sites. Treatment usually involves radiation therapy. Endovascular stenting may help.
   - **Cardiac tamponade:** Can occur secondary to metastatic disease to the pericardium and has been found in 2–21% of patients dying of cancer (Fig. 41-1). Patients with cardiac tamponade usually have a large tumor burden and poor 6-month survival. The diagnosis of a malignant cardiac tamponade is suspected clinically in the hypotensive patient with muffled heart sounds, elevated neck veins, and an enlarged cardiac silhouette on chest x-ray. It is most commonly seen in lung and breast

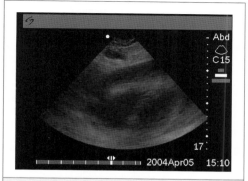

Figure 41-1. Ultrasound of pericardial effusion leading to cardiac tamponade.

carcinomas and lymphoma. Treatment involves pericardial drainage. Emergency physician bedside ultrasound is the best way to make the diagnosis and to guide drainage.

- **Infections:** Because all patients with tumors are by definition immunocompromised, the variety of potential infections is unlimited. Immune status may be further compromised by chemotherapeutic agents. When patients become neutropenic secondary to treatment, any type of infection may occur (bacterial, viral, or fungal), potentially leading to septic shock, adult respiratory distress syndrome, and death. The neutropenic febrile patient should be treated with prophylactic broad-spectrum antibiotics and placed in isolation.

- **Hypercalcemia:** Occurs in approximately 5% of patients followed in a hospital-based oncology practice. Neoplasms that lead to metastatic involvement of the skeletal system are commonly associated with hypercalcemia. Common presenting signs are lethargy, constipation, and altered mental status. Treatment involves hydration with normal saline and agents, such as pamidronate, that act against calcium.

- **SCC:** Occurs in up to 5% of all patients with metastatic disease. The spinal cord or nerve root is directly compressed by an extradural mass, causing secondary neurologic dysfunction. The most common causes of SCC are lung, breast, and prostate cancer and multiple myeloma. The most common presenting symptom is back pain. Any patient with an underlying malignancy who presents with back pain, motor or sensory loss, or incontinence should be considered as having SCC. Prompt diagnosis and treatment can save neurologic function. These patients should undergo emergent magnetic resonance imaging (MRI), including those with negative plain radiographs because up to 40% of patients with SCC may have normal plain radiographs. Treatment is emergent surgical decompression or radiation therapy. Steroids can be used in the emergency department (ED).

Courtheoux P, Alkofer B, Al Refai M, et al: Stent placement in superior vena cava syndrome. Ann Thorac Surg 75:158–161, 2003.

KEY POINTS: SPINAL CORD COMPRESSION

1. Negative plain films do not rule out SCC.

2. Suspicion of SCC is an indication for emergent MRI.

3. Steroids and analgesics are the initial ED treatment.

6. Are these common problems?
Of the life-threatening problems, SCC, infection, and hypercalcemia are relatively common.

7. Which problems are common in patients with an underlying malignancy?
The most common problems are complications of cancer treatment. Each chemotherapeutic agent has side effects, including nausea and vomiting, renal involvement (e.g., cis-platinum), pulmonary toxicity (e.g., bleomycin), cardiac toxicity (e.g., Adriamycin), and diarrhea (e.g., secondary to radiation). These problems are usually treated by the oncologist before the patient leaves the office. Onset of symptoms may be delayed, and the patient may present to the ED for treatment. Other common complications include pain and death.

8. How is an oncologic emergency diagnosed?
The most important element is clinical suspicion. In any patient with an underlying neoplastic process, a complication should be suspected. This includes patients who have been cured of cancer and those with risk factors but no diagnosis.

After concentrating on the ABCs (airway, breathing, and circulation) and vital signs, an extensive history should be taken, followed by a complete physical examination. A presumptive diagnosis should be made and appropriate data obtained.

9. **What symptoms can be related to an underlying oncologic emergency?**
Any presenting symptom can be caused by a neoplastic process. For example, a neoplastic process should be considered in any patient who presents with pain, weakness, dizziness, altered mental status, headache, or seizure. Common ED complaints can be the initial presentation for an oncologic process that has led to SCC (back pain) or intestinal obstruction or perforation (abdominal pain).

KEY POINTS: FEBRILE NEUTROPENIC PATIENT

1. Early antibiotics are helpful.

2. ED antibiotics should be broad spectrum and reflect local infection and resistance patterns.

3. Protective isolation should be used if available.

10. **What treatment is used for patients with oncologic emergencies?**
Treatment is identical to that for patients without an underlying neoplastic process and should be initiated early. Treatment of selected life-threatening problems is provided in Table 41-2.

11. **When should the patient be admitted?**
All patients with life- or limb-threatening disease should be admitted. Patients in whom the diagnosis of an oncologic process is first made in the ED are usually admitted. A special group of patients who need to be admitted are those who lack the resources at home to care for themselves. It is not uncommon for families to give so much of themselves that they need a break, and an admission for respite care is indicated.
For all other patients, it is probably best to discuss the matter with the patient and the primary physician. Most patients with neoplastic processes have a primary oncologist who knows the patient and his or her situation in detail. The emergency physician should balance the medical risks of the current problem with the patient's current needs. Many patients have already spent much time at the hospital and want to spend as much time at home as possible.

12. **Can cancer be cured?**
Modern therapies offer excellent success with medical (testicular cancer, lymphoma, leukemia), surgical (lung, colon, and breast cancer), and combination (radiotherapy and chemotherapy for head and neck, anal cancers) treatments. Many patients today survive long term.

13. **How is a patient with a terminal neoplastic disease treated?**
Often the best treatment for a patient with a terminal malignancy is adequate analgesia, comfort measures, and supportive care. The emergency physician must also deal with issues related to "do not resuscitate" orders in the ED and the out-of-hospital arena.

TABLE 41-2. MANAGEMENT OF SELECTED ONCOLOGIC EMERGENCIES

Clinical Problem	Presenting Symptoms	ED Database	ED Priorities
Superior vena cava syndrome	Plethora Cyanosis Dyspnea Dilated head/arm veins Jugular venous distention Cough Chest pain	Mediastinal mass on chest x-ray	Emergency radiotherapy Consider endovascular stent Consider tissue biopsy Consider chemotherapy Consider surgical debulking
Infection	Fever Varies with source	CBC with differential Urinalysis Chest x-ray Blood cultures Wound culture(s) Catheter culture(s) LP if not contra-indicated	Complete physical exam to locate source Culture all possible sources Protective isolation if neutropenic Begin broad-spectrum antibiotics (varies with known community antibiotic resistance patterns)
Malignant pericardial effusion	Chest pain Cardiac rub Jugular venous distention Distant heart sounds Hypotension	Elevated CVP Low-voltage ECG Cardiomegaly on CXR Pericardial fluid on echocardiogram CVP/PCWP pressure equalization	IV fluid challenge (NS or LR) Drainage Pericardial window (preferred) Pericardiocentesis (ultrasound guided)
Hypercalcemia	Dehydration Constipation Lethargy Altered mental status	Elevated free calcium Abnormal ECG	IV fluid rehydration (NS) Furosemide Pamifronate Consider calcitonin Consider prednisone
Spinal cord compression	Back pain Motor/sensory deficits Incontinence	Spinal x-ray abnormality Image spinal cord (MRI preferred)	Initiate high-dose steroids Analgesics Emergent surgical decompression Emergent radiotherapy

CBC = complete blood count, LP = lumbar puncture, CVP = central venous pressure, ECG = electrocardiogram, CXR = chest X-ray, IV = intravenous, NS = normal saline, LR = lactated Ringer's, PCWP = pulmonary capillary wedge pressure, MRI = magnetic resonance imaging.

BIBLIOGRAPHY

1. Body JJ: Hypercalcemia of malignancy. Semin Nephrol 24:48–54, 2004.
2. Coleman RE: Metastatic bone disease: Clinical features, pathophysiology and treatment strategies. Cancer Treat Rev 27:165–176, 2001.
3. Healey JH, Brown HK: Complications of bone metastases: Surgical management. Cancer 88(12 Suppl):2940–2951, 2000.
4. Sipsas NV, Bodey GP, Kontoyiannis DP: Perspectives for the management of febrile neutropenic patients with cancer in the 21st century. Cancer 103:1103–1113, 2005.
5. Spodick DH: Acute pericarditis: Current concepts and practice. JAMA 289:1150–1153, 2003.
6. Wudel LJ Jr, Nesbitt JC: Superior vena cava syndrome. Curr Treat Options Oncol 2:77–91, 2001.

X. METABOLISM AND ENDOCRINOLOGY

FLUIDS AND ELECTROLYTES

Corey M. Slovis, MD

CHAPTER 42

1. **Why is the study of fluid and electrolytes so difficult?**
   Most people who teach fluid and electrolytes are very educated and talk about things like "the negative log of the hydrogen ion concentration," "idiogenic osmols," and "pseudo-pseudo triple acid-base disturbances." Luckily, this chapter is not written by a person who believes in, or understands, negative logarithms.

2. **What is the anion gap (AG)?**
   The AG measures the amount of negatively charged ions in the serum (unmeasured anions) that are not bicarbonate (HCO_3^-) or chloride (Cl^-). The AG is calculated by subtracting the sum of HCO_3^- and Cl^- values from the sodium (Na^+) value, the major positive charge in the serum. Potassium (K^+) values are not generally used in the calculation because of the huge amount of intracellular potassium (155 mEq) and the relatively low amount of potassium in the serum (only about 4 mEq). The formula for determining AG is as follows:

$$AG = Na^+ - (Cl^- + HCO_3^-)$$

   The normal upper limit for the AG is generally accepted at 8–12, although some centers use 10–14.

3. **Why must AG be calculated each time an electrolyte panel is evaluated?**
   An elevated AG means there is some unmeasured anion, toxin, or organic acid in the blood. If you do not calculate the gap, you could miss one of the only clues to a potentially life-ending disease or overdose. The AG also allows acidosis to be divided into two types: wide gap (AG > 12–14) and normal gap (AG < 12–14).

4. **There are two types of acidosis: wide gap and normal gap. What is a hyperchloremic metabolic acidosis?**
   A hyperchloremic acidosis is just another name for a normal gap acidosis. Just think: If the AG is going to be normal, and the formula for AG = $Na^+ - (Cl^- + HCO_3^-)$, if HCO_3^- goes down, Cl^- has to rise, or, more simply, you become hyperchloremic—hence the name *hyperchloremic metabolic acidosis*.

5. **Is there an easy way to remember the differential diagnosis for wide gap metabolic acidosis?**
   My favorite is taken from Goldfrank and is called **MUDPILES.**
   M = **M**ethanol
   U = **U**remia
   D = **D**iabetic ketoacidosis (DKA) and Alcoholic ketoacidosis (AKA)
   P = **P**araldehyde
   I = **I**NH (Isoniazid) and **I**ron
   L = **L**actic acidosis
   E = **E**thylene glycol
   S = **S**alicylates and **S**olvents

6. **What are the clues to each of the entities in MUDPILES?**
    See Table 42-1.

TABLE 42-1. CLUES TO THE DIFFERENTIAL DIAGNOSIS OF WIDE GAP METABOLIC ACIDOSIS	
Disease	**Clues**
Methanol	Alcoholism, blindness or papilledema, profound acidosis
Uremia	Chronically ill-appearing, history of chronic renal failure, BUN > 100 mg/dL, and creatinine > 5 mg/dL
DKA	History of diabetes mellitus, polyuria, and polydipsia, glucose > 500 mg/dL
AKA	Ethyl alcohol, glucose < 250 mg/dL, nausea and vomiting
Paraldehyde	Alcoholism, distinctive breath, access to this now hard-to-find drug
INH	Tuberculosis, suicide risk, refractory status seizures
Iron	Pregnant or postpartum, hematemesis, radiopaque tablets on abdominal film (unreliable finding)
Lactic acidosis	Hypoxia, hypotension, sepsis
Ethylene glycol	Alcoholism, oxalate crystals in urine with or without renal failure, fluorescent mouth or urine (from drinking antifreeze—unreliable finding)
Salicylates	History of chronic disease requiring aspirin use (i.e., rheumatoid arthritis); mixed acid-base disturbance (primary metabolic acidosis plus primary respiratory alkalosis); aspirin level > 20–40 mg/dL
Solvents	History of exposure or huffing; spray paint on face

AKA = alcoholic ketoacidosis, BUN = blood urea nitrogen, DKA = diabetic ketoacidosis, INH = isoniazid.

7. **What are the causes of narrow gap acidosis?**
    Memorize the mnemonic **HARDUPS.**
    H = **H**yperventilation (chronic)
    A = **A**cetazolamide, **A**cids (e.g., hydrochloric), **A**ddison's disease
    R = **R**enal tubular acidosis
    D = **D**iarrhea
    U = **U**reterosigmoidostomy
    P = **P**ancreatic fistulas and drainage
    S = **S**aline (in large amounts)
    If you do not want to memorize anything, it is important to know that diarrhea, especially in children, and renal tubular acidosis, especially in adults, are the two most common causes of a narrow gap acidosis.

8. **Why should normal saline (NS) or lactated Ringer's (LR) solution rather than 0.5 NS or dextrose in 5% water (D$_5$W) be given to someone who needs volume replacement?**

    Fluid goes into three different body compartments: (1) inside blood vessels (intravascular), (2) into cells (intracellular), and (3) in between the two (interstitial). NS and LR solutions go into all three compartments, and only 25–33% stays in the intravascular compartment. A person who lost 2 U of blood (1000 mL) would need 3–4 L of crystalloid for volume resuscitation. One half NS (0.45 NS) provides only half of what NS or LR provide; each liter of 0.45 NS provides 125–175 mL to blood vessels (versus 250–333 mL for NS and LR). D$_5$W is the worst for trying to give intravascular volume; it puts only about 80 mL per 1000 mL of D$_5$W into the vasculature. The rest goes into cells and the interstitium.

9. **Which solution is better, NS or LR?**

    Both fluids are excellent for early volume replacement.

    NS has a pH of 4.5–5.5 and has a sodium *and* chloride content of 155 mEq/L each. It is acidotic, has an osmolarity of 310, and has a little more sodium than serum and a lot more chloride than serum (155 mEq/L of Cl$^-$ in NS versus about 100 mEq/L of Cl$^-$ in serum). Too much NS too quickly may cause hyperchloremic metabolic acidosis.

    LR is considered more physiologic in that it is much closer to serum in its content. Its sodium content is lower than NS at 130 mEq/L, and its chloride is only 109 mEq/L (versus 155 mEq/L of NS). The solution is called lactated because it has 28 mEq/L of bicarbonate in the form of lactate, which becomes bicarbonate when it is in the body. LR has 4 mEq of potassium (none in NS) and has 3 mEq/L of calcium. Critics of LR do not like all the bicarbonate in it and believe that potassium therapy should be individualized. The bottom line is that neither NS nor LR is better; both are equal in quantities of 2–3 L over 24 hours. Patients with protracted vomiting should be given NS, which is higher in chloride. Patients with severe dehydration and the resultant hyperchloremic metabolic acidosis should be given LR, which has the equivalent of 0.5 ampule of bicarbonate per liter.

10. **What is the most dangerous electrolyte abnormality? What are its five most common causes?**

    Hyperkalemia. It may result in sudden arrhythmogenic death because of its effect on the cells' resting membrane potential. The most common cause of hyperkalemia is often referred to as "laboratory error." Actually, the laboratory does a perfect analysis, but the serum sample has hemolyzed after, or while, it is being drawn.

    The number-one cause of hyperkalemia is **spurious.** The other common causes are as follows:

    - **Chronic renal failure** (the true number-one cause of hyperkalemia)
    - **Acidosis** (potassium moves out of the cell as the pH falls)
    - **Drug-induced** (including nonsteroidal anti-inflammatory drugs, potassium-sparing diuretics, digoxin, angiotensin-converting enzyme inhibitors, and administration of intravenous potassium chloride)
    - **Cell death** (when potassium comes out of injured muscle or red cells); includes burns, crush injuries, rhabdomyolysis, tumor lysis syndrome, and intravascular hemolysis

    Much less common causes of hyperkalemia include adrenal insufficiency, hyperkalemic periodic paralysis, and hematologic malignancies.

11. **What electrocardiogram (ECG) changes are associated with hyperkalemia?**

    The first ECG change seen in hyperkalemia is usually a tall, peaked T wave that may occur as potassium values rise to 5.5–6.5 mEq/dL. Loss of the P wave may follow as potassium levels rise to 6.5–7.5 mEq/dL. The most dangerous ECG finding (generally associated with levels of 8.0 mEq/dL) is widening of the QRS, which may merge with the abnormal T wave and create a sine-wave–appearing ventricular tachycardia.

12. **Summarize the best treatment for hyperkalemia.**
Treatment is based on (1) serum levels, (2) the presence or absence of ECG changes, and (3) underlying renal function. If the patient has life-threatening ECG changes of hyperkalemia (widening QRS or a sine-wave–like rhythm), 10% calcium chloride should be given in an initial dose of 5–10 mL to reverse temporarily potassium's deleterious electrical effects. Most patients with hyperkalemia usually require moving potassium intracellularly, then removing potassium from the body, rather than receiving a potentially dangerous calcium infusion.

13. **How can potassium be moved intracellularly?**
The most effective way is by giving glucose and insulin. Glucose and insulin work by activating the glucose transport system into the cell. As glucose is carried intracellularly, potassium is carried along. The usual dose of glucose is 2 ampules of $D_{50\%}$ (100 mL) and 10 U of insulin. Bicarbonate may be used to drive potassium into the cell, but it is effective *only* in acidotic patients. Usually 1–2 ampules of bicarbonate (44.6–50 mEq of bicarbonate per ampule) is given over 1–20 minutes, depending on how sick or acidotic the patient is. Another method of driving potassium into the cell is use of inhaled beta agonist bronchodilators. Beta agonists may be helpful in a renal failure patient with fluid overload because they may help treat the bronchospasm of pulmonary edema. Intravenous magnesium also drives potassium into the cell, which is advantageous if the patient is having ventricular ectopy but is potentially dangerous if the patient has hypermagnesemia due to chronic renal failure. Magnesium, in a dose of 1–2 g over 10–20 minutes, may, similar to beta agonists, lower serum potassium by 0.5 mEq.

KEY POINTS: HYPERKALEMIA

1. An elevated anion gap should alert you to a potentially serious disease or overdose.

2. Hyperkalemia is asymptomatic; you must check the ECG.

3. The ECG changes seen as potassium rises are a tall peaked T wave, loss of the P wave, and widening of the QRS complex.

4. Bicarbonate only works to lower serum potassium in acidotic patients.

5. Administering glucose and insulin is an effective method to lower serum potassium.

14. **After potassium's electrical effects have been counteracted (if indicated) and potassium has been driven intracellularly, how do you remove it from the body?**
Potassium can be removed from the body by diuresis, potassium-binding resins, and hemodialysis. Diuresis with saline, supplemented by furosemide, is an excellent way to lower total body potassium. Most patients experience renal failure, however, and cannot make much urine, which is how they became hyperkalemic in the first place. Sodium polystyrene sulfonate (Kayexalate) is a sodium-containing resin that exchanges its sodium content for the patient's potassium. Each 1 g of Kayexalate can remove about 1 mEq of potassium from the patient's body. The best method of lowering potassium is by hemodialysis, and it is the method of choice for any severely ill, acidotic, or profoundly hyperkalemic patient.

15. **Discuss the most common causes of hyponatremia.**
Hyponatremia is a serum sodium of less than 135 mEq/dL. Most patients with mild hyponatremia (levels > 125–130 mEq/dL) are on diuretics or have some degree of fluid overload as a result of congestive heart failure or renal failure or liver disease. Diuretic-induced hyponatremia is most common in the elderly. Patients with congestive heart failure, liver failure,

and renal failure develop hyponatremia as a result of secondary hyperaldosteronism. Aldosterone is released because of renal hypoperfusion, resulting in volume overload and dilutional hyponatremia (even in the face of total body sodium excess). Moderate-to-severe hyponatremia (levels < 125 mEq/dL) are most commonly due to the syndrome of inappropriate secretion of antidiuretic hormone (SIADH) and psychogenic polydipsia (compulsive water drinking).

16. **What is SIADH?**
Abnormally high levels of hormone from the posterior pituitary gland, which blocks free water excretion. Normally, when sodium levels fall, levels of antidiuretic hormone (ADH) also decrease, resulting in urinary losses of water (diuresis). In this syndrome, ADH is released inappropriately, and serum sodium levels fall as more excess free water is retained (antidiuresis). The hallmark of this syndrome is relatively concentrated urine, rather than the maximally diluted urine one sees in a water-overloaded patient. Patients cannot be given this diagnosis if they are taking diuretics or have a reason to be water overloaded (i.e., congestive heart failure, chronic renal failure, or liver failure).

17. **What are the classic neurologic signs of hyperkalemia? What are the classic ECG signs of hyponatremia?**
No, not a misprint, just a trick to wake you up after antidiuresing. Potassium causes cardiovascular symptoms via its effects on the ECG (*see* question 11). Sodium causes no ECG changes but does affect the brain because of its effects on osmolality; symptoms include dizziness, confusion, coma, and seizures.

18. **How fast should hyponatremia be corrected?**
There has been much debate over how rapidly (about 2 mEq/h) or how slowly (about 0.5 mEq/h) sodium should be corrected. Patients should be corrected slowly over 1–2 days, and serum sodium should be allowed to rise by no more than 0.5 mEq/h. This approach avoids the possible development of central pontine myelinolysis (which is also called the *osmotic demyelinating syndrome* by some purists), a catastrophic neurologic illness of coma, paralysis, and usually death seen with too-rapid correction.

19. **Should sodium levels *ever* be treated quickly?**
There are some specific indications for raising a patient's sodium rapidly by infusing 3% saline at 100 mL/h for a maximum of 2–3 hours. Patients who have serum sodium levels of significantly less than 120 mEq/L *and* who have acute alterations in mental status, seizures, or new focal findings should have their levels raised about 4–6 mEq/dL over a few hours. Other than these rare patients with severe, symptomatic hyponatremia, slow correction by water restriction, slow infusion of saline, and judicious use of furosemide should be used.

20. **What is osmolality? What is the osmolal gap?**
Osmolality is calculated by multiplying the serum sodium by 2 and adding the glucose (GLU) divided by 18, plus the blood urea nitrogen (BUN) divided by 2.8. Normal is approximately 280–290 mOsm.

$$\text{Osmolarity} = 2 \infty \text{ Na} + \text{GLU}/18 + \text{BUN}/2.8$$

The osmolal gap is determined by using this formula, then asking the laboratory to determine the osmolality by the molal freezing point depression. The difference should be only about 10; if it is more, something else is in the serum (e.g., an alcohol, intravenous contrast media, or mannitol).

$$\text{Osmolal gap} = \text{laboratory-determind osmolarity} - \text{calculated osmolarity}$$

21. **How do you use the osmolal gap in figuring out if someone has ingested methanol or ethylene glycol?**

    If the osmolal gap is elevated, you should measure the patient's serum ethanol level immediately. Because of ethanol's molecular weight, every 4.2 mg/dL of alcohol "weighs" 1 mOsm. If the alcohol level is 100 mg/dL, the patient's osmolal gap should be about 30–35 (about 25 from alcohol, added to the normal osmolal gap, which is about 5–10).

    If there is a higher gap, these unaccounted osmols may represent methanol, ethylene glycol, or isopropyl alcohol. Because isopropyl alcohol causes ketosis without acidosis, acidosis plus an unexplained osmolal gap may mean a life-threatening overdose. Hints to methanol and ethylene glycol overdose appear in answer 6.

22. **What are the most common causes of hypercalcemia? How do they present?**

    Mild hypercalcemia is usually due to dehydration, thiazide diuretics, or hyperparathyroidism. It is often asymptomatic, but mild fatigue, renal stones, or nonspecific gastrointestinal symptoms may be present. Severe hypercalcemia, with levels greater than 2–3 mg/dL above normal, presents as alteration in mental status with the signs and symptoms of profound dehydration.

23. **Describe the emergency treatment of hypercalcemia.**

    Symptomatic hypercalcemia is treated by aggressive volume resuscitation with saline supplemented by furosemide after intravascular volume has been normalized. Once their volume status is normalized, patients should receive approximately 150–200 mL of NS per hour plus enough furosemide to keep urine output at 1 mL/kg or higher. Saline blocks the proximal tubules from absorbing calcium, and furosemide blocks distal tubular absorption. Older patients and patients with impaired cardiac function must be closely followed as they are volume resuscitated and placed on the saline infusion; otherwise, turn to the chapter on congestive heart failure.

BIBLIOGRAPHY

1. Adrogué HJ, Madias NE: Hyponatremia. N Engl J Med 342:1581–1589, 2000.

2. Adrogué HJ, Madias NE: Hypernatremia. N Engl J Med 342:1493–1499, 2000.

3. Ariyan CE, Sosa JA: Assessment and management of patients with abnormal calcium. Crit Care Med 32(Suppl): S146–S154, 2004.

4. Kamel KS, Wei C: Controversial issues in the treatment of hyperkalemia. Nephrol Dialysis Transplant 18:2215, 2003.

5. Hoffman RS: Fluid, electrolyte, acid-base principles. In Goldfrank LR, Flomenbaum NE, Lewin NA, et al (eds): Goldfrank's Toxicologic Emergencies, 7th ed. New York, McGraw-Hill, 2002, pp 364–380.

6. Narins RG, Emmett M: Simple and mixed acid-base disorders—a practical approach. Medicine 59:161–187, 1980.

7. Narins RG, Jones ER, Stom MC, et al: Diagnostic strategies in disorders of fluid, electrolyte and acid-base homeostasis. Am J Med 77:496–519, 1982.

8. Slovis C, Jenkins R: ABCs of clinical electrocardiography: Conditions not primarily affecting the heart. BMJ 324:1320–1323, 2002.

CHAPTER 43

ACID–BASE DISORDERS

Stephen L. Adams, MD, and Morris S. Kharasch, MD

1. **Name the four types of acid-base disorders seen in the emergency department (ED), and give a common example of each.**
   Actually, there are five:
   - Metabolic acidosis (e.g., cardiac arrest)
   - Respiratory acidosis (e.g., chronic obstructive pulmonary disease with carbon dioxide [CO_2] retention)
   - Metabolic alkalosis (e.g., protracted vomiting)
   - Respiratory alkalosis (e.g., hyperventilation syndrome)
   - Mixed acid-base disorder (e.g., respiratory alkalosis and metabolic acidosis, as seen in an adult with salicylate intoxication; metabolic acidosis with respiratory compensation)

2. **What does pulse oximetry contribute to the understanding of the patient's acid-base status?**
   Nothing. Pulse oximetry measures oxygen saturation and does not provide a measurement of acid-base or ventilatory status. Arterial blood gas analysis is necessary to determine acid-base status.

3. **What are the most commonly cited causes of an elevated anion gap?**
   An elevated anion gap, usually indicating a low bicarbonate level, should give the clinician cause to consider the presence of a metabolic acidosis. The differential diagnoses may be remembered by the mnemonic **DR. MAPLES:**
   D = **D**iabetic ketoacidosis (DKA)
   R = **R**enal failure
   M = **M**ethanol
   A = **A**lcoholic ketoacidosis
   P = **P**araldehyde
   L = **L**actic acidosis
   E = **E**thylene glycol
   S = **S**alicylate intoxication
   These are only some of the causes of a metabolic acidosis.

4. **Name some obscure causes of an elevated anion gap metabolic acidosis.**
   Sulfuric acidosis, short bowel syndrome (D-lactic acidosis), nalidixic acid, methenamine, mandelate, hippuric acid salt, rhubarb (oxalic acid) ingestion, and inborn errors of metabolism, such as the methylmalonic acidemias and isovaleric acidemia. Toluene intoxication (glue sniffing) can cause either an elevated anion gap metabolic acidosis or a hyperchloremic metabolic acidosis (no anion gap).

5. **Is the size of the anion gap clinically useful?**
   In one study, an anion gap of greater than 30 mEq/L was usually the result of an identifiable organic acidosis (i.e., lactic acidosis or ketoacidosis). Almost 30% of patients with an anion gap of 20–29 mEq/L had neither a lactic acidosis nor a ketoacidosis.

   Gabow PA, Kaehny WD, Fennessey PV, et al: Diagnostic importance of an increased serum anion gap. N Engl J Med 303:854–858, 1980.

6. **What are some causes of lactic acidosis?**
Shock, seizure, hypoxemia, isoniazid (INH) toxicity, metformin, cyanide poisoning, ritodrine, inhaled industrial acetylene, phenformin ingestion, iron intoxication, ethanol abuse, and carbon monoxide poisoning. Sodium nitroprusside, povidone-iodine ointment, sorbitol, xylitol, and streptozocin are other drugs that have been listed as causing increased lactic acid formation.

7. **How severe is the acid-base disturbance that results from a grand mal seizure? How long does it take to resolve the acidosis?**
A grand mal seizure can result in a profound lactic acidosis. The pH levels may plummet to 6.9 or lower. The acidosis in an uncomplicated seizure usually resolves spontaneously within 1 hour.

Orringer CE, Eustace JC, Wunsch CD, Gardner LB: Natural history of lactic acidosis after grand mal seizures. N Engl J Med 297:796–799, 1977.

8. **Can a patient have a metabolic acidosis without evidence of an elevated anion gap?**
Yes. A patient with a hyperchloremic metabolic acidosis may have no evidence of an elevated anion gap. This condition is caused, in effect, by adding hydrogen chloride to the serum. The fall in serum bicarbonate is offset by the addition of Cl^-; consequently, there is no increased anion gap.

Schwartz-Goldstein BH, Malik AR, Sarwar A, Brandstetter RD: Lactic acidosis associated with a deceptively normal anion gap. Heart Lung 25:79–80, 1996.

9. **How can I remember some of the causes of a normal anion gap metabolic acidosis?**
Use the mnemonic **USED CARP:**
U = **U**reteroenterostomy
S = **S**mall bowel fistula
E = **E**xtra chloride
D = **D**iarrhea
C = **C**arbonic anhydrase inhibitors
A = **A**drenal insufficiency
R = **R**enal tubular acidosis
P = **P**ancreatic fistula

Wilson RF, Barton C: Acid-Base Problems. In Tintinalli JE (ed): Emergency Medicine. A Comprehensive Study Guide, ed 4. McGraw-Hill, New York, 1996, pp 93–107.

10. **In a patient with DKA who is improving with appropriate therapy, why might the measurement of serum ketones show an increase?**
There are three ketone bodies: β-hydroxybutyrate (BHB), acetoacetate (AcAc), and acetone. BHB and AcAc are acids; acetone is not. The proportion of BHB to AcAc depends on the oxidation-reduction status of the patient. A patient who is in DKA on presentation often is severely dehydrated, and the preponderance of ketone bodies may be in the form of BHB. The test by which ketones are noted is the nitroprusside reaction test (Acetest, Ketostix), which measures AcAc and acetone but is not sensitive to BHB. In the patient with DKA, as fluids and insulin therapy are instituted, the amount of BHB converted to AcAc increases, and the nitroprusside reaction, which initially may have been weakly positive or even negative, becomes increasingly positive.

11. **List nine disorders that can cause a hyperketonemic state.**
- Isopropyl alcohol intoxication
- DKA
- Alcoholic ketoacidosis
- Starvation
- Paraldehyde intoxication (pseudoketosis)

- Cyanide intoxication
- Industrial acetylene inhalation
- Hyperemesis gravidarum
- Bovine ketosis
- Stress hormone excess

12. **What may contribute to metabolic acidosis in an abuser of alcohol?**

Ketoacidosis has been well documented in the chronic alcoholic who binges, then presents with nausea, vomiting, abdominal pain, and poor caloric intake. Lactic acid, acetic acid, and indirect loss of bicarbonate in the urine (nonanion gap metabolic acidosis) also may contribute to an alcoholic acidosis.

Adams SL: Alcoholic ketoacidosis. Emerg Med Clin North Am 8:749–760, 1990.

13. **Which electrolyte is affected most commonly by a change in acid-base status?**

Serum potassium. Patients with severe acidosis tend to have elevated serum K^+ levels, whereas patients with severe alkalosis tend to have low serum K^+ levels. A change of pH of 0.10 is consistent with a corresponding change in serum K^+ of about 0.5 mEq/L (range, 0.3–0.8 mEq/L). If the pH is elevated by 0.10, the serum K^+ falls by about 0.5 mEq/L. If the pH is diminished by 0.10, the serum K^+ rises by about 0.5 mEq/L. This concept is well known to clinicians who treat patients who present in DKA. Although the patient's total body K^+ may be severely depleted, initial serum K^+ levels may be elevated in the severely acidotic patient. As the patient is treated appropriately and acidosis resolves, K^+ supplementation is indicated because serum levels may fall precipitously.

14. **What is a pseudometabolic acidosis?**

Underfilling of Vacutainer tubes can cause a significant decline in bicarbonate and an increase in anion gap that may be mistaken for metabolic acidosis. It is theorized that because atmospheric pressure contains less than 5% CO_2, the lower partial pressure of CO_2 over the blood in an underfilled tube causes CO_2 to diffuse out of the venous solution, decreasing the bicarbonate with which it is in equilibrium. Tubes should be filled completely to prevent creating a pseudometabolic acidosis.

Herr RD, Swanson T: Pseudometabolic acidosis caused by underfill of Vacutainer tubes. Ann Emerg Med 21:177–180, 1992.

15. **Are there any potential ill effects of using paper bag rebreathing in the treatment of hyperventilation syndrome?**

Yes. When normal volunteers hyperventilated into a brown paper bag, inspired oxygen was decreased sufficiently so as to endanger hypoxic patients. Paper bag rebreathing therapy probably should not be used unless myocardial ischemia can be ruled out and arterial blood gas analysis or pulse oximetry excludes hypoxia.

Callaham M: Hypoxic hazards of traditional paper bag rebreathing in hyperventilating patients. Ann Emerg Med 18:622–628, 1989.

16. **How does core temperature affect arterial blood gases?**

Uncorrected arterial blood gases yield a falsely elevated pH and a falsely decreased PO_2 and PCO_2 in hypothermia. For every 1°C decrease in body temperature, the pH is elevated 0.015, PCO_2 (mmHg) decreases 4.4%, and PO_2 decreases 7.2% (37°C reference). Hyperthermia decreases the pH and increases the PCO_2 and PO_2 by an equivalent amount. The clinical use of corrected versus uncorrected pH determinations in hypothermia is controversial.

Reuler JB: Hypothermia: Pathophysiology, clinical settings, and management. Ann Intern Med 89:519–527, 1978.

17. **What acid-base alterations are seen commonly in heatstroke?**
Metabolic acidosis (81% of patients in one study) and respiratory alkalosis (55% of patients). The prevalence of metabolic acidosis was associated significantly with the degree of hyperthermia. Of patients, 63% with a rectal temperature of 41°C, 95% with a temperature of 42°C, and 100% with a temperature of 43°C had a metabolic acidosis. This association was not true for respiratory alkalosis. Patients who had a metabolic acidosis had a large anion gap (24 ± 5).

Bouchama A, De Vol EB: Acid-base alterations in heatstroke. Intensive Care Med 27:680–685, 2001.

18. **What disease process can present with an anion gap *higher* than the serum glucose?**
Alcoholic ketoacidosis, a well-known cause of an elevated anion gap metabolic acidosis, may present with hypoglycemia. One case report presented a patient with alcoholic ketoacidosis and a concomitant illness, pneumonia, with an anion gap of 36 and a serum glucose of less than 20 mg/dL. Severe hypoglycemia may cause a lactic acidosis and usually occurs in the setting of a defect in gluconeogenesis, which may be seen in a patient with chronic alcohol ingestion. A concomitant illness commonly is seen in the patient with alcoholic ketoacidosis.

Marinella MA: Alcoholic ketoacidosis presenting with extreme hypoglycemia. Am J Emerg Med 15:280–281, 1997.

KEY POINTS: ACID-BASE DISORDERS

1. Patients with a metabolic acidosis may have an elevated serum K^+ even though they may have a low total body K^+.

2. Patients with alcoholic ketoacidosis should appropriately be treated with crystalloids containing glucose.

19. **How may patients with human immunodeficiency virus (HIV) have an abnormality in the anion gap?**
A patient with HIV may have a low anion gap. Hypergammaglobulinemia, resulting from an increased number of immunoglobulin-secreting B cells because of failure in immunoregulation, has been reported in patients with HIV. Consequently, an elevation of IgG and IgA may occur. The anion gap may be low because of the cationic charge of IgG. One case report described a patient with HIV with lactic acidosis, which should elevate the anion gap, who had a "deceptively" normal anion gap. A patient with hyperlactacidemia and a normal anion gap acidosis should prompt an evaluation of coexisting illnesses that may be responsible for the low anion gap.

Slucher B, Levinson SS: Human immunodeficiency virus infection and anion gap. Ann Clin Lab Sci 23:249–255, 1993.

20. **What is the most common cause of metabolic acidosis in the pediatric population?**
Significant diarrheal illnesses in this population may produce a starvation ketosis.

Cronan KM, Norman ME: Renal and electrolyte emergencies. In Fleisher GR, Ludwig S (eds): Textbook of Pediatric Emergency Medicine, 3rd ed. Philadelphia, Williams & Wilkins, 1993, pp 670–617.

21. **In addition to the toxic alcohols, name two entities causing a metabolic acidosis with an elevated anion gap that have been associated with an elevated osmolal gap.**

Alcoholic ketoacidosis and lactic acidosis. It has been speculated that, in patients with lactic acidosis, organic substances of low molecular weight are released from ischemic tissues, accounting for unmeasured osmols. In alcoholic ketoacidosis, it has been speculated that an increased osmolal gap could be attributed to acetone, an uncharged ketone of low molecular weight that may be elevated if the ketoacidosis is severe and prolonged. The exact pathogenesis of the gap in these two entities is not certain, however. As can be seen, the elevated osmolal gap is not specific for a toxic alcohol ingestion.

Schelling JR, Howard RL, Winter SD, Linas SL: Increased osmolal gap in alcoholic ketoacidosis and lactic acidosis. Ann Intern Med 113:580–582, 1990.

22. **Name a base and an outfielder.**

Al Kaline (Detroit Tigers, 1953–1974; Hall of Fame, 1980).

CHAPTER 44

DIABETES MELLITUS

Jennie A. Buchanan, MD

1. **Describe the physiologic and clinical differences between type I and type II diabetes mellitus.**
   - **Type I disease** (formerly known as insulin-dependent) is characterized by pancreatic beta cell destruction, which causes an absolute insulin deficiency. Patients with type I disease have little or no endogenous production of insulin and often develop diabetic ketoacidosis (DKA) without it. Dietary modifications and oral hypoglycemic agents are inadequate therapy.
   - **Type II disease** (non-insulin-dependent) is characterized by relative insulin resistance. Glucose levels often respond to oral dietary modification and oral hypoglycemic agents; however, insulin is sometimes necessasry to control glucose levels.

2. **What are the diagnostic criteria for diabetes mellitus?**
   Normal fasting plasma glucose is < 100 mg/dL. Impaired fasting glucose is between 100 and 125 mg/dL. Criteria that must be met for the diagnosis of diabetes are a fasting plasma glucose of 126 mg/dL or 2-hour plasma glucose of 200 mg/dL.

   Genuth S, Alberti KG, Bennett P, et al: Follow-up report on the diagnosis of diabetes mellitus. Diabetes Care 26:3160–3167, 2003.

3. **List the physiologic complications of hyperglycemia.**
   - Osmotic diuresis
   - Dehydration
   - Electrolyte abnormalities
   - Coronary artery disease
   - Cerebral vascular disease
   - Peripheral vascular disease
   - Nephropathy
   - Retinopathy
   - Neuropathy
   - Infection secondary to impaired leukocyte function
   - Cutaneous manifestations
   - Ketoacidosis (in type I patients)

   Cydulka RK, Siff J: Diabetes mellitus and disorders of glucose homeostasis. In Rosen's Emergency Medicine Concepts and Clinical Practice, 5th ed. St. Louis, Mosby, 2002, pp 1744–1762.

4. **What types of infections are seen more commonly in diabetics than in other patients?**
   Diabetic patients are more susceptible to urinary tract infections, candidal vaginitis, cystitis, balanitis, pneumonia, influenza, tuberculosis, lower extremity skin and soft tissue infections, and bacteremia.
   Rhinocerebral mucormycosis is a rapidly progressive invasive fungal infection of the nasal and paranasal sinuses. Computed tomography (CT) scan should be obtained to define extent of disease. It is treated with amphotericin B and surgical debridement. The mortality rate is as high as 50%.
   Malignant otitis externa is usually caused by *Pseuodomonas aeruginosa*. Patients present with unilateral otalgia, swelling, and discharge. The external auditory canal is initially affected;

it can then spread to skin and skull. CT scan should be used to image affected regions. Intravenous (IV) antipseudomonal antibiotics and debridement are required for extensive disease.

Emphysematous pyelonephritis and **cholecystitis** are more common in diabetics. Findings include gas on plain film. IV antibiotics and surgical treatment are indicated. The mortality rates even with prompt treatment are 40% and 15%, respectively.

Rush MD, Winslett S, Wisdom KD: Diabetes mellitus. In Tintinalli's Emergency Medicine A Comprehensive Study Guide, 6th ed. New York, McGraw Hill, 2004, pp 1294–1311.

5. **What are the common manifestations of diabetic neuropathy?**
Patients typically present with a peripheral symmetric neuropathy, which often follows a stocking-glove pattern. Symptoms include bilateral pain, hyperesthesia, and anesthesia. It is often treated with amitriptyline, 75 mg at bedtime. Mononeuropathy multiplex affects motor and sensory nerves, often resulting in wrist or footdrop and affecting cranial nerves III, IV, and VI.

6. **Describe the pertinent clinical and laboratory finding of DKA.**
A patient with DKA presents with hyperglycemia; osmotic diuresis with resultant dehydration; polyuria, polydipsia, and polyphagia; weight loss; metabolic acidosis secondary to lipolysis with production of acetoacetate and beta-hydroxybutyrate; tachypnea; Kussmaul breathing; fruity breath odor; and potassium, sodium, chloride, calcium, magnesium, and phosphorus depletion.

Some patients with DKA also complain of nausea, vomiting, or abdominal pain secondary to gastric distention or stretching of the liver capsule. Others may have some degree of altered mentation.

7. **What causes DKA?**
DKA is triggered by insulin deficiency but can also be triggered by infection, stroke, myocardial infarction (MI), pancreatitis, trauma, or pregnancy. DKA is a response to cellular glucose starvation, as insulin is the anabolic hormone produced by the pancreas. The body's catabolic hormones are glucagon, caltecholamines, cortisol, and growth hormone, which increase glucose levels when insulin is absent or minimal. Glucagon and caltecholamines stimulate lipolysis, which breaks down fatty acids. Fatty acids are oxidized to acetoacetate and β-hydroxybutyrate, resulting in a metabolic acidosis.

8. **How does one make the diagnosis of DKA?**
   - Blood glucose > 300 mg/dL
   - Low bicarbonate (< 15 mEq/L)
   - Low pH (< 7.3) with ketonemia or ketonuria

9. **How should DKA be treated in the emergency department (ED)?**
   - **Fluid resuscitation.** Patients often have a deficit of 5–10 L. Normal saline should be administered by giving 2 L in the first 1–2 hours, the next 2 L over hours 2–6, and finally 2 more L over hours 6–12. In children, give 10–20 mg/kg/h of fluid for the first hour, repeated once. Do not give more than 50 mL/kg of IV fluid in the first 4 hours. Fluids should be administered at approximately 1.5 times maintenance for 24 hours.
   - **Insulin.** Initial dosage is 0.1–0.4 U/kg IV bolus followed by 0.1 U/kg/h via IV infusion. Frequent blood sugars should be checked with a goal of dropping the glucose level to 50–75 mg/dL/h.
   - **Potassium replacement.** Serum potassium should be replaced, as insulin and fluids can drop levels profoundly; 20–40 mEq in 1 L bag should help correct the deficit slowly. Goal levels are between 4 and 5 mEq/L.
   - **Phosphorus and bicarbonate.** Therapy is controversial and should be reserved for profound disturbances (phosphorus <1 and pH < 6.9).

- **Glucose.** When serum levels drop below 250 mg/dL, IV fluids should be switched to half normal saline with the addition of 5% dextrose. Insulin requirements should decrease accordingly.
- **Magnesium and calcium.** Levels should be followed and replaced accordingly.

American Diabetes Association: Clinical Practice Recommendations 2002. Diabetes Care 25(Suppl 1), 2002.

10. Do all patients with DKA need to be admitted?
No. Patients with mild DKA, good follow-up, normal vitals, stable lab values, normal mentation, and no other underlying chronic or infectious sources and who able to tolerate oral intake may be discharged from the ED.

11. List the potential complications of therapy for DKA in the ED.
- Hypoglycemia
- Hypokalemia
- Hypophosphatemia
- Adult respiratory distress syndrome
- Cerebral edema

Lebovitz HE: Diabetic ketoacidosis. Lancet 345:767–772, 1995.

12. What is hyperosmolar hyperglycemia nonketotic coma (HHNC)?
HHNC is defined as severe hyperglycemia (usually >600 mg/dL), elevated plasma osmolality (> 315 mOsm/kg), serum bicarbonate > 15 mEq/L, arterial pH > 7.3, and negative serum ketones (can be mildly positive).

13. How is plasma osmolarity determined?

$$Osmolarity(mOsm/kg\ water) = 2(serum\ sodium) + (serum\ glucose/18 + BUN/2.8)$$

where BUN = blood urea nitrogen.

14. What occurs pathophysiologically to cause HHNC?
In the absence of insulin, glucose remains extracellular and creates an osmotic gradient. Extracellular volume expands at the expense of intracellular dehydration. Elevated glucose levels overcome renal filtration, and glucosuria results. Osmotic diuresis occurs as a result of the glucosuria. Along with the loss of free water, there is loss of potassium, often to a profound degree. Why these patients are not ketotic remains controversial. Some authors report that there is inhibition of lipolysis with higher insulin levels than are seen in DKA, whereas others report that free fatty acids are metabolized differently in patients with HHNC.

15. What are the precipitants of HHNC?
Type II diabetes, steroids, propanolol, calcium channel blockers, cimetidine, mannitol, phenytoin, thiazide diuretics, MI, stroke, pancreatitis, infection, and trauma may precipitate this disease. Patients often have concomitant hypertension, renal disease, gastrointestinal bleeding, dementia, and congestive heart failure.

16. What are the four key points in ED management of patients with HHNC?
- **Fluid administration:** 1–2 L of normal saline should be administered initially. Even though fluid deficits can be as high as 10 L, subsequent fluid administration should be judicious in patients with renal, cardiac, or pulmonary disease.
- **Potassium:** Potassium should be repleted at 10–20 mEq/h in patients with normal renal function.

- **Insulin:** Although most patients with HNNC do not receive insulin therapy, patients with acidosis, hyperkalemia, or renal failure need insulin to lower glucose levels and resolve metabolic derangements. A starting dose of 0.15 U/kg of insulin given intravenously, with an infusion rate of 0.1 U/kg/h, is reasonable in these patients.
- **Glucose:** Add to IV fluids when levels are less than 250 mg/dL.

17. **Which patients with HHNC should be admitted to the hospital?**
All patients with HHNC should be admitted. Most require at least 24 hours of monitoring for treatment of electrolyte abnormalities, fluid administration, and evaluation of precipitating causes.

18. **Define hypoglycemia.**
Serum glucose < 50 mg/dL.

19. **Who develops hypoglycemia?**
Patients who are taking hypoglycemic medications are at greatest risk for hypoglycemia. Other risk factors include accidental overdose of insulin or oral hypoglycemics, pentamidine, aspirin, haloperidol, insulinomas, renal failure, sepsis, adrenal insufficiency, sepsis, alcoholism, or heart failure.

20. **Which overdoses of oral hypoglycemic agents do not cause hypoglycemia?**
- Metformin overdose does not cause hypoglycemia because it decreases hepatic production of glucose and increases insulin sensitivity. Instead, symptoms of overdose include nausea, vomiting, abdominal pain, and lactic acidosis. Lactic acidosis may be treated with sodium bicarbonate or hemodialysis.
- Thiazolidinediones increase peripheral tissue glucose use and do not cause hypoglycemia. Hepatoxicity has been reported with these drugs.
- Alpha-glucosidase inhibitors decrease gastrointestinal glucose absorption and do not cause hypoglycemia. Symptoms of overdose include bloating, abdominal pain, and diarrhea.

21. **What are the presenting signs of a patient with hypoglycemia?**
Patients can present with agitation, diaphoresis, tachycardia, decreased level of conciousness, coma, seizures, and even focal neurologic deficits. Symptoms should reverse with administration of glucose. If symptoms do not resolve, seek an alternate diagnosis.
Olson KR: Poisoning and Drug Overdose. New York, McGraw Hill, 2004, pp 93–96.

22. **Which patients with hypoglycemia require admission to the hospital?**
- Patients with persistent altered mental status or hypoglycemia after glucose administration
- Patients who have taken excessive amounts of oral hypoglycemic agents or long-acting insulin
- Patients who are unable to tolerate oral intake
- Patients who are suicidal

23. **Can patients who have been treated for hypoglycemia in the field by paramedics refuse transport?**
Yes. This is a very common scenario. Patients most commonly have taken their normal or recently adjusted dose of insulin and have skipped a meal. If these patients can eat, they may refuse transport. Patients who may have taken an intentional overdose of insulin or oral hypoglycemic agents must be transported.

24. **What is metabolic syndrome X or dysmetabolic syndrome?**
Hyperglycemia, obesity, hypertension, and dyslipidemia.

25. Describe gestational diabetes mellitus.

Gestatinal diabetes usually develops in the second or third trimester and occurs when a woman's pancreatic function cannot overcome the insulin resistance created by the anti-insulin hormones secreted by the placenta during pregnancy. It affects approximately 2.1% of women in the United States but varies according to ethnicity. These woman are at increased risk of developing type II diabetes later in life.

Cousins L: Obstetric complications. In Reece EA, Coustan DR, et al: Diabetes Mellitus in Pregnancy, 2nd ed. New York, Churchill Livingstone, 1995, pp 287–302.

KEY POINTS: DIABETES MELLITUS

1. Infections in diabetics must be aggressively treated because they may spread rapidly.

2. Always measure the serum glucose in patients who are agitated, violent, diaphoretic or comatose to rule out an easily treatable cause of these findings—hypoglycemia.

Acknowledgment

The author gratefully acknowledges the contributions of Christina Johnson, MD, author of this chapter in the previous edition.

CHAPTER 45

THYROID AND ADRENAL DISORDERS

W. Jared Scott, MD, and Michael W. Brunko, MD

1. **Which thyroid-related conditions are considered true emergencies?**
   True emergencies include the two extremes of myxedema coma and thyroid storm. Thyroid disease is quite common, but myxedema coma and thyroid storm occur in less than 2% of patients with thyroid disease. The mortality of thyroid storm and myxedema coma without treatment is 80–100%, and with treatment, it is 15–50%. Rarely, ophthalmologic complications of Graves' disease may also require emergent treatment.

   Manifold CA: Hyperthyroidism, thyroid storm, and Graves' disease, 2005. www.emedicine.com

2. **What is the difference between thyrotoxicosis and hyperthyroidism?**
   - **Thyrotoxicosis** refers to excess circulating thyroid hormone originating from any cause (including thyroid hormone overdose).
   - **Hyperthyroidism** refers to excess circulating hormone resulting only from thyroid *gland* hyperfunction.

3. **What are the most common causes of thyrotoxicosis? How do they present?**
   Excessive thyroid hormone production:
   - Graves' disease (85% of all cases)
   - Toxic multinodular goiter (second most common cause)
   - Exposure to iodine (can precipitate increased hormone production)

   Leakage of thyroid hormone:
   - Subacute thyroiditis (inflammatory condition commonly seen in young women)
   - Radiation-induced inflammation

   Exogenous thyroid hormone administration:
   - Thyrotoxicosis factitia (Munchausen-like; thyroid hormone is taken to cause illness)
   - Thyroid hormone overdose or ingestion of meat containing beef thyroid tissue

4. **What medications can precipitate thyrotoxicosis in the emergency department (ED)?**
   Iodine-containing medications including radiographic contrast material, potassium iodine solution, amiodarone, and large doses of topical povidone-iodine.

5. **What are the common clinical signs and symptoms of thyrotoxicosis?**
   - **Constitutional:** Fatigue, weakness, heat intolerance, diaphoresis, fever, weight loss
   - **Neuropsychiatric:** Tremor, hyperreflexia, apathy, anxiety, emotional lability, psychosis
   - **Ophthalmologic:** Exophthalmos, lid lag, eye dryness
   - **Cardiovascular:** Tachycardia, palpitations, congestive heart failure
   - **Hematologic:** Anemia, leukocytosis
   - **Gastrointestinal:** Diarrhea
   - **Dermatologic:** Hair loss, onycholysis

6. **Is goiter always found in thyrotoxicosis?**
   No. A goiter is not present with exogenous administration of thyroid hormone and apathetic thyrotoxicosis. To complicate matters, a goiter may sometimes be present in hypothyroidism.

This is true in goitrous forms of thyroiditis in which the gland is "burned out," and scar tissue causes gland enlargement.

7. What is apathetic thyrotoxicosis?

A frequently missed presentation of hyperthyroidism seen most commonly in the elderly but present at any age, even in children. The typical patient is 70–80 years old *without* goiter or ophthalmologic findings. The diagnosis should be considered in elderly patients with chronic weight loss, proximal muscle weakness, depressed affect, new-onset atrial fibrillation, or congestive heart failure.

American Association of Clinical Endocrinologists: www.aace.com

8. How can I differentiate thyroid storm from thyrotoxicosis?

No absolute diagnostic criteria exist to differentiate the two, but thyroid storm usually includes (1) exaggerated manifestations of thyrotoxicosis; (2) temperature > 100°F (37.7°C); (3) tachycardia out of proportion to fever; and (4) dysfunction of the central nervous system, cardiovascular system, or gastrointestinal system.

9. What role do thyroid function tests have in making the diagnosis of thyroid storm?

Thyroid function studies in and of themselves are not really very helpful. Although thyroid function tests in a patient with thyroid storm are abnormal, they may not be appreciably different from those with thyrotoxicosis and do not differentiate between the two. The diagnosis is a clinical one. Treatment is initiated based on clinical suspicion without waiting for lab confirmation.

10. What conditions are included in the differential diagnosis of thyroid storm?

Toxicity caused by cocaine, amphetamines, other sympathomimetics, and anticholinergics; alcohol withdrawal syndromes; or infections such as encephalitis, meningitis, and sepsis. A history of thyroid disease or previous thyroid treatment or surgery is helpful in distinguishing thyroid storm from these other conditions.

11. What conditions precipitate thyroid storm?

- Emotional stress
- Infection or serious illness
- Surgery
- Trauma
- Childbirth
- Withdrawal of antithyroid therapy
- Recent thyroid ablation therapy

12. How is thyroid storm treated?

ED management of thyroid storm is essentially the same as for thyrotoxicosis, only more urgent. (See Table 45-1.)

KEY POINTS: THYROID STORM

1. Thyroid disease is extremely common in the emergency department population.

2. Thyroid storm and myxedema coma are true medical emergencies.

3. Include thyroid storm in your differential for toxic ingestions.

4. Treatment for thyroid storm is initiated *without* waiting for laboratory work-up.

TABLE 45-1.   STEP THERAPY OF DECOMPENSATED THYROTOXICOSIS

1. Supportive care
- General: Oxygen, cardiac monitor
- Fever: External cooling, acetaminophen (aspirin is contraindicated because it may increase free T_4)
- Dehydration: Intravenous fluids
- Nutrition: Glucose, multivitamins, including folate (deficient secondary to hypermetabolism)
- Adrenal replacement (depletion secondary to hypermetabolism): Hydrocortisone, 200 mg IV initially, then 100 mg 3 times/day until stable
- Cardiac decompensation (atrial fibrillation, congestive heart failure): Digoxin (increased requirements), diuretics, sympatholytics as required
- Treat precipitating event: Therapy as indicated

2. Inhibition of hormone biosynthesis—thionamides
- Propylthiouracil (PTU),* 1200–1500 mg/day, given as a loading dose of 600–1000 mg followed by 200–250 mg every 4 hours PO, by nasogastric tube, or rectally (also blocks peripheral conversion of T_4 to T_3)

or
- Methimazole, 120 mg/day, given as 20 mg PO every 4 hours (or 40 mg crushed in an aqueous solution rectally) with or without a loading dose of 60–0100 mg

3. Blockade of hormone release—iodides* (at least 1 hour after step 2)
- Lugol's solution, 30–60 drops/day orally divided 3 or 4 times/day

or
- Ipodate (Oragrafin), 0.5–3 gm/day (especially useful with thyroiditis or thyroid hormone overdose)

or
- Lithium carbonate (if allergic to iodine or agranulocytosis occurs with thionamides), 300 mg PO every 6 hours and subsequently to maintain serum lithium at 1 mEq/L

4. Antagonism of peripheral hormone effects—sympatholytics
- Propranolol,* 2–5 mg IV every 4 hours or IV infusion at 5–10 mg/h. For less toxic patients use PO at 20–200 mg every 4 hours (contraindicated in bronchospastic disease[†] and congestive heart failure; digitalize patients with congestive heart failure before starting propranolol)

or
- Reserpine, 2.5–5 mg IM every 4 hours, preceded by 1-mg test dose while monitoring blood pressure (use if beta blocker contraindicated and congestive heart failure and hypotension and cardiac shock not present)

or
- Guanethidine, 30–40 mg PO every 6 hours

IM = intramuscular, IV = intravenous, PO = per os, T_3 = triiodothyronine, T_4 = thyroxine.
*Preferred medication.
[†]Consider esmolol if history of pulmonary disease. Effective dose may be higher than recommended. Begin with 500 mg/kg load over 1 minute, followed by 50 mg/kg/min IV. Repeat load and double infusion as necessary.
American Thyroid Association: www.thyroid.org

13. **How is acute thyroid hormone overdose treated?**
Fatalities are rare with acute ingestion. Toxicity after massive acute overdose usually occurs within 4–12 hours but may be delayed for days, particularly with levothyroxine (T_4) ingestion. Acute overdose management is as usual, including charcoal and work-up for coingestants.

14. **What is Graves' ophthalmopathy?**
Clinical features include eyelid retraction, proptosis, chemosis, periorbital edema, and diplopia with poor eye movement. Eye findings are seen in about half of patients.

15. **When is treatment of Graves' ophthalmopathy an emergent condition?**
Grave's patients with compression of the optic nerve or corneal ulceration require immediate ophthalmologic consultation. Visual blurring that persists with eye closure and diminished color brightness suggest compression of the optic nerve. Severe proptosis can cause keratitis or corneal ulceration presenting as eye pain, photophobia, conjunctival infection, visual loss, and a flare of cells in the anterior chamber. Optic neuropathy is initially treated with high-dose steroids (e.g., prednisone, 1–2 mg/kg per os [PO]). Corneal ulcers, with or without keratitis, require culture and topical antibiotics.

Thyroid Disease Manager: www.thyroidmanager.org

16. **What are the three classes of hypothyroidism?**
Hypothyroidism is simply a deficiency of thyroid hormone.
- **Primary:** Dysfunction of the gland (most common type)
- **Secondary:** Deficiency of thyroid-stimulating hormone (TSH) from the pituitary
- **Tertiary:** Deficiency of thyrotropin-releasing hormone (TRH) from the hypothalamus

17. **What are the most common causes of hypothyroidism?**
Causes include autoimmune and subacute thyroiditis, end-stage Graves' disease, post-thyroidectomy or postirradiation, drug involvement (iodides, lithium, thionamides, amiodarone), heredity, and tumor.

18. **What are the common clinical manifestations of hypothyroidism?**
- **Constitutional:** Cold intolerance, weight gain, hypothermia, weakness, lethargy, hoarse or deep voice, slow speech, drowsiness
- **Neuropsychiatric:** Delayed deep tendon reflexes, dementia, psychosis, paresthesia
- **Cardiovascular:** Angina, bradycardia
- **Respiratory:** Pleural effusion, dyspnea, hypoventilation
- **Musculoskeletal:** Joint pains, muscle cramps
- **Dermatologic:** Cool, dry skin; hair loss; nonpitting edema
- **Gynecologic:** Menorrhagia

19. **What additional features are present in myxedema coma?**
The hallmark clinical features are hypothermia (75%) and coma in a patient with a history of thyroid disease. Laboratory evaluation may reveal anemia, electrolyte abnormalities, hypercarbia, respiratory acidosis, or respiratory failure. Electrocardiogram (ECG) and chest radiograph often show bradycardia and pleural effusion or frank congestive heart failure.

20. **What precipitates myxedema coma in the hypothyroid patient?**
Triggers include pulmonary infection, sedatives and anesthetic agents (including etomidate), cold exposure, trauma, myocardial infarction or congestive heart failure, cerebrovascular accident, and gastrointestinal hemorrhage. Contributing metabolic conditions include hypoxia, hypercapnia, hyponatremia, and hypoglycemia.

21. **What is the treatment for myxedema coma?**
See Table 45-2.

TABLE 45-2. TREATMENT FOR MYXEDEMA COMA

1. Supportive care
  - Airway control, oxygen, IV access, and cardiac monitor (ABCs)
  - Hypotension is treated with crystalloids.
  - Vasopressors as indicated (ineffective without thyroid hormone replacement)
  - Baseline thyroid function studies should be sent.
  - Hypothermia is treated with passive rewarming.
  - Hydrocortisone (because of increased metabolic stress; 100–200 mg IV)

2. Thyroid replacement therapy
  - IV T_4 (4 µg/kg; followed in 24 hours by 100 µg IV, then 50 µg IV until oral medication is tolerated)
  - T_3 (liothyronine), at 20 µg IV followed by 10 µg IV every 8 hours until the patient is conscious (given because of the risk of decreased T_3 generation from T_4 in severely hypothyroid patients)

3. Identify and treat precipitating factors

4. Treat concomitant metabolic abnormalities, including hyponatremia, hypoglycemia and hypercalcemia

ABCs = airway, breathing, circulation, IV = intravenous, T_3 = triiodothyronine, T_4 = thyroxine.
Citkowitz E: Myxedema coma or crisis, 2004. www.emedicine.com

---

22. **What is the significance of a palpable thyroid nodule in an asymptomatic patient?**
Solitary thyroid nodules are a common physical finding in the general population. Most are benign colloid nodules that will disappear over time. Because a small percentage of solitary nodules are thyroid carcinomas, referral for fine-needle aspiration biopsy is indicated for all patients with palpable nodules. Biopsy results identify 70% of nodules to be benign, 5% to be malignant, and the remainder to be cytologically indeterminate with surgical follow-up required.

Hegedus L: The thyroid nodule. N Engl J Med 351:1764–1771, 2004.
Hermus AR, Huysmans DA: Treatment of benign nodular thyroid disease. N Engl J Med 338:1438–1446, 1998.

23. **What is the significance of a nonpalpable thyroid nodule incidentally found on a radiologic study (incidentaloma)? When does it require further work-up?**
Thyroid nodules smaller than 1 cm are usually not detected on physical examination but may be identified incidentally on magnetic resonance imaging, computed tomography, or ultrasound. These types of nodules are quite common and detectable by ultrasound in 30–50% of the general population. Patients do not need to be referred for biopsy unless a nonpalpable nodule is greater than 1.5 cm or a personal history of neck irradiation or family history of thyroid cancer is present. Radiologic findings suggestive of malignancy, such as calcifications, also may warrant

referral. Nodules larger than 1.5 cm should be referred for fine-needle aspiration biopsy on an outpatient basis.

American Thyroid Association: www.thyroid.org

Tan GH, Gharib H: Thyroid incidentalomas: Management approaches to nonpalpable nodules discovered incidentally on thyroid imaging. Ann Intern Med 126:226–231, 1997.

24. How does amiodarone affect thyroid function?
Amiodarone is 37% organic iodine by weight and as such can have many effects on thyroid function. Normal maintenance doses result in iodine loads of 10–20 times the normal dietary requirement of iodine. Chronic use of amiodarone causes either a hypothyroid or a thyrotoxic state in 20–30% of patients. Amiodarone administration also has been cited in the literature as a precipitant of thyroid storm, although not in the setting of acute cardiac resuscitation in the ED.

Harjai KJ, Licata AA: Effects of amiodarone on thyroid function. Ann Intern Med 126:63–73, 1997.

25. What are the adrenal emergencies that I need to worry about?
The most serious adrenal emergency is acute adrenal insufficiency. Hypercortisolemia, or Cushing's disease, is rare, and it is unlikely you will make that diagnosis in the ED.

26. Will I ever need to worry about hypercortisolemia in the ED?
Cortisol excess can lead to psychoemotional disturbances, such as insomnia, mood disorders, mania, depression, and psychosis. If a woman presents with signs of masculinization or a man presents with signs of feminization and the previously mentioned symptoms, think of hypercortisolemia.

27. What adrenal physiology do I need to know?
The primary functions of the glucocorticoid cortisol and the mineralocorticoid aldosterone. Cortisol has essential effects on all organ systems. It influences fat, protein, and carbohydrate metabolism. It affects immunologic and inflammatory responses, bone and calcium metabolism, growth and development, the gastrointestinal tract, and the central nervous system. It is a major mediator of the stress response—affecting the heart, the vascular bed, water excretion, and electrolyte balance. Aldosterone is responsible for maintaining sodium and potassium concentrations and to regulate extracellular volume.

28. How is normal secretion of cortisol controlled?
Cortisol is secreted from the cortex of the adrenal gland in response to direct stimulation by adrenocorticotropic hormone (ACTH). ACTH secretion is stimulated by the hormone corticotropin-releasing factor (CRF) from the hypothalamus. This occurs in a diurnal rhythm, with higher levels secreted in the morning and lower levels in the evening. By negative feedback inhibition, plasma cortisol levels act to suppress release of ACTH.

29. How is secretion of aldosterone controlled?
Primarily by the renin-angiotensin system and the serum potassium concentration. The renin-angiotensin system controls aldosterone levels in response to changes in volume, posture, and sodium intake. Potassium influences the adrenal cortex directly to increase secretion of aldosterone.

30. What are the two types of acute adrenal insufficiency?
Adrenal insufficiency may be due to either destruction of adrenal gland (primary adrenal insufficiency) or inadequate production of ACTH (secondary adrenal insufficiency).

31. List the causes of adrenal insufficiency.
See Table 45-3.

TABLE 45-3. COMMON CAUSES OF ADRENAL INSUFFICIENCY

Primary adrenal insufficiency
- Idiopathic (autoimmune)
- Tuberculosis
- Bilateral adrenal hemorrhage or infarction
- Acquired immunodeficiency syndrome (AIDS)
- Drugs: Adrenolytic agents (metyrapone, aminoglutethimide, mitotane), ketoconazole
- Infections: Fungal, bacterial sepsis
- Infiltrative disorders: Sarcoidosis, hemochromatosis, amyloidosis, lymphoma, metastatic cancer
- Bilateral surgical adrenalectomy
- Hereditary: Adrenal hypoplasia, congenital adrenal hyperplasia, adrenoleukodystrophy, familial glucocorticoid deficiency

Secondary adrenal insufficiency
- Exogenous glucocorticoid administration
- Pituitary or suprasellar tumor
- Pituitary irradiation or surgery
- Head trauma
- Infiltrative disorders of the pituitary or hypothalamus: sarcoidosis, hemochromatosis, histiocytosis X, metastatic cancer, or lymphoma
- Infectious diseases: Tuberculosis, meningitis, fungus
- Isolated adrenocorticotropic hormone (ACTH) deficiency

32. **Which of the causes are the most common causes of primary adrenal insufficiency?**
Tuberculosis and autoimmune destruction account for 90% of the cases of primary adrenal insufficiency.

33. **What is the most common cause of secondary adrenal insufficiency?**
Long-term therapy with pharmacologic doses of glucocorticoid (prednisone, methylprednisolone, dexamethasone) is the most common cause of secondary adrenal insufficiency. These drugs are used to treat a wide variety of medical problems, and if they are used for any significant time, some degree of suppression of the hypothalamic-pituitary-adrenal (HPA) axis occurs.

34. **How long must a patient be treated with steroids to cause suppression of the HPA axis?**
Any patient who is on large doses of steroids (e.g., > 20 mg/day of prednisone) for 2 weeks or more has the potential for long-term suppression of the HPA axis. Severity of adrenal suppression is variable and depends on the dose and potency of the glucocorticoid, the time of day the drug was taken (suppression is greater when taken in the evening), and the potency of the drug. Recovery of the HPA axis may take a few months to a year.

Lamberts SWJ, Bruining HA, de Jong FH: Corticosteroid therapy in severe illness. N Engl J Med 337:1285–1292, 1997.

35. **List some signs and symptoms of primary adrenal insufficiency**
    - Fatigue
    - Weakness
    - Weight loss
    - Anorexia
    - Hyperpigmentation
    - Gastrointestinal symptoms (nausea, vomiting, abdominal pain, and diarrhea)
    - Hypotension (usually with orthostatic changes)

36. **What are the characteristic laboratory findings of primary adrenal insufficiency?**
    Hyperkalemia, hyponatremia, and hypoglycemia are usually present with primary adrenal insufficiency. If the patient is dehydrated, volume depletion may lead to azotemia. A mild metabolic acidosis is often present.

37. **How is the presentation of secondary adrenal insufficiency different from that of primary adrenal insufficiency?**
    In secondary adrenal insufficiency, there is no deficiency of aldosterone secretion. The volume depletion and hypotension are not as severe (unless crisis is present); hyperkalemia is absent, and hyponatremia, if present, is due to water retention and not salt wasting, as in primary adrenal insufficiency. Patients usually have a cushingoid appearance because of long-term glucocorticoid use. If the patient has a pituitary or hypothalamic cause for the adrenal insufficiency, findings may include symptoms of other pituitary hormone deficiencies, such as hypothyroidism and amenorrhea.

38. **What is adrenal crisis?**
    Adrenal crisis often presents in a patient with chronic adrenal insufficiency who undergoes some form of stress, such as an acute myocardial infarction, surgery, or trauma, and is unable to mount a stress response by increasing circulating cortisol levels.

39. **When does acute adrenal crisis usually occur?**
    It usually occurs in response to a major stress, such as acute myocardial infarction, sepsis, surgery, major injury, or other illness in any patient with primary or secondary adrenal insufficiency.

40. **What is the most frequent iatrogenic cause of acute adrenal crisis?**
    Rapid withdrawal of steroids in patients with adrenal atrophy secondary to long-term steroid administration.

41. **Describe the most common clinical features of acute adrenal insufficiency.**
    Patients appear to be profoundly ill. They are significantly volume depleted with hypotension and shock. Nausea, vomiting, and severe abdominal pain, many times mimicking an acute abdomen, are present. Fever may occur as a result of infection or the adrenal insufficiency itself. Central nervous system symptoms of confusion, disorientation, and lethargy may be present.

42. **How is adrenal crisis diagnosed?**
    First, you must always suspect adrenal crisis if a patient has been taking high-dose steroids and presents with the symptoms mentioned. The most useful and practical laboratory test is the **rapid ACTH stimulation test.**

43. How is the rapid ACTH stimulation test performed?

A baseline sample of blood is drawn at time 0 for a cortisol level. Then, 0.25 mg of cosyntropin (synthetic ACTH) is given intravenously. Cortisol levels are checked at 30 minutes, 1 hour, and 6 hours.

Lamberts SWJ, Bruining HA, de Jong FH: Corticosteroid therapy in severe illness. N Engl J Med 337:1285–1292, 1997.

44. Should I withhold treatment until the rapid ACTH stimulation test is accomplished?

No! If your patient is unstable, you can begin treatment using a glucocorticoid that will not cause an increase in measurable cortisol levels. Dexamethasone (6–10 mg) is generally recommended.

Klauer K: Adrenal insufficiency and adrenal crisis. www.emedicine.com

45. How is acute adrenal insufficiency treated?

Intravenous (IV) hydrocortisone (100 mg minimum) and crystalloid IV fluids containing dextrose must be initiated early. A detailed history and examination should be done to attempt to elicit what may have instigated the stress that caused the acute adrenal insufficiency. If a cause is found, supportive and definitive measures need to be instituted in the ED. Mineralocorticoid replacement is usually unnecessary if salt and water replacement is adequate and if the patient receives hydrocortisone—100 mg of hydrocortisone has the salt-retaining effect of 0.1 mg of fludrocortisone.

Cooper MS, Stewart PM: Corticosteroid insufficiency in acutely ill patients. N Engl J Med 348:727–734, 2003.

KEY POINTS: ADRENAL CRISIS

1. Consider adrenal crisis in all hypotensive patients.

2. All patients in adrenal crisis require rapid administration of IV steroids.

3. Dexamethasone may be initiated in adrenal crisis without affecting the cosyntropin (ACTH) stimulation test.

4. Only 2 weeks of chronic steroid use will cause adrenal suppression, making a patient more prone to adrenal crisis.

---

46. What about the patient with chronic adrenal insufficiency who presents to the ED with a minor illness or injury? Should I treat this patient any differently?

Yes. These patients usually require 20–30 mg/day of hydrocortisone. Some also require mineralocorticoid replacement. If these patients experience a minor illness or injury, they should be told to double their daily cortisol dose for 24–48 hours until symptoms improve. Increasing the mineralocorticoid dose is usually not necessary. Follow-up care should be coordinated closely with the primary care physician or endocrinologist. Patients should be told that if nausea or vomiting develops and they are unable to keep down the medication, they should seek immediate medical care.

Oelkers W: Adrenal insufficiency. N Engl J Med 335:1206–1212, 1996.

WEBSITES

1. American Association of Clinical Endocrinologists: www.aace.com

2. American Thyroid Association: www.thyroid.org

3. Citkowitz E: Myxedema coma or crisis, 2004. www.emedicine.com

4. Klauer K: Adrenal insufficiency and adrenal crisis. www.emedicine.com

5. Manifold CA: Hyperthyroidism, thyroid storm, and Graves disease, 2005. www.emedicine.com

6. Thyroid Disease Manager: www.thyroidmanager.org

BIBLIOGRAPHY

1. Beale MB, Belzberg H: Adrenal insufficiency. In Grenvik A (ed): Textbook of Critical Care, 4th ed. Philadelphia, W.B. Saunders, 2000, pp 806–816.

2. Bravermann LE, Burch HB, Wartofsky L: Life-threatening thyrotoxicosis-thyroid storm. Endocrinol Metab Clin North Am 22:263–277, 1993.

3. Jordan RM: Myxedema coma: Pathophysiology, therapy, and factors affecting prognosis. Med Clin North Am 79:185–194, 1995.

4. Loriaux DL, McDonald WJ: Adrenal insufficiency. In DeGroot LJ (ed): Endocrinology, 4th ed, Vol. 2. Philadelphia, W.B. Saunders, 2001, pp 1683–1690.

5. Pimentel L, Hansen KN: Thyroid disease in the emergency department: A clinical and laboratory review. J Emerg Med 28:201–209, 2005.

6. Tietgens ST, Leinung MC: Thyroid storm. Med Clin North Am 79:169–184, 1995.

7. Braverman LE, Utigar RD, Werner SC, et al (eds): Werner and Ingbar's The Thyroid: A Fundamental and Clinical Text, 8th ed. Philadelphia, Lippincott Williams & Wilkins, 2000.

8. Weetman AP: Medical progress: Grave's disease. N Engl J Med 343:1236–1248, 2001.

9. Wogan JM: Selected endocrine disorders. In Marx JA, Hockberger R, Walls R, et al (eds): Rosen's Emergency Medicine: Concepts and Clinical Practice, 5th ed. St. Louis, Mosby, 2002, pp 1770–1785.

SEPSIS SYNDROMES

Stephen J. Wolf, MD, and Sean P. Bender, MD

1. What is SIRS?

Systemic inflammatory response syndrome. As its name implies, it is a syndrome of inflammation not necessarily infection.

KEY POINTS: SIRS CRITERIA (2 OF 4 NEEDED FOR DIAGNOSIS)

1. Temperature $> 38°C$ or $< 36°C$

2. Heart rate > 90 bpm

3. Respiratory rate > 20 breaths/minute or $PaCO_2 < 32$ mmHg

4. Serum white blood cell count $> 12,000$ mm^3 or < 4000 mm^3 or 10% band forms

2. How is sepsis defined?

In the emergency department (ED), sepsis is defined clinically as a syndrome that has the presence of both SIRS and *presumed* bacteremia.

3. What distinguishes sepsis from severe sepsis?

Severe sepsis is sepsis complicated by organ dysfunction. Severe sepsis is now considered to be the most common cause of death in noncoronary critical care units. Approximately 150,000 people die annually in Europe and $> 200,000$ die annually in the United States from sepsis.

4. What is the significance of an elevated lactate level in sepsis?

An elevated serum lactate concentration identifies tissue hypoperfusion in patients who are not hypotensive. Although lactate measurements may be useful and correlate with mortality, they lack precision as a measure of tissue metabolic status.

5. What organ systems can dysfunction, suggesting severe sepsis?

- **Cardiovascular:** Vasodilation, poor myocardial contractility and increased cardiac oxygen demand, systemic hypotension or cardiac ischemia
- **Central nervous system:** Altered mental status
- **Global tissue hypoperfusion:** Elevated lactate ≥ 4.0 mmol/L
- **Hematologic:** Increasing prothrombin time (PT)/international normalized ratio (INR), partial thromboplastin time (PTT), hemolysis and thrombocytopenia, disseminated intravascular coagulopathy (DIC)
- **Liver:** Coagulopathy, jaundice, elevated transaminases

- **Renal:** Acute renal failure determined by increase in blood urea nitrogen (BUN) and creatinine, decreased urine output to less than 0.5 mL/kg/h
- **Pulmonary:** Acute respiratory distress syndrome, respiratory failure, unexplained hypoxia

6. **What is the mortality rate of sepsis versus severe sepsis?**
   The mortality rate of sepsis is 15–20% versus 30–40% mortality for severe sepsis.

7. **What is the primary goal of resuscitation in a septic patient?**
   Aggressive resuscitation to ensure that oxygen delivery meets oxygen demand of tissues affected by the septic state.

8. **What is an easy way to decrease an affected tissue's increased oxygen demand from sepsis?**
   Early appropriate antibiotics. The Institute for Healthcare Improvement recommends initiation of antibiotics within 3 hours of ED presentation.
   Institute for Healthcare Improvement: www.ihi.org/IHI/Topics/CriticalCare/Sepsis/

9. **What are two means of increasing oxygen supply to affected tissues in a septic state?**
   - High-flow supplemental oxygen
   - Early goal-directed therapy (EGDT)

10. **What is the mortality benefit to initiating EGDT in severe sepsis patients?**
    There is a 10–20% reduction in mortality.
    Rivers EP, Nguyen B, Havstad S, et al: Early goal-directed therapy in the treatment of severe sepsis. N Engl J Med 340:207–214, 1999.

11. **What are the goals outlined in EGDT for patients in severe sepsis?**
    During the first 6 hours of resuscitation, the goals of initial resuscitation of sepsis-induced hypoperfusion should include all of the following as part of a treatment protocol:
    - Central venous pressure (CVP): Goal of 8–12 mmH$_2$O
    - Mean arterial pressure (MAP): Goal of $\geq$ 65 mmHg
    - Urine output: Goal of $\geq$ 0.5 mL/kg/h
    - Central venous (superior vena cava) or mixed venous oxygen saturation (SvO$_2$): Goal of $\geq$ 70%
    Shapiro NI, Trzeciak S: Bacteremia, sepsis, and septic shock. In Wolfson AB (ed): Harwood-Nuss' Clinical Practice of Emergency Medicine, 4th ed. Philadelphia, Lippincott Williams & Wilkins, 2005, pp 706–711.

12. **What intervention should be used for a CVP that is less than 8 mmH$_2$O?**
    Intravenous (IV) fluid resuscitation is the first-line treatment and is given in bolus increments over 30 minutes or until CVP is at goal. Use 500–1000 mL of crystalloids or 300–500 mL of colloids boluses, repeated based on response. Caution needs to be used in patients with contraindications to significant volume resuscitation (e.g., patients with congestive heart failure [CHF] or renal failure).

13. **What intervention should be initiated for a MAP that is less than 65 mmHg?**
    After adequate attempts at fluid resuscitation (at least 20–40 mL/kg) to raise the patient's CVP to 8–12 mmH$_2$O, initiate vasopressor support to increase MAP to 65 mmHg.

14. **Does one vasopressor have a proven benefit over another in the setting of severe sepsis?**
    Some evidence suggests that norepinephrine is a better first-line vasopressor than dopamine in the setting of sepsis. Although the jury may still be out on that point, it is agreed that both

dopamine and norepinephrine are good first- and second-line agents for supportive care in sepsis. Epinephrine is associated with higher mortality in animal models and is generally reserved for use if the patient is failing both dopamine and norepinephrine.

15. **What are the implications of a low SvO$_2$?**
This simply means there is a global tissue hypoxia. An SvO$_2$ of less then 70% suggests that the tissue extraction of O$_2$ is greater than the delivery needed to sustain the metabolic demands (i.e., poor perfusion).

16. **What intervention should be initiated for an SvO$_2$ < 70%?**
   - If the SvO$_2$ is less than 70% despite a CVP of at least 8–12 mmH$_2$O and a MAP of at least 65 mmHg, then consider the use of dobutamine for its inotropic properties to help with cardiac pump function, perfusion, and O$_2$ delivery.
   - Additionally, one may consider transfusing packed red blood cells to increase the patient's hematocrit to a level of 30%. This would help increase oxygen-carrying capacity.

17. **What are the drawbacks to transfusion?**
Transfusion of blood is initially helpful. There are, however, several potential drawbacks. Acute transfusion reactions and systemic response to minor antigens and storage breakdown products may further increase the immunocompromised state associated with sepsis. Additionally, the optimal endpoint of transfusion it is unclear.

18. **Is SvO$_2$ a reasonable surrogate measure to superior vena cava oxygen saturation (ScVO$_2$)?**
Recommendations from the latest international sepsis forum suggest that SvO$_2$ from a central line placed in the superior vena cava is a comparable and reliably accurate estimate of the ScVO$_2$ gained from a pulmonary artery catheter, Swan-Ganz catheter.

19. **What are the implications of meeting these goals as quickly as possible?**
There is a clear benefit from aggressively clearing lactate and reversing tissue hypoperfusion in severe sepsis using the goals of EGDT. Rivers et al. demonstrated a 16% decrease in absolute 28-day mortality by implementing EGDT through the first 6 hours of patient presentation to the ED.

20. **How is septic shock defined?**
Septic shock can be defined as severe sepsis with ongoing tissue hypoperfusion refractory to resuscitation.

21. **What is the role of vasopressin?**
Currently, vasopressin is a second- to third-line vasopressor and is reserved for failure of other vasopressors in the setting of septic shock with refractory hypotension. Vasopressin does not confer a mortality benefit and causes extreme peripheral vasoconstriction that may result in digital ischemia.

Institute for Healthcare Improvement: www.ihi.org/IHI/Topics/CriticalCare/Sepsis/

22. **What is the role of activated protein C (APC) in sepsis?**
Recombinant APC (drotrecogin alfa) is a novel sepsis therapy that has demonstrated a 6.1–13% absolute reduction in mortality in some studies. The mortality benefit appears to be highest in those who are the sickest with Acute Physiology and Chronic Health Evaluation II (APACHE II) score > 25.

The use of APC in all septic patients is controversial due to the lack of efficacy in studies of patients with a APACHE II scores < 25 and the expense of the treatment. The cost of each treatment is around $8000.

23. **What is the role of tight glycemic control in sepsis?**
There are data to demonstrate that in critically ill patients there is a 50% reduction in intensive care unit (ICU) mortality from 8% to 4.6% with tightly controlled glucose between 80 and 110 mg/dL. Therefore, it is recommended that an aggressive insulin-controlled glucose protocol be started in critically ill patients in the ED.

BIBLIOGRAPHY

1. Dellinger RP, Carlet JM, Masun H, et al: Surviving sepsis campaign guidelines for management of severe sepsis and septic shock. Crit Care Med 32:858–873, 2004.
2. Rivers EP, Nguyen B, Havstad S, et al: Early goal-directed therapy in the treatment of severe sepsis. N Engl J Med 340:207–214, 1999.
3. Shapiro NI, Howell M, Talmor D, et al: A blueprint for a sepsis protocol. Acad Emerg Med 12:352–329, 2005.

CHAPTER 47

SOFT TISSUE INFECTIONS

Harvey W. Meislin, MD, and David A. Guttman, MD

1. How do I differentiate cellulitis from an abscess?

Cellulitis is a soft tissue infection of the skin and subcutaneous tissue usually characterized by blanching erythema, swelling, tenderness, and local warmth. A cutaneous abscess is a localized collection of pus that results in a painful soft tissue mass that is often fluctuant but surrounded by firm indurated granulation tissue and erythema.

2. What are the causes of cellulitis? How does it progress?

Although most often acute, cellulitis may be subacute or chronic. Minor trauma is often the predisposing cause, but hematogenous and lymphatic dissemination may account for its appearance in previously normal skin. Cellulitis caused by bacterial infection tends to spread radially with associated swelling, whereas nonbacterial or inflammatory cellulitis tends to stay localized. Cellulitis may progress to ascending lymphangitis and septicemia.

3. What are the causes of abscesses? How do they progress?

Abscesses occur on all areas of the body, although they have a predominance for the head and neck, upper extremities, and torso. Abscesses usually are caused by interruptions of the integrity of the protective epithelium, but they may be associated with obstruction of apocrine glands or spread via mucosal involvement in the oral and anorectal areas. Superficial abscesses tend to remain localized and often rupture through the skin if not incised and drained.

KEY POINTS: CELLULITIS VERSUS ABSCESS

1. Abscesses contain pus; cellulitis does not.

2. Fluctuance surrounded by induration signifies fluid, usually pus.

3. There is an increasing incidence of community-associated methicillin–resistant *Staphylococcus aureus* (MRSA).

4. Community-associated MRSA has different sensitivities and susceptibilities to antibiotics than hospital-associated MRSA.

5. Treatment for cellulitis is immobilization, elevation, heat, analgesics, and antibiotics.

6. Simple abscesses can be treated solely with incision and drainage.

4. What is pus? Why is the presence of pus significant?

Pus is a heterogeneous mix of cellular material in various stages of digestion by polymorphonuclear leukocytes (PMNs). These PMNs are drawn to sites of inflammation, infection, or trauma by various chemotactic factors to defend the host against potential pathogens. Abscesses contain pus; cellulitis does not. Although soft tissue infections tend to spread, and abscess and cellulitis may be present in the same anatomic area, the presence of pus defines the diagnosis of an abscess and the need for incision and drainage.

5. **How do I know if pus is present?**
In cutaneous abscesses, a raised painful mass with a fluctuant center surrounded by indurated erythematous tissue signifies the presence of pus. Adjunctive radiographic techniques, such as ultrasound or computed tomography (CT) scan, may be useful for deeper soft tissue infections but are rarely indicated with superficial abscesses. The use of a localizer needle is often helpful, especially in wounds in which the purulence is loculated. Needle aspiration of the involved area with a needle large enough to withdraw thick pus often helps to define the location of purulence for incision and drainage and makes the process more comfortable by decreasing the pressure and pain in the area.

6. **What are the differential diagnoses for cellulitis and abscess?**
The differential is one of bacterial versus nonbacterial infection. The etiologies of nonbacterial cellulitis include arthropod envenomation, chemical or thermal burns, arthritis, and healing wounds. Nonbacterial cellulitis is usually localized and often lacks lymphangitic streaking. The differential diagnosis of abscesses includes sterile abscesses, cutaneously borne bacterial abscesses, and mucous membrane abscesses. Abscesses of the oral and anorectal area usually originate from flora indigenous to those areas. Sterile abscesses, which occur approximately 5% of the time, tend to be associated with drug abuse and subcutaneous injections.

7. **Is it useful to culture cellulitis or abscesses?**
Culturing cellulitis is often futile, with only 10–50% of such efforts yielding successful results. Often there is secondary skin contamination. Culturing can be useful, however, in patients who do not respond to initial management, in patients with recurrent disease, or in patients with sepsis. Culturing the portal of entry may be useful, even if distal to the site of the cellulitis. Culturing of cutaneous abscesses seldom is clinically indicated because normal host defenses tend to contain and localize the process. In diabetics; in patients with acquired immunodeficiency syndrome (AIDS), leukemia, vascular insufficiency, trauma, burns, or recurrent abscess; or when concerned for community-associated MRSA or with failure of initial therapy, Gram stain and culture may be indicated.

8. **What is the yield of blood cultures when treating cellulitis?**
A number of studies have demonstrated that the routine ordering of blood cultures in the emergency department (ED) is not warranted in an immunocompetent host with uncomplicated cellulitis. The impact on clinical management is marginal. One study reported that blood cultures were twice as likely to be contaminated as to be true positives. Blood cultures should be considered prior to starting antibiotic therapy in immunocompromised patients, in those with an exposure to unusual organisms, and in patients with a potentially complicated cellulitis.

9. **What is community-associated MRSA?**
MRSA was first recognized as a community-associated pathogen in the early 1980s. Community-associated MRSA skin and soft tissue infections are spread within the community and are genetically distinct from hospital-associated MRSA infections. Community-associated MRSA has different sensitivities and susceptibilities to antibiotics than hospital-associated MRSA as well.

10. **Who is at risk for acquiring community-associated MRSA?**
The prevalence of MRSA colonization in the community ranges from 0.2–2.8%. Highest rates are seen amongst poor urban populations. There is a high prevalence among injection drug

users as well as in prison populations, athletes sharing equipment, and isolated Native American communities.

11. **Is there a role for routine laboratory studies?**
Laboratory studies are generally not helpful in the treatment of superficial soft tissue infections, unless signs or symptoms of systemic illness are present. These patients are often not systemically ill, and even an elevated white blood cell (WBC) count does not differentiate bacterial from nonbacterial infection, identify the presence of abscess or cellulitis, or show systemic involvement. An exception may be *Haemophilus influenzae* cellulitis, in which WBC counts often exceed 15,000/mm^3 with a left shift, often occurring in children. Laboratory analysis may be useful in the immunocompromised host or in patients who appear to be septic or systemically ill.

12. **Summarize appropriate treatment of soft tissue infections.**
The time-honored treatment for cellulitis is immobilization, elevation, heat or warm moist packs, analgesics, and antibiotics directed toward suspected pathogens. The treatment for cutaneous abscesses is a properly performed incision and drainage, done most commonly with local anesthesia.

13. **Should I routinely prescribe antibiotics for patients with an abscess?**
No. Antibiotics are not indicated in patients with a cutaneous abscess and with normal host defenses. In patients with complications of diabetes, AIDS, leukemia, neoplasms, significant vascular insufficiency, trauma, thermal burns, or suspicion for MRSA, antibiotics should be considered as prophylaxis to prevent spread into local tissues or the bloodstream. Prophylactic antibiotics, although not necessary, could be considered for abscesses of the face, groin, and hand. The selection of antimicrobial agents can be facilitated by knowing the flora associated with the anatomic area involved and if the abscess is from a cutaneous or mucosal process.

14. **How do you treat community-associated MRSA?**
Often simple abscesses can be treated solely with incision and drainage, but when antibiotics are deemed appropriate in the treatment of skin and soft tissue infections, it is no longer recommended to use a ß-lactam such as cephalexin. Antimicrobial susceptibility patterns of MRSA all demonstrate uniform resistance to oxacillin. Susceptibilities appear highest to trimethoprim-sulfamethoxazole, clindamycin, tetracycline, levofloxacin, and vancomycin.

15. **How does the presence of community-associated MRSA change the management of soft tissue infections in the ED?**
All suspected MRSA abscesses should be cultured in the ED prior to starting antimicrobial therapy. Antibiotics active against community-associate MRSA should be used in the treatment of skin and soft tissue infections determined to require antimicrobial treatment.

16. **Are there anatomic areas of significance in a patient with an abscess or cellulitis?**
Cellulitis of the midface, especially in the area of the orbits, must be treated aggressively. The venous drainage of these infections is through the cavernous sinus of the brain, with the potential for causing cavernous sinus thrombosis. In true orbital cellulitis, there must be aggressive intravenous (IV) antibiotic therapy. Often a CT scan is performed to detect abscess formation. *H. influenzae* cellulitis usually occurs in children, resulting in high fevers, high WBC counts, and bacteremia. Perirectal or perianal abscesses that are large or extend into the supralevator or ischiorectal space often need intraoperative management, removing not only the abscess but also the fistulas that are often associated with it. Deep space abscesses of the groin

and head and neck region often must be drained in the operating room because of their proximity to major neurovascular structures.

17. **Are antibiotics always indicated for cellulitis or abscesses?**

The treatment for most abscesses is incision and drainage, and neither antibiotics nor cultures are indicated in patients with normal host defenses as long as the abscess is localized. For abscesses associated with immunocompromised or progressing cellulitis, MRSA, and for abscesses that may be penetrating into deeper soft tissues, incision and drainage, antibiotic therapy, culture, and Gram stain constitute a reasonable initial approach. The choice of antibiotics depends on the anatomic location and the most likely cause of the infection (Table 47-1).

TABLE 47-1. ORAL THERAPY FOR SUPERFICIAL SOFT TISSUE INFECTIONS	
Drug	**Dose**
Group A *Streptococcus*	
Penicillin V (phenoxymethylpenicillin)	250–500 mg q.i.d.
First-generation cephalosporin	250–500 mg q.i.d.
Erythromycin	250 mg-1 g q 6 h
Azithromycin	500 mg × 1 dose, then 250 mg qd × 4
Clarithromycin	500 mg b.i.d.
***Staphylococcus aureus* (not methicillin-resistant *S. aureus*)**	
Dicloxacillin	125–500 mg q.i.d.
Cloxacillin	250–500 mg q.i.d.
First-generation cephalosporin	250–500 mg q.i.d.
Erythromycin (variable effectiveness)	250–500 mg q.i.d.
Azithromycin	500 mg × 1 dose, then 250 mg qd × 4
Clarithromycin	500 mg b.i.d.
Clindamycin	150–450 mg q.i.d.
Amoxicillin-clavulanate	250–500 mg t.i.d.
Ciprofloxacin	500 mg b.i.d.
***Staphylococcus aureus* (community-associated methicillin-resistant) MRSA**	
Trimethoprim (TMP)-sulfamethoxazole (SMX)	160 mg TMP/800 mg SMX b.i.d.
Clindamycin	150–450 mg q.i.d.
Tetracycline	250–500 mg q.i.d.
Linezolid	600 mg b.i.d.
Haemophilus influenzae	
Amoxicillin-clavulanate	250–500 mg t.i.d.
Cefaclor	250–500 mg t.i.d.
TMP-SMX	160 mg TMP/800 mg SMX b.i.d.
Azithromycin	500 mg × 1 dose, then 250 mg q.d. × 4
Clarithromycin	500 mg b.i.d.

b.i.d. = twice a day, q.d. = daily, q 8 h = every 8 hours, t.i.d. = three times a day.

18. **Describe appropriate follow-up care.**

Most patients with simple cellulitis and localized abscesses need to be seen only once or twice in the ED. The packing usually can be removed after 48–72 hours, and the patient can clean the abscess cavity by bathing or showering at home. It is important to ensure that the cellulitis is responding to therapy and, with abscesses, that all pus has been drained and evacuated. Further follow-up is indicated only when the processes are recurrent, when there is no response to therapy, or when the patient is immunocompromised.

19. **Who should be admitted to the hospital?**

Patients who appear septic, are immunocompromised, or are not responding to treatment; patients with soft tissue infections in certain anatomic sites, such as the central area of the face; and patients with infections that potentially may cause airway closure. Examples are sublingual and retropharyngeal abscesses and Ludwig's angina. Close attention must be paid to immunosuppressed patients, who may develop abscesses or cellulitis as secondary infections from gram-negative or anaerobic gas-forming organisms. Abscesses in the perineal area may spread quickly through the fascial planes, resulting in Fournier's gangrene.

20. **Is there an association between abscesses or cellulitis and systemic disease?**

Patients who are immunocompromised or have peripheral vascular disease have a tendency to develop superficial soft tissue infections. Recurrent abscesses in the head and neck or groin regions may be associated with hidradenitis suppurativa, which is a disease of chronic suppurative abscesses of the apocrine sweat glands. Inflammatory bowel disease, diabetes, malignancies, and pregnancy have been associated with a higher incidence of perirectal abscesses. Recurrent abscesses in the perineal and lower abdominal area may signify the presence of associated inflammatory bowel disease. All patients with recurrent soft tissue infections, whether superficial or deep, should be evaluated for underlying systemic disease such as diabetes.

21. **What is the best advice overall for treating cellulitis and abscesses?**

Cellulitis usually responds to antibiotic therapy and immobilization. Cutaneous abscesses usually respond to adequate incision and drainage; antibiotics are not indicated. All soft tissue infections should be observed to ascertain that healing is occurring. Selection of antibiotics, when indicated, is guided by the location and cause of the infection.

22. **What is necrotizing fasciitis?**

A life-threatening and limb-threatening bacterial infection of the fascia often extending to the skin and subcutaneous tissue. Multiple bacteria are usually involved. The most common are gram-positive cocci (*Streptococcus* and *Staphylococcus*), gram-negative organisms (*Enterococcus, Proteus,* and *Pseudomonas*), and anaerobes (*Clostridium, Escherichia coli, Bacteroides fragilis*). Bacteria usually enter the subcutaneous tissue through a break in the skin, often caused by minor or trivial trauma. Blood-borne and postoperative infection may lead to necrotizing fasciitis.

23. **How is necrotizing fasciitis diagnosed?**

The diagnosis should be considered in any patient with a soft tissue infection, who has pain and tenderness out of proportion to the visible degree of cellulitis. It also should be considered in patients without any skin changes who have exquisite muscle tenderness with no obvious reason, such as a history of musculoskeletal trauma. Some patients may have subcutaneous emphysema. Most develop sepsis late in the course, and in severe cases disseminated intravascular coagulopathy develops. Any patient experiencing exquisite tenderness over or adjacent to an area of cellulitis should have a surgical consultation. A soft tissue radiograph may be helpful to visualize subcutaneous emphysema. CT and magnetic resonance imaging (MRI) are helpful when this diagnosis is suspected. Later in the course, the skin may reveal bullous lesions.

KEY POINTS: NECROTIZING FASCIITIS

1. Pain and tenderness are out of proportion to the visible degree of cellulitis.

2. Subcutaneous emphysema may be present.

3. This is a disease requiring early surgical consultation.

24. Why should I get a surgical consultation?

Necrotizing fasciitis is a disease that must be treated with extensive incision, drainage, and debridement of necrotic tissue. Additional therapy includes IV antibiotics and in-hospital supportive care.

25. What is Fournier's gangrene?

A necrotizing subcutaneous infection of the perineum occurring primarily in men, usually involving the penis and scrotum. It most commonly affects individuals who are immunologically compromised or diabetic. Typically, it begins as a benign infection or small abscess that quickly progresses and leads to end-artery thrombosis in subcutaneous tissues. Ultimately, it leads to widespread necrosis of adjacent areas. Any patient complaining of lesions or pain in the aforementioned areas should be approached with this diagnosis in the differential.

26. List the most common (and concerning) organisms found in the following wounds and their accompanying cellulitis.

- **Cat bites:** *Pasteurella multocida* (80%), *Staphylococcus, Streptococcus*
- **Dog bites:** *Pasteurella, Enterobacter, Pseudomonas, Capnocytophaga canimo*rsus (rare, but 25% fatality in immunocompromised)
- **Human bites:** *Streptococcus, Staphylococcus, H. influenzae, Eikenella corrodens, Enterobacter, Proteus*
- **Open water wounds:** *Aeromonas hydrophila, Bacteroides fragilis, Chromobacterium, Mycobacterium marinum, Vibrio*

27. What question must be asked of all patients presenting with cellulitis or abscesses?

When was your last tetanus booster? Current recommendations suggest tetanus-diphtheria toxoid (Td), 0.5 mL IM × 1 if it has been more than 5 years since the previous booster.

BIBLIOGRAPHY

1. Brandt MM, Corpron CA, Wahl WL: Necrotizing soft tissue infections: A surgical disease. Am Surg 66:967–971, 2000.

2. Dong SL, Kelly KD, Oland RC, et al: ED management of cellulitis: A review of five urban centers. Am J Emerg Med 19:535–540, 2001.

3. Frazee BW, Lynn J, Charlebois ED, et al: High prevalence of methicillin-resistant *Staphylococcus aureus* in emergency department skin and soft tissue infections. Ann Emerg Med 45:311–320, 2005.

4. Fridkin SK, Hageman JC, Morrison M, et al: Methicillin-resistant *Staphylococcus aureus* disease in three communities. N Engl J Med 352:1436–1444, 2005.

5. Kilic A, Aksoy Y, Kilic L: Fournier's gangrene: Etiology, treatment, and complications. Ann Plast Surg 47:523–527, 2001.

6. Llera JL, Levy RC: Treatment of cutaneous abscess: A double-blind clinical study. Ann Emerg Med 14:15–19, 1985.

7. Meislin HW, Guisto JA: Soft-tissue infections. In Rosen P, Barkin RM (eds): Emergency Medicine: Concepts Clinical Practice, 5th ed. St. Louis, Mosby, 2002, pp 1944–1957.

8. Meislin HW, Lerner SA, Graves MH, et al: Cutaneous abscesses: Anaerobic and aerobic bacteriology and outpatient management. Ann Intern Med 87:145–149, 1977.

9. Meislin HW, McGehee MD, Rosen P: Management and microbiology of cutaneous abscesses. J Am Coll Emerg Physicians 7:186–191, 1978.

10. Mills AM, Chen EH: Are blood cultures necessary in adults with cellulitis? Ann Emerg Med 45:548–549, 2005.

11. Stevens DL: The flesh eating bacterium: What's next? J Infect Dis 179(Suppl 2):S366–374, 1999.

12. Stone DR, Gorbach SL: Necrotizing fasciitis: The changing spectrum. Dermatol Clin 15:213–220, 1997.

13. Struk DW, Munk PL, Lee MJ, et al: Imaging of soft tissue infections. Radiol Clin North Am 39:277–303, 2001.

CHAPTER 48

SEXUALLY TRANSMITTED DISEASES AND HUMAN IMMUNODEFICIENCY VIRUS (HIV) INFECTION

Catherine A. Marco, MD, and Kerry Broderick, MD

1. **What are the most common sexually transmitted diseases (STDs)?**
   The true incidence of most STDs is unknown because not all cases are reported. The Centers for Disease Control and Prevention (CDC) estimates that 19 million new STD infections occur annually in the United States, nearly half of them among persons aged 15–24 years.

   - **Chlamydia** is estimated to infect 3 million people annually and is a major health problem for young women because of the sequelae of infertility and ectopic pregnancy. In 2002, 834,555 cases were reported to the CDC.
   - The incidence of **gonorrhea** peaked at more than 1 million cases per year in the late 1970s. In 2002, 351,852 cases were reported to the CDC. The rate of gonococcal infections is highest among adolescent girls.
   - **Trichomoniasis** is the most common curable STD in young sexually active women. An estimated 7.4 million new cases occur each year.
   - Approximately 5.5 million annual cases of genital **human papillomavirus** (HPV) are found. More than 30 types of HPV can cause genital tract infection. Genital warts usually are caused by HPV type 6 or 11. Several types are associated with cervical dysplasia.
   - **Genital herpes** occurs in 1 in 5 adolescents and adults.
   - **Syphilis** is on the decline after an epidemic from 1986–1990. In 1996, 52,976 cases were reported, and in 2002, 32,000 cases were reported in the United States. The years 2001–2002 showed a 12.4% increase, and most of these were in males having sex with males (MSM). Syphilis is substantially more common in non-Hispanic blacks than in other ethnic groups.
   - Cases of **HIV**—the most deadly STD—continue to rise. Worldwide, it is estimated that approximately 40 million people are HIV infected, and more than 20 million have died of acquired immunodeficiency syndrome (AIDS). An estimated 850,000–950,000 persons in the United States are living with HIV, including 180,000–280,000 who do not know they are infected. It is estimated that more than 44,000 patients currently live with AIDS in the United States.

   Fleming P, Byers RH, Sweeney PA, et al: HIV prevalence in the United States, 2000. Abstract 11. Presented at the Ninth Conference on Retroviruses and Opportunistic Infections, Seattle, WA, Feb 24–28, 2002.
   Steinbrook R: The AIDS epidemic in 2004. N Engl J Med 352:115–117, 2004.
   www.niaid.nih.gov/factsheets/stdgon.htm

2. **How should I evaluate abnormal vaginal discharge?**
   The first thing to do is to take a complete **sexual history:**
   1. How many partners has she had in the last several months (men or women)?
   2. Has she used protective barriers such as condoms and dental dams with each episode?
   3. Ask about previous STDs.
   4. Obtain a pregnancy test to decide on method of treatment if needed.
      - The appearance of the discharge on **pelvic examination** is important. Always take a sample for wet preparation and potassium hydroxide.

- **Vulvovaginal candidiasis** (not an STD) causes a white, curdlike discharge that clings to vaginal walls. Hyphae are present on potassium hydroxide preparation. Recent antibiotic use is a risk factor for this, as are diabetes and HIV. Treatment is single-dose oral fluconazole or any of the topical imidazoles. Patients frequently treat themselves with an over-the-counter antiyeast product before their emergency department (ED) visit, unaware that the cause of the discharge is an infection other than a yeast infection.

- **Bacterial vaginosis** is not an STD but an alteration of the microbial ecosystem with overgrowth of *Gardnerella vaginalis* and other species. Diagnosis is made by noting clue cells on the wet preparation, and treatment is with metronidazole.

- ***Trichomonas*** vaginitis, the third common cause, is a true STD. It causes a green, frothy discharge, and the cervix may be erythematous and friable (strawberry cervix). Diagnosis is based on finding the motile trichomonads on wet preparation or in urine. Treatment is with metronidazole.

- A discharge with significant leukocytes that does not include yeast, clue cells, or *Trichomonas* may be due to **mucopurulent cervicitis** (MPC).

3. **A sexually active young man presents with dysuria. How likely is it that it resulted from a urinary tract infection?**

About as likely as getting gonorrhea from sitting on a toilet seat. Dysuria in young men almost always is due to urethritis from an STD. The urinalysis will be positive for leukocytes. The likely pathogens include gonorrhea, *Chlamydia, Ureaplasma, Trichomonas,* and herpes simplex virus (HSV). A purulent discharge most likely is caused by gonorrhea, whereas a mucoid discharge most likely is caused by infection with *Chlamydia*. The patient should be tested for both of these pathogens. *Chlamydia* also can infect the urethra of women, and they may present only with dysuria. Consider this diagnosis in a woman with dysuria and no bacteria on urinalysis, and do a pelvic examination.

4. **Are there any single-dose treatment regimens for uncomplicated chlamydial infections?**

Yes, a single 1-g dose of **azithromycin** is an effective treatment for lower tract chlamydial infections, including urethritis and cervicitis. Single-dose therapy is *not* appropriate for upper tract disease, such as epididymitis and pelvic inflammatory disease (PID) or in patients who have had a recent chlamydial infection and may be a failure. This simplified therapy should lead to more effective treatment in noncompliant patients.

www.cdc.gov/std/treatment

5. **Are there suitable oral alternatives to parenteral therapy for gonorrhea?**

Uncomplicated urethral, endocervical, or rectal gonorrheal infections can be treated adequately with a single intramuscular (IM) injection of ceftriaxone (125 mg) or an equivalent third-generation cephalosporin antibiotic. Alternative oral regimens include cefixime (400 mg), ciprofloxacin (500 mg), ofloxacin (400 mg), and levofloxacin (500 mg). Currently, quinolones can be used with confidence to treat most of these infections, but quinolone-resistant *Neisseria gonorrhoeae* (QRNG) is increasing in certain populations, forcing changes in recommended regimens. Azithromycin 2 g as a single oral dose may be used; however, expense and frequency of gastrointestinal (GI) intolerance have limited its use.

www.cdc.gov.std/treatment/Cefixime.htm

6. **What about QRNG?**

Cases of QRNG have been reported from many parts of the world and are becoming widespread in parts of Asia, Pacific Islands, and California. There is also a significant increase in QRNG in homosexual males: 4.9% versus 0.4% in heterosexual males. Ceftriaxone is recommended for treatment in these populations. *Because of possible concomitant chlamydial infections, these patients should be treated with an additional agent to address the* Chlamydia.

Centers for Disease Control and Prevention: Increases in fluoroquinolone-resistant *Neisseria gonorrhoeae* among men who have sex with men. MMWR 53:335–338, 2004.
www.cdc.gov/mmwr/preview/mmwrhtml/mm5316a1.htm

7. **What is the significance of finding MPC in a woman with lower abdominal pain?**
The normal endometrial secretion, as noted on exit from the endocervical canal, should be transparent. The presence of a mucopurulent secretion from the os, which may appear yellow when viewed on a white cotton-tipped swab (positive Q-Tip sign), suggests MPC. MPC, most commonly caused by gonorrhea or *Chlamydia,* is a precursor to upper genital tract infection. (See Chapter 79.)

Centers for Disease Control and Prevention: Sexually Transmitted Diseases Treatment Guidelines 2002. MMWR 51, 2002.

8. **How do I evaluate a sexually active young woman who presents with an acutely swollen, warm, painful right ankle?**
This patient, with acute monarticular arthritis, should be presumed to have a **disseminated gonococcal infection.** This is a syndrome of gonococcal bacteremia that leads to peripheral manifestations of disease, including dermatitis, tenosynovitis, and septic arthritis.
Arthrocentesis should be done on the involved joint, and the fluid should be sent for Gram stain, culture for gonococcus (GC) and regular aerobic cultures, and cell count. GC is cultured from less than 50% of joints. A pelvic examination must be done to culture the cervix for GC. Consider culturing the rectum and urethra. A patient suspected of having disseminated gonococcal infection should be admitted initially and treated with parenteral antibiotics (ceftriaxone, 25–50 mg/kg/day intravenous [IV] or IM in a single daily dose for 7 days).

Centers for Disease Control and Prevention: STD Treatment Guidelines 2002. MMWR 51:40, 2002.

9. **What are the most common causes of genital ulcers?**
Genital ulcers can represent infection with HSV, chancroid, or syphilis. It is difficult to make a diagnosis based solely on history and physical examination. Always ask about travel history and exposure to prostitutes. Genital ulcers are an important risk cofactor for HIV transmission.
- **HSV.** Genital herpes due to HSV is the most common cause of genital ulcers in the United States. Primary HSV infection results in severely ill patients who are toxic with fever, malaise, and inguinal adenopathy. Diagnosis is made by viral culture or antigen testing. HSV is a recurrent disease, and patients may shed the virus while they are asymptomatic. It cannot be cured, but treatment with antiviral agents can shorten the duration of symptoms. Long-term suppressive therapy can prevent outbreaks of ulcers.
- **Chancroid.** Also called *soft sore,* this disease is caused by *Haemophilus ducreyi,* a bacterium that is difficult to culture. Clinically, this syndrome causes a painful nonindurated papule that erodes into an ulcer. Painful inguinal adenopathy is found in more than 50% of cases. Treatment options include single-dose azithromycin or ceftriaxone or 3 days of ciprofloxacin or 1 week of erythromycin.
- **Syphilis.** Primary syphilis presents with a painless indurated ulcer called a *chancre.* Diagnosis is best made by dark-field examination for spirochetes, although this is usually available only in public health laboratories. A Venereal Disease Research Laboratory (VDRL) test should be done on anyone with possible syphilis. Treatment for primary syphilis is penicillin G benzathine, 2.4 million U intramuscularly.

Centers for Disease Control and Prevention: Sexually Transmitted Diseases Treatment Guidelines 2002. MMWR 51, 2002.

10. **What is the Jarisch-Herxheimer reaction?**

After initiation of treatment for syphilis, onset of fever, chills, myalgias, headache, tachycardia, increased respirations, increased neutrophil count, and mild hypotension. This occurs approximately 2 hours after initiation of treatment with peak temperatures at approximately 7 hours, with defervescence at 12–24 hours. This reaction occurs in 50% of primary syphilis, 90% of secondary syphilis, and 25% of early latent syphilis patients. In secondary syphilis patients, the mucocutaneous lesions may become more edematous and erythematous.

11. **Proctitis is a problem primarily seen in men who have sex with men. Discuss the approach and treatment.**

Any individual, male or female, with the onset of acute proctitis symptoms (rectal pain, discharge, tenesmus), who recently has had unprotected, receptive anal intercourse, is at risk for an STD-related problem. These patients should be examined by anoscopy and should be tested for gonorrhea, *Chlamydia,* and HSV. All patients should have serologic testing for syphilis. These patients should have empirical treatment for gonorrhea and *Chlamydia*. If ulcers are apparent on anoscopy, consider empirical antiviral therapy with acyclovir.

12. **Do I need to report STD cases to the health department?**

Yes. Accurate reporting of STDs is essential to national and local STD control efforts. HIV, gonorrhea, and syphilis are reportable infections in every state. Chlamydial infection is reportable in most states. It is the responsibility of each clinician to know his or her local reporting requirements. If you are unsure of what to report about a specific patient, contact your local health department.

13. **What are the important points to address in the discharge instructions for STD patients?**

1. Education about STDs is the responsibility of every ED physician because you may be the only contact the patient has with the medical system.
2. Instruct patients to refer *all* their sexual partners for evaluation and treatment. Some physicians in the United States routinely provide additional antibiotic prescriptions for sexual partners. Although it is well intentioned, it is controversial to provide a prescription for a person you have not interviewed or examined. That person may be allergic to the medication or may have additional infections that you are not treating.
3. All patients should be instructed to avoid sexual contact with their partners until all parties have finished treatment. Because it is unrealistic to expect all patients to follow this advice, explain the importance of using condoms with every sexual contact to avoid further infections and to prevent infection with HIV.

14. **What is the significance of AIDS in the ED?**

Disease caused by HIV infection, ranging from asymptomatic infection to AIDS, with serious, possibly life-threatening complications, is encountered commonly in the ED. Seroprevalence among ED patients varies greatly, depending on the location and type of hospital. Among inner-city ED patients, seroprevalence ranges from 4.2–8.9%. Knowledge of HIV infection and related disease is essential to diagnose and treat disease and to ensure adequate protection of health care workers.

15. **How is the diagnosis of AIDS made?**

AIDS is diagnosed by laboratory evidence of HIV infection and the presence of one of the indicator diseases, some of which are listed in Table 48-1. HIV infection should be suspected in all patients with known risk factors or with presenting symptoms suggestive of opportunistic infection. Questioning the patient directly about risk factors may be crucial to diagnosing HIV-related disease. High-risk behaviors commonly associated with HIV infection include unprotected sexual intercourse, unprotected penetrative sex between men, injection

TABLE 48-1.   AIDS-DEFINING CONDITIONS

Laboratory evidence of HIV infection plus any of the following:

Esophageal candidiasis	Brain lymphoma	HIV wasting syndrome
Cryptococcosis	*Mycobacterium avium* complex	Disseminated histoplasmosis
Cryptosporidiosis	*Pneumocystis carinii* pneumonia	Isosporiasis
Cytomegalovirus	Progressive multifocal	Disseminated *Mycobacterium* retinitis leukoencephalopathy *tuberculosis* disease
Herpes simplex virus	Brain toxoplasmosis	Recurrent *Salmonella* septicemia
Kaposi's sarcoma	HIV encephalopathy	CD4 lymphocyte count $< 200/mL$
Pulmonary tuberculosis	Invasive cervical cancer	

HIV = human immunodeficiency virus.

drug use, a history of receiving a blood transfusion before 1985, and maternal–neonatal transmission.

16. **Should EDs test for HIV?**
Testing for HIV has not been traditionally performed in the ED because of difficulty in maintaining confidentiality and ensuring appropriate reporting and counseling. Recently, several studies have demonstrated feasibility and acceptability of HIV testing in EDs. Several rapid tests are available, including single-use diagnostic system (SUDS), OraQuick, Uni-Gold, Reveal, and Determine. Positive rapid tests may be confirmed in outpatient testing by enzyme-linked immunoassay (EIA) and Western blot (WB). Regardless of whether HIV testing is performed in the ED, outpatient referral for high-risk patients is appropriate.

Kendrick SR, Kroc KA, Couture E, et al: Comparison of point-of-care rapid HIV testing in three clinical venues. AIDS 18:2208–2210, 2004.

Rothman RE, Ketlogetswe KS, Dolan T, et al: Preventive care in the emergency department: Should emergency departments conduct routine HIV screening? A systematic review. Acad Emerg Med 10:278–285, 2003.

Rothman RE: Current Centers for Disease Control and Prevention guidelines for HIV counseling, testing, and referral: Critical role of an a call to action for emergency physicians. Ann Emerg Med 44:21–42, 2004.

www.cdc.gov/hiv/ctr

17. **How do patients with HIV infection present to the ED?**
Patients may present with involvement of virtually any organ system. HIV infection should be suspected in any patient who presents with abnormally severe symptoms of a common disease or with symptoms of opportunistic infection or other debilitating HIV-related disease, such as AIDS wasting syndrome or AIDS dementia. Among AIDS patients, systemic infection or malignancy always must be considered and may present with malaise, anorexia, fever, weight loss, GI complaints, or other symptoms. Because of the wide spectrum of disease related to HIV infection, many specific diagnoses cannot be made definitively in the ED; treatment focuses on recognition of disease, institution of initial therapy, and admission or outpatient follow-up.

18. **What tests should be done for the HIV-positive patient with systemic symptoms?**

In addition to a complete history and physical examination, appropriate laboratory investigations may include electrolytes, complete blood count, blood cultures (aerobic, anaerobic, and fungal), urinalysis and culture, liver function tests, chest radiography, serologic testing for syphilis, blood tests for cryptococcal antigen, and *Toxoplasma* and *Coccidioides* serologies. Lumbar puncture also may be appropriate if no other source of fever is identified.

19. **Explain the significance of fever in these patients.**

Fever may indicate bacterial, fungal, viral, or protozoal infection. The most common causes of fever include HIV-related fever, systemic infections such as *Mycobacterium avium* complex, cytomegalovirus, Hodgkin's disease, and non-Hodgkin's lymphoma.

Many HIV-infected patients with fever may be managed as outpatients. Outpatient management may be attempted if the source of the fever does not dictate admission, if appropriate laboratory studies have been initiated, if the patient is able to function adequately at home (able to ambulate and tolerate oral intake), and if appropriate medical follow-up can be arranged.

20. **What are the common neurologic complications of AIDS?**

The most common acute symptoms are altered mental status, seizures, headache, and meningismus. ED evaluation should include a complete neurologic examination and, when appropriate, computed tomography (CT) or magnetic resonance imaging (MRI) and lumbar puncture. Specific cerebrospinal fluid studies that may be of value include cell count, glucose, protein, Gram stain, India ink capsule stain, bacterial culture, viral culture, fungal culture, *Toxoplasma* and cryptococcal antigen, and coccidioidomycosis titer. The most common causes of neurologic symptoms include *Toxoplasma gondii*, HIV encephalopathy, *Cryptococcus neoformans*, and central nervous system (CNS) lymphoma.

21. **What is HIV encephalopathy?**

Also referred to as "AIDS dementia," it is an organic brain syndrome manifested by decline in attention, cognitive reasoning, speech, motor function, and motivation. HIV encephalopathy is the most common neurologic problem and affects 33–60% of patients. It may be the presenting sign of overt AIDS in 25% of patients. Other causes of dementia and altered mental status must be ruled out.

22. **What are the pulmonary complications of HIV infection? How are they managed?**

Common presenting pulmonary complaints are cough, hemoptysis, shortness of breath, and chest pain. After history and lung examination, arterial blood gases, chest radiography, sputum culture, Gram stain, acid-fast stain, and blood cultures should be obtained if clinically indicated. The most common pulmonary complication is *Pneumocystis* pneumonia, which occurs in 70–80% of seropositive patients and typically presents with dyspnea, nonproductive cough, fever, and weight loss. Rapid institution of therapy with trimethoprim-sulfamethoxazole (TMP-SMX) (weight-based dosing), steroids, dapsone, or pentamidine may prevent excessive morbidity and mortality. Other causes include *Mycobacterium tuberculosis* pneumonia, *Histoplasma capsulatum*, and neoplasm.

ED management includes supplemental oxygen, volume repletion if indicated, and, when appropriate, antibiotic therapy. Admission should be considered for patients with new-onset pulmonary symptoms or patients with a significant deterioration in respiratory status.

Patients with *Pneumocystis* pneumonia should be treated with TMP-SMX, 15–20 mg/kg/day in divided doses. Alternate treatments may be used with primaquine plus clindamycin, or atovaquone, or pentamidine. Patients with hypoxia ($pO_2 < 70$) or a large Aa gradient (>35) should also be treated with corticosteroids (such as oral prednisone 40 mg daily).

Thomas CF, Limper AH: Pneumocystis pneumonia. N Engl J Med 350:2478–2498, 2004.

23. **How should GI complaints be managed?**

Approximately 50% of AIDS patients present with GI complaints at some time during their illness. Esophageal complaints are common and may be most commonly caused by *Candida* esophagitis or herpes simplex esophagitis. Patients with esophagitis should receive a 2-week empiric course of oral antifungal agents, followed by endoscopy if not successfully treated. The most common presenting symptoms are abdominal pain, bleeding, and diarrhea. Diarrhea is the most common GI complaint and is estimated to occur in 50–90% of AIDS patients. Helpful laboratory studies include microscopic examination of stool for leukocytes, acid-fast stain, examination for ova and parasites, and bacterial culture of stool and blood. *Cryptosporidium* and *Isospora* infections in particular are common causes and are associated with prolonged watery diarrhea. Other common infectious agents include *Candida*, Kaposi's sarcoma, *Mycobacterium avium* complex, HSV, cytomegalovirus, *Campylobacter jejuni*, *Entamoeba histolytica*, *Shigella*, *Salmonella*, *Giardia*, *Cryptosporidium*, and *Isospora*. Management should be directed at repletion of fluid and electrolytes and appropriate antibiotic coverage.

Bonacini M: Medical management of benign oesophageal disease in patients with human immunodeficiency virus infection. Dig Liver Dis 33:294, 2001.

24. **What are the common cutaneous presentations of AIDS and how are they treated?**

Kaposi's sarcoma is the most common unique cutaneous manifestation of AIDS. It usually is widely disseminated and may involve mucous membranes. Exacerbation of underlying dermatologic conditions is common in the HIV-infected population. Complaints such as xerosis (dry skin) and pruritus are common and may be manifested before development of opportunistic infections. Xerosis may be treated with emollients and, if necessary, with mild topical steroids. Pruritus may respond to oatmeal baths and, if necessary, antihistamines. Infections, including *Staphylococcus aureus* (presenting as bullous impetigo, ecthyma, or folliculitis), *Pseudomonas aeruginosa* (which may present with chronic ulcerations and macerations), herpes simplex, herpes zoster, syphilis, and scabies, are common and should be treated with standard therapies.

Other dermatologic conditions that occur with increased frequency in HIV-infected patients include seborrheic dermatitis, psoriasis, atopic dermatitis, and alopecia. Dermatologic consultation generally is indicated. Admission may be indicated for patients with any disseminated cutaneous infection requiring IV antibiotics or antiviral agents.

25. **Describe ophthalmologic emergencies that occur in AIDS patients.**

Eye complaints such as change in visual acuity, photophobia, redness, and pain are common and may represent retinitis or invasion of eye or periorbital tissues with a malignant or infectious process. Cytomegalovirus retinitis occurs in 30% of AIDS patients and accounts for most retinitis among AIDS patients. It has a characteristic appearance of fluffy white retinal lesions, often perivascular (sometimes referred to as "tomato and cheese pizza" appearance). Ophthalmology consultation is indicated, followed by treatment with foscarnet or ganciclovir for 2 weeks and long-term maintenance therapy.

Wei LL, Park SS, Skiest DJ: Prevalence of visual symptoms among patients with newly diagnosed cytomegalovirus retinitis. Retina 22:278, 2002.

26. **Should HIV-infected patients receive tetanus and other immunizations?**

According to the U.S. Public Health Service Immunizations Practices Advisory Committee, routine immunization recommendations for diphtheria (DPT); tetanus (Td); and measles, mumps, and rubella (MMR) are unchanged for HIV-infected patients. Smallpox and polio vaccines are not recommended in the HIV-infected population.

27. **How should symptoms of side effects from drugs be managed?**
Reactions to pharmacologic therapy are common in HIV-infected patients and always must be considered as the cause of new symptoms. In one study, 30% of hospitalized patients with HIV disease had an identified probable or definite adverse drug reaction. The most common type of reaction was cutaneous. Certain commonly used pharmaceutical agents cause a particularly high incidence of adverse drug reactions, including TMP-SMX, which has a 65% incidence of adverse drug reactions in AIDS patients, and pentamidine, which has a 50% incidence of adverse reactions. A decision about discontinuing therapy depends on balance between the benefit of the drug and the severity of side effects.

Harb GE, Alldredge BK, Coleman R, Jacobsen MA: Pharmacoepidemiology of adverse drug reactions in hospitalized patients with human immunodeficiency disease. J Acquir Immune Defic Syndr 6:919–926, 1993.

28. **Discuss common ethical problems associated with AIDS.**
Several important ethical considerations are HIV testing in patients and physicians, confidentiality, and resuscitation efforts. Routine testing for HIV is generally not indicated in the ED, and many EDs have adopted strict policies against HIV testing because of difficulties in ensuring adequate confidentiality and availability of counseling. One important exception to this general guideline may include source patients of needlestick injuries. This policy may change as the need for early identification and treatment of patients is shown. Initiation of counseling and referral for testing are recommended for patients at high risk.

Confidentiality regarding HIV-related diagnoses is paramount to providing appropriate patient care. Discretion when discussing the patient's diagnosis and condition with staff members and with the patient's family and friends helps to maintain confidentiality.

Resuscitation of patients with advanced AIDS is somewhat controversial. All appropriate resuscitative procedures should be performed unless advance directives mandate otherwise.

29. **How can health care providers protect themselves from acquiring HIV?**
Health care workers often are exposed to HIV-infected patients and their body fluids. Precautions in handling potentially infectious fluids are crucial. Because HIV infection is often undiagnosed at the time of the ED encounter, the use of universal precautions is strongly recommended, including the appropriate use of gown, gloves, mask, and goggles for procedures with all patients. The Needlestick Safety and Prevention Act of 2000 mandates that safety-engineered devices be used whenever possible and that institutions maintain exposure control plans. With the use of universal precautions, the risk of acquiring HIV infection by occupational exposure is extremely low.

30. **What constitutes high-risk exposure to HIV?**
- Substantial risk from **nonoccupational exposures** are those from an HIV-infected source with blood, semen, vaginal or rectal secretions, breast milk, or any body fluids with visible blood, through the vagina, rectum, eye, mouth, or other mucous membrane, nonintact skin, or percutaneous contact.
- For **occupational exposures**, higher-risk percutaneous exposures associated with an increased likelihood of transmission include deep injuries, visible blood on a device, and injuries sustained when placing a catheter in a vein or artery. Percutaneous exposures that are superficial or involve solid needles are considered lower-risk exposures. High-risk sources are patients with symptomatic HIV, AIDS, acute seroconversion, or high viral load. Patients with asymptomatic HIV or viral load < 15,000 copies/mL are considered lower risk.

Moran GJ: Emergency department management of blood and body fluid exposures. Ann Emerg Med 35:47, 2000.

Smith DK, Grohskopf LA, Black RJ: US Department of Health and Human Services. Antiretroviral post-exposure prophylaxis after sexual, injection-drug use, or other nonoccupational exposure to HIV in the United States: Recommendations from the US Department of Health and Human Services. MMWR 54(RR-2):1–19, 2005.

31. **Should postexposure prophylaxis (PEP) be administered after exposure to blood and body fluids?**

   PEP should be considered following all occupational and nonoccupational exposures. Decisions to treat should be based on the type of exposure, the risk of HIV in the source patient, and careful consideration of the risks and benefits of therapy. PEP is most effective if administered within 30 minutes of the exposure. PEP may consist of a basic regimen (such as zidovudine plus lamivudine) or an expanded regimen for high-risk exposures (such as zidovudine, lamivudine plus either indinavir or nelfinavir). Ideally, each health care institution should have written protocols that are formulated in consultation with occupational medicine and infectious disease specialists for occupational exposures in health care workers and patients with nonoccupational exposures.

   Smith DK, Grohskopf LA, Black RJ: US Department of Health and Human Services. Antiretroviral postexposure prophylaxis after sexual, injection-drug use, or other nonoccupational exposure to HIV in the United States: Recommendations from the US Department of Health and Human Services. MMWR 54(RR-2):1–19, 2005.
   CDC National AIDS Hotline: 1-800-342-2437.
   www.ucsf.edu/hivcntr/PEPline/index.html (or 1-888-448-4911)

32. **What is HAART?**

   Highly active antiretroviral therapy (HAART) is recommended for HIV-infected patients with CD4 counts less than 200/mm or those with symptomatic disease. The use of HAART has led to significant reductions in morbidity and mortality. HAART should be prescribed by infectious disease specialists and typically includes agents such as nonnucleoside reverse transcriptase inhibitors (NNRTIs), such as efavirenz, nucleotide reverse transcriptase inhibitors (NRTIs), such as zidovudine or lamivudine, and protease inhibitors, such as lopinavir or ritonavir. Adverse reactions to HAART are common and may include bone marrow suppression, cutaneous reactions, GI distress, jaundice, nephrolithiasis, abnormal lipid profiles, neuropathy, and others.

   Carpenter CC, Cooper DA, Fischl MA et al: Antiretroviral therapy in adults: Updated recommendations of the International AIDS Society—USA Panel. JAMA 283:381, 2000.
   Palacio H, Li X, Wilson TE, et al: Healthcare use by varied highly active antiretroviral therapy (HAART) strata: HAART use, discontinuation, and naivety. AIDS 18:621–630, 2004.
   Yeni PG, Hammer SM, Hirsch MS, et al: Treatment for adult HIV infection: 2004 recommendations of the International AIDS Society—USA Panel. JAMA 292:251–265, 2004.

KEY POINTS: SEXUALLY TRANSMITTED DISEASES

1. STDs affect 19 million people a year in the United States.

2. Single-dose therapy for *Chlamydia* and GC is very effective for treatment of uncomplicated cervicitis and urethritis.

3. The most common causes of genital ulcers include herpes simplex, chancroid (*Haemophilus ducreyi*), syphilis, and HPV.

4. Patients with suspected *Pneumocystis* pneumonia should be treated with trimethoprim-sulfamethoxazole (weight-based) and corticosteroids (if hypoxic).

5. All patients with high-risk HIV exposure should be considered for postexposure prophylaxis therapy.

CHAPTER 49

TOXIC SHOCK SYNDROME

Bruce Evans, MD, and Gayle Braunholtz, MD

1. What is toxic shock syndrome (TSS)?

TSS describes the constellation of symptoms associated with an exotoxin-mediated immune response to infection. In 1978, Todd et al. reported seven pediatric cases (ages 8–17) in which high fever, headache, confusion, conjunctival hyperemia, and gastrointestinal symptoms were accompanied by a scarlatiniform rash and severe shock. *Staphylococcus aureus* related to phage group 1 was isolated from infected or mucosal sites in these cases, prompting fears that the bacterium was expressing a newly discovered toxin.

> Todd J, Fishaut M, Kapral F, et al: Toxic-shock syndrome associated with phage-group 1 staphylococci. Lancet 2:1116–1118, 1978.

2. Why did a bacterium begin to express a new and deadly exotoxin in the late 1970s?

Todd's report led to additional associations between TSS and *S. aureus*. In retrospect, the syndrome may had been described as early as 1927. Some researchers believe that the syndrome may have been responsible for the plague that ended the Golden Age of Athens.

KEY POINTS: RISK FACTORS FOR TOXIC SHOCK SYNDROME

1. Air-containing foreign bodies (tampon, nasal packing)

2. Recent surgery

3. Postpartum

4. Burns

5. Focal infections

---

3. Who gets TSS?

Menses were associated with 91% of cases reported by 1980, which quickly pointed to the use of new high-absorbency tampons as a risk factor. Such tampons, made with cross-linked carboxymethylcellulose and polyester foam, were thought to provide an ideal environment for the expression of TSS toxin and subsequently were removed from the market.

> Wright SW, Trott AT: Toxic shock syndrome: A review. Ann Emerg Med 17:268–273, 1988.

4. Is tampon use required for the patient to develop TSS?

No. Three of the patients identified in the 1978 report were male. Although the media focused on the association with high-absorbency tampons, clinical interest in the syndrome identified a wide variety of causes in the early 1980s. TSS has been reported in all age groups, in burn and postsurgical patients, after childbirth, and in association with the nasal packing commonly used to control epistaxis.

5. **Describe the pathophysiology of TSS.**
Three stages have been identified in the progression of the syndrome: (1) the local proliferation of toxin-producing bacteria, such as the site of a foreign body; (2) the toxin production, which is thought to require an aerobic environment; and (3) the immune response to the toxin, which sets off the inflammatory cascade and leads to multisystem organ involvement. Air-containing foreign bodies seem to be a common risk factor.

E-medicine: COM/EMERG/topic600.htm

6. **There was heavy media coverage of TSS in the early 1980s because of the high case fatality rate. Has mortality been reduced?**
The initial fatality rate was 13% for the first 55 cases, with white females in the 15- to 19-year-old range thought to be at greatest risk. By 1984, 27% of reported cases were not associated with menses. Nonmenstrual TSS now accounts for about half of all cases. Reanalysis of early cases suggests that significant reporting bias was a factor in the high fatality rate, which is now stable at less than 3%. Also, TSS now may be recognized and treated before the patient becomes ill enough to meet the criteria that define the syndrome.

Hajjeh R, Reingold A, Weil A, et al: Toxic shock syndrome in the United States: Surveillance and update. Emerging Infect Dis J 5:807, 1999.
Wright SW, Trott AT: Toxic shock syndrome: A review. Ann Emerg Med 17:268–273, 1988.
Centers for Disease Control and Prevention: cdc.gov

KEY POINTS: COMMON CHARACTERISTICS OF TOXIC SHOCK SYNDROME ✓

1. Fever

2. Rash

3. Hypotension

4. Diarrhea

5. History of air-containing foreign body, abscess, or recent surgery or childbirth

7. **List the criteria for defining a case of TSS.**
   1. Fever $= 38.9°C$
   2. Diffuse macular erythematous rash
   3. Desquamation, usually of the palms or soles, after 1–2 weeks
   4. Orthostasis or hypotension (with systolic blood pressure < 90 mmHg in adults or less than the sixth percentile in children)
   5. Involvement of three or more of the following organ systems:
      - Gastrointestinal: Vomiting or diarrhea
      - Muscular: Myalgias or elevated creatine phosphokinase (twice normal)
      - Mucous membrane: Vaginal, oropharyngeal, or conjunctival hyperemia
      - Renal: Elevated blood urea nitrogen or creatinine (twice normal) or pyuria in the absence of urinary tract infection
      - Hepatic: Total bilirubin, alanine aminotransferase, aspartate aminotransferase at least twice the upper limit of normal

- Hematologic: Platelets $< 100,000/mm^3$
- Central nervous system: Disorientation or alteration in consciousness without focal neurologic signs (when fever and hypotension are absent)
6. Negative results of the following, if obtained:
   - Blood, throat, or cerebrospinal fluid cultures (blood cultures may be positive for *S. aureus*)
   - Rise in titer to Rocky Mountain spotted fever, leptospirosis, or rubeola

Centers for Disease Control and Prevention: Case definitions for public health surveillance MMWR 39 (RR-13):1, 1990.

8. Describe the rash associated with TSS.

The rash is a macular erythroderma that blanches and is not pruritic. It may be diffuse or localized and often is described as sunburn-like. It appears early in the illness and fades in about 3 days. It may be subtle and can be missed in dark-skinned patients.

Davis JP, Chesney PJ, Wand PJ, et al: Toxic-shock syndrome. N Engl J Med 303:1429–1435, 1980.

9. When is desquamation likely to occur?

Loss of skin, usually of the distal extremities, invariably occurs in survivors 5–12 days after the illness starts. Delayed alopecia and fingernail loss may occur later and seem to depend on the level of hypotension during the acute illness.

10. Given the previously mentioned criteria, list the differential diagnosis.

- Kawasaki disease
- Staphylococcal scalded skin syndrome
- Streptococcal scarlet fever
- Rocky Mountain spotted fever
- Leptospirosis
- Stevens-Johnson syndrome
- Erythema multiforme
- Toxic epidermal necrolysis
- Sepsis
- Colorado tick fever

11. What is streptococcal TSS?

Group A streptococcus (*Streptococcus pyogenes*) can cause a severe systemic reaction similar to TSS. The toxin is similar to that of TSS. Diagnosis requires the isolation of group A streptococci from a sterile or nonsterile site, hypotension, and multisystem organ involvement (at least two or more of the following: renal impairment, coagulopathy causing disseminated intravascular coagulopathy or thrombocytopenia, hepatitis, adult respiratory distress syndrome, necrotizing soft tissue infections, or skin changes similar to those seen in TSS).

Hoge CW, Schwartz B, Talkington DF, et al: The changing epidemiology of invasive group A streptococcal infections and the emergence of streptococcal toxic shock-like yndrome. JAMA 269:384–389, 1993.

Working Group on Severe Streptococcal Infections: Defining the group A streptococcal toxic shock syndrome: Rationale and consensus definition. JAMA 269:390–391, 1993.

12. Summarize the treatment for TSS.

- Supportive care including intravenous fluids for hypotension, with supplemental pressor support as needed
- Identification and removal of the source of infection (tampon, abscess, nasal packing)
- Antibiotics

13. Do antibiotics help?

No prospective studies show that antibiotics alter the severity of the course of TSS. Antibiotics reduce the recurrence rate (which can be 28%), however, and are considered standard care.

Wright SW, Trott AT: Toxic shock syndrome: A review. Ann Emerg Med 17:268–273, 1988.

14. What antibiotics should I use?

Penicillinase-resistant penicillins and **first-generation cephalosporins** are considered the antibiotics of choice. Vancomycin or clindamycin may be used in penicillin-allergic patients. Clindamycin has the added advantage of a direct antitoxin effect. High-dose penicillin is the treatment of choice for streptococcal TSS.

Russell NE, Pachorek RE: Clindamycin in the treatment of streptococcal and staphylococcal toxic shock syndromes. Ann Pharmacother 34:936–939, 2000.

15. Do steroids help control the immune response to the toxin?

Theoretically, steroids should help attenuate the systemic response to the toxin, but there are no prospective data to show they are effective. Steroid use in sepsis still is debated, and steroids are not routinely used in the management of TSS.

Spijkstra JJ, Girbes ARJ: The continuing story of corticosteroids in the treatment of septic shock. Intensive Care Med 26:496–500, 2000.

16. Do all patients with TSS need admission?

Patients in whom TSS is suspected should be admitted because this toxin-mediated disease can progress rapidly. In most patients, the systemic signs of illness (hypotension, fever, and multisystem organ involvement) are present in the emergency department (ED), clearly indicating the need for inpatient supportive care.

KEY POINTS: TREATMENT FOR TOXIC SHOCK SYNDROME

1. IV fluids with pressor support when needed

2. Removal of infectious source

3. Antibiotics

TETANUS, BOTULISM, AND FOOD POISONING

Kevin Dean, MD, and Scott Rudkin, MD, MBA

CHAPTER 50

TETANUS

1. **What is the causative agent of tetanus and its mechanism of action?**
   Tetanus is caused by *Clostridium tetani,* an obligate anaerobic bacteria, with two distinct toxins—tetanolysin and tetanospasmin. The former causes local destruction of viable tissue; the latter is primarily responsible for clinical tetanus. Tetanus enters peripheral nerves and travels in a retrograde fashion to the central nervous system (CNS), where it crosses to presynaptic neurons and disables inhibitory neurotransmitter release (γ-aminobutyric acid [GABA] and glycine). *C. tetani* spores are extremely resilient and can survive at extremes of temperature and humidity, including household disinfectants and boiling in water for several minutes.

2. **What are the forms of tetanus?**
   1. Generalized tetanus involves rigidity and spasm of all muscles in the body, usually starting cranially and proceeding caudally.
   2. Localized tetanus is seen with lower toxin loads and peripheral injuries; spasm and rigidity are limited to the injured body area.
   3. Cephalic tetanus occurs after a head wound and presents as cranial nerve paralysis (most commonly CN VII), and frequently proceeds to generalized tetanus.
   4. Tetanus neonatorum is the most common cause of tetanus worldwide and is caused by poor umbilical hygiene. It is rare in developed countries and is preventable by vaccination.

3. **How is tetanus contracted?**
   Tetanus generally originates from a wound that is grossly contaminated with soil, manure, or rusty metal. It can also develop from burns, ulcers, snakebites, middle ear infections, septic abortions, childbirth, surgery, and intramuscular injections. A prior episode of tetanus is not protective and does not confer lifelong immunity.

4. **What are the presentation and prognosis of neonatal tetanus?**
   Neonatal tetanus presents during the first week of life exclusively in infants of nonimmunized mothers. The bacteria enter through the umbilical cord stump, especially after the application of mud or feces, which is common practice in some developing countries. Symptoms begin as general irritability and poor feeding, which progress to generalized spasms, pneumonia, and pulmonary or CNS hemorrhage. Toxin load is high; mortality is 50–100%.

5. **What is the presentation of generalized tetanus?**
   Initial symptoms include trismus from masseter and parapharyngeal spasm. Patients complain of dysphagia and unilateral or bilateral neck pain. Muscle spasms proceed caudally to involve the paraspinous and abdominal wall muscles. Severe opisthotonos may occur with resultant vertebral fractures. Minor stimuli (light touch, drafts, noises) as well as pain and anxiety may trigger severe spasms. Death usually results from autonomic instability (labile hypertension, dysrhythmias, hyperpyrexia, tachycardia, and even myocardial infarction [MI]), which may present days after onset of symptoms.

6. **How do I treat generalized tetanus in the emergency department (ED)?**
   Initial management involves injection of tetanus immunoglobulin intramuscularly at the site of the wound. Current dosage recommendations vary from 500–6000 IU. This should precede surgical debridement of devitalized tissue to bind and prevent the release of preformed toxin. Penicillin G 4 million units intravenous (IV) q4h is the antibiotic of choice. However, morbidity may be lower with metronidazole 500 mg IV q6h, as penicillin acts as a GABA antagonist and may precipitate seizures. Penicillin-allergic patients may also be treated with doxycycline 100 mg IV every 12 hours. Other alternatives include erythromycin, tetracycline, chloramphenicol, vancomycin, and clindamycin. Cephalosporins do not reliably cover *C. tetani.*

7. **Where should I admit patients with tetanus?**
   Patients with tetanus should be admitted to an intensive care unit (ICU) setting, preferably one in which a dark and quiet environment can be maintained to minimize external stimuli.

8. **What is interval for tetanus vaccine?**
   A primary series is indicated for all patients who have not previously been immunized and consists of three doses, with the second dose given 4–8 weeks after the first, and the third dose given 6–12 months later. Individuals who have received a primary vaccine series should receive a booster every 10 years. More frequent boosters are not needed unless the recipient develops a tetanus-prone wound. In this case, a booster should be given if the last vaccination has been over 5 years prior. Wounds that have devitalized tissue, crush injuries, and contaminated wounds are considered tetanus-prone wounds. The Td formulation, which contains a lower dose of the diphtheria component, should be used in all individuals older than age 7. Consider giving tetanus immunoglobulin in addition to tetanus vaccine to those with grossly contaminated wounds who lack a primary vaccination series.

   Centers for Disease Control and Prevention: Diphtheria, Tetanus, and Pertussis: Recommendations for Vaccine Use and Other Preventive Measures. Atlanta, CDC, 1991.

9. **What is time course of tetanus?**
   The incubation period after exposure ranges from 1–60 days, with an average of 7–10 days. The first week of illness is characterized by muscle rigidity and spasm, followed in a few days by autonomic disturbances that last for 1–2 weeks. Muscle spasms generally subside after 2–3 weeks, but patients may experience persistent stiffness.

10. **What are the side effects of tetanus vaccine?**
    Side effects are generally limited to local reactions including erythema, induration, tenderness, nodule, or sterile abscess at the site of infection. Mild systemic reactions can occur and include fever, drowsiness, "fretfulness," and anorexia, but all are self-limited.

KEY POINTS: TETANUS

1. Tetanus vaccine is safe for pregnant and immunocompromised patients.
2. Patients with tetanus should be admitted to a dark and quiet ICU setting to minimize external stimuli.
3. Penicillin G is the antibiotic of choice.
4. High mortality rate is due to autonomic instability.

11. **Is tetanus vaccine safe for pregnant and immunocompromised patients?**
    Tetanus vaccine is a toxoid (inactivated toxin) and is safe and effective in pregnancy. Vaccination of at-risk pregnant women can help prevent neonatal tetanus. Likewise, it is safe for administration in immunocompromised patients.

BOTULISM

12. **What is the causative agent of botulism? How does it cause disease?**
    Botulism is caused by the toxin produced by *Clostridium botulinum*. This toxin binds to peripheral presynaptic cholinergic membranes, preventing the release of acetylcholine and producing a life-threatening, paralytic illness. Adrenergic synapses are unaffected. By weight, botulism toxin is the most potent toxin known.

13. **State the five ways a patient can contract botulism.**
    1. Adult botulism results from the ingestion of preformed toxin. Most cases are the result of undercooked home-canned food and occur in isolation or in small clusters. Classic adult botulism represents about 25% of the total botulism cases seen in the United States.
    2. Infant botulism is caused by the ingestion of *C. botulinum* spores, which proliferate in the gastrointestinal (GI) tract. It is usually seen between the ages of 2 weeks and 1 year, with a median age of 10 weeks. Although most commonly linked to contaminated raw honey, it has also been shown that changes in gut flora (such as weaning from breast milk) can increase susceptibility. Infant botulism represents about 72% of the total botulism cases seen in the United States.
    3. Wound botulism is caused by the contamination of traumatic wounds with *C. botulinum* spores found in soil. Although this has been reported in rare cases in surgical wounds, it is almost exclusively seen in injection heroin users.
    4. Hidden botulism is an idiopathic form, in which the patient's stool contains *C. botulinum* and the patient has signs and symptoms of clinical botulism, yet no contaminated food or wound can be identified.
    5. Inadvertent botulism is an iatrogenic complication of cosmetic or therapeutic Botox injections. Such patients may present with moderate to severe clinical weakness. This phenomenon has been seen even at Botox doses considered to be therapeutic. Focal neurologic deficits can be seen by craniofacial migration of injected toxin.

14. **What is the differential diagnosis of botulism?**
    Myasthenia gravis, Lambert-Eaton myasthenic syndrome, Guillain-Barré syndrome, tick paralysis, diphteritic neuropathy, and Miller-Fischer variant of Guillain-Barré syndrome.

15. **What is the treatment of classic (food) botulism?**
    Treatment is mostly supportive, including early elective intubation of patients at risk of respiratory failure. Type-specific equine-derived antitoxin is available but cannot reverse existing paralysis and may cause anaphylaxis.

16. **What is treatment for infant botulism?**
    Treatment of infant botulism is mostly supportive care, including intubation and mechanical ventilation if respiratory involvement. Human botulism immunoglobulin (Baby-BIG) is available and has been shown to reduce duration of hospitalization, mechanical ventilation, and tube feedings. Equine-derived antitoxin is immunogenic and is contraindicated in infant botulism.

17. **Are antibiotics indicated for infant botulism?**
No. In fact, aminoglycosides are absolutely contraindicated. They may potentiate neuromuscular blockade and increase duration of symptoms. Additionally, administration of antibiotics in general may cause bacterial lysis in the gut and theoretically increase the free toxin load.

18. **What is the presentation of infant botulism?**
Constipation is often the first presenting symptom. This can be followed by a weak cry, prolonged or poor feeding, hypotonia, and decreased gag or suck reflex. As in adults, infants can develop descending motor weakness, flaccid paralysis, and autonomic dysfunction. Unlike tetanus toxin, botulinum toxin acts peripherally and does not cross the blood–brain barrier, so fever is uncommon, and cerebrospinal fluid (CSF) analysis is normal.

19. **How does a patient with adult botulism present?**
Early symptoms are nonspecific and usually begin 12–36 hours (range, 6 hours to 8 days) after ingestion. These symptoms include nausea, vomiting, weakness, lassitude, and dizziness. The patient then develops anticholinergic symptoms, including extreme dry mouth unrelieved by fluids, decreased lacrimation, constipation, and urinary retention. Neurologic symptoms, which may be delayed 3 days after the appearance of anticholinergic symptoms, most often involve cranial nerves. The patient develops ocular and bulbar symptoms: diplopia, blurred vision, photophobia, dysphonia, and dysphagia. The patient also develops symmetric descending weakness of the extremities, which may progress to involve respiratory muscles.

KEY POINTS: BOTULISM

1. Adult botulism usually presents as nonspecific anticholinergic symptoms followed by symmetric descending paralysis.

2. Infant botulism usually presents as constipation followed by weak cry, prolonged or poor feeding, hypotonia, and decreased gag or suck reflex.

3. CSF analysis in botulism may be normal.

4. Human botulism immunoglobulin (Baby BIG) is available for infant botulism.

20. **Are antibiotics indicated in wound botulism?**
In addition to surgical debridement, antibiotics may be of use in wound botulism, but their use is unproved.

FOOD POISONING

21. **Name the causes of food poisoning.**
Food poisoning is caused by viruses (Norwalk, Calicivirus, Rotavirus), direct bacterial invasion or endotoxins (*Escherichia coli, Vibrio vulnificus, Vibrio parahaemolyticus, Campylobacter, Salmonella, Yersinia enterocolitica*), secreted exotoxins *(Staphylococcus aureus, Shigella,* shellfish-associated algal toxins), toxins innate in food (pufferfish tetrodotoxin, *Aminoides* mushrooms), and parasites (*Giardia lamblia, Entamoeba histolytica*).

22. **What is scombroid and how is it treated?**
Scombroid (histamine fish poisoning), is caused by bacterially contaminated fish, in which high levels of naturally occurring histidine are converted to histamine prior to ingestion. These fish

may have low levels of histamine when fresh, but levels rise as the conversion from histidine to histamine occurs; the fish usually has a normal appearance and odor even after becoming toxic. The disease is generally associated with high levels of histamine (>50 mg/100 g contaminated fish) and can mimic acute anaphylaxis, although it does not represent a fish "allergy." Fish from the scombroid families (e.g. tuna, mackerel, saury) are the most commonly affected fish, although it can also occur with nonscombroid fish, including mahi-mahi, sardines, pilchards, anchovies, herring, marlin, and bluefish. An urticarial rash of the face, neck, and upper chest is the most common presentation. However, symptoms may also include diarrhea, flushing, sweating, headache, nausea and vomiting, burning in the mouth, abdominal pain, dizziness, palpitations, swelling of the mouth and a metallic taste. Treatment with H1 and H2 antagonists is generally effective.

23. **Describe the toxic syndromes associated with ingestion of shellfish.**
    Algal toxins are produced by 40 species of marine algae that contaminate shellfish, crustaceans, and some fish. Clinical syndromes include the following:
    1. **Amnestic shellfish poisoning (ASP)** can present with nausea and vomiting, dizziness, headache, confusion, respiratory difficulty, and coma with loss of short-term memory that may be permanent. The causative agent is domoic acid, a preformed agent found primarily in infected scallops, mussels, and crab. Onset is within 24 hours of ingestion, and treatment is supportive
    2. **Diarrhetic shellfish poisoning (DSP)** is found in mussels, cockles, scallops, oysters, cockles, whelks, and green crabs. Symptoms are characterized by acute onset (within 30 minutes) of diarrhea, nausea, vomiting, and abdominal cramps. Recovery generally occurs within 3 days, and treatment is supportive.
    3. **Paralytic shellfish poisoning (PSP)** causes numbness and tingling around the lips that spreads to the face, head, and neck with onset of 15 minutes to 2 hours of eating affected mussels, clams, oysters, scallops, abalone, crabs, and lobster. Respiratory arrest and death from sodium channel blockade may occur within 24 hours.
    4. **Neurotoxic shellfish poisoning (NSP)** is commonly found in cockles, mussels, and whelks off the coast of Florida and the Gulf of Mexico. Symptoms include numbness of the mouth spreading to the extremities, followed by vomiting, abdominal pain, diarrhea, tachycardia, shortness of breath, and convulsions.
    5. **Ciguatera poisoning** occurs after the ingestion of corral reef fish. Patients have a sensory disorder in which touching cold water causes electric shocklike pain. Other symptoms include muscle pain, itching, vomiting, and diarrhea. Neurologic symptoms may persist for weeks or years following recovery from acute illness.

24. **Describe the clinical course and treatment for puffer fish poisoning.**
    Puffer fish poisoning results from the consumption of tetrodotoxin from the viscera and skin of improperly prepared puffer fish, commonly found in Japan, Singapore, Hong Kong, and Australia. Tetrodotoxin is a sodium channel blocker that acts on both the central and peripheral nervous systems (including autonomic nervous system), causing a rapid ascending paralysis, as well as having a direct effect on the respiratory and vasomotor centers in the medulla oblongata. Patients with severe poisoning may suffer respiratory failure, cardiovascular collapse, coma, and death within 4–6 hours. There is no specific antidote, and treatment is supportive.

25. **Which population of patients is at risk from eating raw oysters?**
    Patients with preexisting liver diseases, including cirrhosis and hemochromatosis, have an 80 times higher risk of invasive *Vibrio* disease and 200 times higher risk of mortality than those without liver disease. Consumption of raw oysters, especially from warmer waters between March and November, has a high incidence of *Vibrio vulnificus* and *Vibrio parahaemolyticus*.

26. **Describe the four stages of *Amanita phalloides* mushroom toxidrome.**
    - **Stage 1:** Latent stage: patient remains asymptomatic for 6–24 hours post-ingestion.
    - **Stage 2:** Acute onset of nausea, vomiting and diarrhea (often bloody), and severe abdominal pain lasting 12–24 hours. This stage may include acid-base disturbances, electrolyte abnormalities, hypoglycemia, dehydration, and even hypotension. Physical exam may be significant for epigastric tenderness and hepatomegaly with normal liver function tests.
    - **Stage 3:** The patient clinically appears to improve over the next 12–24 hours, although liver function tests begin to rise and renal function begins to deteriorate.
    - **Stage 4:** Beginning 2–4 days post-ingestion, the patient develops hepatic and renal failure, with marked rise in liver function tests, cardiomyopathy, hepatic encephalopathy, convulsions, coma, and death.

KEY POINTS: FOOD POISONING

1. *Amanita phalloides* toxic patients may appear to be improving before deteriorating rapidly.

2. Fluoroquinolones may be indicated in severe or bloody traveler's diarrhea.

3. Antibiotics are not recommended in children with bloody diarrhea.

4. Patients with liver disease are at highest risk for *Vibrio* disease from eating raw oysters.

27. **What is the usual time course and geographic distribution of traveler's diarrhea?**
    Destinations of highest risk are Latin America, Africa, the Middle East, and Asia (20–50% prevalence), with southern Europe, China, Russia, and the Caribbean being lower risk (up to 15%). Onset usually occurs on the third day after arrival, with a second episode starting about a week after arrival. However, it may occur anytime and up to 10 days after travel return. It is usually self-limiting with a mean duration of symptoms of 4 days; however, 10% of patients may have symptoms lasting more than 1 week, and 3% may have symptoms that persist more than 1 month. Approximately 20% of individuals afflicted with traveler's diarrhea will have symptoms of dysentery, including bloody stool and fever.

28. **What are some of the more serious complications of traveler's diarrhea? What are the causative agents?**
    - Reiter's syndrome (arthritis, urethritis, conjunctivitis): *Campylobacter jejuni, Salmonella, Shigella, Yersinia enterocolitica*
    - Guillain-Barré syndrome: *C. jejuni,* especially with HLA-B27
    - Hemolytic uremic syndrome (HUS): *Shigella dysenteriae* and enterohemorrhagic *E. coli*
    - Amebic hepatitis and amebic abscesses: *E. histolytica*
    - Bacteremia leading to endocarditis, aortitis, septic arthritis, osteomyelitis: *Salmonella*

29. **Is there any role for prophylaxis against traveler's diarrhea?**
    Patients at high risk for complications, including those with inflammatory bowel disease, insulin-dependent diabetes, heart disease, or immunosuppression, may benefit from prophylaxis. Fluoroquinolones have been shown to have > 90% efficacy in preventing traveler's diarrhea. Ciprofloxacin 500 mg orally (PO) can be started 2 days prior to arrival and taken 1 week after return, up to 3 weeks total. Patients who are otherwise healthy may wish to consider bismuth subsalicylate (Pepto-Bismol, taken as 524 mg four times a day [q.i.d.]) as a nonantibacterial option that has fewer side effects but lower efficacy (approximately 65%).

Increasing resistance to fluoroquinolones has been reported among strains of *C. jejuni* from areas of Southeast Asia (especially Thailand), which may limit their efficacy for travelers to this region. (See Fig. 50-1.)

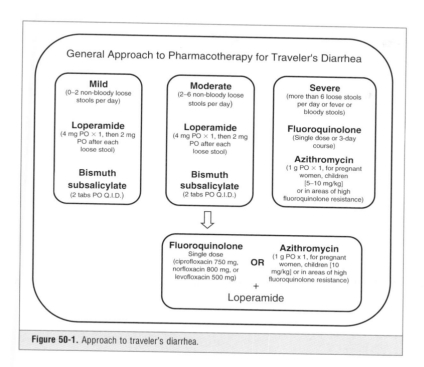

Figure 50-1. Approach to traveler's diarrhea.

30. Should antibiotics be used for bacterial diarrhea?

The use of antibiotics in acute diarrhea remains controversial. Short courses or single-dose regimens of broad-spectrum antibiotics (e.g., ciprofloxacin 750 mg, norfloxacin 800 mg, or levofloxacin 500 mg, as single doses) have been shown to reduce the frequency of stool by 50% and duration of illness to 12–24 hours. Azithromycin (1000 mg PO as a single dose, or weight-based equivalent) can be considered in pregnant women and children, for whom fluoroquinolones are contraindicated. In areas where amebiasis and giardiasis are prevalent, consider metronidazole 500 mg three times a day (t.i.d.) for 5 days. Antibiotic therapy is not generally recommended in children with bloody diarrhea because of the association with enterohemorrhagic *E. coli* (O157:H7) infections, in which antibiotics do not significantly improve outcome, and can promote the development of hemolytic uremic syndrome from increased lysis of organisms with release of endotoxin and Shiga-like toxin.

31. Which diarrhea-producing agent is associated with febrile seizures in children?

Shigella infections in young children can present with high fevers, generalized toxic appearance, abdominal cramps, bloody mucoid stool, and seizures with or without encephalopathy. Other complications include dehydration, hyponatremia, hypoglycemia, and surgical emergencies (e.g., toxic megacolon, rectal prolapse, intestinal perforation). Endemic *Shigella* is responsible for 75% of diarrhea-related deaths in developing countries.

BIBLIOGRAPHY

1. Adachi JA, Ostrosky-Zeichner L, DuPont HL, et al: Empirical antimicrobial therapy for traveler's diarrhea. Clin Infect Dis 31:1079–1083, 2000.
2. Ahasan HAMN, Mamun AA, Karim SR, et al: Paralytic complications of puffer fish (tetrodotoxin) poisoning. Sing Med J 45(2):73, 2004.
3. Ashkenazi S: Shigella infections in children: New insights. Semin Pediatr Infect Dis 15:246–252, 2004.
4. Berger K, Guss D: Mycotoxins revisited. J Emerg Med 28:1:53–62, 2005.
5. Brett M: Food poisoning associated with biotoxins in fish and shellfish. Curr Opin Infect Dis 16:461–465, 2003.
6. Brook I: Tetanus in children. Pediatr Emerg Care 20:48–53, 2004.
7. Casburn-Jones A, Farthing M: Traveler's diarrhea. J Gastroenterol Hepatol 19:610–618, 2004.
8. Cherington M: Botulism: Update and review. Semin Neurol 24:155–163, 2004.
9. Cook TM, Protheroe RT, Handel JM: Tetanus: A review of the literature. Br J Anesth 87:477–487, 2001.
10. Fox CK, Keet CA, Strober JB: Recent advances in infant botulism. Pediatr Neurol 32:149–154, 2005.
11. Gilbert D, et al: The Sanford Guide to Antimicrobial Therapy. Antimicrobial Therapy, Inc.: New York, 2004, pp 43.
12. Goonetilleke A, Harris J: Clostridial neurotoxins. J Neurol Neurosurg Psychiatry 75:35–39, 2004.
13. Hsu SS, Groleau G: Tetanus in the emergency department: A current review. J Emerg Med 20:357–365, 2001.
14. Isbister G, Kiernan M: Neurotoxic marine poisoning. Lancet Neurol 4:219–228, 2005.
15. Lehane L, Olley J: Histamine fish poisoning revisited. Int J Food Microbiol 58:1–37, 2000.
16. Long S: Infant botulism. Concise Rev Pediatr Infect Dis July:707–710, 2001.
17. Niyogi S: Shigellosis. J Microbiol 43:133–143, 2005.
18. Oldfield E: Emerging foodborne pathogens: Keeping your patients and your families safe. Rev Gastroenterol Disord 1(4):177–186, 2001.
19. Sheffield J, Ramin S: Tetanus in pregnancy. Am J Perinatol 21:173–182, 2004.

MOSQUITO- AND TICK–BORNE DISEASES OF NORTH AMERICA

CHAPTER 51

Andrew M. Kestler, MD, MBA

1. Why should I read this chapter?

Mosquitoes are the most important disease vectors worldwide, and ticks are the most important arthropod vectors in North America. West Nile virus and the Lyme disease spirochete are now common endemic pathogens within the continental United States and Canada. In the case of rarer diseases, such as Rocky Mountain spotted fever (RMSF) and tularemia, early recognition and treatment can be life saving. Other diseases, such as dengue fever and malaria, frequently occur in travelers returning from the tropics as well as in recent immigrants who present to emergency departments (EDs) across North America.

2. What are the most important tools in diagnosing these vector-borne diseases?

A detailed history and a skin exam. Many of these illnesses initially present with a nonspecific syndrome of fever, headache, and myalgia. A history of travel, exposure to the vector, or a characteristic rash can provide the key to a difficult diagnosis.

3. Does malaria occur in North America?

Most definitely. The Centers for Disease Control (CDC) was established in Atlanta in 1946 for the specific purpose of controlling malaria in the southeastern United States. Malaria remains endemic in the Caribbean and parts of Mexico. The CDC registered 1402 cases of malaria in the United States for 2003. *Anopheles* mosquito species, the night-biting vector of malaria, are widely found across North America and have recently caused domestic transmission within the United States from one household member to another.

Centers for Disease Control and Prevention: www.cdc.gov/malaria/

4. What causes malaria?

There are four species of the protozoan *Plasmodium*: *Plasmodium falciparum*, *Plasmodium vivax*, *Plasmodium ovale*, and *Plasmodium malariae*. Malaria is usually acquired by the bite of an infected female *Anopheles*, but it also may be transmitted by transfusion of infected blood or from mother to child in utero. *P. falciparum*, the most common and the most life-threatening type of infection, causes virtually all of the 1 million annual malaria deaths worldwide.

Greenwood B, Bojang K, Whitty C, Targett G: Malaria. Lancet 365:1487–1498, 2005.

5. Can malaria be prevented?

Although no one method of protection is 100% effective, proper use of prophylactic medication, bednets, insect repellent, and proper patient education would prevent most cases of traveler's malaria seen in the United States. Travelers should contact a local travel clinic and the CDC Web site when planning a visit to tropical regions or to determine if malaria is endemic in their destination.

Centers for Disease Control and Prevention: www.cdc.gov/malaria

6. Describe the clinical presentation of malaria.

Symptoms develop 10–14 days after *P. falciparum* infection but may be latent for 1 year with *P. vivax*. Patients complain of flulike symptoms, with fever, chills, headache, nausea, vomiting, abdominal pain, cough, and myalgias. Physical examination may reveal jaundice, hepatomegaly, and splenomegaly but is often normal. The presence of significant lymphadenopathy suggests another diagnosis or a co-infection. Anemia, thrombocytopenia, and hemoglobinuria are common laboratory findings. Patients may develop renal failure, pulmonary edema, shock, disseminated intravascular coagulation, profound anemia, acidosis, and hypoglycemia. Cerebral malaria, the most common fatal manifestation of malaria in adults, presents with altered mental status, seizures, and coma.

7. How is malaria diagnosed?

A high index of suspicion is the key to an early clinical diagnosis and survival, because early initiation of treatment is a time-critical action. Definitive diagnosis is established with light microscopy visualization of protozoa on blood smears. Thick blood smears are more sensitive, but thin blood smears are necessary for speciation and calculation of a parasitemia percentage. Repeat blood smears at least three times at 12-hour intervals, although false negatives will still occur. Antigen assay kits also are available.

8. How is malaria treated?

Unless *P. falciparum* infection can be ruled out, prompt treatment should be initiated empirically and the patient admitted. Severe malaria is treated with quinine (intravenous quinidine used in United States), chloroquine if the patient traveled to a chloroquine-sensitive region, and artemesinin compounds (not yet available in United States). All severely ill malaria patients should be admitted to the intensive care unit. Amazingly, most cerebral malaria patients will respond to treatment within 72 hours and may emerge from coma with no neurologic sequelae. Those receiving intravenous medications should receive telemetry monitoring, because quinine, quinidine, and chloroquine cause arrhythmogenic QT prolongation. Combination therapy with clindamycin or tetracyclines is crucial to avoid recurrence and resistance.

Centers for Disease Control: www.cdc.gov/malaria

KEY POINTS: MALARIA

1. Malaria is a common and lethal disease of the returning traveler or recent immigrant.

2. Normal blood smears do not rule out the disease.

3. Begin early empirical treatment in a sick patient with the right travel history.

4. Use quinidine when quinine is not available.

9. What is dengue and where does it occur?

Dengue is a mosquito-borne flavivirus endemic to tropical regions the world over. Only 41 U.S. cases were confirmed by the CDC in 1999 and 2000, but given that many symptoms are nonspecific and that the disease is not reportable on a national level, it is thought to be significantly underdiagnosed and under-reported. Of note, Texas and Hawaii report autochthonous transmission, meaning that the disease was acquired within the state. The principal vector, *Aedes aegypti,* occurs across the southeastern United States.

10. How do dengue fever and dengue hemorrhagic fever (DHF) present?

Many infections, especially in children, are asymptomatic or go unnoticed as a mild febrile illness. Classic dengue fever occurs after 5–6 days of incubation and lasts about 1 week, presenting with fever, retro-orbital headache, nausea, vomiting, arthralgias, and severe myalgias, earning it the nickname of "breakbone fever." A confluent blanching, macular rash is characteristic but only occurs in 50% cases. The illness provides immunity to one of the four virus serotypes, but reinfection with another serotype may lead to the more severe form, DHF. DHF is characterized by capillary leakage and thrombocytopenia, manifesting with dermal and mucosal hemorrhage or pleural and peritoneal effusions. DHF can develop into dengue shock syndrome, which if untreated carries a mortality of more than 40%.

Guzmán MG, Kourí G: Dengue: An update. Lancet Infect Dis 2:33–42, 2001.

11. How do I diagnose and treat dengue fever?

The diagnosis is usually made with enzyme-linked immunosorbent assay (ELISA) serology, which is often negative during the acute illness. Laboratory abnormalities include thrombocytopenia, which occurs frequently even in the absence of DHF, nonspecific elevation of liver enzymes, and hemoconcentration in the case of DHF. Treatment is supportive: fluids and analgesics for dengue fever and intensive care for DHF, which in experienced centers can reduce the mortality below 1%. Nonsteroidal anti-inflammatory drugs (NSAIDs) and aspirin are to be avoided because of platelet inhibition.

12. What is West Nile virus?

The West Nile virus is a flavivirus that is acquired through the bite of *Culex* mosquitoes. Previously endemic in Africa, it first was reported in the United States in an outbreak in New York City in 1999, where it was associated with a die-off of infected crows. Since that time, the disease has spread westward to the Pacific, with a U.S. peak incidence of 9862 in 2003, decreasing to 2470 cases in 2004.

Centers for Disease Control: www.cdc.gov/ncidod/dvbid/westnile

13. What are the symptoms of West Nile infections?

Only one in five infections are symptomatic, and only 1 in 140–320 present with central nervous system involvement. Symptomatic infection with the West Nile virus occurs 3–15 days after exposure. Initial symptoms include fever, headache, weakness, nausea, vomiting, and rash. Those with central nervous system involvement present most frequently with an encephalitic syndrome, for example, altered mental status and/or seizures. Isolated aseptic meningitis also occurs. More rarely, patients suffer polio-type paralysis or Parkinsonian movement disorders. The elderly are at much higher risk for severe disease and death. Neuropsychiatric sequelae occur in more than 50% of those with severe disease.

Solomon T: Flavivirus encephalitis. N Engl J Med 351:370–378, 2004.

14. How is West Nile encephalitis diagnosed and treated?

Diagnosis is made with ELISA antibody assays on serum or cerebrospinal fluid (CSF). Treatment is supportive. Young, nontoxic patients without central nervous system involvement may safely be discharged home.

15. Are ticks a significant vector of disease?

Yes. They are responsible for the greatest variety and number of cases of vector-borne human illness in North America. Tick-transmitted Lyme disease is the most common vector-borne illness in the United States, with more than 21,000 reported cases in 2003. There are two major families of ticks: the hard ticks and the soft ticks (*Ornithodoros*). Hard ticks transmit all tick-borne diseases, with the exception of relapsing fever. Ticks typically spread disease in the summer months, when ticks are actively seeking blood meals, and when most potential human hosts are engaged in outdoor activities.

Centers for Disease Control and Prevention: Summary of Notifiable Diseases-United States, 2003. MMWR 52:1–80, 2005.

16. **List the principal vectors and distribution of tick-borne diseases.**
See Table 51-1.

TABLE 51-1. PRINCIPAL VECTORS AND DISTRIBUTION OF THE TICK-BORNE DISEASES

Disease	Vector	Pathogen	U.S. Distribution	First-Line Treatment
Babesiosis	*Ixodes scapularis*	*Babesia microti*	Northeast	Quinine plus clindamycin
Colorado tick fever	*Dermacentor andersoni*	*Coltivirus*	Western mountains	Supportive
Ehrlichiosis:				
HME	*Amblyomma americanum*	*Ehrlichia chaffeensis*	Southeast, south-central	Doxycycline
HGE	*Ixodes* species	*Anaplasma phagocytophila*	Same as Lyme	Doxycycline
Lyme disease	*Ixodes* species	*Borrelia burgdorferi*	Northeast, midwest, west	Doxycycline
Relapsing fever	*Ornithodoros* species	*Borrelia* species	Western mountains	Doxycycline
RMSF	*Dermacentor* species	*Rickettsia rickettsii*	Nationwide, mostly southeast	Doxycycline
STARI	*A. americanum*	*Borrelia lonestari*	Southern United States	Doxycycline
Tick paralysis	Multiple	Toxins	Nationwide	Tick removal
Tularemia	*A. americanum* and *Dermacentor* species	*Francisella tularensis*	West, south-central	Streptomycin

HGE = human granulocytic ehrlichiosis, HME = human monocytic ehrlichiosis, RMSF = Rocky Mountain spotted fever, STARI = southern tick-associated rash illness.

17. **How is Lyme disease transmitted?**
Ixodes scapularis ticks transmit Lyme disease in eastern and central North America, whereas *Ixodes pacificus* is the vector on the Pacific Coast. Tick nymphs pick up the *Borrelia* spirochetes from mice, then transmit the majority of Lyme infections to people, because their small size makes detection difficult. Transmission of Lyme disease rarely occurs before 48 hours of attachment. Although white-tailed deer do not harbor the disease, they are the preferred hosts of the adult tick. New cases of acute Lyme disease peak between April and September, when nymphs are feeding.

18. **Describe the three clinical stages of Lyme disease.**
    - **Early acute or localized infection.** The classic skin lesion, erythema migrans (EM), develops at the bite site within 3–32 days in 80% of infections. More than 50% of patients will not recall a tick bite. EM expands slowly as an erythematous macule to a size of at least 5 cm and often much larger. Central clearing is common; it is usually painless but at times pruritic. Many individuals will develop systemic flulike symptoms with fever, suggesting some degree of early dissemination. Untreated, EM will typically resolve spontaneously over 3–4 weeks.
    - **Early disseminated disease.** This may occur in untreated individuals days to weeks after the tick bite. Most will have fever and adenopathy, and many will have multiple secondary skin lesions, that are smaller than the initial EM. Lyme arthritis is the most common secondary Lyme manifestation in the United States, arising in 70% of patients with untreated EM. This mono- or oligoarticular process most commonly produces effusions in the knee and other large joints. Neurologic manifestations include cranial neuritis, such as unilateral or bilateral facial nerve palsy (Bell's), and aseptic meningitis. Radiculoneuritis, similar to postherpetic neuralgia, with burning and paresthesias also occurs. Carditis occurs in less than 10% of cases and presents most typically with atrioventricular blocks.
    - **Late or chronic disease.** Late manifestations occur months to years after infection. Lyme arthritis is the most common, presenting in 10% of those with untreated EM. The arthritis typically does not cause joint destruction and may resolve spontaneously after several years. Chronic neurologic disease may include polyneuritis, multiple-sclerosis-like encephalomyelitis (0.1%), and subtle encephalopathy. Chronic dermatitis (acrodermatitis chronicum atrophicans) and keratitis are relatively rare in the United States.

    Stanek G, Strle F: Lyme borreliosis. Lancet 362:1639–1647, 2003.

19. **Does Lyme disease remind you of another spirochetal disease?**
    Primary, secondary, and tertiary phases, and the organ systems involved, are reminiscent of syphilis.

20. **How is Lyme disease diagnosed?**
    The typical EM rash in an endemic area is sufficient for diagnosis. For disseminated disease, ELISA serology is used to detect Lyme antibodies. Suggestive clinical findings are key, because positive serology does not prove active infection in an endemic area. A positive test in an asymptomatic individual is not an indication for treatment.

21. **How is Lyme disease treated?**
    Oral therapy with doxycycline or amoxicillin is effective for early disease and for mild early disseminated disease, such as arthritis. Neurologic and cardiac manifestations (with the exception of an isolated Bell's palsy) typically require parenteral therapy with ceftriaxone over 2–3 weeks, with a good prognosis. Admission to telemetry is recommended in Lyme carditis even for a first-degree atrioventricular block if the PR interval is greater than 300 ms, given the risk of progression. Temporary pacing may be needed for third-degree blocks. Late Lyme disease may not always respond to treatment.

22. **Can Lyme disease be prevented?**
    The only vaccine was removed from the market in 2002. The mainstays of prevention remain avoiding tick exposure (impossible for many outdoor enthusiasts), preventing attachment with protective clothing, and removing ticks promptly if they attach (twice daily tick checks).

23. **An ED patient presents with a tick bite; should you treat prophylactically for Lyme disease?**

Yes and no. If you practice in an endemic area, if you can identify the tick as *Ixodes scapularis*, and if it likely the tick was attached for more than 48 hours (suggested by engorgement, or known exposure time), treatment with a single 200 mg dose of doxycycline is effective in preventing Lyme. If you cannot meet these three conditions, simply give your patient appropriate return precautions.

KEY POINTS: LYME DISEASE

1. Most common vector-borne disease in the United States

2. Classic erythema migrans rash at site of tick bite

3. Heart block, Bell's palsy, and arthritis in advanced disease

4. Positive serology test not diagnostic of infection

5. Treatment: Doxycycline, amoxicillin, or ceftriaxone

24. **What on earth is STARI and what can be done about it?**

STARI stands for southern tick-associated rash illness, because it causes EM just like Lyme disease. It is caused by a nonculturable spirochete, *Borrelia lonestari*, transmitted by the lone star tick, *Amblyomma americanum*. If a patient presents with EM in the southern United States, a Lyme nonendemic area, the diagnosis is likely to be STARI. Treat just as you would early localized Lyme disease.

Centers for Disease Control: www.cdc.gov/ncidod/dvbid/stari

25. **What is relapsing fever?**

Relapsing fever is caused by several *Borrelia* species transmitted by soft ticks. Most cases are linked to stays in rural, rodent-infested cabins, in the mountains of the western United States. Abrupt onset of flulike symptoms (fever, myalgias, headache, and vomiting) occur 2–18 days after exposure. A generalized macular rash or a pruritic eschar at the bite site may develop. After 3 days of fever, symptoms resolve then "relapse" on a weekly basis up to 10 times, with declining severity. Diagnosis is made by detection of spirochetes on stained thick and thin blood smears, or by special culture. The very young and very old suffer increased morbidity and mortality. The disease responds well to doxycycline, penicillin, and erythromycin, but a Jarisch-Herxheimer reaction may occur (malaise and hypotension.)

Ettestad PJ, Voorhees RE, Sewell CM, et al: Tickborne relapsing fever outbreak after a family gathering-New Mexico, August 2002. MMWR 52:809–812, 2003.

26. **What is RMSF?**

RMSF is a life-threatening infection caused by *Rickettsia rickettsii* and transmitted by *Dermacentor*, or dog ticks. Its name derives from its original description in Montana and Idaho in the late 19th century and from the typical petechial rash occurring initially on the wrists and ankles. Currently, the majority of the cases are reported from the southeastern and south-central United States. The rash later involves the palms and soles, then spreads to the trunk, and often progresses into purpuric lesions. About 60% of infections will present with the classic triad of rash, fever, and tick exposure, although the rash is rarely present during the first 3 days of the illness. Abrupt onset fever, severe headache, and myalgias are the most common presenting symptoms, 5–7 days after the tick bite.

Spach DH, Liles WC, Campbell GL, et al: Tick-borne diseases in the United States. N Engl J Med 329:936–947, 1993.

27. **How dangerous is RMSF? What can be done about it?**
Untreated, RMSF mortality hovers around 25%. In 2003, 1091 cases were reported in the United States. The rickettsial pathogen induces a vasculitis that leads to end organ dysfunction, including confusion, respiratory failure, and renal failure, and most typically kills by disseminated intravascular coagulation. Appropriate and timely antibiotics can reduce the mortality to below 5%, but delay is frequent because of the relatively late onset of the characteristic rash. Doxycycline remains the drug of choice, whereas chloramphenicol is recommended for younger children (younger than 8 years). Because antibody production lags behind clinical disease, serology is confirmatory rather than diagnostic. Consider early empiric treatment in the spring and summer in endemic regions.

28. **What are human monocytic ehrlichiosis (HME) and human granulocytic ehrlichiosis (HGE)?**
HME and HGE are tick-borne diseases caused by the rickettsia-like bacteria, *Ehrlichia chaffeensis,* which infects monocytes, and *Anaplasma phagocytophyla* (formerly known as *Ehrlichia phagocytophyla* or *Ehrlichia equi*), which infects neutrophils. HME is transmitted by *A. americanum* in the southeastern and south-central United States, whereas HGE is transmitted by *Ixodes* ticks in a similar distribution to Lyme disease. More than 300 cases of each were reported to the CDC in 2003. Both diseases present with fever and flulike symptoms, progressing to respiratory and renal failure, and coma in severe cases. Rash may occur in HME but not in HGE. Mortality for HGE is higher, because it preferentially attacks older adults. Human immunodeficiency virus (HIV) patients are at much greater risk of severe disease.

29. **How are HME and HGE diagnosed and treated?**
High clinical suspicion is needed in endemic areas during the summer months. Thrombocytopenia, leukopenia, and mildly elevated liver enzymes, in the context of possible tick exposure or bites, are highly suggestive and should prompt treatment in an ill patient. Microscopic examination of buffy coat or peripheral blood may reveal characteristic inclusion bodies in monocytes or neutrophils. Separate serologic and PCR tests exist for HME and HGE but are only useful for confirmation of diagnosis. First-line therapy consists of doxycycline. Chloramphenicol, fluoroquinolones, and rifampin have also been reported to be effective.

Sexton, DJ: Human ehrlichiosis. UpToDate Online 13.1, 2005. (www.uptodate.com)

30. **What is Colorado tick fever?**
Colorado tick fever is caused by an RNA coltivirus transmitted by *Dermacentor* ticks in the western United States. Patients present 3–6 days after a bite, with sudden fever, headache, myalgias, and photophobia. A transient petechial rash may occur. In about 50% of cases, symptoms resolve, then recur after 3 days. Prognosis is excellent, although complications such as encephalitis, meningitis, and pericarditis have been reported. Diagnosis is by serology, although many cases go undiagnosed. Treatment is supportive.

31. **What is babesiosis?**
Babesiosis is a malaria-like illness, caused by the *Babesia microti* protozoan. It is transmitted by *Ixodes* ticks in the northeastern United States but has also been acquired by transfusion. Like malaria, the protozoan infects red blood cells, causing fever, drenching sweats, myalgias, and

headache. Though most disease is mild, life-threatening disease occurs in elderly and asplenic patients. Concurrent infection with Lyme disease occurs in 20%, causing a more severe illness. Diagnosis is made by serology or by detecting ring forms on stained thin or thick blood smears. Treatment typically consists of quinine and clindamycin in combination, although azithromycin and atovaquone together are also effective.

32. What is tularemia?

Tularemia is a caused by *Francisella tularensis,* a virulent gram-negative coccobacillus. Most cases occur in the south-central United States in hunters, through tick bites or contact with infected tissue of rabbits or rodents. The more common ulceroglandular form manifests with an ulcer at the tick bite, painful regional adenopathy, fever, headache, and myalgia. The severe typhoidal form presents with abdominal pain, fever, and prostration without skin and lymphatic manifestations and carries an untreated mortality of 30–60% by septic shock. Transaminitis and patchy pulmonary infiltrates develop in severe disease.

33. How is tularemia diagnosed and treated?

Prompt diagnosis and life-saving treatment depend on a high index of suspicion, because serology and culture results will not be acutely available. Streptomycin remains the drug of choice, but if unavailable, other aminoglycosides (gentamicin and tobramycin), tetracyclines, and chloramphenicol are alternatives

34. What is tick paralysis?

Tick paralysis is a syndrome caused by neurotoxins in the saliva of gravid females of many tick species. Young girls in western North America are at highest risk, especially after prolonged tick attachment. The syndrome usually presents as an ascending paralysis similar to Guillain-Barré, with sparing of sensorium and sensory function. Mortality does occur as a result of respiratory failure. Tick removal usually brings about prompt and complete recovery.

Haas E, Anderson D, Neu R, et al: Tick paralysis-Washington, 1995. MMWR 45:325–326, 1996.

35. What is the proper method for tick removal?

At times, simpler is better: use direct traction with a gloved hand and forceps as close as possible to the tick mouthparts, avoiding twisting. It is not necessary to dig after embedded mouthparts. Cleanse the area well after removal. Please forget every other tick removal method ever imagined.

36. Beside ticks and mosquitoes, do other North American arthropods tranmit disease?

Yes. Fleas transmit plague in the southwestern United States. Deerfly and flea transmission of tularemia has been reported. Body lice transmit *Bartonella quintana,* the cause of trench fever, to the urban homeless. Mites (chiggers) and body lice transmit types of typhus but not in North America.

WEBSITES

1. Centers for Disease Control and Prevention: www.cdc.gov

2. World Health Organization: www.who.int

CHAPTER 52

ARTHRITIS

Catherine B. Custalow, MD, PhD

1. What is arthritis? What are the signs and symptoms?

Arthritis is the inflammation of a joint, which may be characterized as monoarticular (involving a single joint) or polyarticular (involving multiple joints). Patients typically report pain, swelling, redness, and limitation of motion about the involved joint. On examination there may be tenderness, swelling, effusion, erythema, and painful decreased range of motion. Children may present with a limp or may avoid using an extremity.

2. What are the common causes of acute arthritis?

Arthritis has many causes, including infection (bacterial, granulomatous, fungal, or viral), trauma (fracture, overuse), hemorrhage (traumatic hemarthrosis, inherited coagulopathy, or anticoagulant-induced), crystal deposition disease (gout or pseudogout), neoplasm (metastasis), inflammatory conditions (rheumatoid arthritis, rheumatic fever, lupus), or degenerative conditions (osteoarthritis).

3. How can I differentiate between an intra-articular and a periarticular process?

True intra-articular processes typically cause generalized joint pain, joint effusion, tenderness, warmth, swelling, and an increase in pain with both active and passive ranges of motion. Another finding characteristic of an intra-articular process is that the pain increases with axial loading. Periarticular processes, such as bursitis, tendinitis, or cellulitis, tend to have more localized areas of tenderness, no joint effusion or swelling; and the pain may not be reproduced by range of motion in all directions.

4. What other physical findings may be helpful in a patient with arthritis?

A thorough physical exam may provide clinical clues to certain rheumatologic diseases, such as the finding of Heberden's nodes in osteoarthritis, skin lesions in psoriatic arthritis, urethral or cervical discharge in gonococcal arthritis, conjunctivitis in Reiter's syndrome, tophi in gout, or erythema chronicum migrans in Lyme disease.

5. Are x-rays helpful in the diagnosis of arthritis?

Very often the only radiographic evidence of inflammation is soft tissue swelling; however, plain radiographs may reveal foreign bodies, fractures, effusions, osteoporosis, or osteomyelitis. The radiographic changes of degenerative arthritis include asymmetrical joint space narrowing, marginal osteophytes, ligamentous calcifications, and subchondral sclerosis. In advanced gout, there may be "punched out" subchondral and marginal erosions, joint space narrowing, and periarticular calcified tophi.

Schwartz DT, Reisdorff EJ: Fundamentals of skeletal radiology. In Schwartz DT, Reisdorff EJ (eds): Emergency Radiology. New York, McGraw-Hill, 2000, pp 22–24.

6. What is the most important diagnostic test for determining the etiology of acute arthritis?

Arthrocentesis is the most important diagnostic procedure for evaluation of an acutely inflamed joint. Synovial fluid analysis (white blood cell [WBC] count, differential, crystals, Gram stain and culture) provides rapid, critical diagnostic information and should be performed on all patients with an acute joint effusion who have no contraindications. The procedure is simple and safe, and complications are rare when performed under sterile conditions and with proper technique. The procedure may also be therapeutic for the patient with an acutely swollen, painful joint. If infection is suspected in a prosthetic joint, it is recommended that joint aspiration be performed by an orthopedist.

7. **Are the erythrocyte sedimentation rate (ESR) and the C-reactive protein (CRP) useful for the evaluation of acute arthritis?**
No. The ESR and CRP represent the body's acute phase reaction to inflammation and infection. Unfortunately, a normal or elevated ESR and CRP is neither sensitive nor specific enough to confirm or rule out any particular disease. Septic arthritis cannot be excluded based on a normal ESR because false-negative rates may be as high as 20–30%. Therefore, when clinical suspicion is high, a joint should be aspirated regardless of the ESR.

Olshaker JS, Jerrard DA: The erythrocyte sedimentation rate. J Emerg Med 15:869–874, 1997.

KEY POINTS: CAUSES OF ARTHRITIS WITH FEVER

1. Lyme disease

2. Septic joint

3. Reiter syndrome

4. Rheumatic fever

5. Toxic synovitis

8. **In addition to synovial fluid analysis, are there any other laboratory tests that are useful in the evaluation of arthritis?**
The peripheral WBC count is of limited value in diagnosing the etiology of acute arthritis in the emergency department. In fact, only 50% of patients with septic arthritis have a WBC count greater than 10,000 cells/mm.^{3} In suspected disseminated gonococcal infection (DGI), cultures from the urethra and cervix should also be obtained.

Heffner AC. Monoarticular arthritis. In Wolfson AB, Hendey GW, Hendry PL, et al (eds): The Clinical Practice of Emergency Medicine, 4th ed. Philadelphia, Lippincott Williams & Wilkins, 2005, pp 563–568.

9. **How do I interpret the results of the arthrocentesis?**
See Table 52-1 for interpretation of synovial fluid analysis. Usually, synovial fluid from a septic joint has greater than 50,000 WBC/mL, and that from an inflammatory joint will be from 2000–50,000 WBC/mL. Be aware that there is a significant amount of overlap between these conditions. Some patients with septic arthritis have synovial WBC counts less than 50,000/mL, whereas some patients with gout have WBC counts greater than 1000/mL. A high index of suspicion should be maintained when a septic joint is entertained. Gram stain is also critical for the evaluation of synovial fluid and may be positive in up to 75% of nongonococcal septic arthritis and 25% of gonococcal arthritis. Polarized light microscopy is helpful to identify crystals.

Heffner AC. Monoarticular arthritis. In Wolfson AB, Hendey GW, Hendry PL, et al (eds): The Clinical Practice of Emergency Medicine, 4th ed. Philadelphia, Lippincott Williams & Wilkins, 2005, pp 563–568.

TABLE 52-1. SYNOVIAL FLUID ANALYSIS

Diagnosis	Appearance	Total WBC Count (per mm³)	PMN (%)	Mucin Clot Test	Fluid/Blood Glucose (diff.) (mm/dL)	Miscellaneous (Crystals/Organisms)
Normal	Clear, pale	0–200 (200)	<10	Good	NS	—
Group I (noninflammatory; degenerative joint disease, traumatic arthritis)	Clear to slightly turbid	50–4000 (600)	<30	Good	NS	—
Group II (noninfectious, mildly inflammatory; SLE scleroderma)	Clear to slightly turbid	0–9000 (3000)	<20	Good (occ. fair)	NS	Occ. LE cell, decreased complement
Group II (noninfectious, severely inflammatory)						
Gout	Turbid	100–160,000 (21,000)	70	Poor	10	Uric acid crystals
Pseudogout	Turbid	50–75,000 (14,000)	70	Fair-poor	Insuff. data	Calcium pyrophosphate
Rheumatoid arthritis	Turbid	250–80,000	70	Poor	30	Decreased
Group IV (infectious, inflammatory)						
Acute bacterial	Very turbid	150–250,000 (80,000)	90	Poor	90	Positive culture for bacteria
Tuberculosis	Turbid	2,500–100,000 (20,000)	60	Poor	70	Positive culture for *M. tuberculosis*

PMN = polymorphonuclear cells; NS = not significant; SLE = systemic lupus erythematosus; LE = lupus erythematosus. (From Wyngaarden JB, Smith LH [eds]: Cecil Textbook of Medicine, 18th ed. Philadelphia, W.B. Saunders, 1988, p 1994, with permission.)

10. **What is the most serious cause of arthritis?**
    Acute infectious arthritis is by far the most serious cause of acute monoarticular arthritis. It
    can be due to bacteria, mycobacteria, fungi, and viruses, although a bacterial etiology is the
    most common and the most serious. These infections carry a risk of permanent joint damage
    that may occur in as little as 7 days and result in chronic disability. In children, septic arthritis
    can cause epiphyseal damage, resulting in growth impairment and limb length discrepancy. In a
    patient with known chronic arthritis who has suddenly gotten worse, one should consider a
    superimposed infectious or septic cause.

    Heffner AC. Monoarticular arthritis. In Wolfson AB, Hendey GW, Hendry PL, et al (eds): The Clinical
    Practice of Emergency Medicine, 4th ed. Philadelphia, Lippincott Williams & Wilkins, 2005, pp 563–568.

11. **How is acute bacterial arthritis diagnosed and treated?**
    Acute bacterial arthritis is diagnosed in most cases by a synovial fluid count with typical synovial
    fluid counts $> 50,000$ WBC/mm^3, predominantly polymorphonuclear neutrophilic white blood
    cells (PMNs), and a Gram stain positive for bacteria. Treatment is admission to the hospital,
    administration of intravenous (IV) antibiotics, and immediate orthopedic consultation for
    arthroscopic joint drainage, open joint drainage, or daily joint aspirations.

12. **What is the difference between gout and pseudogout?**
    Gout develops when sodium urate crystals precipitate in a joint and initiate an
    inflammatory reaction. Pseudogout is caused by the deposition of calcium pyrophosphate
    crystals. When viewed with polarized light microscopy, gout crystals appear needle shaped
    and negatively birefringent, whereas pseudogout crystals appear rhomboid in shape and
    positively birefringent.

13. **Which joint is most commonly affected in gout?**
    The metatarsophalangeal (MTP) joint of the great toe is the most frequently affected joint (up to
    75%). This type of gout is known as podagra. Other commonly involved joints are the tarsal
    joints, the ankle, and the knee. Gout is polyarticular in as many as 40% of patients.

KEY POINTS: CAUSES OF ARTHRITIS WITH RASH

1. Lyme disease: Erythema chronicum migrans

2. Reiter syndrome: Keratoderma blennorrhagicum

3. Disseminated gonococcal infection: Pustular rash

4. Psoriatic arthritis: Psoriatic lesions

5. Systemic lupus erythematosus: Malar rash

14. **What are the emergency treatment options for gout?**
    Nonsteroidal anti-inflammatory drugs (NSAIDs) are the primary agents used to treat gout.
    Colchicine is effective in treating acute attacks. It may be administered orally at a dosage of
    0.5–0.6 mg every hour until symptoms improve, until diarrhea or vomiting develops, or until the
    maximum dose of 4 mg has been reached. A single IV dose of 1–2 mg of colchicine
    administered over 10 minutes may also be quite effective. Corticosteroids may be administered
    but only after bacterial infection has been ruled out. Drugs that alter serum uric acid levels such
    as allopurinol should not be administered acutely as they can exacerbate the condition.

15. **Why were some of the COX-2 inhibitors removed from the market?**

A newer class of drugs, known as the COX-2 inhibitors, work by inhibiting cyclo-oxygenase-2 and therefore blocking prostaglandin synthesis. It is felt that they are safer on the stomach than many other anti-inflammatory medications. Two of the medications, rofecoxib (Vioxx) and valdecoxib (Bextra), were removed from the market after clinical trials showed an increased risk of heart attack and stroke when taking these medications for a prolonged period of time. Another COX–2 inhibitor, celecoxib (Celebrex) now carries a warning on the label about the risks of cardiovascular events. These medications are still undergoing further scrutiny to determine their safety profile.

16. **Which tick-borne infection causes arthritis?**

Lyme disease, a tick-borne illness caused by the spirochete *Borrelia burgdorferi*, is known to cause arthritis in 60% of untreated patients. In certain endemic areas (now more than 15 states in the United States), the history of a tick bite along with the characteristic annular rash of erythema chronicum migrans and constitutional symptoms is highly suggestive of Lyme disease. The arthritis is usually a manifestation of late-disseminated disease. Although this arthritis usually responds to a course of doxycycline or amoxicillin, some patients develop chronic joint inflammation that does not respond to antibiotics.

Steere AC: Lyme disease. N Engl J Med 345:115–125, 2001.

BIBLIOGRAPHY

1. Lowery DW: Arthritis. In Marx JA (ed): Rosen's Emergency Medicine: Concepts and Clinical Practice, 5th ed. St. Louis, Mosby, 2002, pp 1925–1943.

2. Olshaker JS, Jerrard DA: The erythrocyte sedimentation rate. J Emerg Med 15:869–874, 1997.

3. Steere AC: Lyme disease. N Engl J Med 345:115–125, 2001.

4. Thomas HA Jr, Hartoch RS: Polyarticular arthritis. In Wolfson AB, Hendey GW, Hendry PL, et al (eds): The Clinical Practice of Emergency Medicine, 4th ed. Philadelphia, Lippincott Williams & Wilkins, 2005, pp 568–572.

5. Zink BJ: Bone joint infections. In Marx JA (ed): Rosen's Emergency Medicine: Concepts and Clinical Practice, 5th ed. St. Louis, Mosby, 2002, pp 1925–1943.

CHAPTER 53

SKIN DISEASES

Lela A. Lee, MD, and Joanna M. Burch, MD

1. How are skin lesions best described?

It is helpful to remember dermatologic terms (Table 53-1). Describing in plain terms how the lesions appear is acceptable, however. If you do not remember that a macule is a flat lesion and papules and plaques are raised, you may describe the lesions as either flat or raised. Communication with other care providers may be improved by the use of plain but accurately descriptive terms.

Characteristics helpful in establishing a diagnosis include the following: location and distribution, color, size, presence or absence of scale, contour change (e.g., raised, depressed, pitted), tactile characteristics (e.g., firm, spongy, fluctuant, blanchable or nonblanchable), and apparent depth (e.g., superficial, dermal, subcutaneous).

2. Is photography useful?

Photography of lesions may be the most effective way to convey their appearance. The tactile characteristics are lost with photography, but most other relevant characteristics are retained.

TABLE 53-1.	BASIC DERMATOLOGIC TERMS	
Skin Lesion	**Description**	**Example**
Macule	Flat, circumscribed color change (nonpalpable) <1 cm	Café-au-lait spot
Patch	Flat color change >1 cm	Vitiligo
Papule	Raised lesion <1 cm	Molluscum contagiosum
Plaque	Elevated, flat-topped lesion >1 cm. Lesions with epidermal changes (e.g., scale) would be considered plaques.	Psoriasis
Nodule	Raised lesion with a deeper palpable portion	Erythema nodosum
Vesicle	Raised, usually dome-shaped lesion filled with fluid and <1 cm	Varicella
Bulla	Fluid-filled lesion >1 cm	Bullous pemphigoid
Pustule	Raised lesion filled with exudative fluid, giving it a yellow appearance	Folliculitis
Cyst	Nodule filled with semisolid-to-solid material	Epidermoid cyst
Wheal	Flat-topped, firm, raised, edematous lesion; a hive	Urticaria

3. **What categories of skin conditions are life threatening or associated with life-threatening disease?**
   - Skin diseases resulting in extensive compromise to the cutaneous barrier
   - Skin signs of systemic infection (e.g., meningococcemia)
   - Skin cancers (e.g., melanoma)
   - Urticaria or angioedema with airway compromise
   - Skin signs of vascular compromise (including hemorrhage, emboli, thrombi, and vasculitis)
   - Skin findings of an introduced toxin (e.g., venomous snake bite)
   - Skin signs of physical abuse

4. **List some cutaneous red flags (i.e., skin signs indicating an increased likelihood of disease requiring emergency attention).**
   - Extensive blisters or denuded areas of skin
   - Acute total-body erythema, particularly in the elderly or frail
   - Extensive erythematous eruption in a person who is febrile and systemically ill
   - Petechiae, purpura, and ecchymoses
   - Necrosis
   - Urticaria
   - Isolated, abnormal-appearing mole

5. **What types of skin diseases result in potentially life-threatening compromise to the skin barrier?**
   Most of these are blistering diseases. When the blister breaks, the barrier is removed, and the individual is at risk for infection, fluid and electrolyte imbalance, and difficulties with heat regulation. Skin conditions that can be associated with an extensively compromised barrier include toxic epidermal necrolysis (TEN), Stevens-Johnson syndrome (SJS) (also called *erythema multiforme major*), pemphigus and pemphigus-like chronic blistering diseases, and burns. Patients with erythroderma (total or near-total body erythema) also may have problems with infection, fluid and electrolyte balance, and heat regulation, particularly patients who have significant chronic health problems, such as congestive heart failure. Lesions of the oral cavity may compromise life if they are severe enough to prevent food or fluid intake.

KEY POINTS: PHYSICAL FINDINGS OF LIFE-THREATENING DISEASES WITH COMPROMISE TO SKIN BARRIER

1. Extensive blistering

2. Erythroderma

3. Extensive oral erosions preventing food or fluid intake

6. **Describe the skin findings in meningococcemia, Rocky Mountain spotted fever, toxic shock syndrome, and necrotizing fasciitis.**
   - In **meningococcemia,** lesions may be irregularly shaped petechiae or purpura with dusky centers, located most commonly on the trunk and extremities. The lesions may involve the palms and soles.
   - In **Rocky Mountain spotted fever,** skin lesions appear at about day 4 of the acute febrile illness. Lesions begin on distal extremities, may involve palms and soles, and spread centripetally. After a few days, the lesions become petechial or purpuric. In practice, this eruption may be difficult to distinguish from that of meningococcemia.

- Patients with **toxic shock syndrome** may have a scarlatiniform eruption, edema of the face and extremities, conjunctival erythema, and erythema of the oral or genital mucosa. There is desquamation of the hands and feet 1–2 weeks later.
- **Necrotizing fasciitis** is characterized by a rapidly progressive erythema with development of duskiness and frank necrosis. There may be blisters. The overlying skin change is often mild compared with the necrosis occurring underneath.

7. **Describe the skin findings of common or distinctive childhood exanthems.**
   - **Scarlet fever** occurs in children between the ages of 2 and 10 years. Red macules and papules start on the neck and usually spread to the trunk and extremities. The skin may have a rough *sandpaper* feel on palpation and sometimes can be petechial. Erythema is usually most intense in the axillae, groin, and abdomen. Patients may exhibit Pastia's lines, which are petechiae in a linear pattern along the major skin folds. Palms and soles characteristically are spared. The face appears flushed with a circumoral pallor. Desquamation usually occurs as the eruption resolves in 1–3 weeks.
   - **Staphylococcal scalded skin syndrome** begins as faint erythema on the face, neck, axilla, and groin in a child younger than 5 years, usually following upper respiratory symptoms. The skin is tender, and crusting may occur around the mouth, eyes, and neck. The skin separates through the epidermis with even slight rubbing, leaving a red, moist surface underneath (Nikolsky's sign). Mucous membranes are not involved. In neonates, the entire body is involved, whereas in infants and children the upper body is affected preferentially.
   - **Varicella** presents with abrupt onset of crops of faint macules that progress through several stages. The macules become edematous papules, then vesicles over 24–48 hours. Often there is a small vesicle on a larger erythematous macule, described as a "dew drop on a rose petal." The vesicles develop moist crusts and leave shallow erosions. Lesions tend to begin centrally and spread to the extremities. The palms, soles, and mucous membranes frequently are involved. Characteristically, lesions in multiple stages of development (macules, papules, vesicles, crusts, erosions) are present in the same patient. The number of lesions ranges from 10 to 1500 (average 300). The lesions are usually pruritic. In general, lesions heal without scarring, although scarring may occur in some instances.
   - **Erythema infectiosum (fifth disease)** is a parvovirus B19 infection that results in intense erythema on the bilateral cheeks ("slapped cheeks"). After the facial erythema, a pink-to-red macular eruption develops with a reticular or *lacy* appearance. Although most children have the facial eruption with the slapped cheeks appearance, a few exhibit only the pink, lacy eruption on the body. The macular eruption tends to *reappear* with stimulation of cutaneous vasodilation, such as warm baths, exercise, or sun exposure. This can last for 4 months. Some patients develop a petechial eruption of the distal hands and feet with parvovirus B19 infection. This is the "purpuric gloves and socks syndrome."
   - **Roseola (exanthem subitum)** is a disease of infants and toddlers caused by infection with human herpesvirus 6. After 2–3 days of sustained fever, abrupt defervescence is followed by a pink maculopapular eruption. Periorbital edema sometimes is seen.
   - **Hand-foot-and-mouth disease** exhibits an abrupt onset of a few scattered papules that progress to oval or linear vesicles with an erythematous rim. As the name suggests, most lesions occur on the oral mucosa, palms, and soles. The oral lesions appear as small, discrete, whitish-gray erosions. Coxsackieviruses cause this eruption.
   - **Kawasaki disease** is typified by an irritable child with conjunctival injection and slightly swollen, distinctly red lips. The hands may be edematous or desquamating. The skin findings ar nonspecific and variable, ranging from macules, maculopapules, to vesicles. The child must meet the clinical criteria of fever for 5 or more days plus four of five of the following: (1) nonpurulent conjunctivitis, (2) mucosal changes, (3) edema or desquamation of the distal extremities, (4) exanthem, and (5) cervical lymphadenopathy.

Gable EK, Liu G, Morell DS: Pediatric exanthems. Prim Care 27:353–369, 2002.

8. **What is erythema multiforme (EM)?**

EM is usually an eruption of acute onset that is characterized by multiple, fixed red papules. Because the keratinocyte is the target of inflammatory insult, there is keratinocyte necrosis or apoptosis, manifest clinically as a central dusky center. The characteristic lesion is the "target lesion": a papule with a central dusky zone and an outer zone of erythema. It is typical for the majority of EM lesions to be erythematous, whereas only a few lesions are truly target like. Some lesions may develop vesicular changes in the center, due to intense necrosis.

EM frequently follows herpes simplex infection. Mucous membranes usually are spared or affected mildly. Lesions are found on the dorsal hands and extensor extremities, and palms and soles frequently are involved. Although there may be some systemic symptoms, EM is not usually debilitating and generally is managed on an outpatient basis. The eruption may recur after subsequent episodes of herpes simplex. Antiviral therapy is useful only as suppressive therapy to prevent herpes simplex recurrences. Treatment is usually reassurance or oral antihistamines to treat any burning and itching associated with the eruption. Topical or oral steroids are not indicated.

9. **Which disease is most often mistaken for EM?**

Acute urticaria. Urticarial lesions may be annular with concentric color changes and may occur on the palms and soles. Usually, urticarial lesions have a pale edematous center with an erythematous border, whereas EM lesions tend to have dusky centers. Lesions in urticaria are transient (<24 hours), whereas the target-like lesions of EM are fixed and can be present 1 week or more. Urticarial lesions clear with subcutaneous epinephrine, whereas EM lesions do not.

Zuberbier T, Greaves MW, Juhlin L, et al: Management of urticaria: A consensus report. J Invest Dermatol Symp Proc 6:128–131, 2001.

10. **What is the most common clinical presentation of an cutaneous adverse drug reaction?**

Exanthematous (morbilliform, maculopapular, or urticarial) eruptions are the most common presentation of a cutaneous adverse drug reaction. These reactions are generally thought to be immunologically mediated, type IV hypersensitivity reactions in which part of the drug acts as a hapten that gets presented to T lymphocytes by Langerhans' cells in the skin, leading to a complicated inflammatory cascade. The eruption is characterized by erythematous macules and papules that are usually widespread and symmetrically distributed. Lesions can sometimes show central clearing, often leading to the incorrect diagnosis of EM. The eruptions usually begin 7–14 days after the onset of the new medication, but in the cases of rechallenge, time to onset can be shorter. Treatment includes stopping the offending drug and prescribing antihistamines for symptomatic relief of pruritus.

Revuz J, Valeyrie-Allanore L: Drug Reactions. In: Bolognia JL, Jorizzo JL, Rapini RP (eds): Dermatology. London, Mosby, 2003, pp 336–344.

11. **What are the drugs most often implicated in exanthematous drug eruptions?**

Aminopenicillins, sulfonamides, cephalosporins, and anticonvulsants.

12. **What is the main diagnosis in the differential of exanthematous drug eruptions?**

Viral exanthems are often clinically and histologically indistinguishable from morbilliform drug eruptions. History of recent drug administration or symptoms of viral illness will help distinguish. Peripheral blood eosinophilia favors drug eruption. In children, 10–20% of exanthematous eruptions are drug induced, whereas 50–70% are drug induced in adults.

13. **Will a skin biopsy of an exanthematous eruption help me find the cause of the eruption (which drug, or drug versus viral)?**

No. The histologic pattern in exanthematous eruptions on the skin is the same regardless of the specific cause. Skin biopsy will not help to distinguish viral from drug exanthematous eruptions and does not provide information regarding which drug is the cause if the patient is taking multiple medications.

14. **What clinical signs should prompt consideration of a more serious adverse drug reaction?**
Facial edema; marked peripheral blood eosinophilia; hepatosplenomegaly; hemorrhagic and tender mucous membrane lesions; painful, dusky papules or plaques; or blistering and sloughing of the skin should prompt consideration of the serious drug reactions.

15. **Describe the signs and symptoms of the most serious drug eruptions.**
Three severe adverse drug reactions that can result in death are SJS, TEN, and drug reaction with eosinophilia and systemic symptoms (DRESS). (See Table 53-2.)

French LE, Prins C: Toxic epidermal necrolysis. In Bolognia JL, Jorizzo JL, Rapini RP (eds): Dermatology. London, Mosby, 2003, pp 323–329.

Ghislain PD, Roujeau JC: Treatment of severe drug reactions: Stevens-Johnson syndrome, toxic epidermal necrolysis and hypersensitivity syndrome. Dermatol Online J 8(1):5, 2002.

Roujeau JC, Kelly JP, Naldi L, et al: Medication use and the risk of Stevens-Johnson syndrome or toxic epidermal necrolysis. N Engl J Med 333:1600–1607, 1995.

KEY POINTS: TIME TO ONSET FOR CUTANEOUS DRUG ERUPTIONS

1. DRESS syndrome begins 2–6 weeks after the responsible drug is started.

2. One to three weeks are required for the development of SJS and TEN.

3. Four to fourteen days are required for exanthematous drug eruptions.

16. **Which skin cancers require urgent attention?**
In general, **melanoma** requires the most urgent diagnosis and treatment. Surgical removal of melanoma before it has metastasized can be life saving.

17. **How do I recognize a melanoma?**
Some characteristics that help identify lesions at higher risk to be melanoma are irregularity of pigmentation; irregular shape of the border; and presence of red, white, or blue-black color. An underemphasized finding that can be extremely helpful is a difference in appearance between the lesion in question and the patient's other moles. A brown macule on a fair-skinned person should be viewed with suspicion if the person does not have other similarly pigmented lesions, even if the brown macule is regularly pigmented, small, and perfectly round. A history of change in a mole is a risk factor, as is personal or family history of melanoma.

KEY POINTS: CUTANEOUS FEATURES CONCERNING FOR MELANOMA

1. Different from patient's other pigmented lesions

2. Recent changes in size, shape, and color

3. Markedly irregular borders

4. Markedly irregular pigmentation with colors of red, white, or blue

5. Areas of pigment regression

6. Any *one* of these may be an indicator of melanoma without the other features being present

TABLE 53-2. SIGNS AND SYMPTOMS OF THE MOST SERIOUS DRUG ERUPTIONS

	Causes	Clinical Signs/Symptoms	Mortality Rate	Treatment
SJS	Drugs (70–90%): antibacterial sulfonamides, anticonvulsants, NSAIDs, allopurinol *Mycoplasma pneumoniae* infection	Prodrome 1–14 days before the onset of mucosal involvement is common (fever, malaise, headache, sore throat, rhinorrhea and cough.) Acute eruption with red to dusky, tender papules at times targetoid with potential for blistering/ sloughing (usually <10% of the body surface area [BSA] involved) Extensive, hemorrhagic necrosis of two or more mucous membranes (mouth and eye most common)	5%	Prompt withdrawal of drug Supportive care (wound care in a IC or burn unit setting if sloughing of skin prominent, enteral nutrition, fluid/electrolyte replacement, pain management, monitoring for infection) Steroid use is controversial; some evidence that steroid use results in worse prognosis; if part of treatment should be started very early in the course.
TEN	Drugs (95%): antibacterial sulfonamides, anticonvulsants, NSAIDs, allopurinol	Onset with fever and tender skin several days before blistering/sloughing begins Painful, dusky red macules appear, become dusky, then confluent with islands of sparing, then blisters/sloughing of the skin begins (usually >30% BSA involved). Mucous membrane involvement in 90% of cases Poor prognostic factors include increasing age, delay in withdrawal of offending agent, and greater extent of epidermal attachment.	30–35%	*Prompt withdrawal of drug Supportive care in an intensive care burn unit setting (see SJS section) The following are used in treatment of TEN, but efficacy is controversial: intravenous immunoglobulin, systemic steroids (see SJS section)

Continued

TABLE 53-2. SIGNS AND SYMPTOMS OF THE MOST SERIOUS DRUG ERUPTIONS—CONT'D

	Causes	Clinical Signs/Symptoms	Mortality Rate	Treatment
DRESS	Drugs: anticonvulsants, sulfonamides, allopurinol, minocycline, dapsone, gold salts	Fever and a morbiliform skin eruption are the most common presenting features. The eruption then becomes edematous with follicular accentuation. Facial edema is a hallmark of DRESS. Lymphadenopathy, eosinophilia, and atypical lymphocytosis are common features. Visceral inflammation (hepatitis most common)	10%	Prompt withdrawal of the drug Systemic steroids (severe cases with visceral inflammation although efficacy unproven in controlled clinical trials) Topical steroids (milder cases for cutaneous manifestations)

*Garcia-Doval I, LeCleach L, Bocquet H, et al. Toxic epidermal necrolysis and Stevens-Johnson syndrome: does early withdrawal of causative drugs decrease the risk of death? Arch Dermatol 136: 323–327, 2000.

18. **Which spider bites can cause a necrotic reaction?**
Only a few species of spiders in North America produce bites that lead potentially to skin necrosis. Of these, bites of the brown recluse (*Loxosceles reclusa*) and the hobo spider (*Tegenaria agrestis*) are important because they may be fatal. The range of the brown recluse is limited, with the center of the endemic area being around eastern Arkansas, western Tennessee, and southern Missouri and the radius being several hundred miles in every direction. Outside the endemic area, brown recluse bites are uncommon, although they may occur because the spider may be transported on clothing or in boxes. The range of the hobo spider is the northwest United States and western Canada. Other *Loxosceles* species may cause necrotic reactions, and many of these spiders live in the deserts of the southwest United States. If one is outside an endemic area, the diagnosis of necrotic reaction to spider bite should be made with caution.

Sams HH, Dunnick CA, Smith ML, King LE Jr: Necrotic arachnidism. J Am Acad Dermatol 44:561–573, 2001.

19. **What skin lesions may be confused with a necrotic reaction to a spider bite?**
Necrotizing fasciitis, ecthyma, pyoderma gangrenosum, vasculitis, and clotting disorders. Erythematous reactions to stings or bites, such as bee stings or tick bites, occasionally may be confused with early reactions to spider bites.

20. **Describe common benign skin conditions that mimic melanoma.**
   - **Seborrheic keratoses** are extremely common benign lesions that usually first appear in middle age. They are growths of keratinocytes rather than pigment cells, but the keratinocytes may take up pigment and look alarmingly dark or irregularly pigmented. The scaling produced by the seborrheic keratosis may be so compact that it is difficult to discern, but detection of this rough scaling helps considerably in distinguishing this lesion from melanoma.
   - **Venous lakes** are vascular growths that often appear on the helix of the ears and on the lips of older persons with sun damage. The purple color may mimic that of a melanoma. Pressing firmly on the lesion drains much of the blood from the lesion and reveals it as a vascular growth.

21. **Describe common benign skin conditions that mimic purpura resulting from systemic disease.**
   - **Solar purpura** is common on the forearms and backs of hands of persons who have chronic sun damage. Large areas of purpura may be evident and may have occurred with minimal, sometimes unnoticeable trauma. Solar purpura is restricted to chronically sun-damaged skin and is particularly common in patients on long-term systemic steroid therapy.
   - **Schamberg's purpura** is a benign condition characterized by petechiae primarily on the lower legs. The lesions tend to be pinpoint, nonpalpable, and extremely numerous. By contrast, purpuric lesions of leukocytoclastic (*hypersensitivity*) vasculitis tend to be slightly larger in diameter (often 2–4 mm), and frequently some of the lesions are palpable. (Although leukocytoclastic vasculitis sometimes is referred to as *palpable purpura*, it is common to find that most lesions are flat and only a few are palpable.)

22. **Describe common skin conditions that mimic cellulitis.**
   - A **kerion** caused by fungal infection in the scalp (tinea capitis) may be so intensely inflamed that it is mistaken for cellulitis. Because a kerion may produce permanent, scarring alopecia, it is important to recognize and institute therapy early. Kerions occur almost exclusively in children.
   - **Stasis dermatitis** sometimes may be confused with cellulitis. Stasis dermatitis is usually bilateral, whereas leg cellulitis is more often unilateral. Stasis dermatitis is characterized by

scaling and mild-to-moderate erythema. If the erythema is fiery red, the redness is rapidly progressive, the patient is systemically ill, or there is a leukocytosis, cellulitis may be the presumptive diagnosis.

- **Allergic contact dermatitis**, such as poison ivy dermatitis, may result in lesions that are intensely inflamed. The distribution of the lesions often suggests an exogenous cause. In plant dermatitis, linear erythema, often with blisters, is an indicator of where the plant has brushed against the skin. Antibiotic creams containing neomycin are another relatively common cause of allergic contact dermatitis. Because antibiotic creams often are used on wounds, it is easy to understand how allergic contact dermatitis caused by the cream may be mistaken for a wound infection.

23. **In which disease associated with leg ulceration is débridement generally contraindicated?**
    Pyoderma gangrenosum.

24. **When should patients with dermatitis (eczema) be treated with systemic steroids?**
    Systemic steroids generally should not be given to patients with chronic dermatitis. Systemic steroids, although inexpensive and easy to use, do not correct what is often the underlying problem, that of a faulty skin barrier. This is especially the case when the skin is dry. Patients taking systemic steroids also may exhibit a rebound of disease when the steroids are tapered. Patients with acute dermatitis that is expected to be self-limited may be given systemic steroids if the severity of disease merits and there are no contraindications. An example is severe poison ivy dermatitis.

25. **Should steroids be used for psoriasis?**
    Systemic steroids are generally considered to be contraindicated for the treatment of psoriasis, because severe rebound with generalized pustular psoriasis may occur following withdrawal of the steroid.

26. **What are the divisions of the classes of topical corticosteroids? On which areas of the skin are they appropriately applied?**
    - **Low-potency** topical corticosteroids (class 6 or 7 topical steroids, such as 1% and 2.5% hydrocortisone, 0.05% desonide) are appropriate to use on the face, axillae, groin, breasts, and genitalia, where the skin is thinner and more prone to cutaneous side effects.
    - **Moderate-potency** topical corticosteroids (class 4 or 5 topical steroids, such as 0.025% fluocinolone, 0.1% triamcinolone, 0.2% hydrocortisone valerate) are useful on the neck and body, avoiding the more sensitive areas mentioned previously. This class is given most appropriately as first-line therapy for skin conditions diagnosed in the emergency department (ED).
    - **High-potency** topical corticosteroids (class 2 or 3 topical steroids, such as 0.05% fluocinonide, 0.1% halcinonide, 0.25% desoximetasone) should not be applied to the face, breasts, genitalia, axillae, or groin. Topicals in this class are more likely to produce cutaneous side effects if used diffusely or for long periods (>2 weeks). This class should be prescribed only if moderate-potency topical corticosteroids have not been effective or if the condition is limited to the particularly thick skin of the palms and soles.
    - **Superpotent** topical corticosteroids (class 1 topical steroids, such as 0.05% clobetasol, 0.05% betamethasone dipropionate in optimized vehicle, 0.05% halobetasol, 0.05% diflorasone) usually are reserved for chronic, recalcitrant conditions, often of the palms and soles. The risk of cutaneous side effects is greatest with this class, and this class of steroid should be dispensed in a continuity-of-care rather than an ED setting.

27. Does the vehicle of the topical corticosteroid affect potency?

Yes. The same corticosteroid may be significantly more or less potent, depending on the vehicle. For example, 0.1% mometasone cream is classified as medium potency, class 4, whereas 0.1% mometasone ointment is high potency, class 2. In general, ointments are most potent, followed by gels, emollients, creams, lotions, solutions, and sprays.

XII. ENVIRONMENTAL EMERGENCIES

LIGHTNING AND ELECTRICAL INJURIES

Lee W. Shockley, MD

"To stand against the deep dread-bolted thunder? In the most terrible and nimble stroke of quick, cross lightning?"
—William Shakespeare, *King Lear,* Act 4, Scene 7

"Electricity is really just organized lightning."
—George Carlin

LIGHTNING

1. **True or false: A lightning strike is always fatal.**
   False. Lightning is a surprisingly inefficient killer. The mortality may be as low as 10–30%.

2. **True or false: It is dangerous to touch victims of lightning because they retain a charge.**
   False. Are you kidding? Did you see that in a cartoon?

3. **True or false: During a thunderstorm, get into a car because the rubber tires will insulate it.**
   False. You are safer inside a car than out during a thunderstorm but not because of the tires. Think about it. The lightning bolt just passed several kilometers through the air to get to the ground. It won't be intimidated by 6 inches of rubber (or the rubber soles of your tennis shoes, for that matter). The real reason that the car is safer is the metal skin of the body. It acts as a Faraday cage, allowing electromagnetic flow over the outer surface, isolating the occupants. Now, of course, that may not protect the occupants from the flash, thunderclap, splash current (see later), or induced electromagnetic currents through the interior.

4. **True or false: Lightning strike victims typically suffer extensive burns.**
   False. The "crispy critter" phenomenon is largely untrue. Victims do not burst into flame and become reduced to a pile of ashes. Of the lightning strike victims who have burns, only 5% have deep or significant burns. Lightning most often flashes over a victim with few, if any, burns.

5. **True or false: If a victim of lightning is not killed outright, he or she will likely be fine.**
   False. The majority of victims suffer some sequelae. These complications can include neurologic, psychiatric, cardiac, pulmonary, otic, ophthalmologic, and musculoskeletal disorders.

6. **True or false: People are safe from lightning if they are indoors.**
   False. Maybe safer, but a significant number of lightning injuries occur to people who are inside buildings. One mechanism for this is a side flash through plumbing, telephones, and electrical appliances connected to the outside of the building by metal conductors.

7. **True or false: One should treat lightning victims as one would high-voltage electrical victims.**

False. Lightning and high-voltage electrical injuries can have very different effects and require different treatment approaches. For example, high-voltage injuries often produce deep burns that may require fluid resuscitation and even fasciotomy. These victims often have renal failure from myoglobinuria. If they are in cardiac arrest, it is often ventricular fibrillation. In contrast, lightning victims rarely have deep burns that need fluid resuscitation and fasciotomy. Their kidneys are rarely affected. If the lightning strike victim is in cardiac arrest, it is typically asystole (unless he or she is also hypoxic).

8. **True or false: Lightning never strikes twice in the same place.**

False. The Empire State Building in New York is struck about 23 times a year; once, it was struck eight times in 24 minutes. Virginia Park Ranger Roy C. Sullivan, the "human lightning conductor," was the world record holder for the most lightning strikes. From 1942 to 1977, he was struck seven times. He killed himself in September 1983. The professional golfer Lee Trevino has been struck twice. Mr. Trevino's advice: "If you are caught on a golf course during a storm and are afraid of lightning, hold up a 1-iron. Not even God can hit a 1-iron."

9. **Is a lightning bolt an alternating current (AC) or a direct current (DC)?**

Gotcha, trick question! It is neither. It is a unidirectional current impulse (technically neither AC nor DC, although the closest model would be a large DC discharge). It is very high voltage (100 million to 2 billion volts), very large current (20,000–300,000 peak amps), and very high energy (1 billion joules or 280 kilowatt hours). The bolt is also very hot: 8000–25,000°C (the surface of the sun is *only* 6000°C). The good news is that it's a very short duration phenomenon (0.1–1 msec). The energy released in a lightning bolt is more electrical energy than is produced by all of the electrical generators in the United States at that instant. However, because it is such short duration, it is only enough energy to light a single light bulb for about a month. The energy is dissipated as light, heat, sound, and radio waves.

10. **What the hell was Ben Franklin doing with that kite experiment?**

First of all, you should understand that Franklin was not a stupid man. He was an accomplished printer, author, statesman, diplomat, philanthropist, scientist, and inventor. His inventions included swim fins, bifocals, watertight bulkheads for ships, the Franklin wood stove, an odometer, and *the lightning rod*. People were familiar with static electricity before Franklin's day, but there was debate as to whether lightning was static electricity on a very large scale or some sort of "fire in the sky." His kite experiments, although incredibly dangerous, did show that lightning was electric. This finding led directly to his development of the lightning rod.

11. **How common is lightning?**

There are up to 8 million lightning flashes worldwide each day. Across the globe, there are 2000 active thunderstorms right now. Those storms produce 100 cloud-to-ground strikes per second. In the United States, there are 50–300 lightning fatalities every year.

12. **Where do lightning injuries occur?**

In 40% the location goes unreported. Of those that are reported, 27% happen in open fields and recreation areas; 14% happen under trees; 8% are water-related (boating, fishing, swimming); 5% happen on golf courses; 3% are related to the use of heavy equipment and machinery; 2.4% are telephone related, and 0.7% are related to radio transmitter and antennae. Central Florida is thunderstorm alley with the greatest number of thunderstorm days in the United States. The top five states in terms of lightning injuries are Florida, Michigan, Pennsylvania, North Carolina, and New York. The top five states in terms of lightning deaths are Florida, Michigan, Texas, New York, and Tennessee.

13. **I want to appear as if I read this whole chapter. Is there one number to memorize that will impress my friends and colleagues?**

Sure, try 70%:

- Thunderstorms that happen between noon and 6 pm = 70%
- Thunderstorms that happen in June, July, or August = 70% (June, 21%; July, 30%; August, 22%)
- Lightning victims who survive = 70% (although this may be as high as 90%)
- Survivors with sequelae = 70%
- Singular victims = 70% (fatal singular victims as high as 91%; victims in couples = 15%; victims in groups of 3 or more = 15%)

14. **What is a fulgurite? What phenomenon does it illustrate?**

The word is from Latin, meaning "lightning stone." When lightning strikes the ground, it can spread out underground for up to 60 ft (20 m) in radial horizontal arcing. Depending on soils characteristics, there can be enough heat generated to fuse silica into branching configurations. These stones are the fulgurites. It is important to understand that the electrical energy from a lightning strike dissipates through the ground. If a person were standing near by with one foot closer to the strike epicenter than the other, a current can travel up one leg and down another. This is known as a stride voltage or step voltage injury. This phenomenon can account for multiple victims of a single strike who are not in immediate proximity to each other.

15. **Does lightning ever hit airplanes? What happens?**

Yes, and usually not much. There are at least 160 lightning strikes on aircraft annually. Typically, these strikes happen at 10,000–15,000 ft, in rain and light turbulence, within a cloud and near the freezing level. Because the aircraft skin is metal, the lightning almost always "flashes over," leaving only minor damage. However, the blast effect of the thunderclap can interrupt jet engines; the bright flash can temporarily blind pilots, and the induced electromagnetic field can disrupt avionics and communication equipment—just what you don't want at 10,000–15,000 ft, in rain and light turbulence, within a cloud and near the freezing level. There have been a few aircraft lost to fuel vapor explosions within the fuel tanks induced by lightning.

16. **How does lightning come about?**

First of all, a large charge separation must occur within a cloud, turning it into a giant "battery" or capacitor. This occurs from hailstones and raindrops settling at various rates in a convectively active cloud. Charged particles get "stripped off," and the cloud separates into a dipole or tripole. Most often, the cloud base becomes negatively charged. In response, an "induced shadow" of positive charged forms on the ground. The potential between the ground and the cloud can be as great as 7500 volts per inch. Lightning is initiated by the formation of a "stepped leader," a zigzag, short, stepped, downward series of branching ionized plasma channels. At the same time, a positively charged "pilot stroke" arises from the ground. When the two meet at about 50–100 m above the ground, the "return stroke" is initiated. This is what we think of as the lightning bolt.

It is a high-voltage, high-current, high-velocity discharge that travels up the plasma channel. There is an average of four to five return strokes.

17. **How about thunder?**

Thunder is an acoustic wave caused by the sudden heating of the air. This can cause a pressure rise up to 10 atm. The sound of thunder is rarely heard over 10 miles away and has a lower pitch at greater distances.

18. **What are the mechanisms of lightning injury?**

- Direct strike or contact. This occurs when the victim is in direct contact with the lightning or an object or structure that is struck by lightning. It usually results in the highest mortality and morbidity.

- Splash or side flash. Lightning arcs from an object to a nearby person.
- Step or stride voltage. The lightning current strikes the ground, then spreads out, as in the fulgurite example. Current moving underground can cause an induced current, up one leg and down another. This is a reason for multiple victims of a single strike.
- Rising upward streamer. This newly described mechanism happens with an injury from the rising positively charged streamer, which does not connect with a pilot stroke to create the plasma channel that allows return strokes, what we think of as a lightning bolt.
- Blunt trauma and blast trauma. Blast trauma may occur from the thunderclap. Common findings from this blast include pulmonary contusions, tympanic membrane rupture, and conductive hearing loss. A victim may also be "thrown" by diffuse muscle contractions.
- Secondary trauma and burns from fires. Trauma from falls or falling objects and thermal burns from ignited clothing, heated metal, and burning surroundings can also complicate lightning trauma.

19. **What is the "flashover phenomenon"?**
Given the short duration of a lightning bolt, current is often conducted over the skin without penetration. When this happens, it significantly lowers the mortality of a direct strike victim from 85% with signs of penetration to 40% without.

20. **I'm treating a farmer who was found unconscious in his field after a thunderstorm. He has no recollection of what happened. How can I tell if he was struck by lightning?**
Quick, put down this book, and go look at his skin and look in his ears. His memory of the events won't help; in fact, it is said that 100% of direct-strike victims have amnesia. However, arborescent superficial erythema (known as Lichtenberg's flowers, ferning, arboration, or fractals) is pathognomonic for lightning. Unfortunately, it is seen in only seen in 20% of confirmed cases and fades away over hours. It is not a true burn but the effect of a strong electromagnetic field on wet skin. In addition, there may be partial-thickness linear or punctate burns in moist areas. The ears? Tympanic membrane rupture occurs in 50% of victims. Tinnitus is also common and usually resolves in hours to days. Seven to 12% of victims experience temporary hearing loss, and a few have permanent hearing loss.

21. **The farmer is also tachycardic, hypertensive, with cool, pale skin, and diminished peripheral pulses. Although awake, he seems unable to move his extremities. Why?**
He is likely suffering from "lightning paraplegia" (keraunoparalysis or Charcot's paralysis). It is probably primarily due to intense adrenergic stimulation, vasospasm, and hypoperfusion, not direct nerve injury. If that is the case, it typically resolves. However, you should be wary of occult injuries and diligent in your work-up.

22. **I have been taught that at multiple casualty incidents (MCIs), I should allocate resources to victims who are not breathing and not moving *only after* I have taken care of those with signs of life. Is that rule applicable in a lightning strike MCI?**
No. Lightning strike is the one exception to the usual MCI triage rule. The first priority should go to those who are not breathing and not moving. The reasons are that only those who present in cardiac arrest are at high risk of dying. Bystander cardiopulmonary resuscitation (CPR) doubles survivability from about 24% without CPR to 50% with CPR. Those who have not arrested have little chance of dying, and so in this case the first priority goes to "the dead."

23. **Which organ systems can be damaged by lightning?**
See Table 54-1.

TABLE 54-1.   LIGHTNING INJURIES BY ORGAN SYSTEM

System	Injury
Cardiac	Asystole, ventricular fibrillation (from hypoxia), arrhythmias, nonspecific ST-T changes, ST elevation, T wave inversion, hypertension, tachycardia, acute myocardial infarction (rare)
Respiratory	Apnea from inhibition of the brain stem respiratory centers, hypoxia, pulmonary contusions and hemorrhage, hemothorax, pneumothorax
Nervous	Loss of consciousness, coma, transient aphasia, confusion, disorientation, amnesia, autonomic dysfunction (with loss of pupillary function), coagulation of brain substance, epidural and subdural hematomas, intraventricular hemorrhage, skull fractures, seizures, transient or permanent paralysis, EEG abnormalities, extrapyramidal symptoms, sensory disturbances, SIADH, cerebral edema, ataxia, vertigo, cerebral artery thrombosis, spinal atrophic paralysis
Psychiatric	Hysteria, phobias, psychosis, depression, posttraumatic stress disorder, "storm apprehension," memory impairment, personality changes
Skin	Feathering, linear burns, punctate burns, true thermal burns
Musculoskeletal	Dislocations, fractures, muscle necrosis (rare)
Renal	Myoglobinuria (rare)
Gastrointestinal	Gastric atony, ileus, perforations (uncommon)
Ophthalmologic	Mydriasis, loss of light reflex, anisocoria, Horner's syndrome, cataracts (in 20% of victims within 3 years)
Otologic	Tinnitus, hearing loss, ruptured tympanic membranes

EEG = electroencephalographic, SIADH = syndrome of inappropriate antidiuretic hormone.

24. **What should be the disposition of lightning victims?**
All patients with cardiac abnormalities (including abnormal electrocardiograms [ECGs]), neurologic findings, or significant burns require hospital admission. Patients with associated trauma or burns may need admission, depending on the extent of the injury. All others may be discharged. It is prudent to arrange for ophthalmology follow-up in 6 months and otolaryngology and psychiatry follow-up, as needed.

25. **What's the "30-30 rule"?**
It is a lightning safety recommendation. If you see lightning and cannot count to 30 before hearing thunder, you are in danger and should seek shelter. This is based on the flash-to-bang method of determining your distance from a lightning strike: the time between the lightning flash and the thunderclap in seconds divided by five is the distance in miles. Further, you shouldn't resume outdoor activities until at least 30 minutes after the last flash of lightning is seen and the last clap of thunder is heard. *"If you see it, flee it; if you hear it, clear it."*

ELECTRICAL INJURIES

26. What is the epidemiology of electrical injuries?
There are about 800–1000 injuries from high-voltage electricity per year in the United States. Between 3% and 4% of burn center admissions are for electric burns. Serious electrical burns carry 40% mortality. Electrical injuries follow a bimodal age distribution with a peak in children younger than 6 years and another peak around age 20. The first peak represents children "exploring" electrical cords, wall sockets, or extension cord outlets. This second peak represents occupational accidents (one third of them are electric workers, and one third are construction workers). In fact, electrocution is the fifth leading cause of occupational death.

27. What are the basic physics of electricity?
Electricity is simply the flow of electrons. The electromotive force moving those electrons from high concentration to low concentration is voltage (V). The number of electrons flowing is known as current or amperage (I). Resistance to the electron flow (R) is a property of the medium through which they pass, measured in ohms (O). These three factors are related in Ohm's law: $I = V/R$.

28. What factors determine nature and severity of the injury seen in electrical accidents?
The most harmful effects of electricity on the body are heat related. The heat generated is related to the current, tissue resistance, and duration of contact:

$$\text{Heat} = (\text{amperage})^2 \times \text{resistance} \times \text{time}$$

Because amperage is squared, it contributes the most to tissue injury. However, in real accidents, the amperage is often unknown. Therefore, we use voltage as an approximate indicator because high voltages are usually associated with high amperages. Voltages are classified as:
- High = 1000 volts or more
- Low = less than 1000 volts

KEY POINTS: DIFFERENCES IN LIGHTNING AND HIGH-VOLTAGE ELECTRICAL INJURIES

1. Duration: Instantaneous (lightning) versus prolonged contact (electrical)

2. Energy: 1 billion volts (lightning) versus 1000–10,000 volts (electrical)

3. Current: ~DC (lightning) versus AC (electrical)

4. Shock wave: Present in thunder (lightning) versus absent (electrical)

5. Flashover: Present (lightning) versus absent (electrical)

6. Cardiac effect: Asystole (lightning) versus ventricular fibrillation (electrical)

7. Burns: Minor and superficial (lightning) versus deep with iceberg phenomenon (electrical)

8. Urinary failure: Rare (lightning) versus myoglobinuric (electrical)

9. Fasciotomy: Rarely indicated (lightning) versus common and early (electrical)

29. **What do the terms "threshold for sensation," "let go threshold," and "ventricular fibrillation threshold" mean?**

   In contradistinction to DC, in which there is an unchanging direction of current flow, AC is an electric source that changes its direction of current flow as a particular frequency. Human tissues, particularly muscles, respond well to AC frequencies between 40 and 150 Hz (cycles per second). In the United States, we just happen to supply our homes with exactly that: household current is 60 Hz, 110–120 volts. The threshold for sensation is the minimum current that is perceptible, about 1–4 mA. Between 8 and 22 mA, AC can cause tetanic muscle contractions to the degree that one may not be able to let go of the electric source. This phenomenon, obviously, is very dangerous because it prolongs the time of contact, thus producing more injury. The ventricular fibrillation threshold (50–100 mA) is not much higher than the let go threshold.

30. **How is tissue resistance related to injury?**

   Nerves offer the least resistance and, therefore, allow the deepest penetration but the least heat injury. Blood vessels have the next most resistance, then mucous membranes, muscle, skin, tendon, and fat. The tissue with the greatest resistance is bone. Because of its high resistance, it suffers the greatest heat injury but the least penetration.

   Interestingly, the resistance of skin can be highly variable, depending on its thickness, vascularity, and degree of hydration. The thick, dry skin of callused feet and hands is much more resistant (100,000 ohms) than thin, wet skin (2500 ohms). Immersion in water further drops skin resistance to 1500 ohms. When high-resistance skin is injured by electricity, the heat produces burns. As the skin chars, it loses resistance and allows for penetration.

31. **Which organ systems can be damaged by electrical injury?**

   See Table 54-2.

TABLE 54-2. ORGANS DAMAGED BY ELECTRICAL INJURY	
System	Injury
Skin	Thermal burns such as entrance and exit wounds (typically in AC burns, the entrance and exit burns look similar; in DC burns, the entrance is smaller than the exit), flexor crease burns, mouth commissure burns (risk of delayed bleeding from labial artery when the eschar separates)
Cardiac (the most frequent causes of immediate death from electrical injury)	Cardiac arrest from asystole (DC) or ventricular fibrillation (AC), atrial and ventricular ectopy, atrial fibrillation, first-degree and second-degree heart blocks, bundle-branch blocks, and QT interval prolongation, nonspecific ST-T changes (common), acute myocardial infarction (rare)
Vascular	Hemorrhage, arterial and venous thrombosis, ischemia, progressive necrosis (from "skip" lesions in which the current, presumably, skips from traveling within the blood column to traveling within the wall of the vessel)

Continued

TABLE 54-2.	ORGANS DAMAGED BY ELECTRICAL INJURY—CONT'D
System	**Injury**
Nervous	CNS or peripheral; immediate or delayed, loss of consciousness, amnesia, confusion, disorientation, concentration and memory problems, apnea or respiratory depression, seizures, paralysis, paresthesias, motor nerves more commonly injured than sensory, poor rate of recovery
Musculoskeletal	Muscular pain, muscle necrosis (rhabdomyolysis), compartment syndrome, tendon rupture, dislocations (one of the few mechanisms for posterior shoulder dislocations), fractures, "electroporation" or the formation of cell membrane pores in bone, aseptic necrosis, periosteal burns, "bone pearls" (osteoschisis)
Respiratory	Inhibition of the brain stem respiratory centers
Gastrointestinal	Hollow visceral and solid visceral injury (both rare), stress ulcers
Renal	Rhabdomyolysis and myoglobinuria, acute tubular necrosis, renal failure, hyperkalemia, hypocalcemia, hyperglycemia, acidosis
Ophthalmologic	Cataracts (6–24 months after the incident), corneal burns, intraocular hemorrhage and thrombosis, retinal edema, retinal detachment, uveitis, optic nerve atrophy
Pregnancy	Spontaneous abortion (fetal death rate is 73%), oligohydramnios, IUGR (amniotic fluid and fetal tissues conduct 200 times more than dry, intact adult skin)

AC = alternating current, CNS = central nervous system, DC = direct current, IUGR = intrauterine growth retardation.

32. **What are some prehospital considerations in the treatment of electrical injuries?**
Rescuer safety is the first priority. Rescuers should not become victims, even if that means taking time to turn off the power source before approaching a victim. The essentials of resuscitation are the ABCs (airway, breathing, circulation). It's prudent to assume traumatic injuries and immobilize the spine. Arrhythmias are treated in the standard manner. Two large-bore intravenous (IV) catheters should be established, and aggressive fluid replacement should to be started.

33. **My patient is a 24-year-old, 75-kg man who was working on a high-voltage line when he received a shock. He has a burn on his palm where it contacted a wire and another burn on his knee where it was in contact with a ladder. These two burns together are about 2% of his total body surface area (TBSA). How much IV fluid should he receive?**
Traditional burn formulas for calculating volume repletion, such as the Parkland formula (4 mL × weight in kg × %BSA), are not applicable to electrical injuries because the surface damage does not reflect the degree of deeper tissue damage. The surface burn is just the "tip of the iceberg." For this reason, electrical injuries are closer correlated with crush injuries than thermal burns. IV fluids should be administered at a rate to ensure a urine output of 1–2 mL/kg/h (for this patient 75–150 mL of urine per hour). The objective of early, aggressive fluid resuscitation is to prevent renal failure secondary to rhabdomyolysis.

34. **Who gets admitted, and who goes home?**
See Table 54-3.

TABLE 54-3. CRITERIA FOR ADMISSION AND DISCHARGE	
Admit (Consider Burn or Trauma Center)	**Discharge***
Major burns, circumferential burns, significant hand burns	Asymptomatic low-voltage injury
	No ECG findings
Patients requiring CPR	No significant burns
High voltage, especially transthoracic path	*Ophthalmology follow-up in 6 months
Abnormal ECG, arrhythmias	*ENT, psychiatry follow-up as needed
Loss of consciousness	
Neurologic abnormalities	
Hypoxia, myoglobinuria	
Mouth commissure burns (because of problems with feeding and bleeding from the labial artery)	
Obstetric consultation is recommended for all pregnant patients	

CPR = cardiopulmonary resuscitation, ECG = electrocardiographic, ENT = ear, nose, and throat.
*If discharged, these follow-up arrangements should be provided.

35. **What are some of the pearls, pitfalls, and tips of lightning and electrical emergencies?**
   1. Rescuers should not become victims.
   2. Start with the ABCs.
   3. Assume the presence of spinal injury.
   4. Remember the iceberg phenomenon.
   5. Bystanders should administer CPR.
   6. Search for occult trauma.
   7. Hydrate high-voltage electric shock victims early.

8. Lightning MCI priority goes to the "dead."
9. Reduce lightning risk by:
   - Avoiding thunderstorms, being the tallest "target," holding a "lightning rod," touching conductors
   - Seeking shelter indoors or in a car
   - Staying away from groups (especially people who know CPR—they are your potential rescuers).
   - Holding feet together and crouching down to reduce your stride potential

WEBSITES

1. National Lightning Safety Institute: www.lightningsafety.com/

2. Lightning Injury Research Program: www.uic.edu/labs/lightninginjury/

3. Lightning and Atmospheric Electricity Research at GHCC: thunder.msfc.nasa.gov/primer/

BIBLIOGRAPHY

1. Arnoldo BD, Purdue GF, Kowalske K, et al: Electrical injuries: A 20-year review. J Burn Care Rehabil 25:479–784, 2004.

2. Bailey B, Gaudreault P, Thivierge RL, Turgeon JP: Cardiac monitoring of children with household electrical injuries. Ann Emerg Med 25:612–617, 1995.

3. Baker R: Paraplegia as a result of lightning injury. BMJ 4:1464–1466, 1978.

4. Brighton P: Lightning injuries revisited. Ann Emerg Med 26:264–265, 1994.

5. Carleton SC: Cardiac problems associated with electrical injury. Cardiol Clin 13:263–266, 1995.

6. Celik A, Ergun O, Ozok G: Pediatric electrical injuries: A review of 38 consecutive patients. J Pediatr Surg 39:1233–1237, 2004.

7. Centers for Disease Control and Prevention: Lightning-associated deaths—United States, 1980–1995. MMWR, 47:391–394, 1998.

8. Cherington M: Lightning injuries. Ann Emerg Med 25:516–519, 1995.

9. Cherington M, Mathys K: Deaths and injuries as a result of lightning strikes to aircraft. Aviat Space Environ Med 66:687–689, 1995.

10. Cherington M, Yarnell PR, London SF: Neurologic complications of lightning injuries. West J Med 162:413–417, 1995.

11. Cooper MA: Emergent care of lightning and electrical injuries. Semin Neurol 15:268–278, 1995.

12. Cooper MA, Andrews CJ, Holle RL, Lopez RE: Lightning injuries. In Auerbach PS (ed): Wilderness Medicine, 4th ed. St. Louis, Mosby-Year Book, 2001, pp 73–110.

13. Duff K, McCaffrey RJ: Electrical injury and lightning injury: A review of their mechanisms and neuropsychological, psychiatric, and neurological sequelae. Neuropsychol Rev 11:101–116, 2001.

14. Duis HJ, Klasen HJ, Reenalda PE: Keraunoparalysis, a "specific" lightning injury. Burns Incl Therm Inj 12:54–57, 1985.

15. Espaillat A, Janigian R Jr, To K: Cataracts, bilateral macular holes, and rhegmatogenous retinal detachment induced by lightning. Am J Ophthalmol 127:216–217, 1999.

16. Fahmy FS, Brinsden MD, Smith J, Frame JD: Lightning: The multisystem group injuries. J Trauma 46:937–940, 1999.

17. Fish R: Electric shock. Part I: Physics and pathophysiology. J Emerg Med 11:309–312, 1993.

18. Fish R: Electric shock. Part II: Nature and mechanism of injury. J Emerg Med 11:457–462, 1993.

19. Fish RM: Electric injury. Part I: Treatment priorities, subtle diagnostic factors, and burns. J Emerg Med 17:977–983, 1999.

20. Fish RM: Electric injury. Part III: Cardiac monitoring indications, the pregnant patient, and lightning. J Emerg Med 18:181–187, 2000.

21. Fontanarosa PB: Electric shock and lightning strike. Ann Emerg Med 22:378–387, 1993.

22. George EN, Schur K, Muller M, et al: Management of high voltage electrical injury in children. Burns 31:439–444, 2005.

23. Jain S, Bandi V: Electrical and lightning injuries. Crit Care Clin 15:319–331, 1999.

24. Koumbourlis AC: Electrical injuries. Crit Care Med 30(11 Suppl):S424–S430, 2002.

25. Lee RC: Injury by electrical forces: Pathophysiology, manifestations, and therapy. Curr Probl Surg 34:677–764, 1997.

26. Martinez JA, Nguyen T: Electrical injuries. South Med J 93:1165–1168, 2000.

27. Milzman DP, Moskowitz L, Hardel M: Lightning strikes at a mass gathering. South Med J 92:708–710, 1999.

28. O'Keefe Gatewood M, Zane RD: Lightning injuries. Emerg Med Clin North Am 22:369–374, 2004.

29. Price TG, Cooper MA: Electrical lightning injuries. In Marx JA, Hockberger RS, Walls RM (eds): Rosen's Emergency Medicine: Concepts and Clinical Practice, 5th ed. St. Louis, Mosby, 1998, pp 2010–2020.

30. Wetli CV: Keraunopathology: an analysis of 45 fatalities. Am J Forens Med Pathol 17:89–98, 1996.

31. Zehender M: Images in clinical medicine. Struck by lightning. N Engl J Med, 330:1492, 1994.

32. Zimmermann C, Cooper MA, Holle RL: Lightning safety guidelines. Ann Emerg Med 39:660–664, 2002.

CHAPTER 55

SUBMERSION INCIDENTS

Jedd Roe, MD, MBA

1. **Define terms associated with submersion accidents.**
Traditional nomenclature applied to submersion incidents has included the following:
- **Drowning** is death by suffocation from submersion in liquid.
- **Near drowning** is survival (at least temporarily) after a submersion event.
- **Immersion syndrome** is sudden death after submersion in very cold water, probably secondary to vagally mediated asystolic cardiac arrest.
- **Wet drownings** are those in which aspiration of water occurred during the event; 80–90% of drownings are classified as wet drownings.
- **Dry drownings** are those in which asphyxia is caused by laryngospasm without aspiration.
In an effort to simplify classification, the use of the term **submersion incident** has been adopted to encompass any adverse event suffered by a patient through submersion in a liquid.

2. **How many people drown?**
Each year in the United States, more than 4000 people die from drowning (>400,000 worldwide). It is the third leading cause of accidental death in all ages. Drowning is the second leading cause of accidental death in persons between 5 and 44 years old, exceeded only by motor vehicle fatalities. An estimated 50,000 persons annually survive a submersion event.

3. **Who drowns and why?**
The incidence of drowning peaks in two groups—teenagers and toddlers. In **teenagers** (ages 15–24), nearly 80% of drowning and submersion victims are male. Teenage boys are victims because of risk-taking behavior during swimming, boating, diving, or other water-related activities. Alcohol is a contributing factor in more than 60% of all teenage drownings.
   Of all drowning victims, 40% are younger than 4 years. **Toddlers** are at risk because of their inherently inquisitive nature and their physical inability to extricate themselves from hazards such as pools, buckets, tubs, toilets, or washers. Inadequate supervision, even for brief moments, is the primary cause of drowning in toddlers. One always must consider the possibility of abuse when evaluating a child drowning victim, because inflicted submersions account for 1.5–8% of all events for children younger than age 5. An estimated 59% of drownings in persons younger than 1 year occur in bathtubs, and 56% of these are a result of child abuse.
   Other risk factors in all age groups are as follows:
- Inability to swim
- Seizures
- Trauma
- Ethanol
- Hyperventilation
- Substance abuse
- Hot tubs/spas
- Hypothermia
- Cardiovascular or cerebrovascular disease
- Child abuse/neglect
- Diabetes
- Suicide

   In the United States, 50,000 new pools are added annually to the 4.5 million pools that already exist. The increasing prevalence of hot tubs, pleasure craft, and outdoor sports has increased greatly the number of persons at risk of drowning. Of drownings, 90% occur tantalizingly close to safety, within 10 yards.

Feldhaus KM: Submersion. In Marx JA (ed): Rosen's Emergency Medicine: Concepts and Clinical Practice, 5th ed. St. Louis, Mosby, 2002, pp 2050–2055.

4. **What kills a drowning victim?**

Historically, emphasis has been placed incorrectly on the significance of drowning in salt water versus fresh water because of presumed differences in the pathophysiology of the aspirated water. In fresh-water aspirations, the hypotonic fluid was thought to diffuse into the circulation, increasing blood volume and decreasing the concentration of serum electrolytes. This also causes a loss of surfactant and results in alveolar collapse. Sea water was thought to pull fluid into the alveoli, decreasing the blood volume and increasing the electrolyte concentrations. This transudated fluid would cause a pathologic effect on pulmonary alveolar membranes, causing noncardiogenic pulmonary edema. In humans, such pathologic changes have rarely been seen in patients who have survived to hospital arrival. It has been suggested that a person must ingest 22 mL/kg to cause electrolyte changes, and it is unusual that submersion victims take in more than 3–4 mL/kg.

Of submersion victims, 10–20% have not aspirated water, and most victims of submersion do not aspirate enough fluid to cause a significant alteration in blood volume or electrolytes or a life-threatening pulmonary shunt secondary to perfusion of fluid-filled alveoli. Death is most often the result of asphyxia caused by laryngospasm and glottis closure. Although this mechanism is less common, more successful resuscitations (80–90% of all patients) occur in this group of patients. The aspirated water is a significant pulmonary irritant and contaminant, however, that may increase intrapulmonary shunting, resulting in hypoxemia.

Newman AB: Submersion incidents. In Auerbach PS (ed): Wilderness Emergency Medicine, 4th ed. St. Louis, Mosby, 2001, pp 1340–1365.

5. **What happens in a drowning?**

The first event is an unexpected or prolonged submersion. The victim begins to struggle and panic. Fatigue begins, and air hunger develops. Reflex inspiration ultimately overrides breath holding. The victim swallows water, and aspiration occurs, causing laryngospasm that may last for several minutes. Hypoxemia worsens, and unconsciousness ensues. If the victim is not rescued and resuscitated promptly, central nervous system damage begins within minutes.

6. **Describe the presenting symptoms.**

The presenting pulmonary symptoms are varied. The patient may be completely asymptomatic, have a mild cough, show mild dyspnea and tachypnea, or be in fulminant pulmonary edema. The clinical spectrum of central nervous system findings may range from confusion or lethargy to coma. Some patients may be found in cardiac arrest.

7. **What is the pulmonary pathophysiology?**

The central clinical feature of *all* submersion incidents is hypoxemia caused by laryngospasm or aspiration. The PO_2 decreases; the PCO_2 increases, and there is a combined respiratory and metabolic acidosis. If the patient is successfully resuscitated, the recovery phase often is complicated by aspirated water or vomitus. Aspiration can cause airway obstruction by particulates, bronchospasm by direct irritation, Acute respiratory distress syndrome (ARDS) due to pulmonary edema from parenchymal damage, atelectasis from loss of surfactant, and pulmonary bacterial infections. Some patients may later develop pulmonary abscesses or empyema.

Salomez F, Vincent JL: Drowning: A review of epidemiology, pathophysiology, treatment, and prevention. Resuscitation 63:261–268, (2004).

8. **How is the cardiac system affected in drowning?**

Cardiac decompensation and arrhythmias are caused by hypoxemia and complicated by the ensuing acidosis. The heart is relatively resistant to hypoxic injury, and successful resumption of cardiac activity is common, but severe central nervous system damage often occurs. Response of the heart to therapy, particularly antiarrhythmic medications, may be limited by hypoxia, acidosis, and hypothermia. Primary therapy is aimed at reversal of these three problems.

9. **What is the prehospital treatment?**
The most important part of treatment of a near-drowning victim is delivered in the prehospital phase with immediate resuscitation. If a submersion victim has appropriate airway management and ventilation is rapidly established, anoxic brain injury is avoided, and prompt and full recovery is anticipated. The patient without rapid airway management and ventilation suffers irreversible anoxic brain injury and either is unresponsive to resuscitation or has a progressively deteriorating course after initial resuscitation. Therapy must correct hypoxia, associated acidosis, and hypotension as rapidly as possible. Establish a patent airway using appropriate cervical spine precautions if indicated because diving injuries often are associated with cervical spine injury. Apply a nonrebreather oxygen mask to patients with spontaneous respirations. Initiate bag-valve-mask breathing or endotracheal intubation if indicated. Correct hypoxia and acidosis by hyperventilation with 100% oxygen. Intravenous (IV) access is needed.

Of particular note is that there is no convincing evidence for the effectiveness of postural drainage maneuvers, and their use is not recommended.

10. **When is endotracheal intubation indicated?**
Any person with altered mentation or an inability to protect the airway needs intubation. In the initially stable patient, an inability to maintain a pO_2 greater than 60–90 mmHg with high flow oxygen by nonrebreather mask indicates that extensive pulmonary compromise or ARDS may exist, and early airway management with positive-pressure ventilation and positive end-expiratory pressure is appropriate to decrease intrapulmonary shunting.

One important point is to determine if the submersion event may have occurred as a result of diving into water. This patient may have suffered a cervical spine injury, and appropriate precautions should be taken with in-line stabilization of the neck during intubation.

11. **If aspiration is suspected, what treatment is needed?**
Pulmonary treatment is supportive. Close observation for signs of a developing pulmonary infection or ARDS is needed. Some cases with significant aspirations may require bronchoscopy to remove particulate matter and tenacious secretions. Bronchodilator therapy with beta agonists is appropriate if bronchospasm is evident.

12. **Does a normal chest radiograph rule out pulmonary injury?**
No. A normal chest radiograph may be seen in 20% of cases. Typical findings include perihilar infiltrates and pulmonary edema, although these classic descriptors of ARDS (noncardiogenic pulmonary edema) may take hours to develop.

13. **Is there a role for prophylactic antibiotics or glucocorticoids?**
When contaminated water is involved (e.g., sewage), prophylactic antibiotics may be considered. In all other instances, prophylactic antibiotics are of no proven benefit. Glucocorticoids are of no proven benefit.

14. **Is there an indication for the use of sodium bicarbonate during resuscitation?**
No. Respiratory and metabolic acidosis should be treated by mechanical ventilation and hyperventilation.

15. **Discuss the approach to patients with a decreased level of consciousness or coma.**

Hypoxic injury leads to cerebral edema and a concomitant rise in intracranial pressure. Although there was initial enthusiasm for treatment of presumed elevated intracranial pressure with the usual modalities of muscle paralysis, hyperventilation, mannitol, barbiturate coma, hypothermia, and steroids, more recent studies have shown no improvement in outcome with these therapies. Supportive care is the mainstay of therapy. Be attentive to the possibility of cranial or spinal injuries in all boating or diving injuries. Do not forget the possibility of suicide or child abuse. If the history is in doubt, assume a cranial and a cervical injury. The possibility of toxicologic conditions also should be investigated with appropriate toxicologic screens performed.

16. **Are glucocorticoids, barbiturate coma, or induced hypothermia indicated?**

In the case of glucocorticoids and barbiturate coma, *no*. These therapies are unproven and remain controversial. However, therapeutic hypothermia has recently been shown to be of benefit in cardiac arrest, and case reports have suggested similar outcomes for victims of submersion.

Williamson JP, Illing R, Gertler P, et al: Near-drowning treated with therapeutic hypothermia. Med J Aust 181:500–501, 2004.

17. **What is unique about cold-water submersion?**

Cases in which victims of prolonged submersion in cold water have been resuscitated successfully without apparent neurologic sequelae are reported occasionally. The number remains small, however. Sudden submersion in cold water theoretically induces the mammalian diving reflex, in which blood is shunted from the periphery to the central core. The induced hypothermia causes a decrease in metabolic demand, reducing potential hypoxic injury from prolonged asphyxia. Cold water does have potentially deleterious effects. Most significant are the induced cardiac irritability from hypothermia, exhaustion, and altered mental status. Resuscitation of hypothermic near-drowning victims should be continued until patients are adequately rewarmed or to the level required for therapeutic hypothermia (see Chapter 56).

18. **When should resuscitative efforts be withheld?**

Generally, all patients should receive initial resuscitative efforts. One child recovered successfully from a 66-minute submersion in cold water, and other studies have reported that patients requiring cardiopulmonary resuscitation (CPR) in the field may make a full recovery. When their core temperature has normalized and therapeutic efforts remain unsuccessful, patients can be pronounced dead.

19. **What is the disposition of a submersion victim?**

All submersion victims deserve aggressive in-hospital resuscitation until all reasonable efforts prove futile and the patient is near normothermic. All other submersion victims require close observation. Some respiratory complications of drowning are delayed in presentation and usually appear within 8 hours. A patient with any respiratory complaints or symptoms, chest radiograph abnormalities, or a demonstrated oxygen requirement should be monitored closely in a hospital for at least 24 hours. Similarly, any patient who received resuscitative efforts or had a reported loss of consciousness, cyanosis, or apnea should be monitored closely. Patients without any symptoms and completely normal evaluation may be discharged after 6–8 hours of observation with instructions to return immediately if respiratory distress ensues.

KEY POINTS: SUBMERSION INCIDENTS

1. Toddlers and teenagers are most at risk for death due to submersion.

2. Prehospital treatment is critical and directed at correcting underlying hypoxia.

3. A normal chest radiograph does not rule out pulmonary injury.

4. All asymptomatic victims of submersion must be observed at least 6–8 hours prior to discharge.

5. Many submersion incidents are preventable.

---

20. **What are the most important factors in estimating prognosis?**

The most important factor in determining outcome is the patient's response to resuscitation as measured by serial neurologic examinations. Poor prognostic factors include a Glasgow Coma Scale score less than or equal to 5, prolonged submersion (>5 minutes), delay in initiating CPR, pH less than 7.0, water temperatures of greater than 10°C (77°F), and asystole on arrival to the emergency department (ED). Patients who arrive aware and alert have a 100% complete neurologic recovery, whereas 95% of arousable patients with altered mentation have a complete neurologic recovery.

Szpilman has proposed a clinical classification based on the analysis of 1831 cases of submersion seen in Brazil over a 19-year period. The classification is based on clinical findings in the field, and the mortalities are shown in Table 55-1.

Szpilman D: Near-drowning and drowning classification: A proposal to stratify mortality based on the analysis of 1,831 cases. Chest 112:660–665, (1997).

TABLE 55-1.	SZPILMAN CLASSIFICATION OF NEAR-DROWNING AND DROWNING	
Grade	Clinical Findings	Mortality Rate (%)
1	Normal pulmonary auscultation ± cough	0
2	Rales or crackles in some lung fields	0.6
3	Crackles in all fields without hypotension	5.2
4	Crackles in all fields with hypotension	19.4
5	Respiratory arrest without cardiac arrest	44
6	Cardiopulmonary arrest	93

21. **Can we prevent submersion incidents?**

Many of the factors contributing to death by submersion *are* preventable and can be directed at those groups at risk, particularly children. Efforts can be directed at the following:

- Fencing of private and public swimming pools
- The use of personal flotation devices
- Improving supervision of infants and young children near water
- Increasing public knowledge of the risks of the day's water conditions
- Understanding the limitations of personal health conditions
- Stressing the separation of alcohol from water-related activities.

WEBSITE

Shepard S, Martin J: Submersion injury, near drowning:
www.emedicine.com/emerg/topic744.htm

BIBLIOGRAPHY

1. Feldhaus KM: Submersion. In Marx JA (ed): Rosen's Emergency Medicine: Concepts and Clinical Practice, 5th ed. St. Louis, Mosby, 2002, pp 2050–2055.

2. Newman AB: Submersion incidents. In Auerbach PS (ed): Wilderness Emergency Medicine, 4th ed. St. Louis, Mosby, 2001, pp 1340–1365.

3. Olshaker JS: Submersion. Emerg Med Clin North Am 22:357–367, 2004.

4. Salomez F, Vincent JL: Drowning: A review of epidemiology, pathophysiology, treatment, and prevention. Resuscitation 63:261–268, 2004.

5. Williamson JP, Illing R, Gertler P, et al: Near-drowning treated with therapeutic hypothermia. Med J Aust 181:500–501, 2004.

CHAPTER 56

HYPOTHERMIA AND FROSTBITE

Daniel F. Danzl, MD

HYPOTHERMIA

1. **What is accidental hypothermia?**
   An unintentional decrease in core temperature to less than *35* °C (95 °F). The preoptic anterior hypothalamus normally maintains a diurnal temperature variation within 1 °C.

2. **What factors are important in the epidemiology of hypothermia?**
   Primary accidental hypothermia results from direct exposure to the cold. Secondary hypothermia is a natural complication of many systemic disorders, including sepsis, cancer, and trauma. The mortality of secondary hypothermia is much higher. Outdoor exposure is not the only threat to thermostability. Many victims are found indoors, in particular, the elderly.

3. **How is body temperature normally regulated?**
   The normal physiology of temperature regulation is activated by cold exposure, producing reflex vasoconstriction and stimulating the hypothalamic nuclei. Heat preservation mechanisms include shivering, autonomic and endocrinologic responses, and adaptive behavioral responses. Although acclimatization to heat stress is efficient, humans can't acclimate to a "three-dog night."

KEY POINTS: COMMON MECHANISMS OF HEAT LOSS

1. Radiation

2. Conduction

3. Convection

4. Respiration

5. Evaporation

4. **Describe the common findings in mild, moderate, and severe hypothermia.**
   - **Mild hypothermia** (32.2–35°C [90–95°F]) depresses the central nervous system and increases the metabolic rate, pulse, and amount of shivering thermogenesis. Dysarthria, amnesia, ataxia, and apathy are common findings.
   - **Moderate hypothermia** (27–32.2°C [80–90°F]) progressively depresses the level of consciousness and the vital signs. Shivering is extinguished, and arrhythmias commonly develop. The QT interval is prolonged, and a J wave (Osborn wave) may appear at the junction of the QRS complex and ST segment. Patients become poikilothermic and cannot rewarm

spontaneously. A cold diuresis results from an initial central hypervolemia, which is caused by the peripheral vasoconstriction.

- **Severe hypothermia** (27°C [80°F]) results in coma and areflexia with profoundly depressed vital signs. Carbon dioxide production decreases 50% for each 8°C fall in temperature; there is little respiratory stimulation.

5. **What three factors predispose to hypothermia?**
   - Decreased heat production
   - Increased heat loss
   - Impaired thermoregulation

6. **What decreases heat production?**
   Decreased heat production is common (1) at the age extremes, (2) with inadequate stored fuel, or (3) with endocrinologic or neuromuscular inefficiency. Neonates are poorly adapted for cold, even without being subjected to emergent deliveries and resuscitations. The elderly have progressively impaired thermal perception. Anything from simple hypoglycemia to more severe malnutrition represents a threat to the core temperature. Examples of endocrinologic failure include myxedema, hypopituitarism, and hypoadrenalism.

7. **What are the common causes of increased heat loss?**
   Increased heat loss results mainly from exposure or dermatologic problems that interfere with the skin's integrity. Iatrogenic causes include emergency childbirth, cold infusions, and heat-stroke treatment.

8. **How is thermoregulation impaired?**
   Impairment is via central, peripheral, metabolic, or pharmacologic mechanisms. A variety of central nervous system processes affect hypothalamic function. Traumatic or neoplastic lesions, degenerative processes, and congenital anomalies induce hypothermia. Acute spinal cord transection extinguishes peripheral vasoconstriction, which prevents heat conservation. The abnormal plasma osmolality common with metabolic derangements, including diabetic ketoacidosis and uremia, is an additional cause. Innumerable medications and toxins can impair central thermoregulation when present in either therapeutic or toxic doses.

9. **When should hypothermia be suspected?**
   The diagnosis is simple when a history of exposure is obvious. The history may not be available or helpful, however, and subtle presentations are far more common in urban areas. Ataxia and dysarthria may mimic a cerebrovascular accident or intoxication. The only safe way to avoid missing the diagnosis is to routinely measure the patient's temperature.

10. **Are there decoys that confuse the physical examination?**
    If there is a tachycardia disproportionate for the temperature, suspect hypoglycemia, hypovolemia, or an overdose. Hyperventilation, which is inappropriate during moderate or severe hypothermia, suggests a central nervous system lesion or one of the systemic acidoses, such as diabetic ketoacidosis or lactic acidosis. A cold-induced rectus spasm and ileus may mask or mimic an acute abdomen. Suspect an overdose or central nervous system insult whenever the decreased level of consciousness is not consistent with the temperature.

11. **What options are available to measure the core temperature?**
    Rectal, esophageal, tympanic, and bladder sites can be measured. The rectal temperature may lag or be falsely low if the probe is in cold feces. Esophageal temperature is falsely elevated during heated inhalation. The reliability of tympanic measurements is unclear.

12. **How does temperature depression affect the hematologic evaluation of patients?**
    Anemia is masked because the hematocrit increases 2% per 1°C drop in temperature. Do not rely on leukocytosis to predict sepsis because the leukocytes often are sequestered. There are no safe predictors of values. The increased viscosity seen with cold hemagglutination often results in either thrombosis or hemolysis, and a type of disseminated intravascular coagulation syndrome can occur. Coagulopathies are not reflected by the deceptively normal prothrombin or partial thromboplastin time or International Normalized Ratio because these tests are done routinely on blood rewarmed to 37°C.

13. **Should arterial blood gases be corrected for temperature?**
    No. Correction implies acidosis is beneficial. An uncorrected pH of 7.4 and pCO_2 of 40 mmHg confirm acid-base balance at all temperatures.

14. **What is the key decision regarding rewarming?**
    The primary initial decision is whether to rewarm the patient passively or actively. Passive rewarming is noninvasive and involves simply covering the patient in a warm environment. This technique is ideal for previously healthy patients with mild hypothermia.

15. **What conditions mandate active rewarming?**
    - Cardiovascular instability
    - Temperature < 32.2°C (90°F)
    - Age extremes
    - Neurologic or endocrinologic insufficiency

16. **What is core temperature afterdrop?**
    The commonly observed continued drop in core temperature after initiation of rewarming. There are two causes: (1) temperature equilibration between tissues and (2) the circulatory return of cold peripheral blood to the core.

17. **Are there unique considerations with active external rewarming?**
    The external transfer of heat to a patient is accomplished most safely when the heat is applied directly to the trunk. In chronically hypothermic patients, rapidly rewarming the vasoconstricted extremities may overwhelm a depressed cardiovascular system and result in cardiovascular collapse. Monitoring in a heated tub can be difficult, and vasoconstricted skin is burned easily by electric blankets. Forced heated air rewarmers are commonly used.

18. **What constitutes active core rewarming?**
    Techniques that deliver heat directly to the core. Options include heated inhalation, heated infusion, lavage, and extracorporeal rewarming.

19. **When is airway rewarming indicated?**
    Heated, humidified oxygen is always helpful and can be administered via mask or endotracheal tube. Heat transfer is not as significant by mask, but respiratory heat loss is eliminated while the patient is rewarmed gradually.

20. **What are the techniques for heated irrigation?**
    Heat transfer from irrigation of the gastrointestinal tract is minimal. Irrigation should be considered only in severe cases and in combination with other techniques. Thoracostomy tube irrigation with two tubes is a more efficient alternative in severe cases. Intravenous (IV) fluids heated to 40–42°C are particularly helpful during major volume resuscitations.

21. **When should heated peritoneal lavage be considered?**
Double-catheter peritoneal lavage can efficiently rewarm seriously hypothermic patients. This invasive technique generally should be reserved for severely hypothermic and unstable patients. Infuse 2 L of isotonic dialysate at 40–45°C, and suction after 20 minutes.

22. **When is extracorporeal rewarming indicated?**
Cardiopulmonary bypass, continuous arteriovenous and venovenous rewarming, and hemodialysis can be life saving in cardiac arrest situations. Patients with completely frozen extremities, severe rhabdomyolysis, and major electrolyte fluxes are also easier to manage in this manner.

23. **What are the contraindications to cardiopulmonary resuscitation (CPR) in accidental hypothermia?**
CPR should be initiated unless do-not-resuscitate status is verified, lethal injuries are identified, any signs of life are present, or the chest wall is frozen and cannot be compressed. Because a profoundly hypothermic patient may appear dead, and because vital signs may be difficult to obtain, a cardiac monitor should be applied for at least 60 seconds to ensure that there are no signs of life.

24. **Are there unique pharmacologic considerations during hypothermia?**
Protein binding increases as body temperature drops, and most drugs become ineffective. Pharmacologic manipulation of the pulse and blood pressure generally should be avoided.

25. **What is the significance of atrial and ventricular arrhythmias?**
Atrial arrhythmias normally have a slow ventricular response. They are innocent and should be left untreated. Preexistent ventricular ectopy may resurface during rewarming and can confuse the picture. Ventricular arrhythmia treatment is problematic, because bretylium is no longer available. If the patient is in ventricular fibrillation, only one defibrillation attempt (2 J/kg) is indicated until the core temperature exceeds 30°–32°C.

FROSTBITE

26. **What is frostbite?**
Frostbite is the most common freezing injury of tissue. It occurs whenever the tissue temperature decreases to less than 0°C. Ice crystal formation damages the cellular architecture, and stasis progresses to microvascular thrombosis.

27. **Which factors predispose to frostbite?**
Tissue rapidly freezes when in contact with good thermal conductors, including metal, water, and volatiles. Direct exposure to cold wind (wind-chill index) quickly freezes acral areas (fingers, toes, ears, nose). A variety of conditions can impair the peripheral circulation and predispose to frostbite. Constrictive clothing and immobility reduce heat delivery to the distal tissues. Vasoconstrictive medications, including nicotine, can exacerbate cold damage, especially when coupled with underlying vascular conditions, such as atherosclerosis.

28. **What peripheral circulatory changes precede frostbite?**
Humans possess a *life-versus-limb* mechanism that helps prevent systemic hypothermia. Arteriovenous anastomoses in the skin shunt blood away from acral areas to limit radiative heat loss.

29. **Before frostbite occurs, what other cutaneous events take place in the prefreeze phase?**

    As tissue temperatures decrease to less than 10°C, anesthesia develops. Endothelial cells leak plasma, and microvascular vasoconstriction occurs. Crystallization is not seen as long as the deeper tissues conduct and radiate heat.

30. **What happens during the freeze phase of frostbite?**

    The type of exposure determines the rate and location of ice crystal formation. Usually, ice initially forms extracellularly, causing water to exit the cell and inducing cellular dehydration, hyperosmolality, collapse, and death.

31. **Immediately after thawing, what may occur?**

    In deep frostbite, progressive microvascular collapse develops. Sludging, stasis, and cessation of flow begin in the capillaries and progress to the venules and the arterioles. The tissues are deprived of oxygen and nutrients. Plasma leakage and arteriovenous shunting increase tissue pressures and result in thrombosis, ischemia, and necrosis.

32. **What is progressive dermal ischemia?**

    This is an additional insult to potentially viable tissue that is partially mediated by thromboxane. Arachidonic acid breakdown products are released from underlying damaged tissue into the blister fluid. The prostaglandins and thromboxanes produce platelet aggregation and vasoconstriction.

33. **What delayed physiologic events occur?**

    Edema progresses for 2–3 days. As the edema resolves, early necrosis becomes apparent if nonviable tissue is present. Final demarcation often is delayed for more than 60–90 days. Hence the aphorism, "Frostbite in January, amputate in July."

34. **What are the symptoms of frostbite?**

    Sensory deficits are always present, affecting light touch, pain, and temperature perception. *Frostnip* produces only a transient numbness and tingling. This is not true frostbite because there is no tissue destruction. In severe cases, patients report a "chunk of wood" sensation and clumsiness.

35. **What imaging techniques might help assess frostbite severity?**

    Routine radiography at presentation and later at 4–10 weeks post injury may demonstrate specific abnormalities. Scintigraphy may predict tissue loss and monitor the efficacy of treatment. Magnetic resonance angiography can also predict tissue demarcation.

36. **What are chilblain (PERNIO)?**

    Repetitive exposure to dry cold can induce chilblain (cold sores), especially in young women. Pruritus, erythema, and mild edema may evolve into plaques, blue nodules, and ulcerations. The face and dorsa of the hands and feet are commonly affected.

37. **What is trench foot?**

    Prolonged exposure to wet cold above freezing results in trench foot (immersion foot). Initially, the feet appear edematous, cold, and cyanotic. The subsequent development of vesiculation may mimic frostbite. Liquefaction gangrene is a more common sequela, however, with trench foot than with frostbite.

38. **How should frostbite be classified?**

    Classification by degrees as is done with burns is unnecessary and is often prognostically incorrect. Superficial or mild frostbite does not result in actual tissue loss; deep or severe frostbite does.

39. What do the various signs of frostbite indicate?

The initial presentation of frostbite can be deceptively benign. Frozen tissues appear yellow, waxy, mottled, or violaceous-white. Favorable signs include normal sensation, warmth, and color after thawing. Early clear bleb formation is more favorable than delayed hemorrhagic blebs. These result from damage to the subdermal vascular plexi. Lack of edema formation also suggests major tissue damage.

40. How should frozen tissues be thawed?

Rapid, complete thawing by immersion in 40–41°C circulating water is ideal. Reestablishment of perfusion is intensely painful, and parenteral narcotics are needed in severe cases. Premature termination of thawing is a common mistake because an incomplete thaw increases tissue loss. Never use dry heat or allow tissues to refreeze. Rubbing or friction massage may be harmful.

KEY POINTS: COMMON SEQUELAE OF FROSTBITE

1. Paresthesias

2. Hyperhidrosis

3. Thermal misperception

4. Epiphyseal damage

5. Nail deformities

41. What steps should immediately follow thawing?

- Handle tissues gently, and elevate the injured parts to minimize edema formation.
- If cyanosis is still present after thawing, monitor the tissue compartment pressures.
- Consider streptococcal and tetanus prophylaxis.
- Avoid compressive dressings, and use daily whirlpool hydrotherapy.
- Consider phenoxybenzamine (Dibenzyline) in severe cases.
- Whenever possible, defer surgical decisions regarding amputation until clear demarcation is demonstrated.
- Magnetic resonance angiography may predict demarcation earlier than clinical demarcation.

42. How are blisters treated?

Clear blisters may temporarily be left intact or sterilely aspirated. After debridement, apply antibiotic ointment or a specific thromboxane inhibitor, topical aloe vera (Dermaide). When coupled with systemic ibuprofen. this strategy can minimize accumulation of arachidonic acid breakdown products. In contrast, hemorrhagic blisters should be left intact to prevent tissue desiccation.

43. Are any ancillary treatment modalities really helpful?

A variety of antithrombotic and vasodilatory treatment regimens have been tried, including medical and surgical sympathectomies. These modalities, plus dextran, heparin, and a variety of anti-inflammatory agents, have not conclusively increased tissue salvage.

WEBSITES

1. www.hypothermia.org

2. www.emedicine.com

CHAPTER 57

HEAT ILLNESS

Brandon H. Anderson, MD, and David J. Vukich, MD

1. **What area of the brain is considered the body's thermostat for heat regulation?**
   The anterior hypothalamus.

2. **List the four methods of transferring heat from the body to the environment.**
   - **Radiation.** Infrared energy is radiated directly into the environment.
   - **Conduction.** Whenever the body touches a surface that is cooler than itself, heat is transferred to that object by conduction.
   - **Convection.** Air moving over the surface of the skin, even imperceptibly, carries heat away.
   - **Evaporation.** The water in perspiration changing from its liquid state to its gaseous state is the most effective means of heat loss to the environment.

3. **List the three organ systems primarily responsible for heat loss.**
   - **Skin.** Vasodilatation allows skin blood flow to increase 25–30 times from baseline, making the surface of the skin the primary location of heat loss.
   - **Cardiovascular system.** Increased cardiac output and vasoconstriction of the renal and splanchnic vasculature allow for the increase in skin blood flow.
   - **Respiratory system.** In humans there is a small, almost negligible amount of evaporative cooling through respiration.

4. **What is the most efffective method of cooling in humans? How does high humidity affect this method?**
   Evaporation of perspiration is the primary and most effective method of cooling, normally releasing 1 kcal for each 1.7 mL of perspiration. As humidity rises, perspiration evaporates more slowly, accumulating in clothing or rolling off the body. Less and less cooling is accomplished, and, eventually, at very high humidity, perspiration becomes totally ineffective.

5. **What is the range of heat illness manifestations, from least to most serious?**
   - **Heat edema.** Seasonal, transient, dependent extremity swelling, nuisance only
   - **Heat syncope.** Results from volume depletion, peripheral vasodilatation, and decreased motor tone. Usually responds to oral/intravenous (IV) fluids
   - **Heat cramps.** Painful, easily treated, acclimation occurs
   - **Heat exhaustion.** Serious but no organ damage, mild hyperpyrexia
   - **Heatstroke.** Critical, organ damage, significant mortality, markedly elevated body temperature

   Lugo-Amador N, Rothenhaus T, Moyer P: Heat-related illness. Emerg Med Clin North Am 22:315–327, 2004.

6. **What are heat cramps? How are they treated?**
   Heat cramps are painful contractions of the larger muscle groups of the body, usually the calves and thighs, that occur during or shortly after strenuous exercise in the heat. These cramps are

usually caused by the replacement of water without adequate salt, resulting in a hyponatremic state in the muscles and, eventually, painful large muscle contractions.

The treatment of choice is fluid and electrolyte replacement by oral and/or IV administration of normal saline. Changes in mental status or fever are not associated with heat cramps and indicate more serious heat illness.

7. **Define heat exhaustion.**

   Heat exhaustion is a more serious heat syndrome caused by either **water depletion** or **salt depletion** in the face of heat stress. It results in nausea, vomiting, light-headedness, mild hyperpyrexia, and signs of dehydration with only minimally altered mental status. The salt depletion type arises when fluid losses are replaced with only water, with subsequent hyponatremia and relatively decreased intravascular volume. The water depletion type is more dangerous, progressing rapidly to dehydration and heatstroke if not reversed. The prognosis for both types is good if treated promptly.

8. **How is heat exhaustion treated?**

   Cooling is the primary therapy, and this is accomplished simply by removing the patient from the heat source to recover in a cool area with oral rehydration. IV fluids are required in patients who are vomiting, have abnormal vital signs, or show clinical signs of dehydration. Serum electrolyte levels should be determined, and those results should guide subsequent fluid therapy and electrolyte repletion if needed.

9. **Define heatstroke.**

   Heatstroke is defined clinically by a core body temperature above 40°C (104°F) accompanied by central nervous system (CNS) abnormalities such as delirium, seizures, and coma. If left untreated, renal failure, disseminated intravascular coagulation (DIC), hepatic dysfunction, and ultimately fulminant multisystem organ failure will result.

   Bouchama A, Knochel J: Heat stroke. N Engl J Med 346:1978–198, 2002.

10. **What is the basic pathophysiologic mechanism for heatstroke?**

    Heatstroke results from a failure of the body's thermoregulatory mechanisms to dissipate body heat, causing markedly elevated body temperature and resulting in multisystem organ damage and failure. The source of heat stress is exogenous. The risk for developing heatstroke increases when the heat index (how it "really feels" when air temperature is combined with humidity) is 105°F (40.5°C) or greater. Conditions such as volume depletion, impaired cardiac reserve, systemic vasoconstriction from concurrent illnesses, and drugs that cause anhydrosis (i.e., anticholinergics, phenothiazines) significantly impair the body's ability to dissipate heat and put patients at risk for developing heat stroke.

    There are three mechanisms in which excessive heat stress can damage the body:
    - Heat is directly toxic to cells. Temperatures above 42°C (107.6°F) can produce cellular injury and death in just a few hours.
    - Heat stress results in a release of inflammatory cytokines and endotoxins that interfere with normal thermoregulation and vascular tone.
    - Elevated temperatures cause injury to vascular endothelium, resulting in increased permeability, activation of the coagulation cascade, and DIC.

    These mechanisms cause a systemic inflammatory response syndrome, which results in multiorgan sytem failure in which CNS dysfunction predominates.

    Bouchama A, Knochel J: Heat stroke. N Engl J Med 346:1978–1988, 2002.

11. **How do marathon runners and well-trained athletes prevent heat stroke during exercise?**

    During exercise, these individuals can tolerate extreme core temperatures, sometimes as high as 41.6°C (106.9°F)! They do this through a process known as acclimation. Over several weeks, the body can adapt to extreme heat environments by improving cardiac performance, expanding plasma volume, and enhancing the renin-angiotensin-aldosterone system, increasing the ability to retain salt and prevent volume depletion.

12. **Describe the types of heat stroke. How are they manifested?**

Heatstroke may be categorized as classic or exertional. **Classic heatstroke** usually involves an elderly or debilitated patient, in an urban setting without access to air conditioning, who is exposed passively to significant thermal stress. These persons generally do not have the ability to remove themselves from the heat and are exposed to it over many hours or days. Their ability to respond to the heat stress is compromised, and their normal thermoregulatory mechanisms are overwhelmed. These victims frequently have been perspiring for a prolonged length of time, and they are extremely dehydrated. Other groups at risk are the very young (age <4 years); those with cardiovascular diseases, neurologic diseases, or endocrine disorders; and those with previous heatstroke.

Exertional heatstroke occurs in a younger, usually physically fit population with normal thermoregulatory systems. Because of severe exogenous heat stress and concomitant exertional heat production, the body's heat loss mechanisms are rapidly overwhelmed. Frequently, these victims are not dehydrated and may be wet with perspiration when they are seen. Nonetheless, their body temperatures are elevated significantly.

Both forms of heat illness are associated with significant changes in mental status and involvement of multiple organ systems.

Lu KC, Wang JY, Lin SH, et al: Role of circulating cytokines and chemokines in exertional heatstroke. Crit Care Med 32:399–403, 2004.

13. **Which medications increase the risk of heatstroke?**

Psychotropics (i.e., haloperidol), anti-Parkinson's agents, tranquilizers (i.e., phenothiazines), and diuretics all increase the risk of heatstroke. Caffeine, alcohol, and illicit drugs (i.e., ecstasy, cocaine) also lower the threshold for developing heat illness.

14. **Which organ systems are primarily affected in heatstroke?**

All organ systems may be affected, but four predominate:

- **Central nervous system.** Altered mental status is always present, sometimes with posturing, paralysis, or seizures. As the hyperpyrexia continues, coma eventually may ensue.
- **Cardiovascular system.** High-output congestive heart failure, pulmonary edema, and, eventually, complete cardiovascular collapse occur.
- **Hepatic system.** Central lobular hepatic necrosis occurs with high temperatures.
- **Renal system.** Exertional heatstroke frequently leads to rhabdomyolysis and acute tubular necrosis. These effects are less common with classic heatstroke.

15. **What abnormal laboratory values are expected with heatstroke?**

Although nearly all organ systems and laboratory values eventually may be affected, elevation of hepatic enzymes is consistent and can occur early. Urinalysis frequently shows elevated specific gravity, many cells, and, in exertional heatstroke, myoglobin and lactic acidosis. Complete blood cell count (CBC) and clotting studies may indicate DIC, and creatine phosphokinase (CPK) may be significantly elevated.

Hassanein T, Razack A, Gavaler J, Van Thiel DH: Heatstroke: Its clinical and pathological presentation with particular attention to the liver. Am J Gastroenterol 87:1382–1389, 1992.

16. **State the primary goal in the treatment of heatstroke.**

In addition to supporting the **ABCs** (airway, breathing, and circulation), the most important therapeutic goal is to lower the patient's body temperature to less than 101°F (38.8°C) within 1 hour. Morbidity and mortality are directly related to the duration of hyperpyrexia.

17. **Have any medications been shown to accelerate cooling and improve outcome in heat stroke?**

No pharmacologic agents have been proven to be beneficial in managing heat stroke. Although dantrolene sodium has been postulated to accelerate cooling rates, no studies have shown it to be effective. The routine use of antipyretic agents has not been evaluated. Excessive shivering and seizures should be treated with benzodiazepines. New research using immunomodulators show promising results in animals but have yet to be studied in adults.

Hadad E, Cohen-Sivan Y, Heled Y, Epstein Y: Clinical review: Treatment of heat stroke: Should dantrolene be considered? Crit Care 9:86–91, 2005.

KEY POINTS: HEAT STROKE

1. Heat stroke is defined as a core body temperature $> 40°C$ and central nervous system dysfunction.

2. The most effective means of cooling the body is through evaporation.

3. Rapid core temperature reduction is the most important aspect of treatment for heat stroke and is directly related to morbidity and mortality.

4. Heat stroke can be viewed as causing a systemic inflammatory response syndrome resulting in multisystem organ failure with central nervous system dysfunction predominating.

18. **Describe the most effective means of lowering the body temperature in heatstroke.**

The rapid cooling of heatstroke patients can be achieved by either immersion therapy or evaporation. Evaporation tends to be the most practical and effective in the emergency department (ED) setting. Treatment should begin immediately. The patient must be removed from the thermal heat stress, disrobed, and wrapped in wet towels during transport. In the ED, warm water mist is applied to the patient's exposed skin with a handheld spray bottle. While this is being done, a fan or fans should be directed for continuous airflow over the moistened skin surface, dramatically enhancing evaporation. Although simple, this method is effective at reducing body temperature. Ice packs may be applied to the groin and axilla but must be monitored to avoid cold damage to the skin.

Ice water baths or extremely cold cooling surfaces are effective but are controversial in the emergency setting. There is a risk of vasoconstriction of the periphery that can cause reflex shivering and greatly inhibit the ability of the body to lose heat. Internal or invasive cooling methods, such as gastric lavage, bladder irrigation, or peritoneal lavage, should be used only after there has been no response to external treatment.

Armstrong LE: Whole body cooling of hyperthermic runners: A comparison of two field therapies. Am J Emerg Med 14:355–358, 1996.

Hadad E, Rav-Acha M, Heled Y, et al: Heat stroke: A review of cooling methods. Sports Med 34:501–511, 2004.

19. **What is the prognosis for heatstroke?**

Prognosis varies greatly with the person's age and the setting of the heatstroke. The literature reveals that young military recruits who are treated aggressively have almost no mortality, whereas inner-city elderly persons with heatstroke have a high mortality rate ($>50\%$). Poor prognostic indicators include delay in cooling, coma lasting longer than 2 hours, elevated creatinine kinase, elevated lactate dehydrogenase, elevated liver enzymes, hypotension, and prolonged prothrombin time. Recovery of CNS function during cooling is a favorable prognostic sign.

CHAPTER 58

ALTITUDE ILLNESS AND DYSBARISMS

Jeffrey Druck, MD

1. What are the three disease states that comprise high altitude illness?
High altitude illness is comprised of three distinct clinical entities: acute mountain sickness (AMS), high-altitude pulmonary edema (HAPE), and high-altitude cerebral edema (HACE).

2. What are the symptoms of AMS?
AMS is defined as the presence of a headache in the setting of recent ascent to high altitude with one of the following additional complaints: anorexia, nausea, vomiting, fatigue, weakness, dizziness, lightheadedness, or difficulty sleeping. It is an entirely clinical definition.

> The Lake Louise Consensus on the Definition and Quantification of Altitude Illness. In Sutton JR, Coates G, Houston C (eds): Hypoxia and Mountain Medicine. Burlington, Queen City Press, 1992.

3. How quickly do symptoms of AMS develop? What elevation is the minimum elevation at which one can see AMS?
Usually, symptoms begin within 6–10 hours of ascent. The minimum elevation at which AMS has been documented is 2000 m (6562 ft).

> Gallager SA, Hackett PH. High altitude illness. Emerg Med Clin North Am 22:329–355, 2004.

4. How do I treat AMS?
AMS is usually a self-limited disease that resolves with acclimatization (usually within 24 hours); the real concern is for further progression to HACE or developing HAPE with further ascent. Treatment is tailored to the severity of the symptoms and includes descent, acetazolamide (250 mg b.i.d.), supplemental oxygen, and dexamethasone.

KEY POINTS: TREATMENT FOR ALL TYPES OF HIGH-ALTITUDE ILLNESS

1. Descent (best treatment)

2. Supplemental oxygen

3. Hyperbaric therapy

5. What is the number-one risk factor for AMS?
Age. Although controversial, in one study, subjects younger than 25 years were 2.6 times MORE likely to develop AMS than those older than 55 years. Studies on young children show no increased risk, so it appears the effect is more attributable to older age being productive. Additional predisposing factors associated with AMS are as follows:
- Rate of ascent
- Exertion on arrival
- Elevation attained

- Previous history of AMS
- Duration of stay at altitude
- Cold temperatures

6. **Is there any treatment that will prevent AMS?**
The easiest way to prevent AMS is by minimizing risk. Slow ascent, avoidance of sedatives (alcohol included), and decreased physical activity on arrival minimize risk. Data support using either acetazolamide at 125 mg b.i.d. starting the day prior to ascent and continuing for 2 days at maximum altitude, or dexamethasone at 4 mg b.i.d. for the same regimen. The data on *Gingko biloba* use reducing AMS are controversial and are not supported at this time.

Basnyat B, Gertsch JH, Johnson EW, et al: Efficacy of low dose acetazolamide (125 mg BID) for the prophylaxis of acute mountain sickness: A prospective, double-blind, randomized, placebo controlled trial. High Alt Med Biol 4:45–52, 2003.

Chow T, Browne V, Heilson HL, et al: Gingko biloba and acetazolamide prophylaxis for acute mountain sickness: A randomized, placebo-controlled trial. Arch Intern Med 165:296–301, 2005.

Gertsch JH, Basnyat B, Johnson EW, et al: Randomised double-blind, placebo controlled comparison of Gingko biloba and acetazolamide for prevention of acute mountain sickness among Himalayan trekkers: The prevention of high altitude illness trial (PHAIT). BMJ 328:797, 2004.

KEY POINTS: PREVENTION FOR ALL TYPES OF HIGH-ALTITUDE ILLNESS

1. Slow ascent

2. Limitation of exertion

3. Avoidance of sedatives

4. Acetazolamide or dexamethasone

7. **What is the definition of HACE?**
HACE is a clinical diagnosis defined by a change in consciousness and associated ataxia in the setting of ascent to altitude. Cerebral edema is often present on computed tomography (CT) scans, and death results from brain herniation.

8. **When does HACE occur?**
The onset of HACE usually occurs 3–5 days after arrival to elevation.

9. **What is the treatment for HACE?**
Treatment includes immediate descent, supplemental oxygen, and dexamethasone. If descent is not an option, hyperbaric therapy (simulating descent) is an option; other modalities, such as diuretics or acetazolamide, are untested and are of unproven benefit.

10. **Is there anything that will prevent HACE?**
Because HACE is thought to be one point on the spectrum of altitude illness (HACE, HAPE, and AMS), anticipatory methods for HACE are identical to methods for the avoidance of AMS.

11. **What is HAPE?**
HAPE is defined as two of the following symptoms:

- Dyspnea at rest
- Cough
- Weakness or decreased exercise tolerance
- Chest tightness or congestion
  and two of the following signs:
- Crackles or wheezing in at least one lung field
- Central cyanosis
- Tachypnea
- Tachycardia

in the setting of a recent gain in altitude. HAPE is thought to be noncardiogenic pulmonary edema resulting from failure of the alveolar–capillary barrier. Cold stress and exertion increase pulmonary arterial pressure, which contributes to an increase in pulmonary edema.

12. **When does HAPE occur?**
Usually, HAPE occurs within 1–3 days of arrival at altitude and is rare beyond 4 days.

13. **How do I treat HAPE?**
Descent, supplemental oxygen, and/or hyperbaric therapy are the mainstays of treatment. Temporizing measures aimed at decreasing pulmonary artery pressures (nifedipine and expiratory positive airway pressure masks) have been shown to help, but the recovery period from HAPE is measured in days, so definitive therapy is highly recommended. Beta agonists that promote alveolar fluid clearance may also be beneficial. Other vasodilators such as nitric oxide and sildenafil are currently being researched. In contrast with HACE and AMS, dexamethasone has no effect.

Sartori C, Allemann Y, Duplain H, et al: Salmeterol for the prevention of high altitude pulmonary edema. N Engl J Med 346:1631–1636, 2002.

Schoene RB, Roach RC, Hackett PH, et al: High altitude pulmonary edema and exercise at 4,400 meters on Mount McKinley. Effect of expiratory positive airway pressure. Chest 87:330–333, 1985.

14. **Is there any preventative therapy for HAPE?**
Nifedipine has been shown to decrease the recurrence of HAPE in patients with previous HAPE; acetazolamide is recommended, but no data are available on the prevention of HAPE with that drug. In general, the principles designed to decrease the incidence of AMS (slow rate of ascent, decreased activity at altitude, no sedatives) are also true for HAPE.

Oelz O, Maggiorini M, Ritter M, et al: Prevention and treatment of high altitude pulmonary edema by a calcium channel blocker. Int J Sports Med 13:S65–S68, 1992.

15. **Do you ever see HAPE, HACE, or AMS at the same time?**
HACE is thought to be "end stage" AMS, so you do not see both at the same time. HACE almost always occurs in association with HAPE, but you can see HAPE without any signs of AMS or HACE.

16. **Which form of altitude illness is most common? Which is most deadly?**
The incidence of altitude illnesses depends on the altitude achieved in the group studied:
- AMS: Incidence, 15–70% (most common); mortality rate, 0%
- HACE: Incidence, 1–2%; mortality rate, unknown because of usually coexistent HAPE
- HAPE: Incidence: 1–15%; mortality rate, as high as 44% (most deadly)

Bezruchka S: High altitude medicine. Med Clin North Am 761:1481–1497, 1992.

17. **What is dysbarism?**
Dysbarism refers to pressure-related diseases but is commonly limited to diseases resulting from diving injuries (underwater pressure changes). This category includes disease related

specifically to pressure changes and the physical effects (middle ear barotrauma, pneumothorax, arterial gas embolism, pneumomediastinum, and barosinusitis) as well as disease related to "bubble formation" (pulmonary decompression sickness, spinal decompression sickness, and "the bends").

18. **How much pressure does a diver experience at 33 ft underwater?**
Each 33 ft, or 10 m, is equivalent to 1 atmosphere. Because sea level is equivalent to 1 atmosphere, 33 ft underwater is 2 atmospheres, which is equal to 29.4 psi or 1520 mmHg.

19. **What are the bends?**
"The bends," also known as caisson's disease (after caisson workers, who work in pressurized underwater chambers), is one of the more common forms of dysbarism. It occurs when nitrogen precipitates in tissues, causing muscle and joint pain.

20. **When would you see someone with the bends?**
People experience the bends when they ascend too rapidly from diving underwater.

21. **Why would nitrogen precipitate in tissues?**
According to Boyle's law of gasses, pressure is inversely proportional to volume ($P_1V_1 = P_2V_2$). Add into this mixture that Henry's law states that the amount of gas in solution is directly proportional to the partial pressure of that gas. Thus, with increased pressure underwater, the volume of gas decreases, and the amount of gas in solution (dissolved) increases. However, with rapid ascent, gas will expand and come out of solution, resulting in increased gas bubble size and possible precipitation in tissues. With a slow ascent, the gradual increase in bubble size and slow change in amount of gas in solution allow the gasses to remain dissolved in circulating blood and expelled through the respiratory system.

22. **What is nitrogen narcosis?**
As stated previously, the amount of each gas that goes into solution in the blood increases with increased pressure (or increased depth, because increased depth causes increased pressure). With nitrogen the largest component of air, a large amount of nitrogen goes into solution in the blood, ever increasing with increasing pressure. This high concentration of nitrogen causes an anesthetic-like effect that causes lack of motor control and inappropriate behavior, and eventually causes unconsciousness. Nitrogen narcosis usually is seen at depths of 100 ft or more. To avoid nitrogen narcosis, alternative decreased nitrogen containing mixtures are recommended for dives greater than 100 ft.

23. **What is MEBT?**
MEBT stands for middle ear barotrauma. MEBT occurs when the pressure of the water on the tympanic membrane during descent is not equalized by the eustachian tube. Usually, a diver will mechanically increase the pressure in his or her middle ear by forcing air through the eustachian tube to equilibrate the pressure across the tympanic membrane; if this does not occur, the increased external pressure will cause pain until rupture of the tympanic membrane eventually occurs, which may cause severe vertigo.

24. **How would one get a pneumothorax with ascent?**
If a diver held his or her breath to go underwater to 33 ft (2 atm), the volume in the lungs would decrease to half the prior volume (1 atm × normal lung volume = 2 atm × {1/2} normal lung volume). If he or she is scuba diving and replaces that lung volume back to normal, with ascent, he or she could double the lung volume (2 atm × normal lung volume = 1 atm × 2 normal lung volume). If there is nowhere for this additional gas to escape (i.e., breath holding), the lung may rupture, causing a pneumothorax to develop.

25. **What is AGE?**

AGE stands for arterial gas embolism; this condition occurs when overexpanding gas ruptures an alveolus and the gas is forced into the pulmonary vasculature. The gas then is distributed through the arterial system, with typical symptoms of loss of consciousness, apnea, and cardiac arrest. It is the second most common cause of diving-related deaths.

Neuman TS: Arterial gas embolism and decompression sickness. News Physiol Sci 17:77–81, 2002.

26. **What about the movies that show people bleeding from their eyes when diving? Does that really happen?**

With typical diving masks, an artificial air space is created in front of the eyes. When a diver descends, this air space is subject to the same gas laws, with the volume of air in the mask decreased by one half at 1 atmosphere underwater (effectively 2 atmospheres), one third at an effective 3 atmospheres, and so forth. This pressure change creates a vacuum effect in the mask, which can cause petechial hemorrhage, subconjunctival hemorrhage, and even optic nerve damage, termed facial barotrauma. The usual way divers avoid this problem is by wearing a mask that encompasses their nose and then equalizing the pressure by blowing air into their mask.

Shockley LW: Scuba diving and dysbarism. In Marx JA (ed): Rosen's Emergency Medicine, 5th ed. St. Louis, Mosby, 2002, chapter 137.

KEY POINTS: TYPES OF DCS

1. Type I: Skin DCS (skinny bends) and musculoskeletal DCS (the bends).

2. Type II: Pulmonary DCS (the chokes), spinal cord DCS, CNS DCS.

27. **What is DCS?**

DCS stands for decompression sickness, the term that describes the diseases that occur when gas (usually nitrogen) precipitates out of solution. The earliest form of DCS is the bends, the disease that presents as limb and joint pain. Prior thought was that the bends resulted from gas precipitation within joints themselves, but further research has shown that the gas distension occurs along ligaments and tendon sheaths. Other components of DCS include pulmonary DCS ("the chokes"), skin DCS (skinny bends), and spinal cord DCS. Type I DCS includes skin and musculoskeletal symptoms; type II DCS includes all other symptoms.

28. **What are the chokes?**

The chokes is the common term for pulmonary DCS. Pulmonary DCS manifests as cough, shortness of breath, and chest pain resulting from venous gas embolism in the pulmonary artery.

29. **What are the skinny bends?**

Skinny bends refers to cutaneous DCS, which is the appearance of a diffuse, reticulated, blotchy rash caused by endothelial damage from bubbles, resulting in blood extravasation. It can also refer to a syndrome of cutaneous itching that only appears in the artificial environment of a hyperbaric chamber.

30. **What is spinal cord DCS?**

Spinal cord DCS is a syndrome characterized by ascending paraesthesias and paralysis resulting from venous outflow obstruction by venous gas emboli in the epidural plexus of the spinal cord.

31. **Is there a central nervous system (CNS) form of DCS?**

Yes. It commonly presents with headache, blurred vision, dysarthria, diplopia, and inappropriate behavior. The exact mechanism of CNS DCS is poorly characterized; there was some thought that it was caused by venous gas embolism going across a patent foramen ovale (PFO), but the incidence of PFOs in patients with CNS DCS is equivalent to the general population.

32. **How do you tell the difference between CNS DCS and AGE?**

One main point is that loss of consciousness is uncommon with CNS DCS. However, because both are treated the same way, there is little use in distinguishing between the two.

33. **How are dysbarisms treated?**

In general, DCS and AGE should be treated with immediate recompression in a hyperbaric oxygen chamber. The longer the delay to treatment, the higher the morbidity and mortality. Acute pressure-related injuries (pneumothorax, pneumomediastinum) should be treated with standard therapy, whereas tympanic membrane rupture and inner ear disturbances should be referred to an otolaryngologist. Facial barotrauma victims should be assessed for more serious injuries, but there usually is no further treatment needed. The best way to treat dysbaric injuries is to prevent them.

34. **Is there anything that makes a particular person susceptible to DCS?**

It was thought that increased age or weight might be factors that made one susceptible to DCS, but recent studies fail to show any relationship.

Webb JT, Pilmanis AA, Balldin UI, et al: Altitude decompression sickness susceptibility: Influence of anthropometric and physiologic variables. Aviat Space Environ Med 76:547–551, 2005.

35. **Is there anything that I can do to reduce my risk of DCS?**

Slow ascent is the key. There are some data that show a decrease in the incidence of DCS in a rat model with exercise 20 hours prior to diving, but further research needs to be done. Nitric oxide also shows promise, but further studies may help in determining efficacy.

Wisloff U, Richardson RS, Brubakk AO: Exercise and nitric oxide prevent bubble formation: A novel approach to the prevention of decompression sickness? J Physiol 553:825–829, 2004.

EVALUATION OF FEVER IN CHILDREN YOUNGER THAN THREE

CHAPTER 59

Anna Olson, MD

1. **What is fever?**
   Fever is generally defined as a rectal temperature $\geq 38.0°C$ (100.4°F). Multiple studies evaluating the accuracy of parental reporting of fever (with or without benefit of thermometer use) suggest this is a reliable indicator of the presence of fever. This means fever at home should be evaluated as carefully as fever at triage. That said, however, be aware that measured "fevers" often fall shy of the 38.0°C mark, as when parents say, "She had a fever of 99.2 degrees."

2. **How should temperature be measured in young children?**
   The most reasonable and accurate method is the rectal temperature. Oral temperatures are not generally attempted in young children, for obvious logistical reasons. Axillary and tympanic temperatures are unreliable and should not be used, despite the ease with which they may be obtained.

3. **Is it safe to measure temperatures rectally?**
   Many parents, and even health care providers, are anxious about doing this. British studies investigating safety and efficacy demonstrate an extremely low rate of rectal injury (on the order of 1/100,000), despite widespread misconceptions and reluctance to use this method.

4. **What is a serious bacterial infection (SBI)?**
   SBI is defined as culture-proven cerebrospinal fluid (CSF) infection, urinary tract infection (UTI), or bacteremia or focal pneumonia by radiograph. Many also include cellulitis under the heading of SBI.

5. **Does it matter *how much* fever the child has?**
   SBI is found in 7–9% of children with temperature of 38.0–39.9°C. Mounting evidence suggests that higher fevers are associated with a higher rate of SBI. Hyperpyrexia (temperature $\geq 40.0°C$) may be associated with SBI rates as high as 38%. Any child who appears toxic should be evaluated for SBI, regardless of the temperature.

   Stanley R, Pagon Z, Bachur R: Hyperpyrexia among infants younger than 3 months. Pediatr Emerg Care 21:291–294, 2005.

6. **What is meant by "toxic-appearing"?**
   Toxic children may be pale, lethargic, or limp. They may show evidence of poor perfusion (such as cyanosis or peripheral vasoconstriction with mottling), or changes in respiratory drive such as tachypnea or shallow breathing. They may fail to interact with their environment (as evidenced by poor or absent eye contact, poor feeding, or failure to respond to caregivers or objects in their view). These children are gravely ill and need immediate resuscitation and evaluation.

KEY POINTS: SIGNS OF TOXICITY

1. Lethargy

2. Cyanosis

3. Tachypnea

4. Poor tone

5. Failure to respond to caregivers

7. **Which antipyretics work best for children?**
   Studies show that acetaminophen (15 mg/kg) and ibuprofen (10 mg/kg) have similar efficacy, and both work well for getting febrile children to defervesce.
   Pearl: Most children's elixirs contain half the amount of an adult tablet per teaspoon (5 mL). For example, an adult tablet of ibuprofen contains 200 mg, whereas the children's elixir contains 100 mg/5 mL.

8. **What is the most common cause of antipyretic failure?**
   Underdosing, either by dose or by schedule. Parents may not know the child's weight, fail to calculate an appropriate dose, or be unfamiliar with units of measure (such as "teaspoon"). It is also common for parents to believe that antipyretics should "cure" the fever, and they may complain "I gave her the medicine and it helped for a while, but the fever just came right back." Parental education and provision of an oral syringe frequently help with this issue.

9. **What is wrong with baby aspirin—it is for babies, right?**
   Exposure to aspirin has been associated with the development of Reye's syndrome (encephalopathy and acute liver failure), particularly in children with viral infections. This syndrome, although rare, carries a high mortality rate (20–50%, depending on how quickly it is recognized and how aggressively it is treated.) Although some pediatric conditions (such as juvenile rheumatoid arthritis and Kawasaki disease) may involve treatment with aspirin, its use in children with fever of uncertain origin should be strictly avoided.

10. **Is there any good reason *not* to treat a fever?**
    No. There is nothing to be gained from allowing a fever to run its course unchecked. Children with fever feel crummy, feed poorly, and worry their caregivers; the quickest way to make them feel better is to bring that fever down.

11. **What causes febrile seizures?**
    Febrile seizures are associated with a family history and with very high fevers. There has been a great deal of discussion about whether these seizures are associated with rate of rise, rather than absolute temperature, but there is no evidence to support this. Although benign, they are very frightening for child and parent, and both are likely to need a great deal of reassurance. For more information, see Chapter 60.

    Zensky W: Pediatric febrile seizures. Available at www.emedicine.com/EMERG/topic376.htm, October 2004.

12. **Does careful administration of antipyretics prevent recurrence of febrile seizures?**
    No. There is no sense in unnecessarily burdening parents who don't have any control over seizure recurrence. You should warn them of the possibility (about one third have a second

febrile seizure) and reassure them they are not at fault. Advise them that children feel better when fever is treated, but be clear about the fact that their antipyretic administration is not going to stop a seizure. This becomes especially important in the event of recurrence, because most parents are *already* inclined to blame themselves.

13. **How should tiny babies with fever be evaluated?**

Febrile infants (temperature $\geq 38.0°C$) younger than 1 month get a full sepsis work-up. Little deliberation is required: urinalysis and culture (by catheterization or suprapubic aspiration), complete blood count and culture, lumbar puncture (LP), chest radiograph, and stool analysis for white blood cell (WBC) count and culture (if there is a history of diarrhea). They should receive intravenous (IV) antibiotics and be admitted to the hospital.

   Note: Age cut-offs for fever evaluation are based on **gestational age** not age since birth. This means that a 32-week premature infant born 6 weeks ago is still considered to be younger than 1 month.

14. **What happens after the magic one-month mark?**

In infants 1–3 months with no obvious source of fever, follow the algorithm in Figure 59-1.

   Baraff LJ: Clinical policy for children younger than three years presenting at the emergency department with fever. Ann Emerg Med 42:546–549, 2003.

15. **What about older infants and young children?**

From 3–36 months for a fever with no source, follow the algorithm in Figure 59-2 (and note the difference in concerning temperature).

   Baraff LJ: Clinical policy for children younger than three years presenting at the emergency department with fever. Ann Emerg Med 42:546–549, 2003.

16. **How do we decide whether to do an LP in older babies and young children?**

In children who are nontoxic with a low suspicion for central nervous system (CNS) infection, the LP may be deferred if parents are willing to accept the small risk ($\sim 1/1000$) of missed meningitis. Be aware that many of the classic signs of meningitis (Brudzinski's sign, Kernig's sign, neck stiffness, bulging fontanelle) are frequently absent and highly unreliable in young children.

17. **What if the child has a fever source, or one is found during the work-up?**

If the source *completely* explains the clinical presentation, stop looking and treat it. If not, complete the evaluation as described previously. Be aware that urinary tract infections and bacteremia may coexist with minor respiratory infections or otitis media.

18. **Must we always follow the guidelines, or is there room for clinical judgment in there somewhere?**

A study of more than 3000 febrile infants seen by almost 600 pediatricians throughout the United States demonstrated that selective testing by experienced clinicians in office-based practice was as effective in appropriately identifying and treating SBI as rigid adherence to clinical guidelines. Understand two things, however. First, pediatricians are forced to be fastidious in their choice of testing because they generally don't have the resources to do the full recommended work-up in every child they see. Second, office-based practitioners have the safety net of emergency care, which emergency physicians, as the last line of defense, lack.

   Pantell RH, Newman TB, Bernzweig J, et al: Management and outcomes of care of fever in early infancy. JAMA 291:1203–1212, 2004.

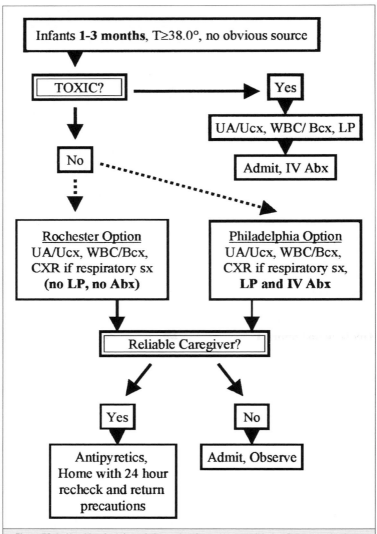

Figure 59-1. Algorithm for infants 1–3 months of age. Abx = antibiotics, Bcx = blood culture, CXR = chest x-ray, LP = lumbar puncture, UA = urinalysis, Ucx = urine culture, WBC = white blood cell count.

19. **What if the child looks great, can he or she go home?**
    Nontoxic-appearing children older than 1 month who meet low-risk criteria may be discharged home with return precautions and close follow-up. This, of course, presumes they have a reliable caregiver, a tenable social situation, and reasonable access to transportation.

20. **What are low-risk criteria?**
    The two sets of low-risk criteria used most often are the Rochester and Philadelphia criteria. Both presume the child is previously healthy and well appearing at the time of evaluation.

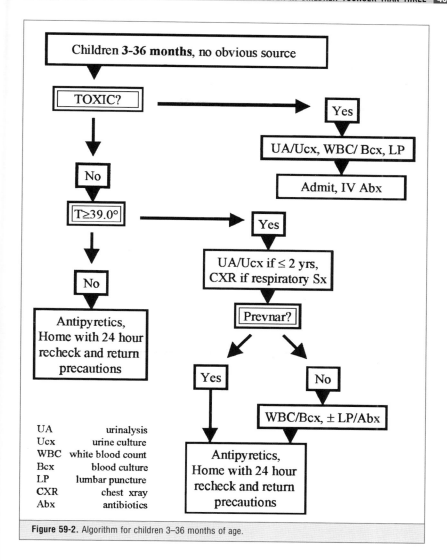

Figure 59-2. Algorithm for children 3–36 months of age.

Rochester criteria
- WBC $\geq$5k/μL and $\leq$15k/μL with absolute band count (ABC) $\leq$1500/μL
- Urine WBC $\leq$10/high power field (hpf)
- Stool WBC $\leq$5/hpf (in infants with diarrhea)
- Note: No LP performed

Philadelphia criteria
- WBC $\leq$15k/μL with band-to-neutrophil ratio <0.2
- Urine WBC $\leq$10/hpf
- CSF WBC $\leq$8/hpf
- Negative CSF Gram stain
- Stool and chest radiograph negative (if obtained)

21. **What is the risk of occult bacteremia?**

This has long been viewed as an important consideration in febrile work-ups. Although true bacteremia certainly constitutes an SBI, new data gathered since the widespread use of heptavalent pneumococcal vaccine suggest that, at least for properly vaccinated children between 2 and 36 months, this is a remote risk, affecting fewer than 1% of well-appearing febrile children younger than 3 years. This risk is low enough that routine blood cultures are no longer recommended for properly vaccinated children older than 3 months.

   Stoll ML, Rubin LG: Incidence of occult bacteremia among highly febrile young children in the era of the pneumococcal conjugate vaccine. Arch Pediatr Adolesc Med 158:671–675, 2004.

22. **What antibiotic should be used in the event that empiric coverage is deemed appropriate?**

   <28 days
   - Ampicillin, 50–100/kg IV every 4–6 hours
   - Gentamicin, 2.5 mg/kg IV every 8 hours (dose-adjusted for gestational age)
   - Acyclovir, 10 mg/kg IV every 8 hours (dose/schedule-adjusted for gestational age)

   28 days–3 months
   - Ampicillin, 50 mg/kg IV every 6 hours
   - Cefotaxime, 50 mg/kg IV every 6 hours

   >3 months or well-appearing/dischargeable
   - Ceftriaxone, 50–75 mg/kg IV/intramuscular (IM) × 1

23. **What about children with fever and rapidly progressive petechial rash?**

This is disseminated meningococcemia until proved otherwise. Patients with this type of infection may go from perfectly well to perfectly dead in just a few short hours, so go straight for the big guns, and do not waste any time.
   - Cefotaxime, 75 mg/kg IV every 6 hours *immediately*
   - Vancomycin, 15 mg/kg IV every 6 hours *immediately*

BIBLIOGRAPHY

1. Bachur RG, Harper MB: Predictive model for serious bacterial infections among infants younger than 3 months of age. Pediatr 108:311–316, 2001.
2. Baraff LJ: Clinical policy for children younger than three years presenting at the emergency department with fever. Ann Emerg Med 42:546–549, 2003.
3. Gorelick MH, Hoberman A, Kearney D, et al: Validation of a decision rule identifying febrile young girls at high risk for urinary tract infection. Pediatr Emerg Care 19:162–164, 2003.
4. Hsiao AL, Baker MD: Fever in the new millennium: A review of recent studies of markers of serious bacterial infection in febrile children. Curr Opin Pediatr 17:56–61, 2005.
5. McCarthy P: Fever without apparent source on clinical examination. Curr Opin Pediatr 17:93–110, 2005.

CHAPTER 60

SEIZURES IN INFANCY AND CHILDHOOD

Patricia A. Braun, MD

1. **What are some common causes of pediatric seizures?**
   - Fever
   - Subtherapeutic anticonvulsant levels
   - Infection
   - Trauma (epidural and subdural hematoma)
   - Metabolic abnormalities (hypoglycemia, hypoxia, electrolyte abnormalities, hypocalcemia)
   - Toxins (intoxication or ingestion, drug withdrawal)
   - Neoplasms or mass

2. **Is it really a seizure?**
   Consider some other possibilities, as listed in Table 60-1.

TABLE 60-1. THINGS THAT MIMIC SEIZURES	
Pseudoseizure	Movements thrashing rather that clonic: brief/absent postictal period
Paroxysmal vertigo (toddler)	Child frightened and crying; no loss of awareness; staggers and falls
Breathholding spell (18 mo to 3 yr)	Loss of consciousness and generalized convulsion always provoked by child crying
Syncope	Loss of consciousness with onset of dizziness; slow collapse to the floor
Cardiogenic syncope	Abnormal ECG/Holter monitor finding; episodic loss of consciousness without convulsive movement
Tics	Involuntary, nonrhythmic, repetitive movements not associated with impaired consciousness
Paroxysmal dyskinesias	Precipitated by sudden movement or startle; remains alert
Shuddering attacks	Brief shivering spells; remains aware
Migraine (confusional)	Headache or visual changes that may precede attack: family history of migraine: autonomic or sensory changes that can mimic focal seizure
Narcolepsy	Sudden loss of tone secondary to cataplexy; no postictal state

Adapted from Murphy JV, Dehkharghani F. Diagnosis of childhood seizure disorder. Epilepsia 35(Suppl 2):S7-S17, 1994.

3. **What components of the history are important?**
   - Obtain details of the actual event: Was this a generalized seizure, or did it start as a focal seizure? How long did it last? Was there incontinence, tongue biting, or a postictal period?
   - Inquire about possible factors that could have caused the seizure. A careful questioning for accidental or nonaccidental head trauma is essential. Is there a possibility of an ingestion? Has the child been ill with fever? Is the child prone to breath holding, or does he or she have pulmonary disease with resultant hypoxia? Is the child taking seizure medications?
   - Determine the past medical history and whether there is a family history of seizures. The perinatal history should be obtained.
   - Assess the child's current neurologic status to determine whether or not it is at baseline.

4. **What about the physical examination?**
   A careful neurologic examination establishes any focal deficits and determines new versus old findings. Always look for evidence of head trauma and trauma to the rest of the body, which may clue you in to the possibility of abuse. Do a funduscopic examination, looking for retinal hemorrhages, a sign of abuse. In febrile seizures, look for the source of the fever.

5. **Do different causes of seizures need to be considered in the neonate?**
   Seizures in neonates must be evaluated more aggressively than those in older children. Causes of neonatal seizures include the following:
   - Hypoxic-ischemic encephalopathy: 35–42%
   - Intracranial hemorrhage or infarction: 15–20%
   - Central nervous system (CNS) infection: 12–17%
   - CNS malformation: 5%
   - Metabolic abnormalities (hypoglycemia, hypocalcemia, pyridoxine deficiency, toxins or drug withdrawal): 3–5%
   - Other inborn errors of metabolism: 5–20%

   Scher MS: Seizures in the newborn infant: Diagnosis, treatment and outcomes. Clin Perinatol 24:735–772, 1997.

6. **Is the work-up for neonatal seizures different than for seizures in older children?**
   Yes and no. In neonates consider evaluation of glucose, calcium, and electrolytes; plasma amino acids, urine organic acids, and ammonia, lactate; and lumbar puncture, computed tomography (CT), and electroencephalogram (EEG).

7. **What is a febrile seizure?**
   A benign event usually occurring between the ages of 6 months and 5 years that is associated with fever but is without evidence of intracranial infection or another defined cause. The peak incidence occurs at 18 months. The etiology is thought to be attributed to the maturing brain's susceptibility to fever. A febrile seizure usually occurs within the first 24 hours of a febrile illness. There should be a return to a normal neurologic state after the seizure.

   Waruiru C, Appleton R: Febrile seizures: An update. Arch Dis Child 89:751–756, 2004. adc.bmjjournals.com

8. **Are all febrile seizures the same?**
   No. Febrile seizures can be divided into two types:
   - A **simple febrile seizure** is a generalized, tonic-clonic seizure that lasts fewer than 15 minutes, occurs only once in a 24-hour period in a febrile child who does not have a CNS infection or abnormality, and spontaneously resolves.
   - A seizure becomes a **complex febrile seizure** if it is prolonged (>15 minutes), focal, or recurs within a 24-hour period.

   Committee on Quality Improvement, Subcommittee on Febrile Seizures, American Academy of Pediatrics: Practice parameter: The neurodiagnostic evaluation of the child with a first simple febrile seizure. Pediatrics 97:769–775,1996. Available at www.pediatrics.org.

9. **Is there a genetic predisposition to developing febrile seizures?**
Yes, there is a familial component to febrile seizures because 10–20% of younger siblings of patients who have had a febrile seizure also go on to have a febrile seizure and there is a family history of febrile seizures in 25–40% of patients.

  Knudsen FU: Febrile seizures: Treatment and prognosis. Epilepsia 41:2–9, 2000.

10. **What is the work-up of the child with a simple febrile seizure?**
See Fig. 60-1.

KEY POINTS: EVALUATING CHILDREN WITH FEBRILE SEIZURES

1. Simple febrile seizures typically are benign events.

2. Children presenting with a simple febrile seizure should carefully be evaluated for the source of the fever.

3. Meningitis should always be either clinically ruled out or ruled out by lumbar puncture if indicated.

4. Given the absence of meningeal signs in children younger than 18 months, strongly consider performing a lumbar puncture.

5. Diagnostic laboratory tests, neuroimaging, and EEG should never be routine.

---

11. **What is the likelihood of further febrile seizures?**
The risk of a recurrence is about 30%, even within the same febrile illness. The risk is higher if the first seizure occurs in a child younger than 12 months, if the febrile seizure is a recurrence, or if there is a family history of febrile seizures. The majority (75%) of recurrences happen within the first year after the initial febrile seizure.

  Baumann RJ. Duffner PK: Treatment of children with simple febrile seizures: The AAP practice parameter. Ped Neurol 23:11–17, 2000.
  Hirtz DG: Febrile seizures. Pediatr Rev 18:5–8, 1997.

12. **Is there a way to prevent febrile seizures?**
In 1999, the American Academy of Pediatrics recognized that simple febrile seizures are a benign and common occurrence and stated that although there are a few therapies effective at preventing the recurrence of febrile seizures, the potential side effects of these drugs do not commensurate with the benefit. Antipyretic medicines alone are not effective in preventing the recurrence of simple febrile seizures, although they may make the patient feel more comfortable.

  Baumann RJ, Duffner PK: Treatment of children with simple febrile seizures: The AAP practice parameter. Pediatr Neurol 23:11–17, 2000.
  Committee on Quality Improvement, Subcommittee on Febrile Seizures, American Academy of Pediatrics: Practice parameter: Long-term treatment of the child with simple febrile seizures (AC9859). Pediatrics 103:1307–1309, 1999.
  Waruiru C, Appleton R: Febrile seizures: An update. Arch Dis Child 89:751–756, 2004.

13. **Does a febrile seizure predict the development of epilepsy?**
Only a few children who have had a febrile seizure go on to develop epilepsy. Children who have a family history of epilepsy, who have a history of preexisting neurologic disease, or who had a

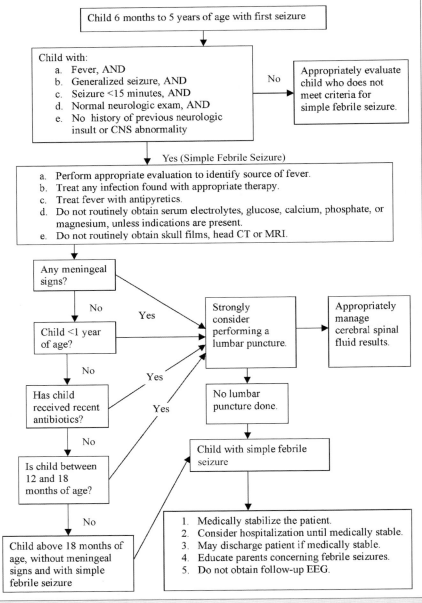

Figure 60-1. Evaluation of child with simple febrile seizure. CT = computed tomography, EEG = electroencephalogram, MRI = magnetic resonance imaging. (Adapted from Committee on Quality Improvement, Subcommittee on Febrile Seizures, American Academy of Pediatrics: Practice parameter: The neurodiagnostic evaluation of the child with a first simple febrile seizure. Pediatrics 97:769–775, 1996. Available at www.aap.org/policy/neuro.htm.)

complex febrile seizure are more likely to develop epilepsy. Without these risk factors, a child has a 1% chance of developing epilepsy, compared with a less than 1% chance for children who have never had a febrile seizure.

Knudsen FU: Febrile seizures: Treatment and prognosis. Epilepsia 41:2–9, 2000.

14. **Which children should be considered for anticonvulsant therapy?**
Because fewer than 50% of children with a single seizure have a second seizure, prophylaxis is not indicated in the emergency department (ED). Complex febrile seizures, particularly if prolonged, and an abnormal neurologic status are risk factors for the development of later epilepsy. However, there is little evidence that the use of antiepileptics reduces the risk of developing epilepsy.

Waruiru C, Appleton R: Febrile seizures: An update. Arch Dis Child 89:751–756, 2004.

KEY POINTS: LONG-TERM TREATMENT OF CHILD WITH FEBRILE ILLNESS

1. Febrile seizures are more likely to recur the earlier the age at which the first febrile seizure occurs or if there is a family history of seizures.

2. Few children (1%) with simple febrile seizures go on to develop epilepsy.

3. Few therapies are effective at preventing the recurrence of febrile seizures, and the potential side effects of these drugs do not commensurate the benefit.

4. Antipyretics are ineffective at preventing seizure recurrence, although they may make the child feel better.

---

15. **What infections cause seizures?**
Meningitis and encephalitis are associated with seizures but, as discussed earlier, should be accompanied by other signs. Worldwide, neurocysticercosis is a common cause of seizures. *Shigella* gastroenteritis provoked seizures in 45% of patients via their endotoxins. These seizures are by definition not febrile seizures.

16. **What is status epilepticus?**
Continuous seizure activity or recurrent seizures lasting at least 30 minutes without the recovery of consciousness between attacks.

17. **How should status epilepticus be treated?**
See Table 60-2.

18. **What are the advantages of lorazepam over diazepam?**
Lorazepam is a longer acting benzodiazepine than diazepam because it is less lipophilic and does not redistribute as quickly. It may have a 12- to 24-hour duration of action. When delivered per os (PO) or intramuscular (IM), lorazepam's peak serum concentration is reached in 30–120 minutes. When given intravenous (IV), the onset of action is 1–5 minutes. Lorazepam may be given intravenously, 0.05–0.1 mg/kg/dose and may be repeated at 0.05 mg/kg/dose × 1 in 10–15 minutes (maximum dose of 4 mg/dose). The injectable product may also be administered rectally.

Gunn VL, Nechyba C (eds): The Harriet Lane Handbook, 16th ed. St. Louis, The Johns Hopkins Hospital, Mosby, 2002, pp 658–659.

TABLE 60-2.	TREATMENT OF STATUS EPILEPTICUS	
Time	**Management**	
Immediately	Airway/breathing/circulation	
	a. High flow oxygen/secure airway	
	b. Establish IV access	
	c. Obtain blood glucose/consider other necessary lab tests (complete blood count, electrolytes, drug levels)	
	d. Treat hypoglycemia/hyponatremia	
	IV Access	**No IV Access**
Immediately	1. Lorazepam IV (0.05–0.1 mg/kg dose) maximal dose = 4 mg *or*	1. Diazepam (parenteral solution) (0.5 mg/kg/dose PR) (use tuberculin syrnge)
	2. Diazepam IV (0.1–0.5 mg/kg/dose) maximal dose = 5mg	
10 minutes	1. Repeat lorazepam (0.05–0.1 mg/kg/dose) maximal dose = 4 mg	1. Paraldehyde 0.4 ml/kg/dose PR (deliver with olive oil)
>10 minutes	1. Phenytoin IV (15 mg/kg/dose) *or*	**Place intraosseous line**
	2. Phenobarbitol IV 20 mg/kg/dose Infused at a rate no faster than 1 mg/kg/min.	1. Administer lorazepam (0.05–0.1 mg/kg/dose) through IO maximal dose = 4 mg *or*
		2. Repeat paraldehyde (0.4 mg/kg/dose)
Continuing seizure	□ Intubation	
	□ General anesthesia	
	□ Neuromuscular blockade	
	□ Correct possible causes (hyperglycemia, INH toxicity, intracerebral mass, infection)	

Modified from The Status Epilepticus Working Party: The treatment of convulsive epilipticus in children. Arch Dis Child 83:415–419, 2000.

CHAPTER 61

ACUTE RESPIRATORY DISORDERS IN CHILDREN

Joan Bothner, MD

1. **What are the signs and symptoms of respiratory distress in a child?**

   The signs and symptoms are shown in Figure 61-1. Arterial blood gases are of limited clinical value and show only mild hypoxemia (as does pulse oximetry), until exhaustion causes hypoventilation. Hypercapnia and respiratory acidosis necessitate immediate intervention. Basically, the clinical state of the child should dictate intervention, with the most important parameter being mental status. A young child who does not cry is not being "good"—he or she is in big trouble.

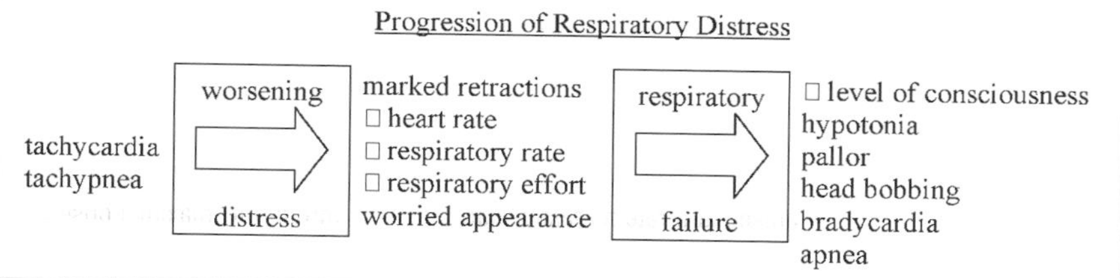

Figure 61-1. Signs and symptoms of respiratory distress in children.

2. **Why are airway problems more serious in pediatric patients than in adults?**

   There are several important differences between the adult and the pediatric airway. The child's tongue is large, easily displaced, and the most common cause of airway obstruction in the obtunded child. The narrowest portion of the pediatric airway is at the cricoid ring, making obstruction with subglottic pathology more likely than in adults. The most significant contribution to increased resistance with obstruction is the small radius of the pediatric larynx (resistance is inversely related to the fourth power of the radius, or 1 mm of swelling in an infant airway causes big problems). A healthy child can tolerate moderate-to-severe airway obstruction and maintain tidal volume almost to the point of exhaustion, at which time hypoxemia, hypercapnia, and acidosis progress rapidly, leading to cardiorespiratory arrest.

3. **How can I determine where the problem is?**

   Supraglottic lesions, such as epiglottitis, present with inspiratory stridor, a prolonged inspiratory phase, and a muffled cry or voice. Glottic lesions lead to high-pitched inspiratory stridor and a voice that is weak or hoarse. Subglottic lesions cause expiratory stridor with a normal voice and a brassy cough. A child who assumes the sniffing position has a significant upper airway obstruction, as does the child who is dysphagic or drools. Expiration should be passive; active expiration with a prolonged expiratory time, recruitment of the accessory muscles, wheezing, and a tripod position is significant for severe lower airway obstruction. All patients who breathe noisily do not have asthma, and with a few seconds of observation one should be able to differentiate between upper and lower airway obstruction.

4. **The child is in trouble. What do I do?**

Ensuring an adequate airway is the first priority. Supplemental oxygen should be provided, and the child needs to be allowed to assume a position of comfort. Remember, almost all children can be bag-valve-mask ventilated. Oral intubation is the method of choice in a child requiring assisted ventilation. Endotracheal tube (ETT) size can be estimated in children older than 2 years by adding 16 to the child's age in years and dividing by 4. An alternative method is by using a length-based tape, which provides a more accurate estimation of correct ETT size than does the child's age. Uncuffed tubes generally are used in children younger than 8–10 years because of the anatomic narrowing of the airway at the level of the cricoid cartilage. A smaller tube and stylet need to be readily available. Assume all children have just eaten, and pay careful attention to aspiration prevention. Also essential are a large, working suction catheter and cricoid pressure. ETTs are uncuffed up to size 5.5. Nasogastric tubes are essential because children are diaphragmatic breathers and cannot ventilate with a stomach full of air.

5. **What are common causes of upper airway obstruction in children?**

See Table 61-1.

6. **Discuss the signs and symptoms of croup, who gets it, what causes it, and what the physician can do for it.**

Croup, or laryngotracheobronchitis, is the most common cause of infectious acute upper airway obstruction. Ten percent require admission, and 1–5% require intubation. The mean age of affected patients is 18 months, with a slight male predominance, and there is a seasonal increase in cases in autumn and early winter. The classic presentation is a history of a mild upper respiratory infection, followed by increasing stridor with worsening at night. Temperature elevation may be significant. Laboratory data are useless. X-rays are not indicated. Treatment includes humidified air or oxygen and steroids, although there is limited evidence to say humidification is beneficial. Antibiotics have no role.

7. **Who needs nebulized epinephrine?**

Aerosolized epinephrine, given via nebulizer, is indicated for children with stridor at rest or with marked increase in work of breathing, and it has been shown to decrease airway obstruction. Racemic epinephrine containing L-isomers and D-isomers historically has been used, but L-epinephrine alone has been shown to be just as effective; 0.5 mL of 2.25% racemic epinephrine is equivalent to 5 mL of 1:1000 L-epinephrine. Maximal effect of nebulized epinephrine is seen within 30 minutes, with a rebound to baseline at 2 hours in some patients. Patients should be observed for 2–3 hours after receiving nebulized epinephrine before being discharged. Criteria for admission include continued stridor at rest, cyanosis, or other signs of significant respiratory compromise, dehydration, questionable follow-up, and possibly extremes of age. Intubation rarely is needed, but remember to have a smaller ETT available.

8. **What about steroids and croup?**

The use of steroids results in clinical improvement and has been shown to decrease the need for hospitalization. Decrease in symptoms occurs within 6 hours even in children with mild-to-moderate croup, and treatment with steroids decreases return emergency department (ED) visits by 50%. Oral dexamethasone has been shown to be as effective as intramuscular (IM) dexamethasone. Dosing of dexamethasone in published studies in outpatients varies from 0.15 mg/kg to 0.6 mg/kg with a maximal dose of 8 mg. Most studies used the 0.6 mg/kg dose. There is no evidence to suggest that repeat dosing is indicated or helpful. Nebulized budesonide also has been studied but has not been shown to be of any benefit over dexamethasone. Steroids should be considered for any child who presents to the ED with croup.

Bjornson CL, Klassen TP, Williamson J, et al: A randomized trial of a single dose of oral dexamethasone for mild croup. N Engl J Med 351:1306–1313, 2004.

TABLE 61-1. CAUSES OF UPPER AIRWAY OBSTRUCTION

	Etiology	Age Range	Onset	Toxicity	Drooling	Treatment
Croup	Parainfluenza, type 1, influenza A and B, RSV, rhinovirus	6 mo–3 yr	URI prodrome	Mild	Absent	Mist, steroids, aerosolized epinephrine
Epiglottitis	*Haemophilus influenzae,* group A beta-hemolytic *Streptococcus, Staphylococcus aureus, Streptococcus pneumoniae,* viruses	3–7 yr	Acute	Marked	Frequent	Airway management, antibiotics
Retropharyngeal abscess	Multiple: anaerobes	Infancy–6 yr	URI, sore throat	Variable	Variable	Antibiotics, drainage
Bacterial tracheitis	*S. aureus, H. Influenzae, S. pneumoniae, Branhamella catarrhalis* after viral insult	≥3 yr	"Croup" prodrome	Moderate	Usually absent	Airway management, antibiotics

URI = upper respiratory infection.

9. **What is epiglottitis?**
   Epiglottitis is a bacterial cellulitis of the supraglottic structures, most notably the lingual surface of the epiglottitis. It has a rapid onset with a high fever, significant toxicity, drooling, dysphagia, stridor, preference for the sitting position with the head extended, and no cough. The incidence of epiglottitis decreased significantly after the introduction of the conjugate *Haemophilus influenzae* type B vaccine. Radiographic evidence of epiglottitis includes a swollen epiglottis (the thumb sign), thickened aryepiglottic folds, and obliteration of the vallecula.

10. **What is the appropriate management of a patient with suspected epiglottitis?**
    Do not agitate the child in any way. Do not send the child for radiographs. Start high-flow oxygen via a nonrebreather bag reservoir mask, if possible. Blood work, intravenous (IV) lines, and antibiotics can wait in a child in distress. Antibiotics need to be effective against *H. influenzae*; cefuroxime, ceftriaxone, and cefotaxime are recommended. If a child obstructs, bag-valve-mask ventilation should be attempted first. Elective intubation in the ED is never indicated.

11. **What about bacterial tracheitis (membranous laryngotracheobronchitis)?**
    Bacterial tracheitis is an uncommon but significant cause of acute upper airway obstruction. Radiography may show subglottic narrowing with irregular intratracheal densities and clouding of the tracheal air column. Airway management and broad-spectrum antibiotics are the mainstay of therapy. Endoscopy is the diagnostic method of choice; findings include edema of the supraglottis, ulceration, and pseudomembrane formation in the trachea. Because of tenacious secretions, some affected patients require intubation and meticulous suctioning.

12. **What are retropharyngeal space infections?**
    Retropharyngeal space infections rarely cause true upper airway obstruction, but there is an increase in incidence of these infections, which seems to correlate with culture-positive group A beta-hemolytic streptococcal abscesses. About 90% of all cases occur in patients younger than 6 years. Symptoms include dysphagia, drooling, fever, neck pain, stridor, irritability, and varying degrees of respiratory distress. A common finding is significant posterior cervical adenopathy. This infection is believed to arise from an extension of an acute infection of the ear, nose, or throat with spread to the retropharyngeal space. Trauma to the nasopharynx (e.g., from accidents with pencils) is also a predisposing factor. Cellulitis, or inflammation of the lymph nodes in the prevertebral space, occurs first with progression to abscess formation and suppuration.

13. **How are they diagnosed?**
    Diagnosis can be difficult in young children. Lateral neck films are diagnostic (90% sensitivity) but can be difficult to interpret, depending on the phase of respiration and neck position. Findings include increase in the width of the prevertebral space to greater than the anteroposterior width of the adjacent cervical vertebral body, anterior displacement of the airway, and loss of the normal step-off at the level of the larynx. Air-fluid levels are seen after abscess formation (Fig. 61-2). Computed tomography (CT) scanning is highly sensitive and is used to differentiate abscess from phlegmon or soft tissue cellulitis.

14. **How are they managed?**
    Treatment includes hospital admission, parenteral antibiotic therapy, and incision and drainage if an abscess is present. Most children do not need acute airway intervention. The most common presentation is a young child who appears mildly toxic, has an upper respiratory infection and a fever, and is alert, but who is holding his head stiffly and slightly extended. Extension of the neck seems to be most painful, versus pain with flexion as seen in meningitis. This diagnosis can be difficult to make, and a high index of suspicion often pays off.

15. **When should a foreign body be suspected?**

Most patients who present with foreign-body aspiration are younger than 3 years and rarely are younger than 5 months; most are male. A history of an aspiration event is lacking in 30–50% of patients. The most commonly aspirated object is food, and most ends up in the esophagus or in the lower airways. Signs and symptoms depend on the site of obstruction. Endoscopy is diagnostic.

16. **How are suspected foreign bodies managed in pediatric patients?**

Immediate management depends on the degree of respiratory distress, but it should be minimal unless respiratory failure is imminent. Basic life support measures should be tried first. If unconsciousness occurs, direct

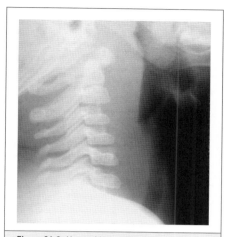

Figure 61-2. X-ray of lateral neck showing thickening of prevertebral space.

laryngoscopy should follow with attempted removal of the foreign object with Magill forceps if it can be visualized. If this fails, bag-valve-mask ventilation and intubation should be attempted, which ideally push the offending object into a bronchus. If the child cannot be intubated, a needle cricothyroidotomy should be performed.

17. **What is bronchiolitis, what causes it, and what are the risk factors?**

Bronchiolitis is a viral infection of the bronchioles characterized by inflammation, edema, and mucus and cellular debris accumulation, which causes bronchiolar obstruction and ventilation-perfusion mismatching. It is seen most frequently in children between the ages of 3 and 6 months, and is the most common lower respiratory tract infection in infants. Respiratory syncytial virus (RSV) is responsible for 70% of cases, and almost all cases in the winter months. Parainfluenza (peaks in the summer), adenovirus, and influenza cause most other cases (Tables 61-2 and 61-3).

TABLE 61-2. RISK FACTORS FOR BRONCHIOLITIS	
Daycare	Male sex
Young age (< 6 mo)	Not breast-feeding
Crowded living conditions	Passive smoke exposure
Lower socioeconomic status	

18. **What are the clinical signs and symptoms?**

Tachypnea, wheezing, nasal flaring, and retractions. These symptoms are usually preceded by 1–2 days of rhinorrhea, cough, or low-grade fever. Auscultation may reveal diffuse wheezing, prolonged expiration, and rales. Findings of more severe disease include hypoxemia, inability to feed, irritability, and lethargy. Young infants may present with apnea only.

TABLE 61-3. RISK FACTORS FOR SEVERE RSV DISEASE
Congenital heart disease
Primary pulmonary hypertension
Cystic fibrosis
Chronic lung disease—bronchopulmonary dysplasia
Congenital or acquired immunodeficiency
Major congenital anomalies
Prematurity <32 weeks
Prematurity <36 weeks and age <6 months
Age <6 weeks

RSV = respiratory syncytial virus.

19. **What laboratory or other evaluation should you do in a patient with bronchiolitis?**

Infants with classic bronchiolitis do not need any laboratory or radiologic evaluation. Chest x-ray (CXR) findings are nonspecific and include hyperinflation, a flattened diaphragm caused by air trapping, parahilar peribronchial infiltrates and atelectasis. The best reason to order a CXR is to rule out other causes of first-time wheezing, including foreign body, congenital airway anomalies, congestive heart failure, or bacterial pneumonia in patients with a confounding clinical picture. Routine CXRs should not be obtained. Fever is a common finding in infants with bronchiolitis; infants with bronchiolitis are at very low risk for serious invasive bacterial infection, and routine complete blood count (CBC), lumbar puncture, or blood culture is not warranted. The incidence of urinary tract infection (UTI) in febrile infants with RSV is similar to that in infants with fever without a source (5–10% in some studies), so in highly febrile (temperature $> 39°C$) infants with bronchiolitis, a catheterized urine specimen for culture should be considered. Routine nasal washes for RSV assay are not indicated because the results do not impact clinical care. Exceptions would be infants at high risk for severe disease.

20. **What is the role of bronchodilators and other agents in the treatment of bronchiolitis?**

A recent systematic review of the literature concluded that there is little evidence to support routine use of beta$_2$ agonist bronchodilators such as albuterol, steroids, epinephrine, or ribavirin. Studies reviewed were underpowered to detect statistically significant outcome differences and few collected data on outcomes that are of great clinical importance, such as impact of therapies on need for or duration of hospitalization. Common practice, however, is to initiate a trial of a beta agonist nebulizer in the ED, because 20–30% of patients with bronchiolitis will have a beneficial response. Nebulized epinephrine has also been used in the ED environment, has been shown to be favorable compared with albuterol among outpatients in some studies, but has not been evaluated for efficacy or safety with regards to home use after discharge.

Hartling L, Wiebe N, Russell K, et al: A meta-analysis of randomized controlled trials evaluating the efficacy of epinephrine for the treatment of acute viral bronchiolitis. Arch Pediatr Adolesc Med 157:957–964, 2003.

King VJ, Viswanathan M, Bordley WC, et al: Pharmacologic treatment of bronchiolitis in infants and children: A systematic review. Arch Pediatr Adolesc Med 158:127–137, 2004.

KEY POINTS: ACUTE RESPIRATORY DISORDERS IN CHILDREN

1. In children, the absence of cough and the presence of agitation and drooling are highly predictive of epiglottitis, whereas presence of a cough strongly suggests croup.

2. Absence of a positive history often delays diagnosis; foreign bodies should be suspected in children with evidence of airway obstruction who do not respond to appropriate interventions.

3. Less than 20–30% of infants with bronchiolitis will respond to inhaled beta agonist or epinephrine therapy. Response should be carefully assessed and treatment continued only in patients with a clearly positive benefit.

4. Observation of the child often offers the best clue to localization and severity of an acute respiratory problem before a cold stethoscope touches his or her chest.

---

21. Is there a role for steroids in bronchiolitis?

Steroids have no proven benefit in the acute management of bronchiolitis and are not recommended.

22. List the admission criteria for bronchiolitis.
- Consider for age younger than 2 months
- Hypoxemia on room air
- History of apnea
- Inability to self-hydrate by feeding
- Respiratory distress
- Underlying chronic cardiopulmonary disorders (see Table 61-2)

23. How are bronchodilators used in the management of acute asthma?

Selective beta$_2$ agonists are the mainstay of medications to reverse bronchospasm. Delivery of albuterol by nebulizer or meter-dosed inhaler with a spacer has been shown to be equally clinically effective, although delivery by nebulizer has remained the preferred route in the ED setting. A mouthpiece should be used with the nebulized route to ensure maximal deliver to the lungs. Albuterol is a racemic mixture of the R and S isomers of the compound, which have bronchodilatory and bronchoconstrictive properties. Levalbuterol, the pure R isomer, has not, in large clinical trials, been demonstrated to be significantly more effective and is more costly. In children with moderate-to-severe asthma, inhaled anticholinergic therapy (ipratropium bromide) has also been shown to decrease severity and hospitalization rate when given in conjunction with beta$_2$ agonists (albuterol).

24. When and how should steroids be administered?

Controlling inflammation is the cornerstone of asthma treatment. Dose is 2 mg/kg as a load orally (maximum 80 mg), followed by 2 mg/kg/day divided twice daily for the next 4 days. Oral prednisone has been shown to be as effective as IV methylprednisolone in the initial management of children with asthma, and the oral route is preferred. An alternative to prednisone is dexamethasone. At a dose of 0.6 mg/kg (maximum, 16 mg) as initial treatment followed by the same dose in 12–24 hours, dexamethasone has shown similar efficacy, improved compliance, and fewer side effects compared with 5 days of prednisone in children with mild asthma symptoms. Studies on sicker populations are pending.

25. **During an exacerbation of asthma, when should a chest radiograph be obtained? What are the typical findings?**
A chest radiograph is not indicated in the routine evaluation of a child with asthma but should be obtained if pneumonia, pneumothorax, pneumomediastinum, or foreign body is suspected clinically. Chest radiographs commonly show hyperinflation, atelectasis, and peribronchial thickening, indicating lower airway obstruction. Pneumothorax is rare. Pneumomediastinum is more common in older children (age >10 years), whereas infiltrates are more common in younger children.

26. **Outline the initial assessment, evaluation, and treatment of an asthma exacerbation in the ED.**
Step 1. Initial assessment
- Evaluate vital signs with pulse oximetry, use of accessory muscles, retractions, alertness, auscultation, and peak expiratory flow rate (PEFR) in patients older than 5 years.
- Consider use of an asthma score for objective assessment and reassessment of the patient.
Step 2. Initial treatment
- Administer oxygen as needed to keep saturation in the normal range.
- Administer nebulized albuterol every 20 minutes or continuously, depending on severity. Dose is 0.15 mg/kg every 20 minutes × 3, or 10 mg/hr continuously.
- Administer nebulized ipratropium bromide with albuterol 0.5 mg with each albuterol nebulizer × 3 doses.
- Give oral steroids at 2 mg/kg, with maximal dose of 80 mg. Consider dexamethasone. Give parenterally only if the child is unable to tolerate oral medication.
Step 3. Repeat assessment
- If PEFR is greater than 70% baseline and there is no wheezing, retractions, or accessory muscle use, observe the patient for at least 1 hour after the last nebulized treatment.
Step 4a. Discharge
- Discharge home with a reliable caretaker, patient education, medications, and follow-up instructions.
- Medications should include albuterol, nebulized or inhaled every 4 hours as needed for wheezing; and prednisone, 2 mg/kg/day divided once or twice daily for a total of 5 days; or dexamethasone, one dose of 0.6 mg/kg the following day.
Step 4b. Continued therapy: Incomplete or poor response
- Continuous albuterol by nebulization
- Atrovent 0.5 mg every 4 hours
- Frequent reassessment of patient
- Continued poor response: IV terbutaline, magnesium, venous blood gas (VBG), intensive care unit (ICU) admission
Step 5. Admission criteria
- Unable to wean to every-2-hour nebulizer therapy
- Hypoxemia by pulse oximetry

27. **What about magnesium?**
The mechanism of action of IV magnesium is not known but is hypothesized to be the counteraction of calcium ions to prevent bronchial smooth muscle contraction. The benefit in patients with mild to moderate exacerbations is unclear, and its use should be reserved for those patients nonresponsive to albuterol and steroids. Dose is 75 mg/kg IV (maximum of 2 gm).

Rowe BH, Bretzlaff JA, Bourdon C, et al: Magnesium sulfate for treating exacerbations of acute asthma in the emergency department. The Cochrane Library, Vol. 3, 2005.

28. **Does aminophylline have any use?**
Aminophylline does not have a role in the routine management of the pediatric asthma patient. IV aminophylline has been shown to improve lung function in children within 6 hours of

treatment in those with severe asthma exacerbations who have received bronchodilators and steroids, but does not reduce symptoms, number of nebulizer treatments, or length of stay. There is insufficient evidence to assess the impact on pediatric intensive care unit (PICU) admission and mechanical ventilation.

Mitra A, Bassler D, Goodman K, et al: Intravenous aminophylline for acute severe asthma in children over two years receiving inhaled bronchodilators. The Cochrane Library, Vol. 3, 2005.

29. What about parenteral beta agonists?

Use of systemic beta agonists is controversial, and few well-designed studies have evaluated their use. They should be considered in patients with severe exacerbations who have failed to respond to maximal inhaled therapy. Options include subcutaneous terbutaline or epinephrine. Terbutaline is the drug of choice for IV therapy; dose is an initial bolus of 10 μg/kg followed by a continuous infusion starting at 0.5 μg/kg/min. Inhaled therapy should not be interrupted, and the patient requires close monitoring of cardiac function and serum potassium levels.

30. What should I do if my patient is going into respiratory failure?

Consider treatment with magnesium, terbutaline, and epinephrine. If intubation is necessary, ketamine, which stimulates the release of catecholamines causing bronchodilation, is a good choice for sedation (dose: 2 mg/kg IV). If ketamine is given, atropine should also be administered to decrease airway secretions. A paralytic agent should then be given using a rapid-sequence protocol.

31. What initial ventilator settings would you recommend for a child with asthma and respiratory failure who requires mechanical ventilation?

Mechanical ventilation of the intubated asthma patient should involve permissive hypercapnia. A slow rate (8–12 breaths/min) provides adequate time for exhalation, preventing breath stacking and the potential for pneumothorax. Positive end-expiratory pressure should be avoided to prevent further risk of barotrauma. Continued sedation and neuromuscular blockade usually are indicated.

CHAPTER 62

PEDIATRIC GASTROINTESTINAL DISORDERS AND DEHYDRATION

Mark E. Anderson, MD

1. **What are the most common causes of acute abdominal pain in children?**

The most common cause of acute abdominal pain in children is nonspecific abdominal pain, and a definitive cause may never be identified. Appendicitis is a common cause (32%) of abdominal pain in children and is a differential consideration of abdominal pain, regardless of age. Other causes are grouped more easily according to patient age. In infants younger than 2 years, causes include colic, gastroenteritis, viral illness, and constipation. Older children may experience pain caused by functional disorders, gastroenteritis, constipation, urinary tract infection, appendicitis, pelvic inflammatory disease, ectopic pregnancy, and inflammatory bowel disease. Uncommon but serious causes of abdominal pain include intussusception, volvulus, pancreatitis, diabetes, Meckel's diverticulum, sickle cell disease, leukemia, lymphomas, and testicular or ovarian torsion.

Barkin RM, Caputo GL, Jaffe DM, et al: Pediatric Emergency Medicine, 2nd ed. St. Louis, Mosby, 1997.

Paajanen H, Somppi E: Early childhood appendicitis is still a difficult diagnosis. Acta Pediatr 85:459–462, 1996.

Rothrock SG, Skeoch G, Rush JJ, et al: Clinical features of misdiagnosed appendicitis in children. Ann Emerg Med 20:45–50, 1991.

KEY POINTS: PEDIATRIC ABDOMINAL PAIN

1. Age is *everything* in pediatric abdominal pain.

2. Presentation may vary from the "classic" presentation.

3. Consider unique pediatric issues such as intussusception in the appropriate clinical scenario.

2. **How should I approach the work-up of a pediatric patient with abdominal pain?**

Children pose a unique challenge, as they may be unable to articulate their complaints; however, careful observation of a child while talking with the caregiver can be elucidating. When possible, allow a child to describe his or her complaints by asking age-appropriate questions. An adolescent should be given more independence and the opportunity to answer some questions, especially those pertaining to sexual activity, without the caregiver present. History from the caregivers and the patient should address acuteness; progression; timing; quality; location; radiation; severity; effect on physical activity; aggravating or alleviating factors; and associated problems, such as fever, nausea, vomiting, diarrhea, dysuria, vaginal discharge, and menstrual history. The physical examination should include vital signs and temperature, determination of hydration status, a chest examination, a thorough abdominal examination (auscultated bowel sounds, palpable masses, tenderness, guarding, or rebound), an external genital examination, and a rectal examination. A pelvic examination should be done in all pubescent girls with lower quadrant abdominal pain or symptoms of pelvic disease. Ancillary data may include urinalysis, urine pregnancy test, complete blood cell count, electrolytes, amylase, cultures for *Neisseria gonorrhoeae* and *Chlamydia trachomatis,* and diagnostic imaging including a chest radiograph.

3. **List the most common causes of gastrointestinal (GI) bleeding in children.**
Common causes of GI bleeding are differentiated most easily by determining upper versus lower GI bleeding, then by grouping according to patient age.

Upper GI bleeding produces positive nasogastric aspirates and generally develops from a site above the ligament of Treitz. It may present as hematemesis, coffee-ground emesis, or melena.

- **Neonates:** Idiopathic, ingested maternal blood, gastritis, esophagitis, peptic ulcer disease, bleeding diathesis
- **Infants:** Idiopathic, gastritis, esophagitis, peptic ulcer disease, foreign-body ingestion, caustic ingestion
- **Children:** Esophageal varices, esophagitis, peptic ulcer disease, foreign-body ingestion, caustic ingestion

Lower GI bleeding is distal to the ligament of Treitz and may present as hematochezia or melena.

- **Neonates:** Benign anorectal lesions, upper GI bleeding, milk allergy, midgut volvulus
- **Infants:** Benign anorectal lesions (anal fissure), intussusception, Meckel's diverticulum, infectious diarrhea, upper GI bleeding, milk allergy, lymphonodular hyperplasia of the colon
- **Children:** Juvenile colonic polyps, benign anorectal lesions, intussusception, Meckel's diverticulum, infectious diarrhea, upper GI bleeding, inflammatory bowel disease (In small children, massive GI bleeds may lead to shock before the onset of hematemesis or melena.)

4. **How does the character of blood help determine the location of GI bleeding?**
- Bright red hematemesis: Little or no contact with the gastric secretions, usually active bleeding at a site at or above the cardia of the stomach
- Coffee-ground hematemesis: Altered by gastric secretions
- Melena and tarry stools: Requires blood loss greater than 50–100 mL in 24 hours and usually originates proximal to the ileocecal valve
- Streaks of blood on stool: Lesion in rectal ampulla or in the anal canal
- Hematochezia: Brisk hemorrhage or hemorrhage distal to the ileocecal valve

5. **What causes newborn jaundice? When is it worrisome?**
Newborns physiologically become jaundiced to the face and upper chest in the first few days of life as the liver begins to conjugate bilirubin. Physiologic newborn jaundice should not exceed a rise of 5 mg/dL per day of life and should consist of unconjugated bilirubin. The conjugated portion should not exceed 20% of the total, and the newborn infant should not appear jaundiced in the first day of life. Entities that may result in red blood cell hemolysis, such as glucose-6-phosphate dehydrogenase deficiency or neonatal sepsis, among others, may present as jaundice.

6. **Do jaundice emergencies exist?**
Yes. Dangerous elevation in serum bilirubin can result in a neonatal encephalopathy that may or may not reverse completely. Deposition of bilirubin in vulnerable areas of the brain, such as the basal ganglia, can cause the irreversible syndrome of kernicterus. Prompt diagnosis, pediatric consultation, and institution of therapy (phototherapy, exchange transfusion) can protect the newborn from significant morbidity. Minutes matter!

Maisels J: Jaundice in a newborn: Answers to questions about a common clinical problem. Contemp Pediatr 22(5):34–40.

KEY POINTS: NEONATAL JAUNDICE

1. Follow-up, follow-up, follow-up—ideally within 24 hours.

2. Physiologic jaundice is a diagnosis of exclusion.

3. Suspicion of jaundice should be confirmed with an objective test.

4. Kernicterus or acute bilirubin encephalopathy is generally irreversible.

7. **How should constipation be managed in the outpatient setting?**
Generally, disimpaction is necessary before the initiation of long-term therapy for constipation. This can be accomplished with one or two enemas, using smaller or *junior* enemas for younger children. Long-term therapy involves the addition of free water to the diet and fiber-rich or bulk foods. In some cases, mineral oil or another mild stool softener can be used to prevent the formation of hardened stool. Encopresis, or involuntary stooling behavior, can be a sign of constipation or of a behavioral problem. Such children should be referred to a primary care provider for ongoing management.

8. **What serious entity can present as constipation in infants and children?**
Apparent constipation in an infant can be an early manifestation of Hirschsprung's disease, wherein a portion of the large bowel, usually the distal segment, is devoid of ganglion cells, rendering the bowel incapable of coordinated motility. In its severe form, toxic megacolon, this can be life threatening. Diagnosis is made on colonic suction biopsy demonstrating the absence of ganglionic cells in the affected portion of bowel.

9. **What are the symptoms of an esophageal foreign body?**
A normal infant investigates objects by placing the object in his or her mouth. This normal developmental behavior can cause an airway or esophageal foreign body. Most swallowed items pass through the GI tract when the object is moved into the stomach, and parents can be advised to expect a surprise in the infant's stool over the ensuing few days. On acute presentation, an airway foreign body must be suspected and ruled out. Extra airway noise is an ominous sign and should alert the practitioner to prepare for urgent airway manipulation or consultation to help manage the foreign body. The upper airway in an infant or child is more funnel shaped than the adult airway, and foreign objects typically are lodged in the upper airway; this causes stridor, or a high-pitched inspiratory noise.

10. **Using a posteroanterior film, how can I determine whether a coin is in the esophagus or in the trachea?**
A coin in the esophagus lies in the frontal plane and usually appears as a full circle on a posteroanterior film. A coin in the trachea lies in the sagittal plane because the incomplete cartilage rings of the posterior trachea offer more space with less resistance, and the coin usually appears end-on. The presumed location should be confirmed by obtaining a lateral film and noting if the foreign body is in or behind the tracheal air column.

11. **When should a foreign body of the GI tract be removed?**
Any foreign body causing symptoms should be removed. Foreign bodies also should be removed if they appear lodged in the esophagus. Some clinicians advocate observing ingested coins for 24 hours in the hope of spontaneous passage, provided that the patient is truly asymptomatic. A conservative approach is the general rule when objects have cleared the

esophagus, and GI passage can require days to weeks. Follow-up is important, and parents should be instructed to return with concerns about the child's abdominal pain, fever, vomiting, and hematemesis or melena.

12. **Describe the typical findings in appendicitis.**

The classic presentation is crampy, periumbilical pain that gradually shifts to the right lower quadrant over 4–12 hours. After the onset of pain, associated symptoms include nausea and vomiting, anorexia, and mild fever. The patient may prefer to lie on his or her side with flexion at the hips. Physical examination may reveal decreased bowel sounds, maximal tenderness at McBurney's point (located 4–6 cm from the iliac crest on a line drawn between the iliac crest and the umbilicus), and positive psoas or obturator signs. Laboratory analysis may show an elevated white blood cell count with a left-shifted differential. Younger children are more likely to have perforated appendicitis (almost 100% of patients <1 year old). This can be a difficult diagnosis to make in a young child or infant because the classic presenting symptoms and signs often are not present.

13. **What is intussusception?**

Intussusception occurs when a portion of bowel telescopes into a neighboring segment, compromising the vascular integrity of the involved bowel. Intussusception is rare in children younger than 3 months and also decreases in frequency after 3 years of age. The classic presentation is with intermittent irritability in a child. The periods of irritability may be associated with the child drawing his or her legs up to the chest. Intussusception also can present simply as altered mental status. Older individuals with intussusception may have a pathologic lead point, such as lymphadenopathy from lymphoma, Meckel's diverticulum, or Henoch-Schönlein purpura. These cases also are more likely to recur. Males are affected more often than females, and the incidence is about 1–4 cases in 1000 live births. The treatment is prompt reduction either by a radiologist with air contrast or barium enema or surgical reduction.

14. **What is Meckel's diverticulum?**

A persistence of the omphalomesenteric duct remnant. This is the most common congenital malformation of the intestine, occurring in 2–3% of the population. It is approximately 2–3 cm long and, in 50% of cases, contains heterotopic tissue (gastric mucosa, pancreatic tissue, or endometrium). It usually is found on the antimesenteric border of the distal small bowel, approximately 90 cm proximal to the ileocecal valve. Only about 5% of patients become symptomatic, most often boys, with a peak incidence at 2 years of age. The presence of gastric mucosa is associated with the formation of bleeding ulcers in the diverticulum, which usually present as painless rectal bleeding. A Meckel's diverticulum also may present as an obstruction secondary to intussusception or volvulus formation.

15. **How is hypertrophic pyloric stenosis best diagnosed?**

The classic clinical presentation is in a first-born 2- to 6-week-old male infant with progressive projectile, nonbilious emesis and failure to gain weight if symptoms are prolonged. Examination findings may include visible peristaltic waves, dehydration, and a palpable olive-shaped mass. Diagnosis can be confirmed by ultrasound of the hypertrophied pylorus or by an upper GI barium swallow showing a narrowing of the distal antrum and pylorus (*string sign*). Many authors recommend starting with a barium swallow because this provides the ability to diagnose other problems that may be considered in the differential diagnosis of hypertrophic pyloric stenosis (e.g., reflux, antral web, pylorospasm, malrotation). The availability of these procedures in children is institution-specific and may factor into the decision regarding which diagnostic test to order.

16. **What are the typical electrolyte abnormalities in hypertrophic pyloric stenosis?**
    The projectile vomiting of hypertrophic pyloric stenosis typically causes a hypochloremic, hypokalemic metabolic alkalosis. Any combination of electrolytes can be seen with this diagnosis, and the associated laboratory findings are nonspecific.

17. **What is a volvulus?**
    A twisting of the bowel on its own axis, causing a closed-loop intraluminal obstruction and occlusion of its blood supply. More commonly seen in children older than 1 year and involving gastric, midgut, transverse, or sigmoid colonic tissue, patients typically present with abdominal pain and vomiting. On examination, the child may have abdominal distention and a palpable abdominal mass.

18. **What are the usual causes of diarrhea in infants and children?**
    Most diarrheal illness in pediatric patients is viral and self-limited in otherwise healthy individuals. The cause is largely seasonal for the viral agents. Rotavirus is a common agent and is noteworthy as a cause of multiple (10–20) loose, watery stools per day. With this degree of fluid loss, attention to hydration status is the mainstay of outpatient and inpatient treatment. Bacterial sources also may cause profuse, watery diarrhea, but the presence of pus or mucus in the stool may help delineate these from viral causes. *Shigella* is noteworthy for the associated tenesmus and small-volume squirts of diarrhea. Fevers can be seen with viral and bacterial causes, but the associated discomfort of the child may be worse with invasive bacterial enteritis.

19. **A 10-month-old infant presents with a high fever and an associated 2-minute generalized tonic-clonic seizure; peripheral white blood cell count is 11,000/mL with 30% segmented forms and 40% bands; the child has notable watery diarrhea. What is the most likely diagnosis?**
    Shigella infection.

20. **How should diarrhea be managed?**
    The patient's hemodynamic stability should be assessed quickly and treated if necessary. The decision to rehydrate orally or intravenously is made by assessing the patient's degree of dehydration (recent urine output, mental status changes, compensated or decompensated shock). Fluid losses amounting to moderate or severe dehydration (easy to calculate if a recent weight is known or documented) require aggressive intravenous fluid therapy while monitoring the patient closely. Infants and children may improve rapidly, then show interest in taking fluids orally. Because most diarrheal illnesses are viral in nature, no specific therapy is indicated. The presence of gross blood should alert the physician to the possibility of hemolytic-uremic syndrome, and stool should be cultured in this instance. Microscopic blood can be present with viral and bacterial causes. The presence of pus or mucus should prompt a stool culture. Empiric antibiotics are not indicated if the patient is not immunocompromised, very young, or very ill. Certain bacterial causes, such as *Shigella,* require antibiotic treatment generally because this agent is so contagious. Conversely, *Salmonella* generally does not require specific treatment, and careful attention to prevent additional fecal and oral spread is the mainstay of therapy.

21. **What are the three major categories of dehydration?**
    - Isotonic
    - Hypotonic or hyponatremic
    - Hypertonic or hypernatremic

22. **What is oral rehydration therapy? When is it appropriate?**
    The administration of small volumes of oral fluid solution (Pedialyte, Rehydralyte, Infalyte) containing glucose and electrolytes to reverse dehydration. The oral glucose in these solutions

facilitates absorption of sodium and water across the mucosal cells of the small intestine. This process may take 4–8 hours and may be instituted in any patient with mild-to-moderate dehydration who can tolerate oral fluids, even if the patient continues to have diarrhea. Instruct the parent or provider to offer sips of fluid frequently, and give precautions to monitor closely for urine output and changing mental status. Infants and children who fail a trial of oral rehydration subsequently may be treated with intravenous fluids.

23. How is intravenous therapy administered?

In pediatric fluid resuscitation, isotonic fluids such as normal saline or lactated Ringer's are given in 20 mL/kg aliquots over short periods of time. Infants and children have extremely elastic cardiovascular systems and can constrict their vasculature to a degree greater than the adult. A child in compensated shock (with normal blood pressure) may require repeat boluses. Dextrose-containing fluids should not be given to children as volume expanders because the solute load to the kidneys can cause further diuresis. Hypoglycemia should be tested for specifically, using a serum glucose measurement device or a rapid colorimetric dipstick. In the setting of hypoglycemia, the infant or child is treated with 2–4 mL/kg of dextrose 10% (if <3 months old) or dextrose 25% (if >3 months old). Obtain a follow-up serum glucose measurement after administering the dextrose.

24. How do I calculate maintenance intravenous therapy?

- 10 kg: 4 mL/kg/hr
- 10–20 kg: Add the above amount to 2 mL/kg/hr for each kg over 10
- 20 kg: Add the above amount to 1 mL/kg/hr for each kg over 20
  A child weighing 26 kg should receive 66 mL/hr [(10 × 4) + (10 × 2) + (6 × 1) = 66 mL/hr] of 5% dextrose one-half normal saline with 20–30 mEq of potassium/L. Alternatively, maintenance 24-hour fluids are 100 mL/kg for the first 10 kg, 50 mL/kg for the next 10 kg (10 to 20 kg), and 20 mL/kg for greater than 20 kg. Divide this result by 24 to get an hourly fluid rate.

25. How is hypernatremic dehydration treated?

Initial treatment is aimed at establishing hemodynamic stability. A volume expansion of 20–30 mL/kg body weight of fluid may be necessary to achieve stability. Subsequent therapy aims to slowly establish normal serum sodium values over the following 48–72 hours. The process involves calculating the free water deficit, accounting for fluid already administered, and adding in maintenance requirements. Careful attention to electrolytes and administered fluid is important to prevent sequelae as the serum sodium corrects. Irreversible neurologic damage may result if the serum sodium is corrected too quickly.

26. How should hyponatremia be corrected?

If the patient is symptomatic with seizures and has severe hyponatremia (usually a sodium level <120 mEq/dL), a hypertonic solution of 3% saline may be administered carefully at 4 mL/kg until symptoms resolve. Use hyperosmolar sodium with caution and generally only in the setting of documented or strongly suspected hyponatremia. Otherwise, the preferred solution is 0.9% saline to correct the deficit no faster than 15 mEq/dL every 24 hours.

27. How do I estimate the amount of total body fluid deficit?

A child's fluid deficit is estimated by multiplying weight in kilograms by the estimated percentage of dehydration (10 kg × 10% = 100 mL). If a recent weight is available, the acute weight loss generally represents fluid losses.

28. State the major complications of dehydration.

Shock and acute renal tubular necrosis. In severe cases, renal vein thrombosis or dural sinus thrombosis can occur.

29. **Do umbilical hernias need surgical consultations?**

    Rarely. Most regress without treatment, although some may persist until school age. Incarceration of umbilical hernias is unusual. Covering the hernia and reducing it (e.g., with tape, coins, straps) does not change the natural course. Surgical consultation may be warranted if there is no resolution by school age or if cosmesis is a concern.

CHAPTER 63

PEDIATRIC INFECTIOUS DISEASES

Roger M. Barkin, MD, MPH, and Elaine Norman Scholes, MD

1. Are infectious diseases important to recognize in the pediatric patient?
Infectious diseases account for a significant percentage of pediatric visits to the emergency department (ED) for acute illness. Although most conditions are self-limited and infrequent, some infections are significant in that they may be multisystem or life threatening or require consideration in the differential diagnosis of many presenting complaints.

2. What is the mechanism of spread of measles (rubeola)?
By direct contact with infectious droplets or airborne dissemination.

3. What is the incubation period for measles?
From exposure to the onset of symptoms, 8–12 days. It is 14 days from exposure to the onset of the rash. Patients are contagious 1–2 days before they become symptomatic and 4 days after the rash appears.

4. List the common signs and symptoms of patients with measles.
- High fever is found.
- Three Cs: Conjunctivitis, coryza, cough may be observed.
- Rash: Discrete red maculopapular rash first appears on the forehead, becoming coalescent as it spreads down the trunk to the feet by the third day of the illness. The rash fades in the same head-to-feet pattern as it appeared.
- Koplik's spots: 1- to 3-mm bluish white spots on a bright red surface that appear first on the buccal mucosa opposite the lower molars. They are a pathognomonic exanthema of measles. They appear approximately within 48 hours after the onset of symptoms. The spots may spread to involve the buccal and labial mucosa and disappear on the second day after the onset of the rash.
- Photophobia may be noted.

5. Name the complications of measles.
Otitis media and bronchopneumonia. Encephalitis may occur as well.

6. What is subacute sclerosing panencephalitis?
A rare degenerative central nervous system disease caused by a latent measles infection, occurring an average of 10 years after a primary measles illness. Patients have progressive intellectual and behavioral deterioration and convulsions. This disease is not contagious.

7. Describe the exanthem seen in rubella. Why is it also called 3-day measles?
Numerous discrete rose-pink maculopapules first appear on the face and, as in rubeola, spread downward to involve the trunk and extremities. The rash on the face fades on day 2, and the rash on the trunk becomes coalescent. By the third day, the rash disappears, which is why rubella is also called *3-day measles*. Rubella is now rarely reported in the United States secondary to the efficacy of immunizations.

8. **What are Forschheimer spots?**
   Pinpoint red macules on the soft palate seen early in rubella; however, in contrast to Koplik's spots, they are *not* pathognomonic.

9. **What is the incubation period for mumps, and when is the patient contagious?**
   The incubation is 12–18 days. The patient is contagious 1–2 days (up to 7 days) before the onset of parotid swelling. Patients are no longer infectious 7–9 days after the onset of parotid swelling.

10. **List the major complications of mumps.**
    - Meningoencephalitis in 0.5% of cases
    - Orchitis after puberty with secondary sterility (rare)
    - Arthritis, renal involvement, thyroiditis, mastitis, and hearing impairment (all rare)

11. **Describe the characteristic rash in erythema infectiosum.**
    Erythematous ears and a maculopapular rash on the cheeks that coalesce to form the characteristic *slapped-cheek appearance* is classic. The rash spreads to the extremities 1–2 days later with a reticular, lacelike pattern caused by central clearing of the confluent rash. Human parvovirus B19 is the causative agent.

12. **What is the typical progession of findings of roseola (erythema subitum)?**
    Typically, a child between 6 months and 2 years old (up to 4 years old) presents with a history of high fever of 3 days' duration and mild symptoms, if any. The fever abates abruptly, followed by the appearance of a macular rash on the trunk and thighs. It is caused by human herpesvirus–6.

13. **What is the incubation period for varicella (chickenpox), and when are patients infectious?**
    The incubation period is 10–20 days. From 1–2 days before the appearance of the rash until no new lesions are forming (usually 7–10 days after the appearance of the rash). Children are generally not considered to be infectious once the lesions are crusted and dry.

14. **Name the mode of transmission and the cause of infectious mononucleosis (IM).**
    IM is transmitted through direct and prolonged contact with oropharyngeal secretions. It is caused by the Epstein-Barr virus.

15. **List the clinical manifestations of IM.**
    - Fever lasting 1–2 weeks
    - Lymphadenopathy (usually nontender, no overlying erythema, most often bilateral cervical location, with epitrochlear nodes being suggestive of IM)
    - Tonsillopharyngitis (usually an exudate is present—need to obtain a throat culture to exclude group A streptococci)
    - Spleen or liver enlargement
    - Young children: May also have rashes, abdominal pain, upper respiratory infections with cough, failure to thrive, and early-onset otitis media

16. **Which parenteral antibiotic is correlated with a rash in older children and adults with IM?**
    Amoxicillin, by an unknown mechanism of action, can cause a rash in patients with IM.

17. **What are the hematologic findings in IM?**
    A relative lymphocytosis of greater than 50% of all leukocytes and a relative atypical lymphocytosis of 10% of leukocytes are the typical findings, although the relative percentage of atypical lymphocytes in children may be lower than in adults.

18. **What are heterophil antibodies?**

Serum IgM antibodies with the capability to agglutinate horse (better than sheep or bovine) erythrocytes. The ability to absorb to beef red blood cells but not guinea pig kidney distinguishes heterophil antibodies in IM from both Forssman antibodies (found in normal serum) and the antibodies in serum sickness. A heterophil antibody titer greater than 40 with a good clinical history for IM strongly supports the diagnosis. It is positive in 90% of cases of IM, with few false-positive results except in young children, in whom Epstein-Barr virus serology is needed to establish the diagnosis.

19. **What is the monospot test?**

This qualitative, rapid slide test is used to detect serum heterophil antibodies in IM. It is positive in 70% of patients during the first week of illness and in 85–90% of patients during the third week. In children younger than 4 years, this test may be negative because of lower levels of detectable heterophil antibodies requiring the more sensitive Epstein-Barr virus serology to be done.

20. **Describe the treatment of uncomplicated IM.**

Supportive therapy and rest are the mainstays of treatment, with emphasis on analgesia for sore throat, headaches, and myalgias; oral fluids to prevent dehydration secondary to discomfort with swallowing; and a decrease in normal activity. Acetaminophen and ibuprofen may be useful.

21. **Summarize the complications of IM.**

Respiratory
- Airway obstruction due to tonsillar hypertrophy
- Sinusitis
- Pneumonia

Hematologic
- Thrombocytopenia
- Hemolytic anemia
- Granulocytopenia

Neurologic
- Encephalitis
- Cerebellar ataxia
- Guillain-Barré syndrome
- Transverse myelitis
- Bell's palsy

Cardiac
- Pericarditis
- Myocarditis

Eye
- Optic neuritis
- Uveitis, keratitis

Other
- Splenic rupture
- Chronic disease

22. **What is the role of corticosteroids in the treatment of IM?**

Steroids may reduce the risk of progression to upper airway obstruction by reducing edema and hyperplasia of the lymphoid tissue. There is usually improvement in 6–24 hours after administration.

23. **How long does the patient need to worry about the risk of splenic rupture?**
Although rare, rupture of the spleen usually occurs during the second or third week of the illness. Patients must avoid contact sports while the spleen is enlarged. Follow-up examinations determine when it is safe to play contact sports.

24. **What are the most common findings associated with botulism in children?**
Botulism results from ingestion of preformed toxins (e.g., canned vegetables), ingestion of spores in infant botulism (honey), or spore contamination of open wounds. One third of the 100 annual cases in the United States are food borne; the remainder are cases of infant botulism. *Clostridium botulinum* produces a neurotoxin that blocks the presynaptic release of acetylcholine after an incubation period of 12–48 hours. Clinically, patients develop symmetric descending paralysis with weakness and equal deep tendon reflexes associated with a normal sensorium. Pupils are fixed and dilated with oculomotor paralysis, blurred vision, diplopia, ptosis, and photophobia. Associated findings may include slurred speech, nausea, vomiting, constipation, vertigo, dry mouth, dysphagia, and urinary retention. Dyspnea and rales, progressing to respiratory failure, may be noted.

Shapiro RL, Hatheway C, Swerdlow DL: Botulism in the United States: A clinical and epidemiologic review. Ann Intern Med 129:221–228, 1998.

25. **Are there specific measures that should be initiated in the patient with botulism?**
Initial management must focus on support, airway maintenance, and monitoring. Botulism equine antitoxin should be administered and is available from the Centers for Disease Control (404-639-3670/2888) or from local state health departments.

26. **What are the distinct clinical presentations of diphtheria?**
Corynebacterium diphtheriae, an unencapsulated, club-shaped gram-positive bacillus, produces an exotoxin that results in four patterns of clinical findings. The pharyngeal-tonsillar complex consists of a sore throat, fever, vomiting, dysphagia, and malaise associated with a gray, closely adherent pseudomembrane. Respiratory obstruction may develop. Less common presentations include laryngeal diphtheria with hoarseness and loss of voice; respiratory tract edema may lead to obstruction. Serosanguineous nasal discharge may persist for weeks, usually without systemic findings. A sharply demarcated ulcer may develop on the skin with a membranous base. This latter cutaneous form is found mostly in the tropics but may present in alcoholics and lower socioeconomic populations. The diagnosis is confirmed by Löffler's medium and tellurite agar cultures and Gram stain.

Galazka A: The changing epidemiology of diphtheria in the vaccine era. J Infect Dis 181(Suppl 1):S2–S9, 2000.

KEY POINTS: PEDIATRIC INFECTIOUS DISEASES

1. Infectious diseases represent the most frequent cause of ED visits for children. It is important to different self-limited from life-threatening conditions.

2. Infections in children are often age specific, and their management must reflect the child's age and concurrent medical conditions.

3. Immunizations have changed the pattern of infectious diseases in children.

4. Multisystem infections in children often present with dermatologic findings but require management of potential complications.

27. **How is a child with diphtheria treated?**
After ensuring stability of the airway and absence of associated cardiovascular dysfunction secondary to myocarditis, antitoxin should be initiated after intradermal or conjunctival tests for horse serum sensitivity. Concurrently, antibiotics should be initiated with penicillin or with erythromycin in a penicillin-allergic patient. Carriers should be treated with antibiotics.

28. **What clinical findings must be present to make the diagnosis of Kawasaki's disease?**
It is a multisystem disease occurring predominantly in children younger than 5 years, Kawasaki's disease also is known as *mucocutaneous lymph node syndrome.* The cause is thought to be related to lymphotropic retrovirus, although the epidemiology is undefined. The syndrome is triphasic in clinical presentation. An acute febrile episode (temperature >38.5°C for at least 5 days) is accompanied by the appearance of five major diagnostic criteria, at least four of which must be present for confirmation of the typical presentation.
   1. Bilateral, nonexudative conjunctivitis usually occurs within 2 days of the onset of fever and lasts up to 2 weeks.
   2. Mouth lesions appear 1–3 days after onset and possibly last for 1–2 weeks. Mouth lesions include erythema, fissuring, crusting of the lips; diffuse oropharyngeal erythema; and strawberry tongue.
   3. Peripheral extremity lesions begin after 3–5 days and last 1–2 weeks. The hands and feet may be indurated. Erythema of the palms and soles is present; desquamation of the tips of fingers and toes occurs 2–3 weeks after the onset of illness.
   4. Erythematous, polymorphous rash occurs concurrently with the fever and spreads from the extremities to the trunk. It usually disappears within 1 week.
   5. Enlarged lymph nodes are present, usually cervical and greater than 1.5 cm.

   Committee on Rheumatic Fever, Endocarditis and Kawasaki's Disease of the American Heart Association Council on Cardiovascular Disease in the Young. Circulation 105:2115, 2002.

29. **What is the most significant complication of Kawasaki's disease?**
The most significant complication is **coronary artery disease** caused by arteritis, aneurysm, or thrombosis. Other findings include diarrhea, vomiting, hydrops of the gallbladder, leukocytosis, cough, proteinuria, arthritis, meningismus, and cerebrospinal fluid pleocytosis. Treatment includes anti-inflammatory agents (i.e., aspirin) and in some cases intravenous (IV) immune globulin.

   Sato N, et al: Selective high dose gamma-globulin treatment in Kawasaki disease: Assessment of clinical aspects and cost effectiveness. Pediatr Int 41:1–7, 1999.

30. **What infectious conditions should be considered in a child presenting with diffuse erythroderma?**
Several acute infectious entities may present with diffuse erythroderma: a scarlatiniform rash caused by group A streptococcus, *Staphylococcus aureus,* or a viral illness; scalded skin syndrome (*S. aureus*); toxic epidermal necrolysis or erythema multiforme caused by a variety of infections and drugs; Kawasaki's disease; toxic shock syndrome (*S. aureus*); and leptospirosis.

31. **Summarize the clinical characteristics of a patient with toxic shock syndrome.**
See Chapter 49.

32. **Describe the three stages of clinical progression of a child with pertussis.**
Pertussis (or whooping cough) is caused by *Bordetella pertussis,* a gram-negative coccobacilli, occurring in all age groups. It peaks in late summer and early fall with an incubation period of 7–10 days. Initially, patients have respiratory complaints of fever, rhinorrhea, and conjunctivitis

lasting 2 weeks (catarrhal). The **paroxysmal phase** follows; severe cough, hypoxia, unremitting paroxysms, and vomiting may occur for 2–4 weeks. Apnea, pneumonia, pneumothorax, seizures, and hypoxia may complicate the illness. In the **convalescent phase**, there is an associated residual cough.

33. **What are the typical stages of Reye's syndrome?**
Reye's syndrome is an uncommon, acute, noninflammatory encephalopathy with altered level of consciousness, cerebral edema without perivascular or meningeal inflammation, and fatty metamorphosis of the liver, probably secondary to mitochondrial dysfunction. It is a multisystem disease that probably has many associated causes, the findings often being referred to as *Reye-like syndrome.* Salicylate ingestion has been incriminated, especially when occurring in association with chickenpox or influenza. It is uncommon. Clinically, patients present with a respiratory or gastrointestinal prodrome followed in several days with an encephalopathic picture that is marked by behavioral changes and a deteriorating level of consciousness. Progression of brain stem dysfunction occurs in a cephalocaudal pattern:

0   Alert, wakeful
I   Lethargy. Follows verbal comments, normal posture, purposeful response to pain, brisk pupillary light reflex, and normal oculocephalic reflex
II Combative or stuporous, inappropriate verbalizing, normal posture, purposeful or nonpurposeful response to pain, sluggish pupillary reaction, and conjugate deviation on doll's eye maneuver
III Comatose, decorticate posture and decerebrate response to pain, sluggish pupillary reaction, conjugate deviation on doll's eye maneuver
IV Comatose, decorticate posture and decerebrate response to pain, sluggish pupillary reflexes, and inconsistent or absent oculocephalic reflex
V   Comatose, flaccid, no response to pain, no pupillary response, no oculocephalic reflex

WEBSITES

1. Centers for Disease Control and Prevention: www.cdc.gov

2. American Academy of Pediatrics: www.aap.org

BIBLIOGRAPHY

1. Barkin RM, Rosen P (eds): Emergency Pediatrics, A Guide to Ambulatory Care, 6th ed. Philadelphia, Mosby, 2002.
2. Feigin RD, Cherry JD (eds): Textbook of Pediatric Infectious Diseases, 5th ed. Philadelphia, W.B. Saunders, 2003.
3. Mandell GL, Douglas RG, Bennett JE (eds): Principles and Practice of Infectious Diseases, 6th ed. Philadelphia, Churchill Livingstone, 2004.
4. Pickering LK (ed): Report of the Committee on Infectious Diseases, 26th ed. Elk Grove Village, IL, American Academy of Pediatrics, 2003.

CHAPTER 64

EMERGENCY DEPARTMENT EVALUATION OF CHILD ABUSE

Anna Olson, MD

1. **What is child abuse?**

   Simply, it is any action or omission that may result in harm to a child. The specifics of abuse, of course, are somewhat nebulous, clouded by significant differences between families and between cultures:

   - **Physical abuse**, or nonaccidental trauma (NAT), is any intentional injury or direct trauma to a child.
   - **Emotional abuse** may include name-calling, intimidation, and harassment.
   - **Neglect** includes denial of basic needs such as food, shelter, clothing, love, or protection.
   - **Sexual abuse** is any involvement of immature children (up to 18 years of age) in acts that they do not fully understand and to which they cannot consent and may include acts of voyeurism and exposure as well as more obvious acts such as fondling and penetration.

2. **How common is abuse?**

   In 2002, nearly 900,000 cases of child abuse were reported (approximately 10% of which were sexual abuse), yielding a rate of 12.3 per 1000. This, however, is likely a gross underestimation. A 1995 Gallup Pole titled "Disciplining Children in America" found parents admitted to knowledge of abuse (both physical and sexual) at 10–15 times the previously mentioned rate. Abused children are over represented in the population presenting for evaluation in the emergency department (ED), so rates are higher there as well.

   Newton AW, Vandeven AM: Update on child maltreatment with a special focus on shaken baby syndrome. Curr Opin Pediatr 17:246–251, 2005.

3. **Who is at risk?**

   Child abuse or neglect may occur in any home and is not bound by socioeconomics, race, religion, culture, ethnicity, or education. That said, there are certain factors that increase a child's risk:

   - Children with special needs (including developmental delay, behavioral disorders, and even giftedness) are at increased risk, as are those with chronic medical conditions. Children who are poorly bonded (such as children in nonmarried or blended-family homes) are at risk as well.
   - Parental factors increasing risk to children include lower level of education, lack of social support, economic, marital, or relationship stressors, parental history of family violence, and substance abuse.

4. **What are the "red flags"?**

   Special care should be given when history does not correlate well with presentation (as when the described mechanism would be unlikely to produce the injuries seen or is not plausible given the developmental age of the child), when significant delays in seeking care are noted, and when there are multiple injuries in various stages of healing. Another red flag is frequent ED visits, but be aware that, in large cities especially, this may be camouflaged by use of multiple EDs.

5. **Do children lie about this stuff?**
   Children lie to get out of trouble, not into it. If they tell you they are being abused, they are. Children are often reluctant to disclose, in part because they are aware, on some level, of the amount of upheaval and "trouble" that is likely to result. For this reason, disclosure followed by retraction or partial retraction should be viewed as the norm and should *not* decrease the suspicion for abuse. Fabrications regarding abuse are very rare and may be a warning sign of other difficulties in the home.

6. **What happens if abuse is suspected and not reported?**
   It is the physician's ethical and legal responsibility to report suspected child abuse. The legal requirement to report is actually meant, in part, to relieve the physician of the burden of making the decision as to whether or not to report. Our colleagues in social work and law enforcement are well trained to deal with these situations; let them help us help these children.

7. **What if the physician is wrong?**
   The Federal Child Abuse Prevention and Treatment Act (CAPTA) provides immunity from civil and criminal liability for those making reports in good faith. Keep in mind that failure to find sufficient evidence to prosecute does not necessarily mean the physician was wrong in his or her suspicions. For more information on what happens after suspected abuse is reported, visit the Web site for the Department of Health and Human Services Administration on Children, Youth, and Families, Children's Bureau (www.acf.hhs.gov/ programs/cb/index.htm).

8. **Which sorts of confounders may confuse a work-up for possible child abuse?**
   - Coagulation disorders (Studies are easily obtained if caregivers suggest this is causative.)
   - Bony fragility syndromes: Osteogenesis imperfecta, rickets, scurvy
   - Cutaneous manifestations of medical or congenital conditions: Purpuric rashes, mongolian spots.
   - Traditional remedies: Coining (vigorous rubbing with a coin results in linear ecchymoses), cupping (circular suction ecchymoses)
   - Sudden infant death syndrome (SIDS)

9. **What types of injuries are generally seen in children presenting for evaluation of NAT?**
   Soft tissue injuries (bruises, bites, burns, cuts), skeletal injuries (especially long bone fractures), and closed head or neurologic injuries constitute the majority of nonaccidental injuries seen in the ED.

10. **Are there any injuries that are particularly worrisome for abuse or neglect rather than the normal wear and tear of childhood?**
    - Soft tissue injuries: Human bites with an intra-incisor distance greater than 2.5 cm, immersion burns to the extremities or buttocks (especially common in children of potty-training age), loop-shaped bruises suggesting beating with an electrical cord or belt, or an impression of any recognizable object (such as a hair brush or hand)
    - Skeletal injuries: Spiral fractures, corner or bucket-handle fractures, skull, rib, spinous process fractures, multiple fractures of different age, or any fracture at all in a preambulatory child
    - Closed head injuries: Retinal hemorrhage, sudden changes in neurologic status
    - Gestalt: Failure to thrive without identifiable organic cause

KEY POINTS: INJURIES THAT ARE NON-ACCIDENTAL UNTIL PROVED OTHERWISE

1. Bilateral retinal hemorrhage

2. Bite marks

3. Bruises taking the shape of recognizable objects

4. Corner or bucket-handle fractures

5. Any fracture in a preambulatory child

11. What is a corner fracture?

This well-known entity, virtually pathognomonic for NAT, is an epiphyseal-metaphyseal junction fracture. Bucket handle fractures and corner fractures (Fig. 64-1) are architecturally similar but have slightly different appearance on plain film, depending on angle of view and severity. These fractures usually result from violent pulling or twisting of an extremity.

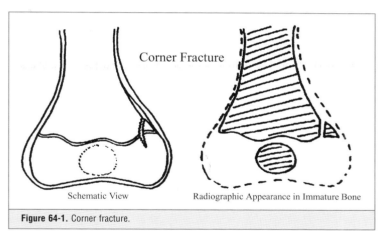

Corner Fracture

Schematic View   Radiographic Appearance in Immature Bone

Figure 64-1. Corner fracture.

12. What is a skeletal survey? What is its purpose?

A skeletal survey is a series of films designed to evaluate each bone individually, used in cases of suspected abuse in preverbal children. It is rarely used in children older than the age of 2. In common practice, a request for a skeletal survey often results in a "babygram," which is a single anteroposterior (AP) view of a young infant whose body is small enough that it will (nearly) fit on a single cartridge of film. Survey films show a significant number of both false positives and false negatives, and additional imaging may be needed. It is always wise to alert your radiologist to your suspicions prior to having him or her read any film, but this is especially true of surveys.

13. How accurate is visual dating of bruises?

Visual dating cannot be relied on to accurately reveal the time elapsed since injury; however, it is very useful for estimating relative ages of multiple resolving ecchymoses. Cutaneous soft tissue injuries go through a fairly predictable progression of colors during the healing process (from red immediately afterwards, through purplish blue to green to yellow to brown, and finally resolving completely). The most important contribution made by visual appearance of bruises may be a suggestion of multiple injuries in various stages of healing, which increases the concern for ongoing NAT.

14. Which types of injuries are most likely to be deadly?
Most NAT fatalities result from closed head injuries. Visceral injuries due to blunt abdominal trauma also factor heavily into pediatric NAT mortality. These injuries include damage to hollow and solid organs, as well as vasculature.

15. What is the most common neurologic injury seen in nonaccidentally injured infants?
Shaken baby syndrome, also called inflicted traumatic brain injury (ITBI), consists of subdural hemorrhage, traumatic brain injury, and retinal hemorrhage. Diagnosis may be difficult, because accurate history is usually lacking. This triad classically occurs from the extreme accelerative forces of shaking alone and does not require impact due to throwing. Mortality estimates range from 25 to 30%, with an estimated 1200–1400 injuries per year. Permanent disability (including blindness, seizure disorder, mental retardation, and cerebral palsy) is seen in the majority of survivors.

Newton AW, Vandeven AM: Update on child maltreatment with a special focus on shaken baby syndrome. Curr Opin Pediatr 17:246–251, 2005.

16. Is there any other way to get those retinal hemorrhages?
Birth trauma may cause retinal hemorrhage, but these usually resolve within 3 weeks. Accidental injury and bleeding disorders may also cause retinal hemorrhages. Studies of infants with pyloric stenosis show that forceful vomiting does not cause these characteristic hemorrhages, nor do attempts at resuscitation, isolated cervical injuries, brief hypoxia, or rough play.

Newton AW, Vandeven AM: Update on child maltreatment with a special focus on shaken baby syndrome. Curr Opin Pediatr 17:246–251, 2005.

17. How can one differentiate between accidental and nonaccidental hemorrhages?
Retinal hemorrhage is much more likely with NAT than accidental injury (60% versus 10%) and is more likely to be bilateral and extend to the periphery.

Newton AW, Vandeven AM: Update on child maltreatment with a special focus on shaken baby syndrome. Curr Opin Pediatr 17:246–251, 2005.

18. What should be done for children reporting sexual abuse?
Ideally, you would have access to a facility with a pediatric assault specialist who may be a physician or a properly trained sexual assault nurse examiner. Children, providing they are medically stable, should be taken there immediately. They should not be made to undergo more than one exam, and care should be given to minimize the number of times they are asked to discuss the assault (or ongoing abuse). This is both compassionate and legally sound, because initial accounts are considered to be the most accurate.

19. But what if no specialist is available?
Do as you would for an adult sexual assault. This means a full physical exam, including genital and rectal exams, evidence collection with care given to protecting the chain of evidence, and pregnancy test (and prophylaxis), if appropriate.

20. **What is the difference between sexual abuse and sexual play?**

Sexual abuse is defined as any sexual activity involving a child who is unable to consent. Sexual play, on the other hand, is defined as unsophisticated acts between preadolescent children fewer than 4 years apart in the absence of coercion, including bribes or threats.

21. **Should a normal physical exam decrease the suspicion of abuse?**

Absolutely not. There will be no physical findings in the vast majority of sexual abuse cases. In fact, one study of gravid adolescent girls found that only 7% could be said to have "definitive evidence for penetrating trauma," despite objective evidence of penetration (pregnancy), and more than 80% had "normal" exams.

Sapp M, Vandeven A: Update on child sexual abuse. Curr Opin Pediatr, 17:258–264, 2005.

22. **What finding would suggest a need for radiographs in a child reporting sexual abuse?**

Bruising around the pelvis suggests use of force, and radiographs should be obtained. Fractures are seen in approximately 5% of children reporting sexual abuse, especially to pelvic rami during forced restraint. Conversely, children being evaluated for physical abuse who are found to have pelvic bruising should be evaluated for sexual abuse as well.

Sapp M, Vandeven A: Update on child sexual abuse. Curr Opin Pediatr, 17:258–264, 2005.

23. **Should child survivors of sex assaults and abuse be treated empirically for sexualy transmitted diseases (STDs)?**

Prophylactic treatment of prepubertal children reporting sexual abuse is not usually indicated, unless the perpetrator is known or presumed to be infected. If abuse is chronic, culture is recommended (followed by treatment if needed.) In cases of acute assault with high-risk exposure, prophylactic antibiotics and pregnancy prevention may be offered as with an adult assault.

Botash AS: Child sexual abuse. E-Medicine: www.emedicine.com/emerg/topic369.htm, October, 2004.

24. **What becomes of children who are abused?**

There are frequently long-term delays in social and psychological development for survivors of childhood abuse. Childhood abuse has been found to be associated with increased rates of suicidality, depression, psychiatric disorders, and substance abuse. It is an independent predictor of future antisocial behavior, with a dose-response curve.

Paz I, Jones D, Byrne G: Child maltreatment, child protection and mental health. Curr Opin Psychol 18:411–421, 2005.

25. **What can we do?**

Most physical injuries in young children heal well; outcome is determined, in large part, by the social management of children in abusive homes. The primary responsibility of physicians suspecting abuse is to report it and to arrange for safe disposition. It is perfectly acceptable (and in fact, imperative) to admit the child, if no safe disposition can be arranged in the community.

BIBLIOGRAPHY

1. Caffo E, Forresi B, Lievers LS: Impact, psychological sequelae and management of trauma affecting children and adolescents. Curr Opin Pediatr 18:422–428, 2005.

2. Minnus R, Bustuttil A: Patterns of presentation of the shaken baby syndrome. BMJ 328:766, 2004.

3. Newton AW, Vandeven AM: Update on child maltreatment with a special focus on shaken baby syndrome. Curr Opin Pediatr 17:246–251, 2005.

4. Sapp M, Vandeven A: Update on child sexual abuse. Curr Opin Pediatr 17:258–264, 2005.

CHAPTER 65

PROCEDURAL SEDATION AND ANALGESIA OF THE PEDIATRIC PATIENT

Joseph Wathen, MD

1. **Why is it called procedural sedation and analgesia or (PSA)?**

   What used to be called "conscious sedation" is now more accurately referred to as PSA. This is defined as using sedatives, dissociative agents, and analgesics alone or in combinations to assist patients in tolerating unpleasant procedures, while maintaining cardiorespiratory function. An **analgesic** treats pain, whereas a **sedative** or **anxiolytic** relieves fear and anxiety. Some analgesics, particularly narcotics, have sedative and analgesic properties, which make them useful in certain procedures.

   > Agency for Healthcare Research and Quality: National guideline clearinghouse. www.guideline.gov
   >
   > Mace SE, Barata IA, Cravero JP, et al: Clinical policy: Evidence-based approach to pharmacologic agents used in pediatric sedation and analgesia in the emergency department. Ann Emerg Med 44:4, 2004.

2. **Do I need sedation and analgesia when performing procedures on children?**

   Children undergoing frightening or painful procedures would benefit from agents providing sedation and/or analgesia. There are many procedures that occur in the emergency department (ED) in which PSA should be considered. These include reduction of fractures or dislocations, laceration repair, incision and drainage of abscesses, burn care, examinations after sexual assault, and diagnostic procedures such as lumbar puncture, computed tomography (CT), or magnetic resonance imaging (MRI). Systemic sedatives or analgesics may not be needed in some older children who can remain calm and when local anesthetics provide adequate pain control. A comforting staff or family member may be the needed calming ingredient. Some emergency departments (EDs) have also employed "child life advocates" for this very purpose.

3. **What is "brutaine"? Should I use it?**

   Brutaine, or simply holding a child down without medications to perform a procedure, although tempting as a fast approach, is not ideal. Using sedation and analgesia helps prevent or reduce crying and thrashing. Not only does PSA allow the provider to have a better chance of actually performing the procedure, it also provides pain control, reduces anxiety, and in some cases results in amnesia for the event. Continuous crying leaves the child, family, and staff exhausted and appears to onlookers as torture. Sometimes, the addition of a sheet wrap or papoose in combination with sedation is needed. The ability to provide PSA for children is an accepted and expected part of emergency medicine.

4. **What are the different levels of sedation?**

   - **Mild sedation** or anxiolysis refers to very little to no depression of **level of consciousness** (LOC). This is the ideal level for procedural sedation in the older child when anxiolysis alone is adequate.
   - **Moderate sedation/analgesia** previously considered "conscious sedation," is a drug-induced depressed LOC in which patients may respond to verbal or tactile stimulation while protecting their airway reflexes. The child is still awake but with droopy eyes and slurred speech. Only minimally painful procedures will be tolerated with this level of sedation (e.g., suture repair).

- **Deep sedation/analgesia** implies a depressed LOC from which the child is not easily aroused and may need airway and ventilatory assistance. This level may be needed for more painful procedures (e.g., fracture reduction).
- **General anesthesia** represents the end of this continuum, which many sedatives can achieve if given in sufficient doses. This is not desirable because of the risk of cardiorespiratory depression, loss of airway reflexes, and aspiration.

American Academy of Pediatrics: Guidelines for monitoring and management of pediatric patients during and after sedation for diagnostic and therapeutic procedures. Pediatrics 89:1110–1115, 1992.

5. **List the ideal characteristics of an agent used for PSA.**
   - Produces effective anxiolysis, even during painful procedures
   - Safe; produces a predictable degree of sedation for a given dose and has minimal effects on airway reflexes and cardiorespiratory status
   - Movement is minimized so that the procedure can be performed
   - Amnesia is provided for the procedure
   - Produces no adverse interactions with other agents that may be used concurrently
   - Is reversible
   - Can be administered painlessly
   - Is titratable, (advantage of intravenous [IV] administration)
   - Has rapid onset, short duration, and rapid recovery (most important)

6. **What routes of administration are available for administrating a sedative?**
   There are several potential routes available for administration of PSA. The route can parallel the depth of sedation needed and the type of procedure to be performed. Routes include oral, transmucosal (nasal, oral mucosal, rectal), intramuscular, intravascular, or inhalational. Intravenous and inhalational routes allow for the important quality of titrating to effect. However, it may be difficult in some pediatric patients to obtain intravenous (IV) access; in those cases in which moderate or deep sedation is needed, the intramuscular (IM) route may be ideal (i.e., IM ketamine). Likewise, if anxiolysis or mild sedation is needed, oral midazolam or transmucosal fentanyl may be sufficient.

7. **What are the key items to ask in the medical history prior to PSA?**
   - When was the last oral intake of liquids and solids (aspiration risk)?
   - Are there allergies to any sedative or analgesic agents?
   - What are the current medications—will there be any interactions?
   - What prior medications (i.e., narcotics) were given if transported in (additive effect)?
   - Any chronic medical problems (i.e., chronic lung disease or airway abnormalities)?
   - Prior complications if received prior sedatives/analgesics or general anesthesia?

8. **Are there guidelines for presedation fasting?**
   In fact, adherence to presedation fasting guidelines is not only difficult in the ED setting but has not been shown to alter the rate of adverse events. The American Society of Anesthesiologists fasting recommendations for **elective procedures** are (1) 2 hours after liquids, (2) 4 hours after breast milk, and (3) 6 hours after infant formula or a light meal. There are, however, no official fasting guidelines for **emergent procedures.** Instead, case by case prudence is suggested. If clinically feasible, delaying PSA after your patient just consumed a large meal is advisable.

Agrawal D, Manzi SF, Gupta R, et al: Preprocedural fasting state and adverse events in children undergoing procedural sedation and analgesia in a pediatric emergency department. Ann Emerg Med 42:636–646, 2003.

Roback MG, Bajaj L, Wathen JE, et al: Preprocedural fasting and adverse events in procedural sedation and analgesia in a pediatric emergency department: Are they related? Ann Emerg Med 44:5:454–459, 2004.

9. **What physical exam findings are important to note prior to PSA?**
Items to note are the presence of airway abnormalities such as large tonsils or adenoids, congenital abnormalities that may have a floppy or anatomically susceptible airway (Down syndrome, Pierre Robin syndrome, Treacher-Collins syndrome, storage diseases), or lower respiratory findings such as wheezing and rales. Obese children may have associated sleep apnea and be at increased risk of a respiratory adverse event. A visual inspection of the open mouth will tell you what the upper airway looks like (Mallampati score) and will remind you to look for loose teeth or dental hardware (retainers, etc.). A careful cardiac and neurologic exam should also be performed.

10. **Are there any patients who should not receive PSA?**
Relative contraindications to procedural sedation in the ED relate to the risk of complications, including aspiration and potential difficulty in managing the airway. Children who may be better candidates for operating room procedures under more controlled conditions include the following:
- Unstable patients, such as children with abnormal mental status or hemodynamic instability
- Infants younger than 6 months
- Children with craniofacial malformations, such as Pierre-Robin syndrome
- Children with cerebral palsy and abnormal swallowing mechanisms
- Children with snoring, stridor, apnea, or abnormal breathing regulation
- Children with seizure disorders
- Children with vomiting or gastroesophageal reflux

KEY POINTS: HOW TO AVOID ADVERSE EVENTS WITH PEDIATRIC PROCEDURAL SEDATION AND ANALGESIA

1. Beware of infants and children with systemic disease processes, obstructive airway disease, or active respiratory infections.

2. Become acquainted and comfortable with PSA drug regimens.

3. Verify that the weight is in kilograms not pounds prior to dosing.

4. Monitor carefully, both with equipment and a dedicated medical staff per American Academy of Pediatrics (AAP) and American College of Emergency Physicians (ACEP) guidelines.

5. Be attentive to the end of the procedure when the painful stimulus is over and the child is more prone to developing respiratory depression.

6. Prior to starting PSA, have advanced airway equipment ready, including suction, oxygen, and *proper-sized* bag-valve-mask.

11. **List the monitoring that should occur with PSA.**
The level of monitoring can parallel the degree of sedation. The best monitor is a skilled, dedicated observer who is not involved in the procedure and who can observe the child's LOC,

response to verbal and physical stimulation, airway patency, respiratory function, and perfusion. Sedated children should not be left unobserved.

Monitoring equipment may include cardiorespiratory monitor, pulse oximetry, capnography, blood pressure cuff, suctioning equipment, proper-sized bag-mask ventilation connected to oxygen source, and proper-sized advance airway equipment (i.e., endotracheal tubes and laryngoscopes).

12. **What are the agents used for pediatric PSA?**
    See Table 65-1.

TABLE 65-1. PSA AGENTS			
Agent	**Dose**	**Route**	**Comment**
Anxiolytics			
Midazolam	0.1 mg/kg	IV,IM	Titrate to effect
	0.3 mg/kg	IN	
	0.5 mg/kg	PO,PR	15 mg max
Sedative analgesics			
Fentanyl	1–3 µg/kg	IV	Avoid rapid or high dose infusion
Morphine	0.1 mg/kg	IV, IM	
Meperidine	1.0 mg/kg	IV, IM	
Dissociative agents			
Ketamine	1–2 mg/kg	IV	Coadminister an antisialagogue
	2–4 mg/kg	IM	Longer recovery
Pure sedatives			
Pentobarbital	4–6 mg/kg	IM	
	2–4 mg/kg	IV	
Etomidate	0.1–0.2 mg/kg	IV	Ultrashort
Propofol	0.5–1.0 mg/kg*	IV	Rapid onset and offset
Methohexital	1 mg/kg	IV	Ultrashort, limited studies
	20–30 mg/kg	PR	
Chloral hydrate	50 mg/kg	PO,PR	Long duration, avoid in newborns
Inhalational agents			
Nitrous oxide	30–50% NO_2	Inhalation	Older children, able to hold mask
Reversal agents			
Naloxone	0.1 mg/kg	IV,IM, ETT	Can repeat every 5 min, 4 mg max
Flumazenil	0.001 mg/kg	IV	Titrate to max of 0.1 mg

PO, oral; PR, rectal; IN, intranasal; IM, intramuscular; IV, intravascular; ETT, endotracheal tube.
*Can be given as a continuous infusion: 25–150 µg/kg/min.

13. **What agents would you use if you needed to obtain a CT scan on a young child?**
Radiologic diagnostic procedures are common and may prove to be difficult to achieve without adequate sedation. The newer CT scanners, however, are faster diagnostic procedures with the ability of being performed without sedatives. If medications are needed, sedatives alone are usually adequate. Potential agents include pentobarbital (Nembutal), midazolam, methohexital, or etomidate. Pentobarbital has been shown to more effectively sedate a child for radiologic imaging (97%) versus midazolam (19%).

Moro-Sutherland DM, Algren JT, Louis PT: Comparison of intravenous midazolam with pentobarbital for sedation for head computed tomography imaging. Acad Emerg Med 7:1370–1375, 2001.
Sacchetti A, Carraccio C, Giardino A, et al: Sedation for pediatric CT scanning: Is radiology becoming a drug-free zone? Pediatr Emerg Care 21:295–297, 2005.

14. **Would the agents used for obtaining a CT scan work for an MRI?**
Obtaining an MRI is less common than that of a CT, but does on occasion occur. MRIs are not particularly rapid events, so the child must remain motionless for a longer time period. The ultra-short acting sedatives would not be the best choice. Instead, agents that can either be continuously infused (propofol) or have a longer duration of action (chloral hydrate) would be preferred.

15. **What are the advantages and disadvantages of propofol for PSA?**

Advantages	Disadvantages
Sedative hypnotic qualities	Can cause apnea
Rapid onset and offset	Hypoxia-hypoventilation, 2–31%
High efficacy	Decreased peripheral vascular resistance
Lipophilic suspension = pain at injection	
Constant infusion for longer procedures	
Needs opiate for painful procedures	

Bassett KE, Anderson JL, Pribble CG: Propofol for procedural sedation in children in the emergency department. Ann Emerg Med 42:773–782, 2003.

16. **What medications would you use for a 2-year-old with a facial laceration?**
This may represent the most common scenario where PSA would be used in the ED. For the majority of the patients, local anesthetics can be provided such as topical lidocaine, epinephrine, tetracaine (LET) or local injection with lidocaine. The difficulty then is reducing the anxiety for the child who sees bright lights and staff bearing down on him or her. Effective sedation can be provided with midazolam administered intravenously, intranasally, or orally. When this does not provide adequate sedation and motion control for a difficult repair (i.e., laceration crossing the vermillion border of the lip), then an agent such as ketamine either IV or IM could be used.

17. **What medications would you consider for a 6-year-old needing reduction of an angulated forearm fracture?**
Fracture reduction is associated with significant pain and anxiety. Both need to be treated. Several options can be effective and include fentanyl or morphine and midazolam, ketamine, or nitrous oxide with a hematoma block. Ketamine has been shown to have fewer respiratory adverse events when compared with fentanyl/midazolam.

Kennedy RM, Porter FL, Miller JP. Comparison of fentanyl/midazolam with ketamine/midazolam for pediatric orthopedic emergencies. Pediatrics 102:956–963, 1998.

18. **What makes ketamine or "kidamine" useful as a PSA agent?**

Ketamine, a dissociative agent causing a trancelike cataleptic state, has become a more commonly used medication for pediatric PSA. It provides strong sedation, analgesia, and amnesia while maintaining cardiovascular stability and protective airway reflexes. Ketamine requires an anti-sialagogue, either atropine or glycopyrrolate, that can be coadministered in the same syringe and given either IV or IM. Onset of action is within a couple of minutes IV and 5–10 minutes IM. Coadministration of midazolam has *not* been shown to decrease recovery agitation or emergent phenomena (vivid dreams, hallucinations, delirium), but it can decrease recovery emesis that occurs in 15–20%. Ketamine, although protective of airway reflexes, may be associated with hypoxia in ~5%, and rarely laryngospasm or apnea.

Green SM, Krauss B: Clinical guideline for emergency department ketamine dissociative sedation in children. Ann Emerg Med 44:5, 2004.

19. **What are the contraindications for ketamine?**

Glaucoma or globe injury, increased intracranial pressure (ICP) or central nervous system (CNS) mass lesion, seizure disorder, hypertension, congestive heart failure, major psychiatric disorder, porphyria, previous adverse reaction, procedures or conditions that can exacerbate laryngospasm (pharyngeal procedures, endoscopy, upper respiratory infections), and age younger than 3 months.

20. **What complications are seen with PSA?**

- With **oversedation,** there is risk for (1) respiratory events: aspiration (from vomiting and loss of airway reflexes), hypoventilation, hypoxia, laryngospasm and apnea; (2) cardiovascular events: hypotension, bradycardia; and (3) vomiting.
- With **postsedation,** there is a recovery period, during which children may vomit, be agitated, be ataxic, and develop dysphoria or other "emergent reactions." In addition, the chance of respiratory depression is increased when the painful stimulus of the procedure is complete. Close observation and parental reassurance are essential. Because of the risks involved, at least verbal informed consent should be obtained and documented.

21. **What are the complications associated with fentanyl?**

Fentanyl is a commonly used narcotic in the ED, as it provides analgesia and sedation with a rapid onset and recovery. However, a few reminders about fentanyl are important. When fentanyl is given rapidly or in high doses, it can cause the *wooden-chest syndrome* (thoracic and abdominal wall rigidity). This muscular rigidity can be reversed by naloxone (Narcan) or with neuromuscular blockade. In addition, fentanyl can cause apnea without the usual concomitant decrease in mental status. Full monitoring is essential, including frequent blood pressures.

22. **Are some agents safer than others?**

Using proper monitoring, most agents can be used, and the adverse events, when noted, can be promptly treated. Seldom are reversal agents needed. Certain drug types used are associated with different adverse event profiles (Table 65-2).

Roback MG, Wathen JE, Bajaj L, et al: Adverse events associated with procedural sedation and analgesia in a pediatric emergency department: A comparison of common parenteral drugs. Acad Emerg Med 12:6:508–513, 2005. Available at www.aemj.org

23. **What reversal agents are available for children?**

For narcotics and benzodiazepines, specific reversing agents are available. Naloxone (0.1 mg/kg intravenously, intramuscularly, or endotracheal, up to 4 mg per dose) reverses narcotic effects, and flumazenil (0.01 mg/kg intravenously, up to 1.0 mg) reverses benzodiazepine overdose.

General measures. Discontinue sedative or narcotic administration. Maintain the airway and provide assisted ventilation, initially with bag-valve-mask ventilation, then with endotracheal

TABLE 65-2. ADVERSE EVENT PROFILES OF SEDATION DRUGS

Sedation Drugs	Respiratory Events* (%, OR†)	Vomiting (%, OR†)
Ketamine alone	6%, 1	10%, 1
Ketamine/midazolam	10%, 1.7	5%, 0.5
Fentanyl/midazolam	19%, 3.7	2%, 0.2
Midazolam alone	6%, 0.9	0.8%, 0.07

*Respiratory events included hypoxia, laryngospasm, and apnea.
†OR represents odds ratio.

intubation if necessary. If poor perfusion or shock is present (e.g., capillary refill time >2 seconds, cool extremities, weak pulses, poor tone), obtain vascular access, and initiate treatment with a bolus infusion of 20 mL/kg of crystalloid solution.

24. **When can I discharge a child home after performing PSA?**
The child should have normal vital signs, be reasonably alert, be able to sit without assistance, take liquids by mouth, and respond to commands given in a normal voice.

CHAPTER 66

NEONATAL RESUSCITATION

Owen P. O'Meara, MD

1. **I am an emergency department (ED) physician. Why should I learn about neonatal resuscitation?**

   Resuscitation of the newborn in the ED is a fact of life, no matter where the hospital is or how big or small it is. Virtually all hospitals that deliver newborns have training programs available to personnel, and the ED staff should be included in these programs. Most mistakes in neonatal resuscitation are made as a result of panic, which can be eliminated by this type of training.

2. **What is the most important thing to learn from this chapter on newborn resuscitation?**

   The most important thing to learn from this chapter is that there are major differences between newborns and all other ages of patients, and these differences alter how resuscitative efforts should proceed with these infants.

3. **How can you tell if a newborn infant needs resuscitative efforts?**

   All infants have some degree of cyanosis after birth due to the low partial pressure of oxygen in utero. The most important criteria for the need for resuscitation are lack of spontaneous activity and respiratory effort along with bradycardia even after stimulation.

4. **What spontaneous activity should you expect in a normal newborn at the time of birth?**

   Almost all infants have a grimace-like facial expression at birth and make some attempt to move the upper and lower extremities. Infants will almost always make an effort to breathe spontaneously and cry within 15–20 seconds following birth.

5. **Define bradycardia in the newborn.**

   A heart rate of less than 100 bpm at 30 seconds following birth.

6. **When should central cyanosis resolve in a healthy newborn following delivery?**

   Central cyanosis and cyanosis of the oral mucous membranes should clear after the first minute of life. Peripheral cyanosis of the hands and feet may persist for several minutes in an otherwise healthy newborn. Peripheral cyanosis restricted to the hands and feet is referred to as **acrocyanosis** and usually has no significance.

7. **After delivery in the ED, what is the first priority in the care of the newborn?**

   The first priority is to prevent body heat loss. The infant must be dried ASAP to prevent evaporative heat loss as well as be placed under a radiant warming unit to lessen loss of radiant heat. These initial steps take only seconds to accomplish and may prevent serious metabolic derangements later. These steps should be taken even prior to the initiation of cardiopulmonary resuscitation (CPR). Following these steps, CPR may proceed.

   Bloom RS, Cropley C: AHA/AAP Neonatal Resuscitation Steering Committee. American Heart Association and American Academy of Pediatrics, 2000.

8. **How do I approach the meconium-stained newborn?**

   Meconium presents a real and serious risk to the respiratory system of the infant if it is aspirated. The material contains noxious substances such as bile acids that can lead to serious obstructive problems for the airways. The initial steps involve the suctioning the mouth and nasopharynx as soon as possible. If it is possible to do this right after the head is delivered but still on the perineum, this should be done. Suctioning of the nasopharynx and mouth should proceed prior to the initiation of positive pressure ventilation of any kind. If the infant is intubated right after delivery, suctioning of the endotracheal (ET) tube should proceed as soon as possible as well.

   Note: By this time, support from the pediatric and neonatal services should be brought into play, if they are available.

   Yoder BA: Meconium stained amniotic fluid and respiratory complications: Impact of selective tracheal suction. Obstet Gynecol 83:77, 1994.

9. **After the infant is dried, suctioned, and placed under the warmer, how do I decide whether further active intervention is needed?**

   If the infant is active, is crying, has a heart rate of greater than 100 bpm, and does not have evidence of central cyanosis, further intervention is seldom needed. If the infant demonstrates apnea, bradycardia, or central cyanosis, then use of bag and mask ventilation must be considered after attempts at stimulation have failed. Most of the time, if the infant is near term gestation, the heart rate will respond quickly to a few effective assisted breaths. The most effective bag for this type of assistance is an infant self-inflating unit connected to wall oxygen. There is currently a great deal of discussion in the literature as to whether 100% oxygen is the safest gas for this type of intervention. For the time being, in the setting of the ED, 100% oxygen is the best choice until this issue is decided.

   If these initial efforts are effective and the infant begins to breath on its own or cry, it is reasonable to simply provide some blow by oxygen while awaiting help from the pediatric staff.

   Saugstad OD: The role of oxygen in neonatal resuscitation. Clin Perinatol 31:3, 2004.

10. **How many infants will require intubation to provide adequate ventilation?**

    Almost all newborn infants can be ventilated with bag-mask technique. Bag-mask ventilation should be done only with equipment designed for newborn and premature infants. Inspiratory pressures of greater than 25 cm of water should be avoided unless efforts are failing. All neonatal bags should be equipped with pressure manometers.

11. **How can I be certain I am ventilating the infant or that the position of the head is correct?**

    During this type of situation, a person should be present whose main job should be to listen for breath sounds and monitor the infant's heart rate. If the operator is the only person present, then watching for chest wall movement is the next best thing. Movement of the infant's head into a sniffing position will often help if breaths are not effective.

12. **When should chest compressions be started in the course of the resuscitative effort?**

    If, after 30 seconds of adequate ventilation, the heart rate remains at less than 80 bpm, then chest compressions should begin. Compressions should be at a rate between about 100–120 per minute. This should be done with no more than two fingers over the sternum. Avoid pressure over the liver, as laceration of the organ can occur. Heart rate should be evaluated about every 30 seconds during the effort. Compressions should be done in between breaths. When a sustained heart rate of greater than 100 bpm is achieved, compressions should be discontinued.

    Burchfield D, Erenburg A, Mullett MD, et al: Why change the compression and ventilation rates during CPR in neonates? Pediatrics 93:1026, 1994.

13. **At what point in this process should obstetrics and pediatrics be notified?**
They should be notified as soon as it is known that there will be a delivery in the ED.

14. **When should I attempt vascular access? What vessel should I use?**
As soon as it is fairly obvious that drugs or volume expanders may be needed, an umbilical venous line should be attempted. It is uncommon for this to be needed. For such events, an umbilical venous tray should always be available in the ED. Remember that there is one umbilical vein and two umbilical arteries.

15. **What drugs should be available for use in newborn resuscitation use, and when should they be given?**
Drugs are rarely needed in the resuscitation of the newborn infant, especially if bag-and-mask ventilation is started early. Usually, no more than two agents are needed.

- **Epinephrine 1:10,000 dilution** is used if there has been no heart beat noted for 6–10 seconds at any point during the event or if heart rate remains less than 60-8- bpm after 30 seconds of bag-and-mask ventilation and chest compressions. The usual dose is 0.1–0.3 mL/kg, either via the ET tube or via the umbilical vein. The drug can be given as frequently as every 5 minutes if bradycardia persists.

- **Volume expanders** may be used via the umbilical vein catheter (UVC) if there is evidence of blood loss from the infant. Rapid volume expansion must be done with caution in infants less than 32 weeks' gestation because of the risk of central nervous system (CNS) bleeding. The usual agents used are normal saline or 5% albumin in a dose of 10 mL/kg. A 4.2% solution of sodium bicarbonate may be used if cardiac arrest has occurred. The usual dose is 2.0 mEq/kg given over 2 minutes. The 4.2% solution is 0.5 mEq/mL.

16. **What is the best means of documentation of the results of resuscitation in the neonate?**
The Apgar score remains the standard, despite some limitations (Table 66-1). The score is calculated at 1 minute and at 5 minutes and at every 5 minute interval thereafter.

American Academy of Pediatrics, Committee on the Fetus and Newborn: Use and abuse of the Apgar score. Pediatrics 78:1148, 1986.

Catlin EA, Carpenter MW, Brann BS, et al: The Apgar Score revisited; influence of gestational age. J Pediatr 109:865, 1986.

TABLE 66-1. APGAR SCORING SYSTEM

Sign	0	1	2
Heart rate (bpm)	Absent	Slow (<100)	>100
Respirations	Absent	Slow, irregular	Good, crying
Muscle tone	Limp	Some flexion	Active motion
Reflex irritability (catheter in nares)	No response	Grimace	Cough or sneeze
Color	Blue or pale	Pink body with blue extremities	Completely pink

GENERAL APPROACH TO POISONINGS

Katherine Hurlbut, MD, and Ken Kulig, MD

1. **List the 15 most common causes of death from acute poisoning reported to poison centers.**
   - Analgesics 59.3%
   - Sedative/hypnotics/antipsychotics 29.7%
   - Antidepressants 24.8%
   - Stimulants and street drugs 20.3%
   - Cardiovascular drugs 14.6%
   - Alcohols 10.9%
   - Anticonvulsants 8.0%
   - Antihistamines 6.8%
   - Gases and fumes 5.5%
   - Muscle relaxants 5.3%
   - Chemicals 3.9%
   - Hormones and hormone antagonists 3.7%
   - Pesticides 3.7%
   - Cleaning substances 2.3%
   - Gastrointestinal (GI) preparations 2.2%

   Note: Despite a high frequency of involvement, these substances are not the most toxic but rather may be the most readily accessible.

   Percentages total more than 100% because multiple substances are involved in some fatal exposures. Percentages are based on the total number of human exposures rather than the total number of substances.

   Watson WA, Litovitz TL, Klein-Schwartz W, et al: 2003 Annual report of the American Association of Poison Control Centers Toxic Exposure Surveillance System. Am J Emerg Med 22:335–404, 2004.

2. **What is the current role of syrup of ipecac in treating acute poisoning?**
   Although syrup of ipecac induces vomiting within 20–30 minutes in most persons who are given therapeutic dose, little poison is removed; there are more effective means of decontaminating the GI tract. Ipecac may have a limited role in treating children at home, who frequently can be given a dose soon after ingestion; however, its use in the prehospital setting is declining. By the time most patients present to a hospital, too much time has elapsed for syrup of ipecac to be of benefit. Its use also delays the administration of activated charcoal, which needs to be given as quickly as possible for maximal benefit.

   American Academy of Clinical Toxicology, European Association of Poisons Centres and Clinical Toxicologists: Position Paper: Ipecac syrup. J Toxicol Clin Toxicol 42:133–143, 2004.

3. **What is the current role of gastric lavage in treating acute poisonings?**
   Gastric lavage has not been shown to alter clinical outcome in large series of patients presenting with overdose. Although serious sequelae of gastric lavage are rare, it carries the risk of aspiration, laryngospasm, and esophageal injury. The risk of injury appears to be greater in uncooperative patients. Endotracheal intubation should precede gastric lavage in patients with altered mental status or the inability to protect the airway. Although lavage can be accomplished without prior tracheal intubation in most patients, airway equipment, including suction, should

be immediately available at the bedside. Placing the patient on the left side in mild Trendelenburg position helps to prevent aspiration if vomiting occurs. Nasogastric tubes are too small to remove pills or large pill fragments; whenever gastric lavage is done, a large-bore tube (36 Fr or 40 Fr in adults) should be placed through the mouth. A bite-block with an oral airway prevents the patient from biting the tube. Proper location of the lavage tube in the stomach must be verified clinically or radiographically before lavage or administration of fluid or charcoal. Deaths have been reported resulting from charcoal instillation into the trachea by nasogastric tube. Gastric lavage generally is reserved for patients with potentially serious or life-threatening overdose who present within 1–2 hours after ingestion.

American Academy of Clinical Toxicology, European Association of Poisons Centres and Clinical Toxicologists: Position Paper: Gastric lavage. J Toxicol Clin Toxicol 42:933–943, 2004.

Pond SM, Lewis-Driver DJ, Williams GM, et al: Gastric emptying in acute overdose: A prospective randomised controlled trial. Med J Aust 163:345–349, 1995.

4. **What is the current role of activated charcoal?**
   Activated charcoal has been shown in numerous studies to be superior to gastric emptying procedures for the treatment of acute overdose. Gastric emptying procedures involve time and some risk to the patient. The time involved in lavaging the patient is time during which drugs are being actively absorbed. By giving a dose of activated charcoal immediately on patient presentation, the most effective means of GI decontamination already has been performed. Not all drugs are adsorbed to charcoal, however. Drugs that are not well adsorbed include lithium, potassium, iron, some metals, and alcohols. Activated charcoal is contraindicated after ingestion of hydrocarbons, because toxicity from gastric absorption is generally not a major concern with these substances, and activated charcoal may induce vomiting, which increases the risk of aspiration pneumonitis. Activated charcoal is also not indicated after ingestion of acids or alkalis, because the primary toxicity associated with these agents is local mucosal burns rather than systemic absorption. Patients with trivial ingestions (generally children) do not require activated charcoal therapy.

American Academy of Clinical Toxicology, European Association of Poisons Centres and Clinical Toxicologists: Position Paper: Single-dose activated charcoal. J Toxicol Clin Toxicol 43:61–87, 2005.

5. **What about the asymptomatic overdose patient?**
   It has been advocated by some that simple observation of asymptomatic overdose patients, with treatment only if symptoms develop, is a management option. Although this approach is safe for many patients who have ingested trivial overdoses, if a patient ingested something quite toxic, an opportunity to prevent absorption may have been lost if nothing is done until symptoms develop. Administering a dose of activated charcoal to all patients with a history of deliberate drug overdose is done easily (although it is often messy) and helps to ensure safe and timely patient disposition. If a reliable history indicates ingestion of substances with minimal toxicity, activated charcoal may not be necessary.

6. **Is there a role for cathartics in treating acute poisoning?**
   The theory behind cathartics is that they speed up GI transit time, allowing activated charcoal to catch up with pills in the bowel and prevent desorption of drug from activated charcoal. Cathartics have not been shown to reduce drug absorption or improve outcome significantly after overdose, but they can cause vomiting, abdominal pain, and electrolyte abnormalities. Use of cathartics is *not* warranted.

7. **What is the current role of whole-bowel irrigation in the treatment of acute poisoning?**
   Whole-bowel irrigation uses a polyethylene glycol electrolyte solution such as GoLYTELY or Colyte, which is not adsorbed, and flushes drugs or chemicals rapidly through the GI tract. This

procedure seems to be most useful when radiopaque tablets or chemicals have been ingested because their progress through the GI tract can be monitored by radiography. It should be considered when toxic amounts of substances that are not well adsorbed by activated charcoal (iron, lithium, heavy metals) are ingested. This procedure also is commonly used when multiple packets of street drugs, such as heroin or cocaine, have been ingested and need to be passed through the GI tract as quickly as possible, and should be considered after overdose of sustained-release products. The limitations of the procedure are that, unless the patient is awake, cooperative, and able to sit on a commode, there is a risk of vomiting and aspiration in addition to the logistical problem of having an unconscious patient in bed with massive diarrhea.

American Academy of Clinical Toxicology, European Association of Poisons Centres and Clinical Toxicologists: Position Paper: Whole bowel irrigation. J Toxicol Clin Toxicol 43:129–130, 2005.

8. What is the role of multiple-dose charcoal in the treatment of acute poisoning?
Multiple-dose charcoal has been shown to enhance the elimination of many drugs that already have been absorbed from the GI tract or that are given intravenously. This process has been called **gastrointestinal dialysis** and has been shown to be effective for theophylline and perhaps phenobarbital poisoning. Numerous other drugs have been shown to have their pharmacokinetics altered by multiple-dose charcoal, but it is not clear if this makes a difference in clinical outcome. Many of these drugs have large volumes of distribution, and increasing elimination of the small amount present in the blood is unlikely to be of benefit. Multiple-dose activated charcoal is used most commonly after overdose of theophylline, phenobarbital, carbamazepine, and quinine.

Vale JA, Krenzelok EP, Barceloux GD: Position statement and practice guidelines on the use of multi-dose activated charcoal in the treatment of acute poisoning. J Toxicol Clin Toxicol 37:731–751, 1999.

9. Is forced diuresis of benefit in the treatment of acute poisoning?
Few drugs are excreted unchanged in the urine so that even increasing urine flow significantly above baseline is unlikely to be of benefit. By manipulating the pH of the urine by infusions of bicarbonate solution along with enhanced urine flow, however, in certain cases drug elimination can be increased. This most commonly is used for salicylates and phenobarbital. By placing three ampules of sodium bicarbonate in 1 L of D_5W along with potassium chloride and infusing this solution at rates sufficient to produce at least a normal urine flow and a urine pH of 7.5 or greater, the elimination of salicylate and phenobarbital can be increased. Intake and output and urine pH should be monitored hourly with a Foley catheter in place. In the presence of pulmonary or cerebral edema, which may occur in severe salicylate intoxication, alkaline diuresis is dangerous and should not be undertaken.

Alkaline diuresis also may work in a similar manner for chlorophenoxy herbicides, but acute poisonings by these agents are rare. The use of high-volume normal saline to treat lithium intoxication is common, and it is important to maintain adequate urine output and serum sodium in this scenario. It is not clear, however, that forced-saline diuresis for lithium intoxication is of extra benefit over simply ensuring normal renal flow.

Proudfoot AT, KrenzeloL EP, Vale JA: Position paper on urine alkalinization. J Toxicol Clin Toxicol 42:1–26, 2004.

10. When are extracorporeal techniques, such as hemodialysis or hemoperfusion, indicated?
Drugs can be removed successfully by extracorporeal maneuvers only if they have relatively small volumes of distribution and are found in significant quantities in the circulation, as opposed to having rapid and thorough tissue distribution. This is the case for only a few drugs. In practice, the toxins most commonly dialyzed after overdose include aspirin, lithium, methanol, ethylene glycol, and perhaps theophylline. Dialysis has the advantage over hemoperfusion in that it is usually easier and faster to get started, and it can correct fluid and electrolyte abnormalities as it removes

drugs. Charcoal hemoperfusion may be more effective at removing drugs that are highly bound to plasma proteins, because the affinity for charcoal may be higher than the affinity for the protein carrier. The disadvantages of hemoperfusion are that it is less widely available, it frequently causes hypocalcemia and thrombocytopenia, and it can result in frequent canister clotting. Drugs for which charcoal hemoperfusion is frequently employed include theophylline, phenobarbital, and a few other less common agents such as paraquat and amatoxin.

11. **How can the diagnosis of a drug overdose be made when the patient is unconscious and history is unavailable?**
The diagnosis of acute overdose is difficult to make sometimes and requires some detective work on the part of the physician. All unconscious patients should receive a rapid bedside serum glucose determination (or intravenous dextrose) and naloxone (Narcan); a positive response to either is diagnostic. Whenever possible, examine the pill bottles available to the patient; it is useful to call the pharmacies where the prescriptions were filled to determine if other prescriptions were filled there for different drugs. Discovering which chemical agents were available to the patient, including street drugs, is always important. If needle track marks are seen, consider street drugs commonly used intravenously, such as opiates, cocaine, and amphetamine. The physical examination is useful in narrowing the diagnosis to a class of drug or chemicals. This concept is commonly called **toxic syndromes** (Table 67-1).

TABLE 67-1.   MOST COMMON TOXIC SYNDROMES

Anticholinergic

Common signs: Agitated delirium, often with visual hallucinations and mumbling speech, tachycardia, dry flushed skin, dilated pupils, myoclonus, temperature slightly elevated, urinary retention, decreased bowel sounds. Seizures and arrhythmias may occur in severe cases.

Common causes: Antihistamines, antiparkinsonism medication, atropine, scopolamine, amantadine, antipsychotics, antidepressants, antispasmodics, mydriatics, skeletal muscle relaxants, many plants (most notably jimson weed)

Sympathomimetic

Common signs: Delusions, agitation, paranoia, tachycardia, hypertension, hyperpyrexia, diaphoresis, piloerection, slight mydriasis, hyperreflexia. Seizures and arrhythmias may occur in severe cases.

Common causes: Cocaine, amphetamine, methamphetamine (and derivatives MDA, MDMA, MDEA), over-the-counter decongestants (phenylpropanolamine, ephedrine, pseudoephedrine). Caffeine and theophylline overdoses cause similar findings secondary to catecholamine release, except for the organic psychiatric signs.

Opiate/sedative

Common signs: Coma, respiratory depression, miosis, hypotension, bradycardia, hypothermia, acute lung injury, decreased bowel sounds, hyporeflexia, needle marks

Common causes: Narcotics, barbiturates, benzodiazepines, ethchlorvynol, glutethimide, methyprylon, methaqualone, meprobamate

Cholinergic

Common signs: Confusion/central nervous system depression, weakness, salivation, lacrimation, urinary and fecal incontinence, GI cramping, emesis, diaphoresis, muscle fasciculations, pulmonary edema, miosis, bradycardia (or tachycardia), seizures

TABLE 67-1.   MOST COMMON TOXIC SYNDROMES—CONT'D
Common causes: Organophosphate and carbamate insecticides, physostigmine, edrophonium, some mushrooms (*Amanita muscaria, Amanita pantherina, Inocybe, Clitocybe*)
Serotonin
Common signs: Fever, tremor, incoordination, agitation, mental status changes, diaphoresis, myoclonus, diarrhea, rigidity
Common causes: Fluoxetine, sertraline, paroxetine, venlafaxine, clomipramine; the preceding drugs in combination with monoamine oxidase inhibitors
GI = gastrointestinal, MDA = methylenedioxyamphetamine, MDMA = 3,4-methylenedioxymethamphetamine.

12. **How can a toxicology screen and other ancillary laboratory tests make the diagnosis of acute poisoning?**
   The blood and urine toxicology screen should be done on any patient who has significant toxicity (persistent altered mental status or abnormal vital signs) and when the diagnosis is uncertain. Alternatives to a full toxicology screen include testing discrete serum levels of the toxins in question, doing a urine qualitative test for drugs of abuse, or drawing specimens but holding them until it is determined that a toxicology screen is definitely indicated.
   More drugs and chemicals are *not* found on typical toxicology screens than *are* found on the screens, although most drugs that commonly are ingested are found on comprehensive toxicology screens. It is important to communicate with the laboratory about which drugs are suspected, which drugs the patient takes therapeutically, and the clinical condition of the patient. Whenever there is a discrepancy between clinical suspicion and findings from the toxicology screen, it is useful to communicate with the toxicology laboratory personnel and determine if other tests are likely to be of benefit. Toxicology screens are expensive, frequently are inexact, and frequently do not give all the information that is expected by the clinician. It is important to interpret toxicology screens carefully and to know which drugs and chemicals were not screened for.

13. **What other studies are useful in the evaluation of a poisoned patient?**
   - An **acetaminophen level** should be obtained in patients with deliberate overdose, because this substance is widely available, frequently involved in overdoses, and causes little in the way of initial symptoms; and treatment with *N*-acetylcysteine is most effective if begun within 8 hours of ingestion.
   - **Nontoxicologic laboratory tests** that are frequently useful include an electrocardiogram (ECG), which can help diagnose overdose of tricyclic antidepressants or cardiac medications; a chest radiograph in patients with pulmonary symptoms or hypoxia, which if demonstrative of acute lung injury would make one think of salicylates or opiates; and, rarely, a kidneys-ureters-bladder (KUB) screen, looking for radiopaque material, which would make one suspicious of ingestion of a heavy metal, iron, phenothiazines, chloral hydrate, or chlorinated hydrocarbon solvents.
   - **Liver function tests** may help to diagnose ingestion of hepatotoxins, such as acetaminophen or carbon tetrachloride late in the course of poisoning.
   - A **urinalysis** may show the presence of calcium oxalate crystals, suggesting the diagnosis of ethylene glycol poisoning.

- The **acid-base status** of the patient is important and should be evaluated in all patients with deliberate overdose. Persistent unexplained metabolic acidosis always should prompt the search for other diagnostic clues to aspirin, iron, methanol, or ethylene glycol poisoning. Many other drugs can cause a persistent, unexplained metabolic acidosis, including the ingestion of acids themselves, cyanide, carbon monoxide, theophylline, and others.
- In the work-up of persistent acidosis, a **serum osmolality** done by freezing point depression can be useful if it is elevated. A difference between the measured osmolality and the calculated osmolality of greater than 10 is always significant, although a normal osmolol gap does not rule out toxic alcohol ingestion.

KEY POINTS: MANAGEMENT OF SUSPECTED TOXIC INGESTION

1. Activated charcoal is sufficient decontamination for most overdose patients.

2. Urine toxicology screens are NOT indicated in patients with normal mental status and vital signs.

3. Serum electrolytes and acetaminophen concentration should be obtained in patients with deliberate overdose.

4. Although there are a few antidotes for specific toxins, most poisoned patients recover with supportive care.

---

14. **Discuss some other useful antidotes for common poisonings.**
    - **Naloxone** and **dextrose** are the most common antidotes and should be given routinely to unconscious overdose patients. Intravenous administration of 2 mg of naloxone that results in awakening of the patient is diagnostic of acute opiate overdose. Small, incremental doses of 0.2 mg can be used if it is suspected that the patient is opioid dependent, because the 2-mg dose of naloxone will precipitate withdrawal. Many drugs and chemicals can cause hypoglycemia, including ethanol, and for this reason dextrose likewise should be given, unless it can be determined quickly that the blood glucose is normal.
    - **Physostigmine** is an antidote for the anticholinergic syndrome. Physostigmine can be used diagnostically and therapeutically when the diagnosis of the anticholinergic syndrome is suspected. It should not be used to treat tricyclic antidepressant poisoning. Seizures and bradyarrhythmias have been reported when used in this setting. A dose of 1–2 mg given slowly intravenously to an adult is usually sufficient.
    - **Digoxin immune Fab (Digibind, Digitab)** is a safe and effective antidote for digitalis glycoside poisoning and can rapidly reverse arrhythmias and hyperkalemia, which can be life threatening. In contrast to naloxone, Digibind does not work immediately, and a full response to therapy may not be seen until approximately 20 minutes after administration. For a life-threatening digitalis overdose when the dose and the serum level are currently unknown, 10 vials of Digibind should be given.
    - **Atropine** and **pralidoxime (Protopam)** are antidotes used for cholinesterase inhibitor toxicity. This group of pesticides includes the organophosphates and carbamates, which commonly are found in household insecticides. Atropine is used to dry up secretions, primarily pulmonary, and pralidoxime is used primarily to reverse the skeletal muscle toxicity of these agents, including weakness and fasciculations.
    - **Flumazenil** is a benzodiazepine antagonist that has been shown to be useful in cases of acute benzodiazepine overdose resulting in significant toxicity. Its use may precipitate

benzodiazepine withdrawal, including seizures. It should not be used when tricyclic antidepressants or other proconvulsants have been coingested with benzodiazepine. The usual adult dose is 0.2 mg followed in 30 seconds by 0.3 mg, followed in 30 seconds by 0.5 mg, repeated up to a total of 3 mg.

- **Ethanol and fomepizole** are alcohol dehydrogenase blocking agents that are used to treat methanol and ethylene glycol poisoning. They prevent the metabolism of methanol and ethylene glycol to their toxic metabolites. Intravenous ethanol is less expensive than fomepizole but is somewhat more difficult to use. The initial intravenous dose is 8 mL/kg of 10% ethanol over 30 minutes, followed by an infusion of 0.8 mL/kg/h in a nondrinker, 1.4 mL/kg/h in an average drinker, and 2 mL/kg/h in a heavy drinker. Blood ethanol concentration should be measured immediately after the loading dose and repeated every hour initially, and the dose adjusted to maintain a blood ethanol of 125 mg/dL. The loading dose of fomepizole is 15 mg/kg intravenously over 30 minutes with subsequent doses of 10 mg/kg every 12 hours. The dose of both agents must be increased in patients undergoing dialysis.
- ***N*-acetylcysteine** is extremely effective in preventing acetaminophen-induced liver injury. It is most effective if administered within 8 hours of ingestion but reduces morbidity and mortality even in patients with acetaminophen-induced acute liver failure. It can be administered orally (loading dose 140 mg/kg, subsequent doses 70 mg/kg every 4 hours) or intravenously (initial dose 150 mg/kg in 200 ml D_5W over 15 minutes, followed by 50 mg/kg in 500 ml D_5W over 4 hours, followed by 100 mg/kg in 1 L D_5W infused over 16 hours).

CHAPTER 68

THE ALCOHOLS: ETHYLENE GLYCOL, METHANOL, AND ISOPROPYL ALCOHOL

Louis J. Ling, MD

1. **Why is it important to understand the metabolism of methanol?**
   The metabolites of methanol are the toxins and depend on alcohol dehydrogenase (ADH) for their conversion from the parent methanol. Ethanol and fomepizole both saturate ADH and greatly slow the metabolism of methanol to the toxic metabolite. Folate is a cofactor in the breakdown of formic acid, and in monkeys (and other primates) folate supplementation maximizes its metabolism and decreases injury. Knowledge of the metabolism directs the treatment.

$$\text{Methanol} \xrightarrow{\text{ADH}} \underset{\text{(toxic)}}{\text{Formaldehyde}} \rightarrow \underset{\text{(toxic)}}{\text{Formic Acid}} \xrightarrow{\text{Folate}} \underset{\text{(nontoxic)}}{CO_2 + H_2O}$$

   Palatnick W, Redman LW, Sitar DS, Tenenbein M: Methanol half-life during ethanol administration: Implications for management of methanol poisoning. Ann Emerg Med 26:202–207, 1995.

2. **List the signs and symptoms of methanol poisoning.**
   Gastrointestinal toxicity
   - Nausea and vomiting
   - Abdominal pain
   Central nervous system toxicity
   - Headache
   - Decreased level of consciousness
   - Confusion
   Ocular toxicity
   - Retinal edema
   - Hyperemia of the disc
   - Decreased visual acuity
   Other toxicity
   - Metabolic acidosis

   Dethlefs R, Naraqi S: Ocular manifestations and complications of acute methyl alcohol intoxication. Med J Aust 2:483–485, 1978.
   Sharma M, Volpe NJ, Dreyer EB: Methanol-induced optic nerve cupping. Arch Ophthalmol 117:286, 1999. Available at archopht.ama-assn.org/content/vol117/issue2/index.dtl.

KEY POINTS: METHANOL

1. Symptoms and acidosis are delayed.

2. Osmolal gap is often absent.

3. Persistent acidosis correlates best with a poor prognosis.

4. Fomepizole, ethanol, and dialysis can all be used to treat the poisoned patient.

3. **Why is it important to understand the metabolism of ethylene glycol?**

As with methanol, ethanol and fomepizole saturate ADH, inhibiting conversion of ethylene glycol into its harmful metabolites. Pyridoxine (vitamin B_6) and thiamine are cofactors in the final steps to form nonharmful end products and should be given to ensure maximal metabolism. Oxalate crystals may not appear until late in the course of the poisoning (Fig. 68-1).

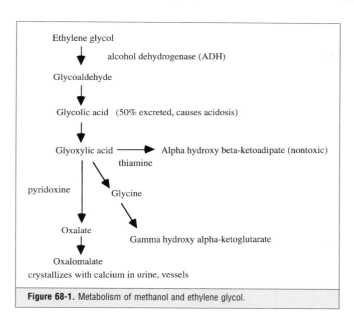

Figure 68-1. Metabolism of methanol and ethylene glycol.

4. **Why are the symptoms of ethylene glycol and methanol overdose often delayed?**

Because the toxicity of methanol and ethylene glycol is the result of toxic metabolites, it may take 6–12 hours for sufficient quantities of these toxic metabolites to appear and cause symptoms. The delay in onset of symptoms is even greater with concurrent ethanol intoxication because the ethanol slows down the rate of methanol and ethylene glycol metabolism, so the appearance of the toxic metabolites is even later.

KEY POINTS: ETHYLENE GLYCOL

1. Symptoms and acidosis are often delayed.

2. Urinary oxalate crystals, fluorescence, early osmolal gap, and metabolic acidosis all suggest ethylene glycol poisoning.

3. Fomepizole, ethanol, and dialysis can all be used to treat the poisoned patient.

5. **How are methanol and ethylene glycol poisonings similar?**

Methanol and ethylene glycol are metabolized initially by ADH. Methanol is metabolized further to formic acid; and ethylene glycol is metabolized to glycolic acid, glyoxylic acid, oxalate, and several nontoxic metabolites. Because of these end products, both poisons result in metabolic acidosis with an anion gap. Because of their low molecular weight, both increase the osmolar gap.

www.emedicine.com/emerg/byname/toxicity-alcohols.htm

6. **What is an anion gap?**

A normal anion gap is the difference between unmeasured anions (e.g., various proteins, organic acids, phosphates) and unmeasured cations (e.g., potassium, calcium, and magnesium). The anion gap can be calculated from the formula:

$$\text{Anion gap} = (Na^+) - (HCO^{-3} + Cl^-)$$

7. **What causes an increased anion gap?**

When metabolic acidosis results from an ingestion or increase of nonvolatile acids, there are increased hydrogen ions with positive charges. Because there is an equal increase in unmeasured negatively charged anions and no increases in chloride, the difference between the measured cations and measured anions is increased, causing an increased anion gap. The normal anion gap is about 6–10 mEq/L. The cause of increased anion gap can be remembered by the mnemonic **A MUD PILES.**

A = **A**lcohol	**P** = **P**araldehyde
M = **M**ethanol	**I** = **I**ron, **I**soniazid (INH)
U = **U**remia	**L** = **L**actate
D = **D**iabetic ketoacidosis	**E** = **E**thylene glycol
	S = **S**alicylate

8. **What is an osmolal gap?**

Small atoms and molecules in solution are osmotically active, and this activity can be measured by a depression in the freezing point or an elevation in the boiling point of the solution. If there is an increase in low-molecular-weight molecules, such as acetone, methanol, ethanol, mannitol, isopropyl alcohol, or ethylene glycol, the osmolality increases more than what is calculated from the usual serum molecules. The difference between the actual measured osmolality and the calculated osmolality is the osmolal gap, and a gap greater than 10 mOsm is considered abnormal.

9. **How is an osmolal gap calculated?**

$2 \times Na^+$ (mEq/L) + glucose (mg/dL)/18 + blood urea nitrogen (BUN) (mg/dL)/2.8 + ethanol (mg/dL)/4.3. The inclusion of the ethanol level excludes patients who have an elevated osmolal gap from ethanol ingestion alone. Using International System (SI) units, the calculated osmolality = $2 \times$ Na (mEq/L) + glucose (mmol/L) + BUN (mmol/L) + ethanol (mmol/L). The calculated osmolality is 285 ± 5 mOsm/L. A toxic ethylene glycol level of 25 mg/dL can be predicted to increase the osmolal gap 5 mOsm/L. Because of the small effects on the osmolality and the imprecision of the measurement, this test is not precise enough to be definitive. A normal osmolal gap does not exclude toxic levels of methanol or ethylene glycol. The laboratory must use the method of freezing-point depression so that volatile alcohols contributing to an osmolal gap are not boiled away during a boiling point elevation procedure.

Glaser DS: Utility of the serum osmol gap in the diagnosis of methanol or ethylene glycol ingestion. Ann Emerg Med 27:343–346, 1996.

10. **What comes first, the anion gap or the osmolal gap?**
    With initial absorption, the small parent molecules cause an early osmolal gap, but with
    metabolism, acidic metabolites are formed causing a late metabolic anion-gap acidosis.

11. **How toxic are methanol and ethylene glycol?**
    Death has been reported after 15–30 mL (1–2 tablespoons) of methanol. Others have
    survived larger ingestions, however. A minimal lethal dose for ethylene glycol is
    approximately 1–2 mL/kg.

    Ford MD, McMartin K: Ethylene glycol and methanol. In Ford M, Delaney K, Ling L, et al (eds): Clinical
    Toxicology. Philadelphia, W.B. Saunders, 2001, pp 757–769.

12. **What is the toxicity of ethylene glycol?**
    Initially, there is central nervous system intoxication and gastrointestinal irritation, which is
    followed by metabolic acidosis. Renal failure occurs frequently and typically is delayed in
    presentation. Cranial nerve deficits are a rare complication.

    Hylander B, Kjellstrand CM: Prognostic factors and treatment of severe ethylene glycol intoxication.
    Intensive Care Med 22:546–552, 1996.

13. **Why is ethylene glycol so dangerous to animals?**
    Ethylene glycol is a frequent cause of death in animals (especially dogs, who drink almost
    anything) who ingest antifreeze. The taste is sweet and a small volume is deadly. The cause of
    death for these animals may not be apparent because toxicity is delayed, and the death occurs
    long after the animal has left the scene.

14. **Why does antifreeze have such a bright color?**
    Antifreeze is a bright color that fluoresces with ultraviolet (UV) light so that leaks from auto
    radiators can be detected more easily. If the mouth and the urine are examined with a UV light,
    fluorescein can be detected in about 30% of patients with an ingestion. A positive test should
    encourage immediate treatment, but a negative test misses two thirds of ingestions.

15. **How should patients with methanol and ethylene glycol poisoning be treated?**
    Airway protection is paramount in patients with decreased level of consciousness or respiratory
    depression. Although gastric lavage might be helpful in large ingestions, small volumes and
    rapid absorption limit its effectiveness. Acidosis (pH<7.2) should be treated aggressively with
    sodium bicarbonate. Ethanol and 4-methylpyrazole (4-MP) are antidotes that competitively block
    the conversion of methanol and ethylene glycol to their toxic metabolites, allowing for
    elimination of the unchanged poison without injury.

    Barceloux DG, Krenzelok EP, Olson K, et al: American Academy of Clinical Toxicology practice guidelines
    on the treatment of ethylene glycol poisoning. Clin Toxicol 37:537–560, 1999.

16. **What are the indications for ethanol or 4-MP therapy?**
    They should be used if ethylene glycol or methanol levels exceed 20 mg/dL; if acidosis is
    present, regardless of drug level; and if there is a history of a toxic ingestion while awaiting
    confirmatory blood methanol or ethylene glycol levels.

17. **How is ethanol treatment started and maintained?**
    1. Maintain an ethanol level of 100–200 mg/dL.
       - Load   0.6–0.8 gm/kg
       - Maintenance   0.11 gm/kg/h
       - Dialysis   0.24 gm/kg/h

2. Oral methods
 - Load
   20–50% solutions for load per nasogastric tube; 2 mL/kg of 50% gives 0.8 gm/kg
 - Use stock pharmacy solution and dilute 1:1
 - Maintain
   0.11–0.13 gm/kg/h
   0.16 mL/kg/h of 95% solutions but dilute with water 1:1 to avoid gastritis and give 0.33 mL/kg/h
 - Increase proportionately with dialysis

3. Intravenous methods
 - Load
   10% concentration (used as standard treatment for stopping labor) in D_5W through a central catheter at 10 mL/kg
 - Maintain
   1.6 mL/kg/h of 10% solution
 - Increase proportionately with dialysis

18. What are the problems with ethanol therapy?

Ethanol can be difficult to give consistently; ethanol blood levels are required to adjust the dose and avoid oversedation. Dialysis requires an increased dose and more blood levels. An infusion can cause pain, resulting in the use of a central catheter. Ethanol may cause hypoglycemia and respiratory depression, especially in children. These patients usually require the close monitoring of an intensive care unit (ICU).

19. What is the role of fomepizole (4-MP)?

4-MP is replacing ethanol as a safe, easy-to-use antidote for methanol and ethylene glycol poisoning. 4-MP acts to inhibit ADH conversion of methanol and ethylene glycol to their toxic metabolites in exactly the same way as ethanol. The dose is 15 mg/kg every 12 hours and is increased to every 4 hours during dialysis. Typical treatment is for 48 hours.

Brent J, McMartin KE, Philips S, et al: Fomepizole for the treatment of ethylene glycol poisoning. N Engl J Med 340:832, 1999.

Brent J, McMartin KE, Philips S, et al: Fomepizole for the treatment of methanol poisoning. N Engl J Med 344:424–429, 2001.

20. What are the advantages of 4-MP over ethanol?

4-MP does not cause sedation and does not require blood testing to ensure a therapeutic range. It is easily given a bolus and does not require ICU management.

21. What are the indications for hemodialysis?

Dialysis used to be the primary treatment for these poisons and should be done in patients with blood levels greater than 50 mg/dL, when the metabolic acidosis is not correctable, with pending renal failure, or with visual symptoms in a methanol overdose. Many clinicians recommend dialysis when blood levels exceed 25 mg/dL, if dialysis is readily available. Treatment with fomepizole often may obviate the need for hemodialysis.

22. What if dialysis is unavailable?

Patients with ethylene glycol poisoning have been treated successfully with 4-MP alone without dialysis if there is no acidosis or renal failure. Because the half-life of ethylene glycol is prolonged, the treatment may be extended, but the invasive treatment of dialysis is avoided. As experience grows, the primary treatment for ethylene glycol may be 4-MP alone with limited dialysis use. In methanol poisoning, 4-MP slows the metabolism and increases the half-life of methanol, which has been measured at 30–52 hours. The use of 4-MP alone would not suffice for these patients.

23. How is isopropyl alcohol poisoning different from methanol and ethylene glycol poisoning?

Isopropyl alcohol is metabolized in the liver to acetone, which results in measurable ketonemia in the serum. Acetone is excreted by the kidney, resulting in ketonuria, and is exhaled through the lungs, giving patients an acetone aroma on their breath. Because these metabolites are not acidic, isopropyl alcohol poisoning does not result in metabolic acidosis and is far less toxic than either methanol or ethylene glycol poisoning.

Burkhart KK, Kulig KW: The other alcohols: Methanol, ethylene glycol, isopropanol. Emerg Med Clin North Am 8:913–918, 1990.

24. What are the symptoms of isopropyl alcohol ingestion?

Isopropyl alcohol, commonly found as rubbing alcohol, has a three-carbon chain rather than a two-carbon chain similar to ethanol. Because of this, it crosses the blood–brain barrier much faster and is about twice as intoxicating as ethanol. Because it commonly is found in concentrated solutions and is more potent, the central nervous system depression can occur rapidly and can continue from residual poison in the stomach. Isopropyl alcohol is much more irritating to the gastric mucosa and often causes abdominal pain, vomiting, and hematemesis.

25. Why is isopropanol so frequently abused?

Isopropanol is easy and legal to obtain and in the form of rubbing alcohol is 70% isopropanol. Unlike consumable beer, wine, and liquor, it is not taxed and is very inexpensive.

26. What treatment is advisable for isopropyl alcohol poisoning?

Generally, patients need observation to watch for respiratory depression similar to that for patients intoxicated with ethanol. An isopropyl alcohol level is roughly equivalent to an ethanol level twice as high. An isopropyl level usually does not add greatly to clinical observation. In the rare, severe instance of coma or hypertension corresponding to isopropyl levels greater than 500 mg/dL, intubation and ventilation may be necessary, and hemodialysis may be helpful because it can greatly enhance removal of isopropyl alcohol from the body. An antidote is not available for isopropyl alcohol (nor is one needed).

KEY POINTS: ISOPROPANOL

1. Symptoms and toxicity are completely different from methanol and ethylene glycol.

2. Ketosis occurs, but acidosis does not.

3. Supportive treatment is adequate in almost all cases.

CHAPTER 69

ALCOHOL-RELATED DISORDERS

John A. Marx, MD

1. **Is a patient who smells of alcohol simply intoxicated?**
   Perhaps, and in most cases, yes. There is a clinically relevant differential of altered mentation in such a patient, however. It is crucial that every patient assumed to be drunk (only) receive careful initial and serial evaluations. This is neither time consuming nor expensive.

2. **List the differential diagnosis for altered mentation.**
   Traumatic
   - Intracranial hemorrhage
   - Hypotension secondary to hemorrhage

   Metabolic
   - Hypoglycemia
   - Hepatic encephalopathy
   - Hypoxia

   Toxicologic
   - Other alcohols
   - Other toxins
   - Withdrawal from other toxins (e.g., sedative-hypnotics)
   - Disulfiram
   - Disulfiram-ethanol reaction

   Infectious
   - Meningitis, meningoencephalitis
   - Brain abscess
   - Sepsis

   Neurologic
   - Postictal state
   - Alcohol withdrawal
   - Wernicke-Korsakoff syndrome

3. **When should an acutely intoxicated patient be intubated?**
   Whenever you think it is indicated. No quantitative determinants (e.g., serum ethanol level) exist that serve as useful guidelines. Hypopnea and hypoventilation are rarely the issue, but the inability of the patient to protect the airway is. The odds against the stomach being empty approach infinity. For patients who are heavily intoxicated but not deemed to require intubation, lateral decubitus positioning is preferred. Restraining a patient supine or prone can be dangerous because of the risk of aspiration and airway compromise.

4. **Which pharmacologic agents are best for management of alcohol withdrawal?**
   The most widely used and time-honored mainstay is the **benzodiazepine** class. Benzodiazepines should be given orally, intravenously, or in combination and titrated by clinical response. No single benzodiazepine has been proclaimed the best agent. Pharmacokinetics, the presence of intermediate metabolites, and mostly physician preference are deciding factors. Patients with mild withdrawal (normal vital signs, no hallucinosis) may be discharged with a 2- to 3-day course of a single agent (e.g., lorazepam, 1–2 mg twice a day). Haloperidol, a butyrophenone, is

an appropriate adjunct for hallucinosis. Theoretical concerns over haloperidol lowering seizure threshold and exacerbating hemodynamic abnormalities in this class of patients have not been substantiated. More severe withdrawal syndromes require increasingly aggressive therapy with these same agents as well as sufficient observation by medical personnel.

5. **Describe an appropriate diagnostic work-up for alcohol withdrawal seizures (AWDS).**

Two issues are germane:

- Is the story consistent with AWDS?
- Is this the initial presentation and work-up for suspected AWDS?

Typically, AWDS occur approximately 6–96 hours after the last drink and in clusters of one to four seizures. The seizures are usually generalized and self-limited. Coincident features of withdrawal may be lacking, and lateralizing findings during the seizure, the postictal state, or both are often present because of underlying structural pathology. In a first-time evaluation, other causes of or contributors to seizures should be sought.

Routine laboratory studies (electrolytes, glucose, magnesium, calcium, toxicologic screen) are rarely useful unless history or physical examination is suggestive. Noncontrast computed tomography (CT) helps guide management. Nearly 10% of patients show traumatic, infectious, vascular, or miscellaneous abnormalities.

Generally, electroencephalography is not integral to the work-up. Lumbar puncture is indicated when meningitis, meningoencephalitis, or subarachnoid hemorrhage is suspected.

Subsequent visits for suspected AWDS demand scrupulous history and physical examination to ensure that other pathologic causes have not developed in the interim. If the presentation matches prior episodes and the findings on current neurologic examination are baseline, no other work-up, including CT, is necessary. Lingering postictal confusion warrants a check of glucose and electrolytes. If the story or examination has changed significantly or is worrisome, the clinician should start from scratch.

Earnest MD, Feldman H, Marx JA, et al: Intracranial lesions shown by CT in 259 cases of first alcohol-related seizures. Neurology 38:1561–1565, 1988.

6. **How should AWDS be managed?**

- **Acute.** Active AWDS are handled in routine fashion (i.e., ensure patient safety and patent airway and administer D_{50}, naloxone, and intravenous benzodiazepines as needed). If diagnostic evaluation is unremarkable, an observation period of at least 6 hours is optimal because additional seizures are common and occur within this period. Use of benzodiazepines in the immediate postseizure observation period and for 2 days thereafter decreases the incidence of additional seizures during this vulnerable time.
- **Chronic.** Patients whose seizures have an elliptogenic focus (e.g., old subdural) should receive anticonvulsant therapy such as **phenytoin.** However, compliance is typically poor, hence the dictum to never bet against a zero phenytoin level in this patient cohort. In the patient with pure AWDS (CT is unremarkable), long-term anticonvulsant therapy is absolutely *contraindicated*. Physicians must resist the pharmacologic imperative to "prescribe something" long-term, unless there is clear justification to do so.

Rathlev NK, D'Onofrio G, Fish SS, et al: The lack of efficacy of phenytoin in the prevention of recurrent alcohol-related seizures. Ann Emerg Med 23:513–518, 1994.

7. **Can AWDS be prevented?**

Data support prophylactic use of benzodiazepines in the acute withdrawal period, particularly in patients with a history of AWDS during abstinence and in patients who sustained suspected AWDS as cause for their being brought to the emergency department (ED) or during their stay there.

D'Onofrio G, Rathlev NK, Ulrich AS, et al: Lorazepam for the prevention of recurrent seizures related to alcohol. N Engl J Med 341:609–610, 1999.

8. **Who is at risk for alcohol-induced hypoglycemia (AIH)? What is the clinical presentation?**

   AIH results from two pathophysiologic processes: insufficient glycogen stores and alcohol-induced impairment of gluconeogenesis. The three groups vulnerable to AIH are chronic alcoholics, binge drinkers, and young children. AIH may occur during intoxication or up to 20 hours after the last drink. Manifestations of neuroglycopenia (headache, depressed mental status, seizure, coma) predominate. Evidence of catecholamine excess, typical of insulin-induced hypoglycemia (tremulousness, diaphoresis, anxiety), is unusual. Two clinical caveats are important. Seizures are a frequent presentation in children. Localized central nervous system signs, including a stroke-like picture (alcohol-induced hypoglycemic hemiplegia), often occur in adults.

9. **What causes alcoholic ketoacidosis (AKA)?**

   This common metabolic disturbance occurs early after heavy binge drinking and is heralded by starvation and vomiting and occasionally shortness of breath (Kussmaul respirations) and abdominal pain. Ketoacidosis results from accumulation of acetoacetate and, particularly, ß-hydroxybutyrate. Because this latter ketoacid is not measurable on routine blood and urine tests, the patient may have trace or absent ketones at presentation. Similarly, as the patient improves and ß-hydroxybutyrate is metabolized to acetoacetate, there may be a paradoxical spike in urine and serum ketones. The wise clinician will not be fooled by this.

   At presentation, serum pH and bicarbonate average 7.1 and 10, respectively. These values vary widely, however, because of the frequently overlapping conditions of withdrawal-related hyperventilation (respiratory alkalosis) and protracted emesis (metabolic alkalosis). When all three are coincident, the result is a triple acid-base disturbance. When in a clinical teaching situation, this allows you to interpret arterial blood gases and electrolytes pretty much any way you wish and still be at least partially correct. Be aware that depressed body stores of potassium and phosphate are typical. In AKA, serum glucose is usually normal or may be low, a distinguishing feature from diabetic ketoacidosis.

10. **How should AKA be managed?**

    Treatment consists of rehydration with dextrose-containing crystalloid, antiemetics if needed, and benzodiazepines as dictated by symptoms of withdrawal. Vitamin, potassium, and phosphate supplementation is indicated. Bicarbonate administration is rarely required, and insulin therapy is proscribed. Normalization of metabolic abnormalities usually follows 12–16 hours of therapy.

11. **What is the relationship between alcohol and metabolic acidosis?**

    - **Ethanol:** Acute ethanol ingestion results in a mild increase in the lactate-to-pyruvate ratio. Clinically significant metabolic acidosis does not ensue.
    - **AKA:** This ethanol abstinence syndrome produces marked elevations in acetoacetate and ß-hydroxybutyrate with resultant and occasionally profound increased anion gap metabolic acidosis. During the correction phase, a non-anion gap, hyperchloremic picture often develops (because some of the bicarbonate-bound ketoacids are excreted in the urine) on the road to normalization.
    - **Ethylene glycol and methanol:** Certain by-products of these highly toxic compounds produce increased anion gap metabolic acidosis. In the suspected alcoholic patient who presents with significant metabolic acidosis, a quick method of distinguishing the presence of ethylene glycol or methanol from AKA is the determination of the osmolal gap. If this exceeds 25 mOsm/Kg, it is 88% specific for the presence of ethylene glycol or methanol.
    - **Isopropyl alcohol:** A significant portion of isopropyl alcohol is metabolized to acetone. This is a ketone but not a ketoacid. Exposure to this alcohol can cause ketosis and ketonuria but not acidosis.

    Almaghamsi AM, Yeung CK: Osmolal gap in alcoholic ketoacidosis. Clin Nephrol 48:52, 1997.

12. **Which coagulopathies should be anticipated in a chronic alcoholic?**

Thrombocytopenia results from direct bone marrow depressant effects of ethanol, folate deficiency, and hypersplenism secondary to portal hypertension. Counts less than 30,000/mL resulting from alcohol usage alone are unlikely. Qualitative platelet defects also may occur.

Hepatocyte loss caused by chronic alcohol abuse depletes all coagulation factors except VIII, particularly II, VII, IX, and X. Alcoholics often have inadequate vitamin K stores because of hepatobiliary dysfunction and poor diet. Additionally, vitamin K is a requisite cofactor for the production of factors II, VII, IX, and X. When faced with gastrointestinal hemorrhage in a chronic alcoholic, an intravenous vitamin K supplementation trial is warranted. The far more likely culprit is hepatocellular destruction, however, for which vitamin K would not be helpful. Vitamin K does not begin to restore factor levels for 2–6 hours after administration. For emergent scenarios, fresh frozen plasma provides immediate factor supplementation.

13. **How should the combative alcoholic patient be managed?**

When the patient or staff is in jeopardy, the first step is mechanical containment of the patient. A sufficient number of competent personnel and restraint devices are necessary. A simple matter such as a closed head injury, hypoxia, or a full bladder may be the source of distress and should be excluded, managed, or relieved.

For chemical sedation, haloperidol is the preferred agent. It can be given quickly (initial dose, 5–10 mg intravenous push) and cause rapid onset of sedation (5 minutes). Repeat doses may be required. This agent is not detrimental to airway patency, ventilation, or hemodynamics. There is a 5–10% incidence of extrapyramidal reactions that usually occur 12–24 hours after administration; this compares very favorably with the obvious dangers of benzodiazepines, narcotics, and paralytic agents. Droperidol, another butyrophenone that has been utilized for sedation, received a black-box warning in 2004 due to reports of QT prolongation and torsades de pointes associated with its usage. As such, its administration is supposed to be limited to patients who fail to show acceptable response to other adequate treatment regimens. In any case, haloperidol and droperidol have been shown to be relatively comparable in efficacy and side effects when given intravenously, the preferred route due to greater rapidity of action.

Schwartz TH Jr, Petrilli R: Droperidol versus haloperidol for chemical restraint of agitated and combative patients. Ann Emerg Med 21:407–413, 1992.

14. **When can an acutely intoxicated patient be safely discharged from the ED?**

From a management perspective, there are two fundamental concerns:

- Acute intoxication obfuscates the verification of certain diagnoses and the exclusion of others.
- A physician who discharges an acutely intoxicated (i.e., incompetent) patient may be held accountable for the actions of that patient subsequent and proximate to discharge from the ED.

The conundrum lies in the definition of **intoxication.** Numerous texts provide tables that match serum alcohol levels with clinical findings. In truth, the degree of clinical intoxication at a specific serum alcohol level is variable in accordance with the patient's chronicity and severity of drinking. A veteran drinker with a level in excess of 500 mg/dL can look less drunk than a teenager at 100 mg/dL. The patient should undergo a scrupulous initial evaluation, then repeated examinations until the physician is comfortable that other medical concerns do not exist.

Documentation of the discharge neurologic examination, including mental status, gait, and the fact that the patient is **clinically sober** is imperative. Particular attention should be paid to any patient in whom abdominal or closed head trauma may have occurred. The patient then may be discharged to an appropriate environment. Serum or breath alcohol determinations sometimes can be helpful at the outset of care but often are unneeded and can be problematic when obtained at discharge.

KEY POINTS: ALCOHOL-RELATED DISORDERS

1. **Airway protection:** Clinical judgment is the key factor in determining whether an acutely intoxicated patient requires airway protection via active airway management. This is true for every patient encountered by the emergency physician.

2. **Phenytoin for prevention of alcohol withdrawal seizures:** This should only be given to patients with clear indication of an elliptogenic focus. Otherwise, its use for prevention of alcohol withdrawal seizures is strictly proscribed.

3. **Haloperidol and the agitated, intoxicated patient:** Haloperidol is an extremely effective agent for the safe and rapid sedation of the combative, intoxicated patient.

4. **Discharge documentation:** The critical determination in the discharge of the patient who presents with acute intoxication is the progression to and documentation of "clinical sobriety."

CONTROVERSIES

15. **Must thiamine be administered before glucose in the alcoholic patient?**
It has been widely held that delivery of glucose to a patient with marginal thiamine reserves would catapult that patient into Wernicke-Korsakoff syndrome. In an alcoholic patient, AIH or hypoglycemia of any cause is a far more likely cause of depressed level of consciousness than is Wernicke-Korsakoff syndrome. The use of a rapid glucose analyzer can avoid unneeded glucose administration to patients considered at risk for inadequate thiamine stores. Wernicke-Korsakoff syndrome develops over hours to days. The precipitous initiation of Wernicke-Korsakoff syndrome by dextrose has not been substantiated. The consequences of neuroglycopenia begin within 30 minutes, can be tremendously morbid, and are easily prevented. In alcoholic patients with known or strongly suspected hypoglycemia, administer glucose and deliver thiamine empirically as soon afterward as possible. Because magnesium is a cofactor of thiamine and because alcoholics are frequently hypomagnesemic, 2 gm of magnesium should be administered intravenously when there is suspicion of Wernicke-Korsakoff syndrome.

16. **Is it dangerous to administer thiamine intravenously?**
Orally administered thiamine may be absorbed poorly in the alcoholic. The intramuscular route is painful and can result in hematomas or abscesses, particularly if the patient's coagulation status is impaired. The experience with intravenous thiamine is enormous, and the safety profile is exceptional. Thiamine may be given as part of fluid hydration and multivitamin preparations. It also can be given by bolus infusion.

Frommer DA, Marx JA: Wernicke's encephalopathy. N Engl J Med 313:637–638, 1985.

17. **Is there a cure for a hangover?**
Probably not, at least not one with solid scientific credentials. There is no shortage of remedies, however, from the well-worn "hair of the dog that bit you" (i.e., start drinking again) to a more recently acclaimed concoction of vitamin B_6, nonsteroidal anti-inflammatories, and hydration. The only sure-fire preventative measure is the avoidance of drinking in the first place.

Wiese JG, Shlipak MG, Browner WS: The alcohol hangover. Ann Intern Med 132:897–902, 2000.

18. **Are there promising agents for terminating alcohol dependence?**

Disulfiram (Antabuse) is a well-known, long-standing agent utilized for intercession in patients with alcohol dependency. It can be effective, but there are numerous side effects, some life threatening, and compliance with the daily regimen is typically poor, mitigating the potential value of this intervention. Recently, intramuscular naltrexone, in a dosage of 380 mg intramuscularly given once every 4 weeks, demonstrated efficacy in reducing the rate of heavy drinking in alcohol-dependent adults over a 6-month interval with an acceptable incidence of mild-to-moderate side effects. However, the optimal duration of this treatment needed to achieve a durable effect while avoiding adverse reactions has not been determined.

Garbutt JC, Kranzler HR, O'Malley SS, et al: Efficacy and tolerability of long-acting injectable naltrexone for alcohol dependence: A randomized controlled trial. JAMA 293:1617–1625, 2005.

19. **Are there specific criteria for the diagnosis of Wernicke-Korsakoff syndrome?**

Yes, recently developed criteria require two of the following four signs to be present:
1. Dietary deficiencies
2. Ocular motor abnormalities
3. Cerebellar dysfunction
4. Either an altered mental state or mild memory impairment

Harper C: The neuropathology of alcohol-specific brain damage, or does alcohol damage the brain? J Neuro Pathol Exp Neurol 57:101, 1998.

BIBLIOGRAPHY

1. Mayo-Smith MF: Pharmacological management of alcohol withdrawal: A meta-analysis and evidence-based practice guideline. American Society of Addiction Medicine Working Group on Pharmacological Management of Alcohol Withdrawal. JAMA 278:144–151, 1997.
2. Swift RM: Direct therapy for alcohol dependence. N Engl J Med 340:1482, 1999.
3. Victor M, Adams RD, Collins GH: The Wernicke-Korsakoff Syndrome. Philadelphia, F.A. Davis, 1971.
4. Wrenn KD, Slovis CM, Minion G, Rotkowski R: The syndrome of alcoholic ketoacidosis. Am J Med 91:119–128, 1991.

CHAPTER 70

ANTIPYRETIC POISONING

James C. Mitchiner, MD, MPH

SALICYLATE POISONING

1. **What are the causes of salicylate overdose?**

   A salicylate overdose may be intentional or accidental. Parental administration of aspirin to a child using adult doses may cause toxicity. Bismuth subsalicylate (Pepto-Bismol), which contains 130 mg/tablespoon of salicylate, is often the culprit. In adults, simultaneous ingestion of proprietary aspirin and prescription medication may lead to unintentional overdose and to the formation of gastric concretions. Liquid methyl salicylate (oil of wintergreen) is especially toxic because of its high salicylate content (1 teaspoon = 7 g of salicylate) and rapid absorption. Dermal application of salicylic acid ointment is a rare cause of acute salicylism. The minimal acute toxic ingestion is 150 mg/kg.

2. **What are the characteristics of a patient who presents with an acute salicylate overdose?**

   Patients may present with nausea, vomiting, tinnitus, vertigo, fever, diaphoresis, and confusion. Hyperventilation may be ascribed mistakenly to anxiety. Patients also may present with headache or chronic pain, which prompted the ingestion of salicylate.

3. **List some common signs of salicylate intoxication.**

   See Table 70-1.

TABLE 70-1. COMMON SIGNS OF ACUTE SALICYLATE TOXICITY	
General	Hyperthermia, dehydration
Respiratory	Hyperventilation, noncardiogenic pulmonary edema
Central nervous system	Confusion, delirium, seizures, coma
Gastrointestinal	Gastrointestinal hemorrhage
Dermatologic	Eyelid petechiae
Laboratory	Acid-base disturbances, azotemia, hyperkalemia or hypokalemia, hypoglycemia (children), elevated CK levels (rhabdomyolysis), coagulopathy

CK = creatine kinase.

4. **Describe the acid-base disturbances.**

   Acute **respiratory alkalosis**, without hypoxia, is due to salicylate stimulation of the respiratory center. If the patient is hypoxic, salicylate-induced noncardiogenic pulmonary edema should be considered. Within 12–24 hours after ingestion, the acid-base status in an untreated patient shifts toward an anion gap **metabolic acidosis.** A mixed respiratory alkalosis and metabolic acidosis typically is seen in adults. In patients presenting with **respiratory acidosis,** concomitant ingestion of a central nervous system depressant should be suspected. **Metabolic acidosis** is the predominant acid-base disturbance in children, in patients who take massive amounts of salicylates, and in patients (adults and children) who have chronic salicylate toxicity (see later).

5. **What are some of the other metabolic disturbances seen in acute salicylate poisoning?**
   The patient may be dehydrated secondary to vomiting or to the diuretic effects of increased renal sodium excretion. Insensible losses are increased in patients with hyperventilation, and water and electrolyte losses may occur through diaphoresis in response to the hyperpyrexic state. Hypokalemia is due to renal excretion and respiratory and metabolic alkalemia (secondary to bicarbonate therapy).

6. **I thought aspirin is an antipyretic. How does it cause a fever?**
   At a cellular level, salicylate poisoning leads to the uncoupling of oxidative phosphorylation. When this occurs, the energy obtained from oxygen reduction and reduced nicotinamide adenine dinucleotide oxidation that normally is captured to form adenosine triphosphate instead is released as heat.

7. **Name some of the hematologic abnormalities.**
   These are rare in an acute overdose. Features include decreased production of prothrombin (factor II) and factor VII, an increase in capillary endothelial fragility, and a decrease in the quantity and function of platelets (i.e., decreased adhesiveness). Significant hemorrhage is unusual.

8. **How is the severity of salicylate overdose assessed?**
   The **Done nomogram** has limited, if any, value, and treatment should be based on serial salicylate levels and clinical reevaluation. Salicylate levels should be repeated several hours apart, *while the patient is still in the emergency department (ED),* so that the trend in the severity of poisoning can be assessed.

9. **Which laboratory tests are indicated?**
   Serial serum salicylate levels (initial and 6 hours later) should be obtained. Arterial blood gases, complete blood cell count, electrolytes, blood urea nitrogen (BUN), creatinine, glucose, prothrombin time, international normalized ratio (INR), and urinalysis also should be considered. If the patient presents less than 6 hours after an acute ingestion, a salicylate level should be repeated at 6 hours. A quantitative acetaminophen level is recommended because many patients confuse these two drugs or mix both kinds in the same bottle.

10. **What is the initial ED treatment for an acute salicylate overdose?**
    If poisoning is through dermal contact, the skin should be washed copiously with tap water. For acute ingestions, isotonic intravenous fluids with bicarbonate (D5W + three ampules of sodium bicarbonate) should be administered. A slurry of activated charcoal and cathartic (sorbitol or magnesium sulfate) should be given orally or by gastric lavage tube at a dose of 1gm of charcoal per kg body weight. Lavage may be useful even if the patient presents several hours after ingestion because large amounts of aspirin may form gastric concretions and delay absorption for 24 hours or longer.

11. **What else needs to be done in the ED?**
    After the patient has responded with diuresis, potassium loss should be replaced with potassium chloride at a dose of 20–40 mEq/L. Patients with hyperthermia should be cooled with a cooling blanket. Documented hypoglycemia should be treated with intravenous D_{50}. Patients with aspirin-induced noncardiogenic pulmonary edema should be treated in standard fashion, with

oxygen, continuous positive airway pressure (CPAP), bi-level positive airway pressure (BiPAP), or intubation and positive end-expiratory pressure (PEEP). Sedation should be avoided because of the risk of respiratory depression leading to respiratory acidosis.

12. Is there a role for repetitive dosing of activated charcoal?
Because of aspirin release from the aspirin-charcoal complex in the gastrointestinal tract and subsequent reabsorption, salicylate levels may not decline significantly after a single dose of activated charcoal. Repeated doses of charcoal may be indicated to enhance elimination.

Hillman RJ, Prescott LF: Treatment of salicylate poisoning with repeated oral charcoal. BMJ 291:1472, 1985.

13. What is the rationale for alkaline diuresis?
Because aspirin is an organic acid, administration of bicarbonate intravenously raises the pH of the blood and *traps* salicylate ion, limiting the amount of salicylate that crosses the blood–brain barrier. Similarly, an alkalotic urine retains salicylate ion, preventing its reabsorption by the renal tubules. The use of forced alkaline diuresis is difficult to attain and has been reported to cause pulmonary edema. It may be achieved by adding three ampules of $NaHCO_3$ to each liter of D5W.

14. Explain the paradox of a decreasing serum salicylate concentration and increasing clinical toxicity.
The serum salicylate level by itself does not reflect tissue distribution of the drug. If the patient's blood is acidemic, salicylate acid remains unionized, and more penetrates the blood–brain barrier, resulting in central nervous system toxicity. Salicylate levels should be interpreted in light of the patient's clinical condition and a concurrent blood pH; an acidotic pH is associated with toxicity regardless of the salicylate level.

15. What are the indications for hemodialysis?
Standard indications include persistent, refractory metabolic acidosis (pH < 7.10), renal failure with oliguria, cardiac dysfunction (congestive heart failure, arrhythmias, cardiac arrest), central nervous system deterioration (seizures, coma, cerebral edema), and an acute salicylate level greater than 130 mg/dL 6 hours after ingestion. Because ingestion of more than 300 mg/kg predicts severe toxicity, a nephrologist should be contacted early in anticipation of the possible need for dialysis.

Fomenbaum NE: Salicylates. In Goldfrank LR, Flomenbaum NE, Lewin NA, et al (eds): Goldfrank's Toxicologic Emergencies, 8th ed. Norwalk, CT., McGraw Hill, 2006, pp 550–564.

16. What are the most common findings in chronic salicylate poisoning?
In contrast to acute salicylate poisoning, chronic salicylism is usually accidental. The principal diagnostic feature is a change in mental status manifested by weakness, tinnitus, lethargy, confusion, drowsiness, slurred speech, hallucinations, agitation, or seizures. Because these signs are common to many other disorders, the diagnosis frequently is missed, resulting in a mortality rate of 25%. Most patients are tachypneic, which is a compensatory response to an anion gap metabolic acidosis. The serum salicylate level may not be elevated, and the Done nomogram is of no use in chronic salicylate ingestions.

Anderson RJ, Potts DE, Gabow PA, et al: Unrecognized adult salicylate intoxication. Ann Intern Med 85:745–748, 1976.

ACETAMINOPHEN POISONING

17. Is there anything new in acetaminophen toxicology?
Yes. The approval by the Food and Drug Administration of the intravenous formulation of *N*-acetylcysteine (NAC) (Acetadote) has given clinicians another choice for administering this valuable antidote.

18. **What are the characteristics of acetaminophen overdose?**
    Acetaminophen is the drug most commonly involved in acute analgesic ingestions, either as a single agent or in combination with various cough, cold, or pain remedies. Early diagnosis of acute (phase I) acetaminophen toxicity is important because early symptoms may be subtle or absent; the onset of hepatotoxicity, the major manifestation, is delayed by several days after ingestion. Failure to recognize and treat toxicity within 16 hours of ingestion results in significant morbidity and mortality. *The main issue in treatment is the prevention of hepatotoxicity.*

19. **Outline the four phases of acetaminophen overdose.**
    See Table 70-2.

TABLE 70-2.	PHASES OF ACETAMINOPHEN TOXICITY		
Phase	**Onset Posting Estion**	**Clinical Characteristics**	**Laboratory Findings**
I	< 24 hours	Anorexia, nausea, vomiting, diaphoresis (patient may be asymptomatic)	Toxic acetaminophen level
II	24–72 hours	Right upper quadrant abdominal pain	Mild elevation in LFTs
III	3–5 days	Jaundice, encephalopathy	Marked elevation in LFTs, coagulopathy, azotemia, hypoglycemia
IV	~ 1 week	Gradual resolution of toxicity	Improvement in laboratory values

LFTs = liver function tests.

20. **What are the initial central nervous system manifestations of acetaminophen poisoning?**
    Gotcha! In the early stages, there are none, and abnormalities in mental status or level of consciousness should be attributed to other drugs (e.g., salicylates, opiates, sedatives) or to other disease states. Hepatic encephalopathy can occur in phase III.

21. **Describe the pathophysiology of acetaminophen toxicity.**
    Acetaminophen is metabolized primarily by the liver. About 90% of it is conjugated with glucuronic or sulfuric acid to form nontoxic compounds that are excreted in the urine. About 2% of the drug is excreted unchanged in the urine. The remainder is metabolized by the cytochrome P-450 mixed-function oxidase system. This involves formation of a toxic intermediary compound, which is conjugated rapidly with hepatic glutathione. The resulting conjugate is metabolized further, and its by-products are excreted in the urine. Because the liver normally has a fixed amount of glutathione, this compound is depleted rapidly in an acute overdose. The toxic intermediary then accumulates, unmetabolized, and binds to the sulfhydryl groups of hepatic enzymes. The result is irreversible centrilobular hepatic necrosis.

22. **How is hepatotoxicity predicted?**
    An acute ingestion of 7.5 gm or more in an adult or 140 mg/kg in a child is generally predictive of hepatotoxicity. The most accurate predictor of hepatotoxicity is the serum acetaminophen level

obtained between 4 and 24 hours after **acute** ingestion. The **Rumack-Matthew nomogram,** which plots serum concentration against hours postingestion, is the standard reference for predicting hepatotoxicity in an acute overdose. Certain drugs, such as cimetidine, compete with acetaminophen for metabolism by the P-450 pathway and theoretically offer some protection from hepatotoxicity. Other drugs, such as phenytoin and phenobarbital, may induce the P-450 enzymes, allowing a greater percentage of acetaminophen to be metabolized to the toxic intermediary and increasing the risk of toxicity.

Hendrickson RG, Bizovi KE: Acetaminophen. In Goldfrank LR, Flomenbaum NE, Lewin NA, et al (eds): Goldfrank's Toxicologic Emergencies, 8th ed. Norwalk, CT, McGraw Hill, 2006, pp 523–543.

23. Are serial serum acetaminophen levels helpful?

If an accurate estimate of the time of ingestion cannot be obtained, the nomogram cannot be used, and serial levels should be obtained. Rising levels indicate potential hepatotoxicity.

24. Why is hepatotoxicity in children rare?

No one knows for sure. Toxicity in children is rare, even when toxic levels of acetaminophen are found. One theory holds that acetaminophen metabolism in children shows a preference for alternative pathways other than the P-450 system. The conversion from juvenile to adult metabolism is believed to occur between 6 and 9 years of age.

25. Which laboratory tests are helpful?

If a serum acetaminophen level is in the toxic range on the nomogram, additional blood should be obtained for a complete blood cell count, electrolytes, BUN, glucose, prothrombin time, INR, and liver function tests. A **limited** toxicology screen also should be ordered, with attention to treatable concomitant ingestions, such as salicylates, opiates, barbiturates, ethanol, and cyclic antidepressants. If the acetaminophen level is within the toxic range, liver function tests, prothrombin time, and INR should be repeated daily while the patient is receiving treatment.

26. Outline the general treatment of acetaminophen poisoning.

If the patient presents within 1 hour of ingestion, gastric lavage should be done. Activated charcoal (1 gm/kg) mixed with sorbitol or magnesium sulfate should be administered by gastric lavage tube. If the patient presents more than 1 hour after ingestion, the charcoal and cathartic should be administered orally without lavage, unless there is another indication for gastric lavage (see Chapter 67). The specific antidote is NAC. This agent is a glutathione substitute with a high therapeutic-to-toxic safety ratio. It should be given orally or intravenously as soon as possible after a toxic acetaminophen level, as predicted by the nomogram, is discovered.

KEY POINTS: ED APPROACH TO ANALGESIC TOXICITY

1. Serial salicylate levels should be used to exclude toxicity prior to admitting the patient to the psychiatric floor.

2. Salicylate levels must be interpreted in light of the patient's clinical condition, the formulation of the drug (pills, capsules or liquids), and the blood pH.

3. The primary goal in the treatment of acetaminophen toxicity is the prevention of hepatotoxicity.

4. The antidote for acetaminophen overdose is *N*-acetylcysteine. It is most effective when given within 10 hours, regardless of whether it is given orally or intravenously.

27. How is NAC administered?
Oral NAC (Mucomyst) is given by mouth or nasogastric tube after diluting it 1:5 with water or juice. This dilution produces a 20% solution, which is given as a loading dose of 140 mg/kg, followed by a maintenance dose of 70 mg/kg every 4 hours for 17 additional doses. If the patient vomits a dose within 1 hour, the dose should be repeated. Antiemetics should be given if vomiting is persistent. The intravenous NAC formulation (Acetadote) is indicated for patients in whom oral NAC is contraindicated (e.g., persistent vomiting, encephalopathy, gastrointestinal bleeding, bowel obstruction, concomitant ingestion with anticholinergic drug). The dose is 150 mg/kg in D_5W over 15 minutes, followed by 50 mg/kg over 4 hours, then 100 mg/kg over 16 hours.

Smilkstein MJ, Knapp GL, Kulig KW, et al: Efficacy of oral *N*-acetylcysteine in the treatment of acetaminophen overdose: Analysis of the national multicenter study 1976–1985. N Engl J Med 319:1557–1562, 1988.

Yip L, Dart RC, Hurlbut KM: Intravenous administration of oral *N*-acetylcysteine. Crit Care Med 26:40–43, 1998.

www.acetadote.com/prescribe.pdf

28. Which route is better for administering NAC—oral or intravenous?
It depends. Compared to the oral route, intravenous NAC is easier to administer, takes less time (20.25 hours versus 72 hours for the oral route), and can be given to patients who are vomiting. Disadvantages include a higher rate of adverse reactions (up to 17%) and greater expense. There is no evidence to date that one route is preferable to the other in terms of reducing the risk of hepatotoxicity.

Prescott L: Oral or intravenous *N*-Acetylcysteine for acetaminophen poisoning? Ann Emerg Med 45:409–413, 2005.

29. Is there a critical window in time to administer NAC?
Yes. Whenever possible, NAC should be given within 10 hours of acute acetaminophen overdose. NAC still may be of benefit if given more than 10 hours after acute ingestion, particularly in patients who have taken extended-release formulations or staggered overdoses, and in patients with persistently toxic acetaminophen levels or elevated liver enzymes. The intravenous route is recommended in these cases.

Prescott L: Oral or intravenous *N*-Acetylcysteine for acetaminophen poisoning? Ann Emerg Med 45:409–413, 2005.

30. Should I be concerned about potential adverse reactions to intravenous NAC?
Yes. The incidence of such reactions is 5–17%, and they tend to occur during infusion of the loading dose. Typical symptoms not requiring therapy include nausea, vomiting, and flushing; mild urticaria can be treated with diphenhydramine. Interruption of NAC therapy is not necessary, but the initial infusion rate should be slowed. Serious reactions, such as bronchospasm, angioedema, and hypotension, require aggressive therapy with antihistamines, steroids, and epinephrine and discontinuation of the NAC.

Bailey B, McGuigan MA: Management of anaphylactoid reactions to intravenous *N*-acetylcysteine. Ann Emerg Med 31:710–715, 1998.

31. What is the acetaminophen-alcohol syndrome?
Alcohol affects hepatic acetaminophen detoxification in two ways: (1) it lowers hepatic glutathione stores, resulting in a reduced capacity to detoxify the toxic intermediate compound, and (2) it induces the cytochrome P-450 system, increasing the proportion of ingested acetaminophen that is converted to the toxic intermediate. Diagnostic findings include a history of acetaminophen ingestion and elevated aspartate transaminase levels (usually >800 IU/L) in patients with known or occult alcohol abuse who regularly take acetaminophen. The diagnosis initially is missed in one third of cases, and the mortality rate is greater than 30%.

Treatment is generally supportive, although NAC has been tried, and liver transplantation is an option.

Johnson SC, Pelletier LL: Enhanced hepatotoxicity of acetaminophen in the alcoholic patient: Two case reports and a review of the literature. Medicine 76:185–191, 1997.

32. What is the treatment for chronic acetaminophen toxicity?
In chronic acetaminophen poisoning, the nomogram is not helpful in predicting toxicity. Repetitive ingestion is thought to be of serious concern only in alcoholics, patients on anticonvulsants, children with febrile illnesses, individuals taking large doses (e.g., >10 gm/day), and patients with symptoms of toxicity. NAC is recommended only for patients with detectable acetaminophen levels and evidence of liver injury.

Lane JE, Belson MG, Brown DK, et al. Chronic acetaminophen toxicity: A case report and review of the literature. J Emerg Med 23:253–256, 2002.

IBUPROFEN POISONING

33. What are the characteristics of ibuprofen overdose?
Ibuprofen is readily available as an over-the-counter medication used in the treatment of mild-to-moderate pain and fever. Rapid absorption leads to peak drug levels within 2 hours. Symptoms usually are seen within 4 hours of ingestion and are more likely to be serious in children. Toxicity is limited in patients who ingest less than 100 mg/kg, whereas patients, primarily children, who ingest more than 400 mg/kg may be at risk for more severe symptoms.

Hall AH, Smolinske SC, Kulig KW, et al: Ibuprofen overdose: A prospective study. West J Med 48:653–656, 1988.
Oker EE, Hermann L, Baum CR, et al: Serious toxicity in a young child due to ibuprofen. Acad Emerg Med 7:821–823, 2000.

34. List the primary symptoms of ibuprofen toxicity.
- **Gastrointestinal toxicity** is manifested by nausea, vomiting, abdominal pain, and hematemesis.
- **Nephrotoxicity** results in acute renal failure.
- **Central nervous system toxicity** (seen mostly in children) includes somnolence, apnea, seizures, and coma.
- **Severe metabolic acidosis** and **thrombocytopenia** have also been described.

35. When should a serum ibuprofen level be obtained?
Because the serum ibuprofen level does not correlate with clinical symptoms, there is no role for this test in decision making.

36. Describe the treatment for ibuprofen toxicity.
Treatment is directed at alleviating symptoms and providing supportive care (see Chapter 67). If hematemesis is present or there is blood in the stool, a nasogastric tube should be placed; if blood is present, the stomach should be irrigated with saline. A limited toxicology screen to search for other readily treatable toxins (salicylates, acetaminophen, opiates, barbiturates, cyclic antidepressants, and ethanol) is recommended. Seizures should be treated with intravenous diazepam. Renal and hepatic function tests should be ordered. Children with ingestions of greater than 400 mg/kg should be observed in the hospital. Forced diuresis, alkalinization, and hemodialysis are not indicated.

CHAPTER 71

OPIOIDS AND SEDATIVE-HYPNOTICS

Corey D. Harrison, MD, and Vikhyat S. Bebarta, MD

1. Isn't abuse of heroin and other opioids decreasing?

Actually, it is just the opposite. The data collected by the American Association of Poison Control Centers (AAPCC), demonstrated an increase from 5% to 13% in opioid-related deaths from 1995 to 2003. Analgesics are the most common killer in toxic ingestions of pharmaceuticals every year since 1995. Opioids represent approximately half of those deaths each year. The Drug Abuse Warning Network in the United States showed a 25% increase in emergency department (ED) visits involving heroin from 1998 to 2002.

> www.aapcc.org
> dawninfo.samsha.gov

2. What do the terms *opium*, *opiate*, *opioid*, and *narcotic* mean?

- **Opium** is a mixture of alkaloids, including morphine and codeine, extracted from the opium poppy.
- An **opiate** is a natural drug derived from opium (e.g., heroin, codeine, and morphine).
- An **opioid** is any drug that has opium-like activity, including the opiates and all synthetic and semisynthetic drugs that interact with opioid receptors in the body (e.g., hydrocodone and oxycodone).
- The term **narcotic** is nonspecific; it refers to any addictive drug that reduces pain, alters mood and behavior, and usually induces sleep or stupor.

3. What is the typical clinical presentation of opioid poisoning?

The classic triad of opioid poisoning is **central nervous system (CNS) depression, respiratory depression,** and **miosis.** Patients who have overdosed on opioids are hyporeflexic and have decreased bowel sounds. They may be hypothermic, cyanotic and mildly hypotensive, and bradycardic.

> Hoffman JR, Schriger DL, Luo JS: The empiric use of naloxone in patients with altered mental status: A reappraisal. Ann Emerg Med 20:246–252, 1991.

4. Do all opioid intoxication cases present with miosis?

No. Mydriasis or normal pupils can occur in conjunction with opioid overdose in the following situations: intoxication of specific synthetic opioids (meperidine, propoxyphene, or pentazocine), diphenoxylate-atropine (Lomotil) ingestion, coingestion of other drugs such as anticholinergics, after the use of naloxone, in the setting of hypoxia, or with use of mydriatic eye drops. Occasionally, phenylephrine, instilled into the patient's nares by paramedics for nasal intubation, may spill into the patient's eyes, causing mydriasis. See Table 71-1 for other non-opioid-related causes of miosis.

5. How should a patient with respiratory compromise by opioid overdose be treated?

Resuscitation takes precedence over the administration of naloxone. The patient's respiration must be supported with a bag-valve-mask until the opioid antagonist is given. If there is an inadequate response to naloxone, the patient should be intubated. Obtain a serum glucose level,

TABLE 71-1. COMMON CAUSES OF NON-OPIOID-RELATED MIOSIS	
Sympatholytic agents	Clonidine, antipsychotics, oxymetazoline, tetrahydrozoline
Cholinergic agents	Organophosphates, carbamates, nicotine, pilocarpine, phencyclidine and similar congeners
Miscellaneous	Pontine infarct, Horner's syndrome

administer oxygen, and consider thiamine administration for a patient with altered consciousness. Activated charcoal should be given to patients with a recent oral opioid ingestion.

6. **What is the appropriate naloxone dose?**
   The recommended initial dose of naloxone for adults and children with severe CNS and respiratory depression is 2.0 mg intravenously. For children younger than 5 years or less than 20 kg, 0.1 mg/kg should be administered. If a patient has CNS depression only, it is reasonable to start with a smaller dose (0.4–0.8 mg intravenous [IV]). If there is no response to a smaller dose, 2.0 mg can be given. For patients who abuse opioids and those who use opioids for chronic pain, 0.1 mg may be used to awaken the patient yet prevent or attenuate withdrawal. Additional doses should be given judiciously in this patient group. Opioid withdrawal is unpleasant to the patient but is not life threatening. It is sensible to titrate the dose of naloxone to reverse respiratory and CNS depression without precipitating withdrawal.

   Dawson AH: Naloxone, naltrexone, nalmefene. In Dart RC (ed): Medical Toxicology, 3rd ed. Philadelphia, Lippincott Williams & Wilkins, 2004, pp 228–230.

7. **Can naloxone be administered by other routes besides intravenously?**
   Yes. If an intravenous venous access cannot be started, naloxone can be given intramuscularly or subcutaneously. A dose of 0.8mg subcutaneously has an equal time to effect as 0.4 mg intravenously. It can be administered through the endotracheal tube, injected sublingually, or given intranasally. Naloxone is not effective orally because of significant first pass metabolism.

   Sporer KA, Firestone J, Isaacs SM: Out-of-hospital treatment of opioid overdoses in an urban setting. Acad Emerg Med 3:660–667, 1996.
   Wolfe T, Barton E: Nasal drug delivery in EMS: Reducing needlestick risk. JEMS 28(12):52–63, 2003.

8. **Do all patients respond to a standard dose of naloxone?**
   No. Larger doses of naloxone may be required to reverse the effects synthetic opioids such as codeine, diphenoxylate-atropine (Lomotil), propoxyphene (Darvon), pentazocine (Talwin), codeine, dextromethorphan, and the fentanyl derivatives. If an opioid overdose is suspected and the patient does not respond to an initial naloxone dose, repeat additional doses until a response is noted or until 10 mg has been given. If there is no response to 10mg of naloxone, it is unlikely that the diagnosis is an isolated opioid overdose.

9. **How long does the clinical effect of naloxone last?**
   The duration of action of intravenous naloxone is 40–75 minutes, although the serum half-life is shorter. Many opioids produce clinical effects that last 3–6 hours. Although the duration of action of most opioids is much longer than that of naloxone, significant resedation is relatively uncommon, particularly with parenteral opioids. Many oral opioids, particularly long-acting agents, have effects that last several hours and may require additional naloxone doses.

10. **Should naloxone be administered empirically to every patient with altered mental status?**
    No. Although naloxone is a safe medication, it is not helpful in every patient who has altered mental status. If a patient presents with an obvious sympathomimetic or anticholinergic

syndrome, this agitated and stimulated patient would not benefit from naloxone. If the diagnosis of an opioid syndrome is obvious and the patient's ventilatory status is adequate, naloxone may stimulate an opioid withdrawal that may be more difficult to handle in a busy ED than a slightly sedated patient.

11. **How should recurrent sedation and respiratory depression resulting from a long-acting opioid be treated?**
A continuous naloxone infusion may be started. Giving repeated doses of naloxone to an opioid-dependent patient may cause the patient to fluctuate between symptoms of withdrawal and CNS depression. A naloxone infusion is made by administering two thirds of the dose needed to reverse the patient's respiratory depression every hour. Multiply the dose by 6.6, mix it into 1 L of D_5W, and run it at 100 mL/h. The infusion can be adjusted accordingly, based on the patient's symptoms of withdrawal or sedation.

Nelson LS: Opioids. In Goldfrank LR, Flomenbaum NE, Lewin NA, et al (eds): Goldfrank's Toxicologic Emergencies, 7th ed. New York, McGraw-Hill, 2002, pp 901–923.

12. **What is nalmefene? Is it better than naloxone?**
Nalmefene is an opioid antagonist with a structure similar to naloxone but with a longer duration of action of 4–8 hours when given intravenously. When compared in a randomized, double-blinded study with naloxone, it had similar clinical outcomes of adverse events. Nalmefene has not become popular in most EDs because of the presumption that prolonged withdrawal symptoms would result from its use. Some opioid abusers may attempt to counter the antagonist by taking large doses of heroin or other opioids. When nalmefene wears off, the patient may be at risk for opioid toxicity. A realistic indication for nalmefene may be with pediatric patients who have an accidental single ingestion and are admitted to the hospital for observation.

Kaplan JL, Marx JA, Calabro JJ, et al: Double-blind, randomized study of nalmefene and naloxone in ED patients with suspected narcotics overdose. Ann Emerg Med 34:42–50, 1999.

13. **What about naltrexone?**
Naltrexone is an oral opioid antagonist with a long duration of action. It is used for long-term detoxification therapy and has no significant role in management of acute opioid toxicity in the ED.

14. **Who should be observed in the ED and for how long?**
Whether or not naloxone has been given, if the ventilatory drive is adequate, most patients can be observed for several hours until appropriately awake and discharged. Occasionally, patients who have recurrent inadequate ventilation necessitating treatment or those who develop complications of opioid use must be admitted. Most patients should be watched for at least 2 hours after narcotic use. Noncardiogenic pulmonary edema almost always occurs during this time period. Most emergency physicians consider a conservative period of 4 hours after the last dose of naloxone adequate in an asymptomatic patient who used a parenteral opioid. This extended period may allow for recognition of potential coingestants and recurrent respiratory depression. Oral opioids, particularly long-acting opioids, such as methadone or long-acting morphine or oxycodone, may require a longer period of observation and likely admission.

Kleinschmidt KC, Wainscott M, Ford MD: Opioids. In Ford M, Delaney KA, Ling LJ, et al (eds): Clinical Toxicology. Philadelphia, W.B. Saunders, 2001, pp 627–639.

15. **What are the signs of opioid withdrawal?**
Signs of withdrawal are anxiety, yawning, lacrimation, rhinorrhea, diaphoresis, mydriasis, nausea and vomiting, diarrhea, piloerection, abdominal pain, and diffuse myalgias. Opioid withdrawal typically occurs 12 hours after last heroin use and 30 hours after last methadone

use. Seizures, dysrhythmias, and other life-threatening complications are not consistent with opioid withdrawal.

16. **How is opioid withdrawal best treated?**
Treatment is symptomatic. Intravenous fluids, sedation, antiemetics, and antidiarrheal agents are the mainstays of treatment. Clonidine, 0.1–0.2 mg orally, may also be helpful. However, a number of published cases describe a concomitant abuse of clonidine, because the user feels it enhances the opioid euphoria. Also, if naloxone was given, the withdrawal symptoms should resolve in 45–75 minutes, when the naloxone effect subsides.

17. **What are body stuffers and packers?**
    - **Body packers** are individuals who carefully pack large amounts of illegal drugs into small, condom-wrapped packets or glass or plastic vials. The vials or packets are sealed and ingested by the carrier along with an antimotility agent. The individual then travels by plane or other vehicle to another location. Body packing is used to transport illegal drugs such as heroin or cocaine to other countries. The individual then defecates the vials or packets and delivers them to the recipient. The packets rarely rupture but can be life threatening if they do.
    - **Body stuffers,** on the other hand, are individuals who quickly ingest ("stuff") poorly wrapped illegal drugs while attempting to evade law enforcement. The wrapping containing the drug is usually referred to as a "baggie." Commonly, it is a much smaller amount of drug than body packers and is loosely wrapped. The drug is typically absorbed quickly, and the patient usually develops symptoms shortly after ingestion.

18. **How should body stuffers/packers be managed?**
For **body stuffers**, a conservative estimate of the time of ingestion should be used (i.e., time of arrival to the ED or transported by ambulance). Body stuffers should receive activated charcoal and be observed in a monitored setting for at least 8 hours. Radiographs are not helpful. If the patient develops symptoms, admission for continued monitoring in an intensive care setting should be initiated.

The packets from **body packers** can be seen on plain abdominal radiographs, radiographs with oral contrast material (Gastrografin), or abdominal CT. Body packers should receive activated charcoal and polyethylene glycol electrolyte solution (Colyte, GoLYTELY) to enhance elimination through the colon. Polyethylene glycol administered through a nasogastric tube at approximately 2 L/h until all packets have cleared. Clear rectal effluent is not a sufficient endpoint to end decontamination. Enemas may be used if the packets are in the distal colon or are felt on digital rectal examination. Occasionally, it may take days for all packets to evacuate. Surgery is rarely needed to remove retained packets. Radiologic testing, such as abdominal CT or radiograph with oral contrast, can be used to determine when all packets have cleared.

Keyes DC: Body packers stuffers. In Dart RC (ed): Medical Toxicology, 3rd ed. Philadelphia, Lippincott Williams & Wilkins, 2004, pp 59–62.
Nelson LS: Opioids. In Goldfrank LR, Flomenbaum NE, Lewin NA, et al (eds): Goldfrank's Toxicologic Emergencies, 7th ed. New York, McGraw-Hill, 2002, pp 901–923.

19. **How useful are toxicologic screens for opioids, and which opioids often are not detected?**
Toxicologic screens are generally not helpful or indicated in the acute management of patients. Opiate screens do not detect methadone or other synthetic opioids, such as fentanyl, pentazocine, meperidine, oxymorphone, oxycodone, and propoxyphene. Ingestion of poppy seeds does not commonly cause a positive screen because the lower limit threshold has been raised. However, with further testing, this erroneous cause of positive screens can be ruled out.

20. **Are there any other tests that should be checked with opioid ingestions?**
Acetaminophen levels should be checked in all patients with opioid ingestions because it is often combined with hydrocodone, oxycodone, propoxyphene, and codeine. A metabolic panel, salicylate level, and electrocardiogram should also be obtained. Serum or urine opioid toxicology screens are of no benefit in acute management and should not be obtained.

21. **What is the most common pulmonary complication of opioid use?**
Noncardiogenic pulmonary edema occurs in 3% of nonhospitalized opioid intoxications, and approximately 50% of all opioid abusers develop it once in their life. The mechanism is unclear, but is thought to be a result of capillary permeability and fluid leak. The patient presents with pink frothy sputum, cyanosis, and rales, and bilateral alveolar infiltrates are seen on the chest radiograph. Naloxone does not reverse the process, and many patients may need bilevel positive airway pressure (biPAP), continuous positive airway pressure (CPAP), or mechanical ventilation. Heroin, methadone, morphine, and propoxyphene have been associated with noncardiogenic pulmonary edema.

Kleinschmidt KC, Wainscott M, Ford MD: Opioids. In Ford M, Delaney KA, Ling LJ, et al (eds): Clinical Toxicology. Philadelphia, W.B. Saunders, 2001, pp 627–639.

22. **Can opioids cause seizures?**
Seizures are rare in therapeutic doses of opioids, but may be seen with an intoxication of the synthetic opioids—meperidine, tramadol, pentazocine, and propoxyphene.

23. **Is it appropriate to give dextromethorphan or meperidine to patients on antidepressant medications?**
No. These combinations of drugs may precipitate life-threatening serotonin syndrome. Meperidine and dextromethorphan, like many cyclic antidepressants and all selective serotonin reuptake inhibitors, inhibit serotonin reuptake.

24. **Which antidiarrheal agent can cause significant toxicity if ingested?**
Lomotil (diphenoxylate 2.5 mg + atropine 0.025 mg). Most overdoses occur in children. Classically, the overdose is a two-phase toxicity:
- Phase 1, anticholinergic symptoms (flushing, dry mouth)
- Phase 2, opioid effects
However, this pattern is uncommon. Delayed presentations have been reported, and all children should be observed in a monitored setting for at least 24 hours.
Loperamide is a nonprescription antidiarrheal agent derived from diphenoxylate. Acute overdoses usually produce only mild drowsiness. It can rarely cause coma, bradycardia, apnea, and miosis.

25. **Which opioid can produce ventricular arrhythmias, a wide QRS complex, mydriasis, and seizures?**
Propoxyphene has a quinidine-like effect that blocks sodium channels similar to cyclic antidepressants. Large doses of naloxone (10 mg) may reverse the CNS depression but not the cardiotoxic effects. Sodium bicarbonate has been used successfully for propoxyphene-induced arrhythmias. Propoxyphene has never been proved to be more effective for analgesia than salicylates, acetaminophen, or codeine.

26. **What are designer drugs? What are the two notorious designer drugs that have been used?**
Designer drugs are substitutes for other chemicals or drugs that are popular with illicit drug users. They are made inexpensively in "underground" laboratories. 3-Methylfentanyl is an analog of fentanyl known as *China white* or *Persian white*. It is 2000 times more potent than morphine and 20 times more potent than fentanyl. It can cause respiratory compromise quickly.

It does not cause the abbreviated "rush" of heroin but instead causes a longer euphoria. Various outbreaks in California, the East Coast, and more recently in Europe have been reported. MPTP (1-methyl-4-phenyl-1,2,5,6 tetrahydropyridine) is a compound that was produced accidentally during the synthesis of MPPP, a meperidine analog. MPTP is cytotoxic for dopaminergic neurons in the substantia nigra. It produces a Parkinson-like syndrome that is permanent and occurs after a single ingestion of MPTP. The symptoms do not respond to typical antiparkinsonism medications.

27. **What over-the-counter cold remedy is sometimes abused by teenagers?**
Dextromethorphan is the D-isomer of codeine. Its metabolite stimulates the release of serotonin and acts at the phencyclidine receptor site, which accounts for its abuse as a hallucinogen. It may present with symptoms of opioid toxicity but more commonly presents with slurred speech, nystagmus, hyperexcitability, and ataxia. Naloxone does not usually reverse the symptoms. Dextromethorphan does not cause false-positive results on urine toxicology screens for opioids, but it may for phencyclidine.

28. **Identify another analog of codeine.**
Tramadol (Ultram) is a synthetic analog of codeine. Overdoses have been associated with seizures, hypertension, respiratory depression, and agitation. The seizures do not respond to naloxone. Although the drug has a low abuse potential, it is not recommended for patients with a history of opioid dependence.

SEDATIVE-HYPNOTICS

29. **What is a sedative-hypnotic?**
Sedatives-hypnotics are drugs that primarily cause relaxation and tranquilization and induce drowsiness and sleep. There is no consistent structural relationship among the agents of this group. In sufficient quantities, all drugs of this group result in CNS depression.

30. **How do sedative-hypnotics cause CNS depression?**
Most sedative-hypnotics, particularly benzodiazepines and barbiturates, cause CNS depression through enhancing the effects of gamma-aminobutyric acid (GABA), an inhibitory neurotransmitter in the brain. Benzodiazepines increase the frequency of the opening of chloride channels associated with GABA. Propofol and barbiturates directly open the chloride channels, potentially causing greater sedation and respiratory suppression.

KEY POINTS: OPIOIDS AND SEDATIVE-HYPNOTICS

1. Sedative-hypnotic intoxication is a diagnosis that should not be made without appropriate measures to rule out other causes of central nervous system depression.

2. In patients with respiratory compromise secondary to opioid intoxication, patient resuscitation takes precedence over opioid antagonists such as naloxone.

3. Flumazenil is an antidote to benzodiazepine intoxication and has no role in the undifferentiated or mixed overdose.

4. The classic triad of opioid poisoning is central nervous system depression, respiratory depression, and miosis.

31. **What medications fall into this category?**
There are three groups: benzodiazepines, barbiturates, and miscellaneous. Some examples of miscellaneous sedative-hypnotics are chloral hydrate, ethanol, and gamma-hydroxy butyrate (GHB). Many of the miscellaneous agents are also pharmaceutical agents. For example, ethanol is used in treatment of methanol and ethylene glycol toxicity, and GHB (Xyrem) is used for narcolepsy.

32. **What is a typical presentation of sedative-hypnotic intoxication?**
Mild intoxication presents with slurred speech, ataxia, and loss of coordination (think of the last party you attended where ethanol was consumed). Moderate to severe intoxication presents with greater CNS depression. Respiratory depression may occur with large ingestions, and is compounded by other agents that suppress respiratory drive, such as opioids or ethanol. Pupils are usually midsize and reactive. Due to the variety of drugs within the class, there are also many symptoms specific to ingestion of individual drugs. Some examples are choral hydrate (pear odor), ethchlorvynol (pulmonary edema, vinyl odor), and glutethimide (anticholinergic effects) (Table 71-2).

TABLE 71-2. CLINICAL PRESENTATIONS OF LESS COMMON SEDATIVE-HYPNOTICS	
Chloral hydrate	Vomiting, ventricular dysrhythmias
Ethylchlorvynol	Vinyl-like odor on breath, prolonged coma, noncardiogenic pulmonary edema
Glutethimide	Cyclic coma, anticholinergic symptoms (tachycardia uncommon), thick secretions
Methaqualone	Hyperreflexia, clonus, muscle hyperactivity
Meprobamate/carisoprodol	Euphoria, concretions in stomach may be seen on radiographs

33. **Don't a lot of overdoses present this way?**
Many overdoses present with CNS depression. However, some intoxications also present with a pattern of symptoms known as a toxidrome (see Chapter 67). Signs of antipsychotic intoxication include sedation and are similar to sedative-hypnotics but also commonly include tachycardia, mild hypotension, and occasionally miosis. CNS depression is also a common presentation of illness other than intoxication. Maintain a broad differential while evaluating these patients for such illnesses as meningoencephalitis, intracranial hemorrhage, hypoglycemia, shock, and sepsis.

34. **How do I make the diagnosis of sedative-hypnotic overdose in a patient with undifferentiated CNS depression?**
See Chapter 67.

35. **Is there a role for drug screens or specific drug levels?**
Not really. Routine drug screens are often not helpful in acute patient management. Because the most important treatment in sedative-hypnotic intoxication is supportive care, recognizing the intoxication pattern is more helpful than toxicology testing.

36. **What is the treatment for sedative-hypnotic overdose?**
Rapid resuscitation is the initial treatment, focusing on the managing the patient's airway, assessing respiratory effort, evaluating circulation and perfusion, and examining for neurologic

deficits. After resuscitation has been completed, initiate gastrointestinal (GI) decontamination, and then exclude other causes for altered mentation, acid-base disturbances, or unstable hemodynamics. GI decontamination with activated charcoal within approximately 1 hour of ingestion should be performed.

37. **How do patients die of sedative-hypnotic overdose?**
Respiratory depression and resultant hypoxia with large ingestions or coingestions is the cause of most deaths.

38. **What is the appropriate way to decontaminate the GI tract?**
See Chapter 67.

39. **Are there specific antidotes for sedative-hypnotic intoxication?**
Flumazenil can be used for benzodiazepine and related medications such as zolpidem.

40. **How does flumazenil work?**
Benzodiazepines and zolpidem act as GABA-A receptor agonists. Flumazenil antagonizes the effects of these drugs by competitively inhibiting the GABA receptor. For a known, severely symptomatic benzodiazepine overdose, 0.2–0.5 mg of flumazenil may be given intravenously in increasing doses to a generally accepted maximum dose of 5 mg. If there is no response with 5 mg, consider another intoxication or coingestant.

41. **Should flumazenil be given empirically to all patients with depressed mental status?**
No. Flumazenil, which is very expensive, may be used for a patient with a pure benzodiazepine overdose causing significant CNS depression or to aid in making this diagnosis. It has no role in undifferentiated or mixed overdose because it can induce seizures and, rarely, life-threatening dysrhythmias. Flumazenil may also induce seizures and withdrawal symptoms in chronic benzodiazepine users. The onset of flumazenil is 1–5 minutes, and duration of effect is 1–4 hours. Sedation will resume after its effects have worn off. Most patients with a benzodiazepine overdose will do well with only supportive care and will not require flumazenil. Contraindications are listed in Table 71-3.

TABLE 71-3.   CONTRAINDICATIONS TO FLUMAZENIL
Prior seizure history
ECG evidence of cyclic antidepressants
Chronic benzodiazepine use
Abnormal vital signs including hypoxia
Coingestants that provoke seizures or dysrhythmias
ECG = electrocardiogram.

42. **What is Rohypnol?**
Flunitrazepam (Rohypnol) is an intermediate to long-acting benzodiazepine not available legally in the United States but is licensed in Europe, Asia, and Central America. It gained notoriety as a "date rape drug" in the late 1980s and early 1990s. Although similar in structure and effects to other benzodiazepines, flunitrazepam imparts greater amnesic and hypnotic effects over other benzodiazepine derivatives. Street names for this drug are *roshay, roofies,* and *roach.* It is not

detected in routine urine toxicology screens. Rohypnol use has decreased in the late 1990s and in 1998–2002 has represented a vanishingly small percentage of drug intoxications that present to EDs.

dawninfo.samhsa.gov

43. What is GHB?

It is an abbreviation for gamma-hydroxybutyrate, which is a naturally occurring human neurotransmitter similar in structure to GABA. GHB has been manufactured and used as a sleep aid, anesthetic, and muscle builder. It is sold on the Internet and abused for its mild sedating and euphoric effects. Although restricted by the Food and Drug Administration in the 1990s, GHB is available again (trade name: Xyrem) as a tightly controlled treatment for narcolepsy. However, it is easily synthesized; recipes and materials are widely available. Congeners, including gamma-butyrlactone and 1,4-butanediol, are metabolized to GHB and have the same effects and are common. After increased frequency of use from 1998 through 2000, presentations of GHB intoxication to EDs has remained relatively steady from 2000–2003.

dawninfo.samhsa.gov.

Lee DC: Sedative-hypnotic agents. In Goldfrank LR, Flomenbaum NE, Lewin NA, et al (eds): Goldfrank's Toxicologic Emergencies, 7th ed. New York, McGraw-Hill, 2002, pp 929–945.

44. How does a GHB overdose present?

Most ingestions of GHB are mild and produce minimal sedation and euphoria. Rarely, patients overdose on GHB and present to the ED with a decreased level of consciousness. In contrast to other sedative hypnotic intoxications, the level of consciousness tends to fluctuate between mild agitation and severe CNS depression. Airway reflexes are usually intact and often hypersensitive. An attempt at direct laryngoscopy may cause the patient to quickly sit up and be agitated for several minutes. Because the clinical effects of GHB usually last less than 6 hours, decisions about airway management should be based on their respiratory status and ability to monitor oxygenation closely in the ED. Although naloxone, flumazenil, and physostigmine have been described as reversal agents in GHB intoxication, no antidote has consistently been shown effective. Death from GHB intoxication is generally from respiratory failure.

Lee DC: Sedative-hypnotic agents. In Goldfrank LR, Flomenbaum NE, Lewin NA, et al (eds): Goldfrank's Toxicologic Emergencies, 7th ed. New York, McGraw-Hill, 2002, pp 929–945.
Snead OC, Gibson KM: Gamma hydroxybutyric acid. N Engl J Med. 352:2721–2736, 2005.

45. What are the effects of GHB withdrawal?

Recreational users of GHB manifest withdrawal symptoms of anxiety, insomnia, disorientation, tachycardia, hypertension, and visual and auditory hallucinations. GHB withdrawal is similar in presentation to benzodiazepine withdrawal, but with greater intensity.

46. How do zolpidem and benzodiazepine overdose differ?

Zolpidem (Ambien) acts similarly to benzodiazepines by binding at the alpha-1 subunit of the GABA-A receptor, and is useful as a sleep aid. Due to its specific affinity for the alpha-1 subunit, zolpidem has minimal muscle relaxant, anxiolytic, and anticonvulsant properties. Therefore, zolpidem intoxication presents with CNS depression, but respiratory depression is uncommon.

47. What is a "Mickey Finn?"

A "Mickey Finn" is a drug-laced drink named for a Mafia-associated bartender from Chicago in the 1920s. Specifically, it refers to a mixture of chloral hydrate and alcohol. Alcohol and chloral hydrate act to potentiate each other's effects, and prolong their duration of effect as they are metabolized via the same pathway. Mr. Finn would use the drink to induce his victims into unconsciousness and then relieve them of all their valuables.

Lee DC: Sedative-hypnotic agents. In Goldfrank LR, Flomenbaum NE, Lewin NA, et al (eds): Goldfrank's Toxicologic Emergencies, 7th ed. New York, McGraw-Hill, 2002, pp 929–945.

CHAPTER 72

MUSHROOMS, HALLUCINOGENS, AND STIMULANTS

Christina E. Hantsch, MD, and Donna L. Seger, MD

MUSHROOMS

1. **What are the symptoms and signs of mushroom poisoning?**
   Many mushrooms contain toxins that cause gastrointestinal (GI) manifestations including nausea, vomiting, and diarrhea. Certain species have toxins that are associated with more severe GI manifestations and/or other characteristic symptoms and signs. (See Table 72-1.)

TABLE 72-1. MANIFESTATIONS OF MUSHROOM POISONING		
Mushroom Species	**Toxin**	**Symptoms and Signs**
Amanita phalloides, *Galerina*	Amatoxins	Delayed onset GI manifestations, hepatic failure
Gyrometra	Monomethylhydrazine	Delayed onset GI manifestations, CNS manifestations, hemolysis
Psilocybe	Muscimol, psilocybin	Anticholinergic (including hallucinations and seizures)
Clitocybe	Muscarine-containing	Cholinergic
Coprinus	Coprine	Disulfiram-like reaction with ethanol

CNS = central nervous system, GI = gastrointestinal.

2. **Which mushrooms toxins cause the most concern?**
   Amatoxins, which are cyclopeptides found in *Amanita* and some *Galerina* species. The classic presentation of amatoxin poisoning includes an initial asymptomatic 6- to 12-hour period followed by GI symptoms. Severe hepatotoxicity becomes evident 24 hours to several days after the initial ingestion.

3. **Do symptoms within 6 hours rule out amatoxin ingestion?**
   No. Not all patients exhibit the classic presentation. In addition, mushroom ingestion often involves more than one species. The possibility of amatoxin ingestion needs to be considered in all cases.

4. **Will boiling mushrooms destroy their toxins?**
   Not always. Although some toxins are heat labile and can be deactivated by heating, amatoxin is not. Amatoxin is the most deadly mushroom toxin, and it is not destroyed by cooking.

5. **Does coingestion of ethanol change the effects of mushrooms?**
   Coprine-containing mushrooms, when consumed in combination with ethanol, cause tachycardia, flushing, nausea, and vomiting. This is the same type of reaction as produced by

disulfiram or metronidazole when combined with ethanol. Symptoms may occur when alcohol is consumed as late as 72 hours after mushroom ingestion. Coprine, similar to disulfiram and metronidazole, inhibits acetaldehyde dehydrogenase activity. Consequent accumulation of acetaldehyde causes the clinical manifestations.

6. **How do I treat someone who has ingested mushrooms?**
   Therapy is primarily supportive including volume resuscitation, seizure control, and treatment of agitation. Identify the mushroom species ingested, if possible, and monitor for delayed onset of symptoms when orellanine, amatoxin, or monomethylhydrazine are ingested. Specific antidote therapy is available for some mushroom toxins.

HALLUCINOGENS

7. **What are hallucinogens?**
   Typically, the term hallucinogen refers to agents that are used recreationally for their mind-altering effects. Many substances (including mushrooms and stimulants) can cause hallucinations, perceptions without any basis in reality, or alterations in the perception of reality.

8. **List some examples of hallucinogens.**
   - Dextromethorphan (DM)
   - *N,N*-Diisopropyl–5-methoxytryptamine (Foxy-Methoxy)
   - Lysergic acid diethylamide (LSD)
   - Marijuana
   - Mescaline
   - 3,4-Methylenedioxymethamphetamine (MDMA, Ecstasy)
   - 1-(1-Phenylcyclohexyl) piperidine (PCP)

9. **DM? Isn't that just cough medicine?**
   Yes, DM is a common ingredient in over-the-counter cough suppressant and cold medications. Therapeutic doses of DM, a synthetic analog of codeine, are generally safe and effective. However, supratherapeutic doses may produce hallucinogenic or dissociative effects. Not surprisingly, DM abuse has become increasingly popular, especially among teenagers. Pill forms, such as Coricidin HBP Cough and Cold (nicknamed "Triple C" due to three Cs on the red tablet) contain 30 mg of DM per pill. Coingredients may also cause clinical toxicity, such as decongestants (anticholinergic or sympathomimetic toxidrome) and acetaminophen (hepatic toxicity.) Pharmacies in many states have placed DM-containing products behind the counter so that patients must sign their name to obtain the product.

   Kirages T, Sule Harsh, Mycyk M: Severe manifestations of Coricidin intoxication. Am J Emerg Med 21: 473–475, 2003.

10. **Name the life-threatening effects of hallucinogens.**
    Seizures, hyperthermia, metabolic acidosis, hypertension, and arrhythmias. Rhabdomyolysis can develop subsequently. The effects of hallucinogens are unpredictable and different with each use. Trauma frequently occurs as a result of the disinhibition and aggressiveness caused by hallucinogen abuse.

11. **Why would you "lick a toad"?**
    Hallucinations are produced by bufotenine, the substance in the skin secretions of Bufo (*Bufo vulgaris, Bufo marinus*) toads. Bufotenine and many other natural toxins have been used for years for hallucinogenic effects. Mescaline is the toxin in peyote, a cactus found in the southwestern United States and Mexico. Psilocybin (4-phosphoryloxy-*N,N*-dimethyltryptamine) is found in some species of mushrooms; *N,N*-dimethyltryptamine (DMT) is in many plants and

seeds. Natural agents (such as these) and their synthetic derivatives are used for hallucinogenic purposes.

12. What is the treatment of hallucinogen toxicity?

Reassurance, a calm environment, and avoidance of further trauma in addition to good supportive care all are important. A benzodiazepine may be given (at times in large doses) to calm agitated patients or to treat seizures. Haloperidol may be considered for patients experiencing primarily the mind-altering effects of hallucinogens. Occasionally, physical restraint, in addition to chemical restraint, may be necessary to protect the patient or staff from harm in cases of severe agitation.

STIMULANTS

13. How should one screen for cocaine?

Cocaine is metabolized rapidly, and detection of the parent compound in blood indicates recent use. The elimination half-life of cocaine after intravenous administration is 45–90 minutes. Cocaine undergoes nonenzymatic degradation to benzoylecgonine and ecgonine methyl ester. These substances are excreted renally and may be present in the urine for several days after the initial exposure. Routine urine drug screens are positive for degradation products of cocaine.

14. What are "free-base" and "crack" cocaine?

Cocaine usually arrives in the United States as a white powder, cocaine hydrochloride (CHCI). This powder is highly water soluble and therefore crosses mucous membranes and intestinal mucosa very quickly. Vaporization requires very high temperatures, so the powder is not suitable for smoking. The powder can be dissolved with sodium bicarbonate (baking soda) or ammonia and water. This solution may subsequently be treated with diethyl ether, decanted, and dried to form "freebase"; or it can be boiled, ice added to reduce the temperature, and dried to form "crack" (so called due to the popping sound that occurs during heating). Freebase and crack are resistant to pyrolysis and can be smoked.

KEY POINTS: MUSHROOMS, HALLUCINOGENS, AND STIMULANTS

1. Mushrooms of the *Amanita* species are associated with delayed onset fulminant hepatic failure produced by amatoxin.

2. Simultaneous cocaine and ethanol use depresses myocardial contractility.

3. Hyperthermia caused by Ecstasy is associated with increased lethality.

4. Cough syrups containing dextromethorphan are popular drugs of abuse.

15. What is the significance of chest pain after use of cocaine?

Pneumothorax or pneumomediastinum may occur after a Valsalva maneuver when cocaine has been smoked. Myocardial infarction has followed intranasal, intravenous, and smoked cocaine, even in young patients with normal coronary arteries. Benzodiazepine is the initial treatment of choice for cocaine-induced chest pain of cardiac origin.

Lange RA, Hillis LD: Cardiovascular complications of cocaine use. N Engl J Med 345:351–358, 2001.

16. **Does coingestion of ethanol change the effects of cocaine?**
Yes. In the presence of ethanol, cocaine is metabolized to cocaethylene, a metabolite that retains the pharmacologic and toxicologic properties of cocaine. Cocaine and ethanol cause synergistic depression of ventricular contraction and relaxation which is greater than the arithmetic sum of the two drugs alone. Simultaneous ethanol ingestion and intranasal cocaine increase peak plasma concentration of cocaine by 20%, compared with intranasal cocaine alone. The increased cocaine concentration is associated with increased euphoria, compared to use of cocaine alone.

Farre M, de la Torre R, Gonzalez ML, et al: Cocaine and alcohol interactions in humans, neuroendocrine effects and cocaethylene metabolism. J Pharmacol Exp Ther 283:164–167, 1997.

17. **What is "Ice"?**
Ice is the smokable form of methamphetamine, named for its appearance of transparent crystals. In contrast to cocaine HCl, this pure base form of methamphetamine HCl evaporates easily at room temperature and is absorbed rapidly from the lungs. Similar to intravenous methamphetamine, it causes immediate euphoric effect but without the risks of intravenous drug administration. The clinical manifestations of methamphetamine are secondary to heightened catecholamine activity and are the same, regardless of the route of administration. Potential adverse effects include hypertension, arrhythmias, intracranial hemorrhage, seizures, and hyperthermia.

Beebe DK, Walley E: Smokable methamphetamine ("Ice"): An old drug in a different form. Am Fam Physician 51:449–453, 1995.

18. **What about Adam and Eve?**
Adam, Ecstasy, E, and XTC are street names for 3,4-methylenedioxymethamphetamine (MDMA). Eve is a street name for MDEA. Originally "designer drugs" and therefore not subject to legalities as they were not scheduled, all designer drugs are now scheduled as analogs and are illegal. Potent releasers of serotonin, and to a lesser extent dopamine, the exact mechanism of action of these agents is not known. MDMA causes long-term neurotoxic damage in brains of experimental animals. Overdose of MDMA or MDEA, both phenylethylamines, clinically resembles amphetamine toxicity. Hyperthermia (caused by the drug, and hot, crowded conditions at the raves [dances]) and seizures are associated with lethality. In addition, Ecstasy use has been associated with severe hyponatremia related to increased water intake during raves and/or increased secretion of antidiuretic hormone. Ecstasy and other designer drugs are not detected on routine urine drug screens.

19. **How should I treat someone with toxicity from stimulants?**
Agitation or seizures can be treated with a benzodiazepine. Large doses may be required. Hyperthermia should be aggressively treated with mechanical cooling measures ("wet and windy"). Hypertension from stimulant toxicity is usually short lived; however, a true hypertensive emergency can be treated with nitroprusside and benzodiazepine. Nitroglycerin and other cardiac interventions may be used in patients with ischemic chest pain from vasoconstriction or myocardial infarction. Beta blockers, such as propranolol, should be avoided because they may potentiate alpha effects and cause coronary artery vasoconstriction.

WEBSITE

United States Drug Enforcement: www.dea.gov

BIBLIOGRAPHY

1. Babu K, Boyer EW, Hernon C, Brush DE: Emerging drugs of abuse. Clin Pediatr Emerg Med 6:81–84, 2005.
2. Diaz J: Evolving global epidemiology, syndromic classification, general management, and prevention of unknown mushroom poisonings. Crit Care Med 33:419–426, 2005.
3. Diaz J: Syndromic diagnosis and management of confirmed mushroom poisonings. Crit Care Med 33:427–436, 2005.
4. Ernst T, Chang L, Leonido-Yee M, Speck D: Evidence for long-term neurotoxicity associated with methamphetamine abuse. Am Acad Neurol 54:1344–1349, 2000.
5. Henning RJ, Wilson LD, Glauser JM: Cocaine plus ethanol is more cardiotoxic than cocaine or ethanol alone. Crit Care Med 22:1896–1906, 1994.
6. Milroy CM: Ten years of ecstasy. J R Soc Med 92:68–72, 1999.

CHAPTER 73

ANTIDEPRESSANTS: CYCLICS AND NEWER AGENTS

Norberto Adame, Jr, MD, and Russ Braun, MD, MPH, MBA

1. **How are antidepressants classified?**

   Antidepressants can be divided into three broad categories that include tricyclic antidepressants (TCAs), monoamine oxidase inhibitors (MAOIs), and newer agents often referred to as atypical, heterocyclic, or second-generation antidepressants.

   Mills KC: Newer antidepressants serotonin syndrome. In Tintinalli JE, Kelen GD, Stapczynski JS (eds): Emergency Medicine: A Comprehensive Study Guide, 6th ed. New York, McGraw-Hill, 2004, pp 1033–1039.

2. **Describe the mechanism of action for each antidepressant drug group.**

   - **TCAs** are classified as secondary or tertiary amines and contain a side chain with a varied number of methyl groups. They inhibit reuptake of neurotransmitters and antagonize postsynaptic serotonin receptors.
   - **MAOIs** block the intracellular, mitochondrial enzyme monoamine oxidase, which normally deaminates biogenic amines, such as epinephrine, norepinephrine (NE), serotonin, and dopamine (DA).
   - The **atypicals** are structurally diverse, but all have the common ability to inhibit presynaptic reuptake of serotonin. Many have additional actions, such as inhibition of DA or NE reuptake and serotonin or alpha-adrenergic blockade.

     For a more detailed summary, see Table 73-1.

   Mills KC: Newer antidepressants serotonin syndrome. In Tintinalli JE, Kelen GD, Stapczynski JS (eds): Emergency Medicine: A Comprehensive Study Guide, 6th ed. New York, McGraw-Hill, 2004, pp 1033–1039.

TABLE 73-1. MECHANISM OF ACTION OF ANTIDEPRESSANTS		
Group	**Mechanism of Action**	**Examples**
Tricyclic	Blocks reuptake of NE	Amitriptyline (Elavil)
Tertiary amine		Doxepin (Sinequan)
Secondary amine		Nortriptyline (Pamelor, Aventyl)
		Amoxapine (Ascendin), protriptyline (Vivactil)
		Desipramine (Norpramin)
Tetracyclic		Maprotiline (Ludiomil)
Dibenzoxazepine		Amoxapine (Ascendin)
Selective serotonin reuptake inhibitors (SSRIs)	Block reuptake of serotonin	Fluoxetine (Prozac), citalopram (Celexa)
		Sertraline (Zoloft), escitalopram (Lexapro)

Continued

TABLE 73-1. MECHANISM OF ACTION OF ANTIDEPRESSANTS—CONT'D		
Group	**Mechanism of Action**	**Examples**

Triazolopyridine
Monocyclic
Monoamine oxidase
    inhibitors (MAOIs)
	Serotonin receptor antagonist
	Blocks reuptake of DA
	Increases CNS NE and
	    DA levels
		Paroxetine (Paxil),
		    fluvoxamine (Luvox)
		Trazodone (Desyrel)
		Bupropion (Wellbutrin)
		Phenelzine (Nardil)
		Tranylcypromine (Parnate),
		    moclobemide
		    (Manerix), isocarboxazid
		    (Marplan)

CNS = central nervous system, DA = dopamine, NE = norepinephrine.

3. **What are the epidemiologic characteristics associated with antidepressant overdoses?**
   Based on the Annual Report of the American Association of Poison Control Centers, the third most common class of drugs associated with fatalities was antidepressants, accounting for 274 deaths. Amitriptyline, either alone or in combination, is the single most commonly implicated agent. There were 101,331 total antidepressant medication exposures, of which 70,253 were treated in a health care facility. The newer antidepressant agents continue to result in numerous deaths.

   Watson AW, Litovitz TL, Klein-Schwartz W, et al: 2003 Annual Report of the American Association of Poison Control Centers Toxic Exposure Surveillance System. Am J Emerg Med 22:335–404, 2003.

4. **Compare the features of the selective serotonin reuptake inhibitors (SSRI) versus TCAs.**
   The SSRIs have fewer side effects, less toxicity, and a larger safety margin. The newer agents have little affinity for DA, gamma-aminobutyric acid, acetylcholine, and alpha-adrenergic receptors; and as a result, there are fewer side effects. Atypicals have little action on cardiac sodium, potassium, and calcium channels and avoid much of the cardiotoxicity. In contrast to MAOIs, SSRIs pose no risk of tyramine-like reactions, and there is no contraindication to the use of indirect sympathomimetics.

   Klein-Schwartz W, Anderson B: Analysis of sertraline-only overdoses. Am J Emerg Med 14:456–458, 1996.

5. **Describe the major side effects of SSRIs.**
   Nausea, diarrhea, headache, agitation, and panic attacks. Long-term use can lead to weight gain.

   Khawaja IS, Feinstein RE: Cardiovascular effects of selective serotonin reuptake inhibitors and other novel antidepressants. Heart Dis 5:153–160, 2003.

6. **What is the serotonin syndrome?**
   The serotonin syndrome is a constellation of signs and symptoms manifesting as altered mental status, autonomic dysfunction (diaphoresis, fever, shivering, diarrhea), and neuromuscular hyperactivity (myoclonus, hyperreflexia, ataxia). Agents reported to cause serotonin syndrome when used in combination includes MAOIs, TCAs, SSRIs, meperidine (Demerol), dextromethorphan, and tryptophan.

   Sporer KA: The serotonin syndrome. Drug Safe 13:94–104, 1995.

7. **What is the treatment of serotonin syndrome?**

Supportive care and early recognition in the emergency department (ED) are paramount. Include cardiac monitoring and laboratory testing for suspected polydrug ingestion. Benzodiazepines are recommended for symptomatic treatment, and they may have a protective role as a result of their inhibitory effects on serotoninergic transmission. Fever may be controlled with acetaminophen and external cooling measures. Cyproheptadine, a first-generation histamine-1 receptor blocker with nonspecific antagonism of serotonin receptors, is recommended for use as treatment of serotoninergic symptoms. Dantrolene should be reserved for use in neuromalignant hyperthermia.

Mills KC: Newer antidepressants serotonin syndrome. In Tintinalli JE, Kelen GD, Stapczynski JS (eds): Emergency Medicine: A Comprehensive Study Guide, 6th ed. New York, McGraw-Hill, 2004, pp 1033–1039.

8. **Describe your approach to a well-appearing patient with a reported history of TCA ingestion.**

A trivial appearing TCA overdose patient may collapse very rapidly. Patients who present with this history should never be allowed to wait for care. In one study, 50% of the patients presenting to the hospital with a history of TCA overdose demonstrated catastrophic deterioration. These patients presented initially with trivial or no signs of poisoning but went on to develop major signs of toxicity within an hour or less.

Callaham M, Kassel D: Epidemiology of fatal tricyclic antidepressant ingestion: Implications for management. Ann Emerg Med 14:29–37,1985.

9. **Name the four mechanisms of TCA toxicity.**

- **Anticholinergic:** The anticholinergic effects of TCA ingestions include supraventricular tachycardia, hallucinations, seizures, and hyperthermia.
- **Quinidine-like:** The quinidine-like effects, manifested by decreased cardiac contractility, hypotension, and ventricular arrhythmias, are characteristic of all type 1a antiarrhythmics (e.g., quinidine, procainamide, and disopyramide).
- **Alpha-adrenergic blockade:** Peripheral-receptor blockade may lead to hypotension.
- **Antihistamine:** Some TCAs (doxepin) are more potent than many of the newer histamine H_1 antagonists. These agents can cause sedation and coma.

Elliott R: Pharmacology of antidepressants. Mayo Clin Proc 76:511–527, 2001.

10. **Summarize the clinical presentations of TCA overdose.**

See Table 73-2.

11. **What is the anticholinergic syndrome?**

Hyperthermia, blurred vision, dry mouth, skin flushing, hallucinations, and tachycardia. These effects may be summarized by the phrase "Hot as a hare, blind as a bat, dry as a bone, red as a beet, and mad as a hatter." Other substances that can cause anticholinergic symptoms are antihistamines, phenothiazines, scopolamine, belladonna, jimsonweed, nightshade, and *Amanita muscaria* mushrooms.

Weisman RS, Goldfrank LR: Goldfrank's Toxicologic Emergencies, 5th ed. 1994, pp 605–606.

12. **What are the Antidepressant Overdose Risk Assessment criteria?**

Multiple studies have used the Antidepressant Overdose Risk Assessment (ADORA) criteria to determine probable outcome. These criteria include QRS interval greater than 0.10 second, arrhythmias, altered mental status, seizures, respiratory depression, and hypotension. Patients are classified as low risk (absence of criteria) or high risk (presence of one of the criteria), based on development of signs or symptoms within 6 hours. One study showed 100% sensitivity in identifying patients who developed significant toxicity problems. If (anticholinergic) signs or

TABLE 73-2.   CLINICAL PRESENTATION OF TCA OVERDOSE

	Cardiovascular	CNS	Anticholinergic
Symptoms	Dizziness	Confusion	Blurred vision
			Dry mouth
Signs	Tachycardia	Delirium	Mydriasis
	Conduction blocks	Agitation	Decreased bowel sounds
	QRS widening	Hyperreflexia	Urinary retention
	Hypotension	Myoclonus	Hyperthermia
	Arrhythmias	Seizures	Hypothermia
	Cardiac arrest	Sedation Coma	

CNS = central nervous system, TCA = tricyclic antidepressant.

symptoms have resolved by 6 hours, patients may be medically cleared for psychiatric evaluation.

Foulke GE: Identifying toxicity risk early after antidepressant overdose. Am J Emerg Med 13:123–126, 1995.

13. **What is the general approach to management of antidepressant overdoses?**
Patient stabilization after an acute ingestion is paramount, including management of the ABCs (airway, breathing, and circulation). Be cautious during stabilization and gastrointestinal decontamination because patients can lose consciousness rapidly, placing them at risk for aspiration. Endotracheal intubation should be considered before gastric emptying in patients with a decreased (or rapidly changing) level of consciousness. As a general guideline, gastric emptying should be performed if TCA ingestion occurred within 1 hour or less prior to arrival to the ED. Single-dose activated charcoal is recommended for gastric decontamination. These patients require constant cardiac monitoring with intravenous access.

Bosse GM, Barefoot JA, Pfeifer MP, Rodgers GC: Comparison of three methods of gut decontamination in tricyclic antidepressant overdose. J Emerg Med 13:203–209, 1995.

KEY POINTS: MOST COMMON CONSIDERATIONS FOR ANTIDEPRESSANT OVERDOSE

1. Consider an acute ingestion a polydrug ingestion until proven otherwise.

2. Alcohol is a common coingestant in acute overdoses.

3. Gastric lavage is rarely indicated; activated charcoal should be administered.

4. Cardiovascular events (dysrhythmias and hypotension) remain the leading cause of fatal outcomes from TCA overdose.

5. Consider serotonin syndrome early in the management of patients taking SSRIs.

14. **What diagnostic testing is helpful with an antidepressant overdose?**

An electrocardiogram (ECG) is essential in the evaluation of a patient with TCA overdose. Any prolongation of the ECG intervals should be considered a sign of TCA cardiotoxicity. Because of the potential for polydrug ingestions with any overdose, you need to consider other toxins. Testing for acetaminophen and aspirin (or anion gap) levels is recommended. A full urine and serum toxicology screen generally is not indicated because of low yield and cost ineffectiveness. Results of toxicology screens are often delayed and rarely change patient management.

Harrigan RA, Brady WJ: ECG abnormalities in tricyclic antidepressant ingestion. Am J Emerg Med 17:387–393, 1999.

15. **TCA toxic changes seen on ECG are primarily the result of what mechanism? What are the ECG changes?**

TCA toxic changes seen on the ECG are due primarily to the myocardial sodium channel blockade. The majority of patients at risk for seizures and arrhythmias will have a QRS complex greater than 0.10 seconds and a rightward shift of the terminal 40 ms in lead aVR.

Harrigan RA, Brady WJ: ECG abnormalities in tricyclic antidepressant ingestion. Am J Emerg Med 17:387–393, 1999.

16. **Summarize the treatment recommendations for cardiovascular system toxicity resulting in dysrhythmias.**

Sodium bicarbonate is the drug of choice for treatment of ventricular tachycardias. The mechanism of action of sodium bicarbonate is thought to be the result of increased sodium conductance through myocardial fast sodium channels and of increased plasma protein binding of TCAs. The dose of bicarbonate is 1–2 mEq/kg and may be repeated to maintain an arterial pH of 7.5. Alkalinization may be maintained through administration of repeated bicarbonate boluses or constant intravenous infusion of sodium bicarbonate added to maintenance fluids. Hypertonic saline and hyperventilation are useful as an adjunctive measure to increase plasma pH.

Burkhart KK: Cyclic antidepressants. In Wolfson AB (Editor-in-Chief): Harwood-Nuss' Clinical Practice of Emergency Medicine, 4th ed. Philadelphia, Lippincott Williams & Wilkins, 2005, pp 1619–1622.

17. **What do I need to know about the pharmacologic treatment of cardiac aryhthmias from TCA overdose?**

Group 1a antiarrhythmics (quinidine, procainamide, and beta blockers) are contraindicated because of their synergistic effects on cell membranes, which enhance antidepressant toxicity. Physostigmine is contraindicated for the treatment of ventricular arrhythmias. Lidocaine is effective for ventricular tachycardia but may decrease cardiac contractility. Phenytoin has been used in first-degree atrioventricular block and intraventricular conduction defects; however, it also has been found by some authors to increase the frequency and duration of ventricular tachycardia. Sinus tachycardia and supraventricular arrhythmias usually do not require any specific treatment beyond supportive care.

Burkhart KK: Cyclic antidepressants. In Wolfson AB (Editor-in-Chief): Harwood-Nuss' Clinical Practice of Emergency Medicine, 4th ed. Philadelphia, Lippincott Williams & Wilkins, 2005, pp 1619–1622.

18. **Describe the management of hypotension associated with cardiovascular toxicity from a TCA overdose.**

Hypotension should be treated initially with intravenous crystalloid boluses up to 20 mL/kg. Vasopressors such as DA and NE may be used. DA may lose some of its effects when epinephrine stores have been depleted in TCA overdoses. Infusion rates should be initiated at dose equal to or greater than 10 μg/kg/min. The lower doses have more beta-adrenergic effects and could worsen the hypotension. NE infusion rates of 1 μg/kg/min have been used successfully when the blood pressure response to DA has been inadequate.

Burkhart KK: Cyclic antidepressants. In Wolfson AB (Editor-in-Chief): Harwood-Nuss' Clinical Practice of Emergency Medicine, 4th ed. Philadelphia, Lippincott Williams & Wilkins, 2005, pp 1619–1622.

19. **How have the newer antidepressant agents helped in the management of clinical depression?**

The newer antidepressants such as fluoxetine (Prozac), citalopram (Celexa), venlafaxine (Effexor), mirtazapine (Remeron), and nefazodone (Serzone) can be used with very little risk of significant cardiovascular and central nervous system (CNS) complications from intentional overdose. The main features reported after an intentional ingestion include sinus tachycardia and drowsiness. Patients may still develop QRS and QTc prolongation, but the risk of developing cardiac arrhythmias is rare.

Kelly CA, Laing WJ, Strachan FE, et al: Comparative toxicity of citalopram and the newer antidepressants after overdose. J Toxicol Clin Toxicol. 42:67–71, 2004.

20. **What other information regarding the overdose of antidepressants is important for expectant management?**

The history or evidence of coingestions should make one very cautious in the management of these patients. Coingestants frequently involve other medications along with alcohol. This clinical scenario makes the possibility of developing fatal cardiac arrhythmias, coma, and death more likely.

Phillips S, Brent J, Kulig K, et al: The Antidepressant Study Group: Fluoxetine versus tricyclic antidepressants: A prospective multicenter study of antidepressant drug overdoses. J Emerg Med 15:439–445, 1997.

BIBLIOGRAPHY

1. Burkhart KK: Cyclic antidepressants. In Wolfson AB (editor-in-chief): Harwood-Nuss' Clinical Practice of Emergency Medicine, 4th ed. Philadelphia, Lippincott Williams & Wilkins, 2005, pp 1619–1622.

CHAPTER 74

HYDROCARBON AND CORROSIVES POISONING

Louis J. Ling, MD, and Stacey Bangh, PharmD

HYDROCARBONS

1. **What are hydrocarbons, anyway?**

   Hydrocarbons are distillation products of crude oil. Although all petroleum distillates are hydrocarbons, all hydrocarbons are not derived from petroleum. Hydrocarbons are classified as follows:
   - **Aliphatic,** which are straight or branched-chain carbon links that are fully or incompletely saturated to hydrogen atoms
   - **Aromatic,** which contain cyclic benzene rings and smell really good
   - **Halogenated,** in which hydrogen atoms have been substituted with halide anions (Br, Cl, F, or I)

2. **What is the biggest danger with hydrocarbon ingestion?**

   The primary concern is aspiration, which may lead to a **chemical pneumonitis.** Swallowing a hydrocarbon may produce gagging and influx of the agent into the trachea, producing acute inflammation, hemorrhage, edema, and loss of surfactant activity. Gastrointestinal (GI) absorption of hydrocarbons plays a minimal role in the development of toxicity.

3. **Which hydrocarbons are most likely to be aspirated?**

   Those with low viscosity and high volatility:
   - **Viscosity** (the ability to spread out) is the property that most increases the risk of aspiration. The viscosity of a hydrocarbon is measured by the time it takes to flow a specified distance through a calibrated diameter, measured in Sabolt seconds universal (SSU) units. Low-viscosity agents (<60 SSU) have less resistance to flow and easily spread over the epiglottis and into the larynx (Table 74-1).
   - **Volatility** refers to the tendency of a liquid to become a gas. Vapors released from highly volatile hydrocarbons (primarily aromatics and those with low molecular weight) displace oxygen and result in hypoxia, especially in enclosed spaces.

4. **What are the signs and symptoms of hydrocarbon poisoning?**

   The severity of symptoms depends on the degree of pulmonary aspiration. Patients may have immediate paroxysmal coughing in an effort to clear the airway. Nausea, emesis, and variable degrees of respiratory distress may occur. Physical signs may be absent initially, yet progress to cyanosis, mottling of the skin, tachycardia, tachypnea, stridor, salivation, grunting, nasal flaring, retractions, hemoptysis, fever, rales, or wheezing. Symptoms may resolve or progress rapidly to significant respiratory distress. Hypoxia may lead to central nervous system (CNS) excitation (hallucinations, agitation, confusion) or CNS depression (lethargy, coma). Poison centers report 1 death in about every 2000 cases.

5. **What types of x-ray changes are seen?**

   Initial chest radiographs may be normal in 60% of patients who later develop symptomatic pulmonary disease. Abnormalities may present within 30 minutes of aspiration and include perihilar densities, extension of interstitial infiltrate, lobar consolidation, linear/basilar

TABLE 74-1. LOW VISCOCITY (EASILY ASPIRATED) VS. HIGH VISCOCITY (NOT EASILY ASPIRATED) HYDROCARBONS

Low Viscocity Hydrocarbons (< 60 SSU)	High Viscocity Hydrocarbons (>100 SSU)
Lamp oil	Wax
Mineral spirits	Paraffins
Kerosene	Jellies
Liquid furniture polish	Greases
Turpentine	Lubricating oils
Naptha	
Gasoline	
Aromatics	

atelectasis, early alveolar infiltrate, and lobar atelectasis. Early (6–8 hours) abnormalities may lead to further progression. Pleural effusions, pneumothorax, pneumomediastinum, pneumopericardium, and pneumatoceles may develop.

6. **How long should a patient with hydrocarbon ingestion be monitored before discharge from the emergency department (ED)?**
Patients who remain asymptomatic, maintain normal oxygen saturations, and have a normal chest x-ray at 6 hours may be discharged, provided that adequate follow-up can be ensured. A 24-hour follow-up for discharged patients should be arranged.

   Klein BL, Simon JE: Hydrocarbon poisonings. Pediatr Clin North Am 33:411–419, 1986.

7. **Which patients should be admitted?**
Symptomatic patients (respiratory, CNS, and GI symptoms mentioned earlier), patients who develop abnormalities on chest radiograph in the first 6–8 hours, or patients who develop desaturation or hypoxemia within 6–8 hours should be admitted. Other reasons for admission may include suicidal intent or ingestion of a hydrocarbon with unique systemic toxicity (i.e., pesticides or carbon tetrachloride).

   Anas N, Namasonthi V, Ginsburg CM: Criteria for hospitalizing children who have ingested products containing hydrocarbons. JAMA 246:840–843, 1981.

8. **Are there any other concerns with hydrocarbon ingestions?**
Hydrocarbons should be assessed for the presence of **CHAMP** additives that may induce additional toxicity:
   - **C** = **C**amphor
   - **H** = **H**alogenated (10 mL of CCl_4 may lead to acute hepatic failure)
   - **A** = **A**romatics
   - **M** = **M**etals
   - **P** = **P**esticides

   Toxic effects may include CNS depression or excitation, bone marrow suppression, hepatic or renal toxicity, and cardiac arrhythmias. Specific hydrocarbons may have unique toxicities requiring antidotal administration (e.g., nitrobenzene leading to methemoglobinemia; methylene blue antidote). Hydrocarbons, when coupled with heavy metals (i.e., lead), may produce heavy metal intoxication. Toxicologic consultation can be obtained to help manage such complicated agents.

9. **How are hydrocarbons abused?**

Hydrocarbons may be poured into a container for **sniffing**, sprayed into a plastic or paper bag for **"bagging,"** or soaked onto a rag for **"huffing."** Inhaled vapors have a rapid onset of action and are well absorbed through the lungs with rapid distribution into the CNS. (*See* Table 74-2.)

Kurtzman T, Otsuka K, Wahl R: Inhalation abuse by adolescents. J Adolesc Health 28:179–180, 2001.

TABLE 74-2. COMMONLY ABUSED HYDROCARBON-CONTAINING PRODUCTS	
Common Sources	**Chemical Ingredients**
Spray paint	Toluene, butane, propane
Gasoline	Benzene, aliphatic and aromatic hydrocarbons
Cigarette lighter fluid	Butane, isopropane
Hair spray, deodorants, room fresheners	Butane, propane
Paint strippers	Methylene chloride
Model glues, rubber cement	*n*-Hexane, toluene, benzene
Varnishes, lacquers, resins	Benzene
Spot remover, typewriter correction fluid	Trichloroethane, trichloroethylene, carbon tetrachloride
Wood glues, lacquer thinner	Xylene

10. **Why do spray paint abusers prefer metallic colored paint?**

The toluene content is higher in metallic-color paints such as gold, copper, and silver.

11. **What are signs and symptoms of hydrocarbon abuse?**

Hydrocarbons may "sensitize" the myocardium to catecholamines, leading to an increased risk of dysrhythmia, especially with sudden exertion (such as running from the police) and augmented by the substance-associated hypoxia. This is known as sudden sniffing death. After acute abuse of hydrocarbons, respiratory irritation, salivation, and erythema may be seen. Slurred speech, diplopia, ataxia, disorientation, and hallucinations occur with larger doses. This may progress to severe CNS depression, coma, seizure, or death. Chronic abuse can lead to cognitive impairment, personality changes, depression, anxiety, and renal and hepatic damage.

Flanagan RJ, Ruprah M, Meredith TJ, et al: An introduction to the clinical toxicology of volatile substances. Drug Safety 5:359–383, 1990.

12. **Is there any special treatment for hydrocarbon abusers?**

Avoiding stimulation of these patients is important. Benzodiazepines should be used for agitation or hallucinations. Avoid catecholamines because they may exacerbate the cardiotoxicity of inhaled hydrocarbons.

KEY POINTS: HYDROCARBONS

1. Aspiration is the biggest danger after ingestion.

2. Patients with ingestions can be observed for 6 hours and discharged if asymptomatic.

3. Exertion can precipitate sudden cardiac death with hydrocarbon inhalant abuse.

CORROSIVES

13. **Which agents are classified as corrosives and can cause injury?**
    - **Alkali** are bases that release hydroxide ions on dissociation in water and are more frequently the reported causes of corrosive burns.
    - **Acids** liberate hydronium ions with water contact. The alkaline and acidic materials may be in either liquid or solid form. The severity of tissue injury from acids and alkali is determined by the substance's pH or pKa, concentration, duration of contact, and volume of contact. A pH less than 2.0 or greater than 12.5 indicates potential for severe tissue damage.
    - **Strong oxidizing agents** such as silver nitrate can also cause corrosive injury.
      See Table 74-3 for a more detailed list.

TABLE 74-3. COMMON ACID- AND ALKALI-CONTAINING PRODUCTS	
Type of Corrosive	**Products**
Acids	Toilet bowel cleaners
	Drain cleaners
	Metal cleaners
	Pool cleaners
	Fingernail primer
	Car battery fluid
	Rust-proofing
Alkali	Household cleaners
	Hair relaxers
	Ammonia
	Bleach
	Drain cleaners
	Oven cleaners
	Dishwasher detergent
	Clinitest tablets
	Cement
Oxidizing agents	Bleach
	Peroxides
	Sanitizing agents
	Corrosion inhibitors
Hydrofluoric acid	Rust removers
	Tire cleaners
	Glass etching

14. **What injuries are caused by ingestion of alkali?**
    Alkali produce **liquefaction necrosis**, with destruction of protein and collagen, tissue dehydration, saponification of fat, and blood vessel thrombosis. Injury is most frequently in the oropharynx and esophagus (Fig. 74-1). Perforation and infection are early causes of morbidity and mortality. Stricture with altered motility is a late complication.

15. **How are injuries classified?**
The injuries are classified by endoscopists according to the degree of penetration:
- **First-degree burns:** Superficial erythema, edema
- **Second-degree burns:** Erythema, blistering, superficial ulceration, fibrinous exudate
- **Third-degree burns:** Deep ulceration, friability, eschar formation, perforation

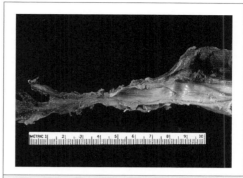

Figure 74-1. Esophagus after ingestion of 35% potassium hydroxide.

16. **What injuries are caused by ingestion of acids?**
Acids produce **coagulation necrosis,** with damage to the columnar epithelium, submucosa, and muscularis mucosa. The injury is covered by a coagulum consisting of damaged tissue and thrombosed blood vessels. In mild-to-moderate cases, this eschar blocks further penetration of acid and protects the deeper muscular layers. This facilitates passage of acid further down the GI tract with frequent involvement of the stomach and occasionally the proximal small intestine. In severe cases, full-thickness injuries with perforation can occur.

17. **Are injuries produced by alkaline caustic agents limited to the esophagus?**
No. Crystal or solid formulations (i.e., drain cleaner) adhere to the mucous membranes, making it difficult to swallow and limiting the injury to the esophagus. Liquid formulations are easily swallowed and are more likely to damage the esophagus and stomach.

Gumaste VV, Dave BP: Ingestion of corrosive substances by adults. Am J Gastroenterol 87:1–5, 1992.

18. **What injuries occur with the ingestion of household ammonia or bleach?**
These common household cleaners generally cause problems only if aspirated or ingested in large amounts. Ingestion of household bleach (sodium hypochlorite) usually produces no injury or only mild esophageal burns. In some patients with vomiting, which re-exposed the esophagus to the sodium hypochlorite, surgery was needed. Large ingestions of household ammonia have caused severe esophageal burns and perforation, adult respiratory distress syndrome, gastric necrosis, airway obstruction resulting from supraglottic edema, and death.

Zarger SA, Kochhar R, Nagi B, et al: Ingestion of corrosive acids: Spectrum of injury to upper gastrointestinal tract and natural history. Gastroenterology 97:702, 1989.

19. **How should the airway be managed?**
Airway management is the first priority because pharyngeal or laryngeal burns can compromise airway patency. Immediate endotracheal intubation can be performed, but blind-nasotracheal intubation should never be done. Cases without stridor need examination to evaluate the hypopharynx, cords, and larynx, with the decision to intubate based on the presence and severity of burns.

20. **What is the treatment for most stable patients?**
Immediate water or milk may dilute the caustic agent, but vomiting must be avoided. Intravenous crystalloids and opioid analgesics may be used for pain control.
- **Alkali:** Gastric evacuation is contraindicated. The efficacy of H_2-blocker drugs is unknown, and antibiotics should be used only for known infection or concomitantly with corticosteroid therapy. Patients with second-degree and third-degree burns should be admitted.

- **Acids:** Gastric emptying with a small nasogastric tube may decrease gastric mucosal exposure and systemic absorption of acids in large ingestions. The patient should remain gastrically intubated for continued decompression. The use of corticosteroids and antibiotics is unproved. Laboratory tests include coagulation studies and blood type and crossmatch.

   E-medicine: Toxicity, caustic ingestions: www.emedicine.com/EMERG/topic86.htm

21. **Which laboratory or radiographic studies should be considered with corrosive ingestions?**
    A complete blood cell count, blood type and crossmatch, arterial blood gases, and disseminated intravascular coagulation panel should be considered in hemodynamically unstable patients or in patients with suspected severe burns or perforation. Chest and abdominal radiographs can aid in the diagnosis of GI perforations by exhibiting free air in the mediastinum or peritoneal cavity. Radiographs may identify ingested batteries or other radiopaque foreign bodies in the GI tract.

22. **What are the indications for emergency endoscopy?**
    Patients with presenting signs and symptoms indicative of upper GI tract burns more serious than first degree should undergo endoscopy within 12–24 hours after ingestion. Endoscopy also aids in lavage and evacuation of any remaining acid from incomplete nasogastric emptying and decompression in acid ingestions. A third-degree burn of the hypopharynx is a contraindication for endoscopy.

    Ramasamy K, Gumaste VV: Corrosive ingestion in adults. J Clin Gastroenterol 37:119–124, 2003.

23. **When is immediate surgical intervention indicated?**
    - **Alkali:** Surgery may be required for life-threatening GI hemorrhage or GI tract perforation, although some esophageal perforations have been managed successfully with drainage and antibiotics. Exploratory laparotomy for direct visualization of the stomach may be necessary when severe gastric injury is suspected and severe esophageal burns preclude gastric endoscopic examination.
    - **Acids:** Immediate surgery is indicated for GI tract perforation and when endoscopy reveals grade 3 burns with full-thickness necrosis of the esophagus or stomach.

24. **What is the big deal with hydrofluoric acid (HF) exposure?**
    HF can cause severe local and systemic toxicity via ingestion, dermal, or inhalation exposure. Delayed presentation of burns and significant metabolic abnormalities associated with the calcium-leeching properties of free fluoride ions can occur. If the acid is of a low concentration ($<12.5\%$), the tissue damage and symptoms may be delayed by 8–12 hours. Strong consideration should be given to admitting and monitoring all moderate-to-significant HF exposures for 24–48 hours to ensure adequate cardiac and electrolyte monitoring.

25. **How can HF cause cardiac arrest?**
    Significant and immediate hypocalcemia, hypomagnesemia, and hyperkalemia may result from 1% burn exposures. It takes less than 10 mL of 100% HF to bind all of the calcium in a 70-kg man. Electrocardiogram (ECG) monitoring for prolonged QT intervals, arrhythmias, and classic ECG findings of hyperkalemia is important. The immediate treatment of hypocalcemia is paramount to ensure patient survival. The intravenous use of large amounts of calcium is indicated until the patient's ECG normalizes and the serum calcium is normal. Do not wait to obtain serum calcium levels on patients to initiate or maintain treatment.

    Chan BS, Duggin GG: Survival after massive hydrofluoric acid ingestion. J Toxicol Clin Toxicol 35:307–309, 1997.

26. **How should HF burns be managed?**
The primary symptom of severe pain can be managed with the application of calcium-based gels made of calcium gluconate in KY Jelly often used in a glove. Local arterial infusions of calcium gluconate in the radial artery can be done to neutralize the fluoride ions in hand exposures.

27. **Is there any specific treatment for HF ingestion?**
Management is essentially supportive. Dilution with milk may be useful until lavage can be performed. The addition of 10% calcium gluconate to the lavage fluid has been suggested.

   Kirkpatrick JJ, Enion DS, Burd DA: Hydrofluoric acid burns: A review. Burns 21:483–493, 1995.

28. **What about treatment for the inhalation of HF?**
There is some evidence that a 2.5% calcium gluconate nebulizer with systemic calcium replacement may be beneficial.

KEY POINTS: CORROSIVES

1. Alkali frequently cause pharyngeal and esophageal burns.

2. Acids frequently cause esophageal and gastric burns.

3. Hydrofluoric acid exposure needs special attention.

CHAPTER 75

BITES AND STINGS

Lee W. Shockley, MD

*Always carry a flagon of whiskey in case of snakebite
and furthermore always carry a small snake.*
—W.C. Fields (1880–1946)

ARACHNIDA (CHIGGERS, SCABIES, SCORPIONS, SPIDERS)

1. **What is a tarantula?**
   It's either (1) a combination of scotch, vermouth, Benedictine, and a lemon twist or (2) the large spiders of the family Theraphosidae and suborder Mygalomorphae ("mygalomorphs"). The largest of these beasties is the South American *Grammostola mollicoma,* with a leg span of up to 27 cm and a body length of up to 10 cm! Mygalomorphs make up less than 10% of all spider species. Not much is known about tarantula venom, although it seems to contain a mixture of hyaluronidase, nucleotides, and polyamines (which act as neurotransmitters to paralyze the prey). On the whole, these bites tend to be of low toxicity in humans with a mild, briefly active venom causing pain, numbness, and lymphangitis. The bites usually do not cause necrosis or serious sequelae. Their little urticating hairs cause skin and mucous membrane irritation with edema and pruritus that can last for weeks. Eye exposure can cause a severe keratoconjunctivitis and ophthalmia nodosa.

2. **What spider bites are likely to be an issue?**
   Although all spiders possess venom, there are two spiders of particular clinical importance in the United States: *Latrodectus* (black widow) and *Loxosceles* (brown recluse or fiddleback). In 2003, the American Association of Poison Control Centers (AAPCC) reported 2739 bites from *Latrodectus* and 2843 from *Loxosceles*. There were no deaths and only 16 major reactions attributed to Latrodectus bites (0.58%). Similarly, one death (0.035%) and 22 major reactions (0.77%) were attributed to *Loxosceles*. The envenomation syndromes of these two spiders are quite distinct (Table 75-1).

   Watson WA, Litovitz TL, Rodgers GC, Jr, et al: 2002 annual report of the American Association of Poison Control Centers Toxic Exposure Surveillance System. Am J Emerg Med 21:353–421, 2003.

3. **What is Mustov's disease?**
   It is a play on words. Although there were 23,201 bites attributed to spiders reported to the AAPCC in 2003, this number is likely to be an inaccurate estimate of the true incidence because (1) these are only the cases that were reported to Poison Control Centers and (2) the effect of **Mustov's disease** (as in, "Doc, I woke up with this. I *must've* been bitten by a spider in my sleep."). It seems that a number of nonbite skin lesions are unfairly blamed on spiders. Mustov's disease is not specific to spider bites.

TABLE 75-1.   COMPARISON OF BLACK WIDOW AND BROWN RECLUSE SPIDERS

Latrodectus: Black Widow	Loxosceles: Brown Recluse
Markings: Red hourglass shape on the ventral abdomen (♀)	**Markings:** Dark, violin-shaped spot anterodorsally
Presentation: Pain at the bite within one hour Target-shaped erythema, swelling, diaphoresis — Diffuse large muscle cramping, including the abdomen (which may mimic peritonitis) — Latrodectisima: characteristic facial muscle spasm, lacrimation, photophobia, and swollen — Headache — Light-headedness — Nausea and vomiting Severe envenomations may result in dysphagia, hypertension, respiratory failure, shock, and coma.	**Presentation:** Typically, an initially mild bite characterized by erythema Bite becomes necrotic over 2–4 days. Systemic reaction may occur in 1–2 days: — Fever — Chills — Vomiting — Arthralgia — Myalgia — Hemolysis — Coagulapathy May result in renal failure and death
Treatment — Wound care — Analgesics, benzodiazepines for spasm — Tetanus prophylaxis — Calcium gluconate (IV) provides only minimal (if any) relief and is no longer recommended. — There is a horse-serum antivenin: administer a test dose, and then, if no severe reactions, 1–2 vials over 30 min (somewhat controversial given the incidence of reactions to the horse serum).	**Treatment** — Wound care — Analgesics — Tetanus prophylaxis — Surgical debridement and possible grafting for lesions greater than 2 cm — Transfusion or dialysis, as necessary — Hyperbaric oxygen therapy, corticosteroids, and dapsone have been advocated by some, but there is no clear evidence of efficacy in humans. — Currently, there is no commercially available antivenin.

Saucier JR: Arachnid envenomation. Emerg Med Clin North Am 22(2):405–422, ix, 2004.

4. **A 5-year-old boy presents with genital itching that started several hours after sitting on the lawn watching a fireworks display. His examination reveals intensely puritic, erythematous papules around his groin. What is this? How can it be treated? (Clue: he had been wearing shorts.)**

Chiggers. They are tiny mite larvae that cause intense pruritus. The diagnosis is based on identifying the characteristic skin lesions in a person with an outdoor exposure. Itching begins within a few hours of exposure, and the papules can enlarge to form nodules in 1–2 days. There may be fever and erythema multiforme. Treatment is with antihistamines and steroids (topical or oral) for the symptoms and lindane, permethrin, or crotamiton for definitive therapy.

5. **What are the distinguishing features of scabies?**

The bites are typically in the web spaces between the fingers and toes (also the penis, face, and scalp in children). They create "burrows" of pruritic, white, thread-like patterns with small gray spots at the closed end, where the parasite rests. Treatment is with a thorough application of permethrin from the neck down and may require a second course of treatment in 2 weeks.

6. **How dangerous are scorpion stings?**

Scorpions have paired venom glands located in the last of the five abdominal segments (the tail). The principal toxins are polypeptides and low-molecular-weight proteins, histamine, and indole compounds (including serotonin). The venom causes an increase in the sodium permeability of presynaptic neurons, which leads to continuous depolarization. Most scorpions that inhabit the United States are of low toxicity. In North America, only the bark scorpion (*Centruroides exilicauda*) is capable of producing systemic toxicity. In 2003, the AAPCC reported 14,417 patients with scorpion stings. There was moderate morbidity in 2.6% of patients, major morbidity in 0.07%, and no deaths.

7. **What are the signs of scorpion envenomation?**

The sting is acutely painful. Systemic manifestations are rare and mainly occur at the extremes of patient age. The principal signs of systemic toxicity are salivation, tachycardia, roving eye movements, opisthotonos, and tongue fasciculations.

8. **What is the treatment for a scorpion sting?**

The recommended treatment of scorpion stings consists mainly of local wound care, analgesia, and possibly benzodiazepines for the neuromuscular symptoms. There is a *Centruroides* scorpion antivenin, but its use is controversial, given the low mortality and morbidity associated with most of these bites. The exception may be in the treatment of young children, however, because the mortality rate among children younger than 5 years with severe scorpion envenomation may be 2.5 times that of adults. The antivenin is not Food and Drug Administration (FDA) approved and is available only in Arizona through Arizona State University.

Foex B, Wallis L: Best evidence topic report. Scorpion envenomation: Does antivenom reduce serum venom concentrations? Emerg Med J 22:195–197, 2005.

FORMICOIDEA (ANTS)

9. **I have a patient who received multiple stings from fire ants. What do I do?**

Don't panic. Treatment is the same as for a bee sting. Fire ants swarm during an attack, and each sting contributes to the total antigen load. The individual stings result in papules that may evolve to sterile pustules within 24 hours. Local necrosis and scarring may occur.

HYMENOPTERA (BEES AND WASPS)

10. What types of reactions occur from Hymenoptera stings?
There are four types of reactions:

- The **toxic reaction** is a nonantigenic response to the venom characterized by local irritation at the sting site and, potentially, vomiting, diarrhea, light-headedness, and syncope. There may also be headache, fever, drowsiness, involuntary muscle spasms, edema without urticaria, and occasionally convulsions. Local toxic reactions are treated with supportive care, including cool packs and analgesics.
- **Anaphylactic reactions** are most commonly seem in Vespidae stings (wasps, hornets, yellow jackets). These reactions can range from mild to fatal and occur from 15 minutes to 6 hours after the sting. These reactions are treated like any other allergic reaction.
- **Delayed reactions** present as a serum sickness-like syndrome 10–14 days after the sting. The delayed reactions are treated with antihistamines and corticosteroids.
- **Unusual reactions** reported after *Hymenoptera* stings include encephalitis, neuritis, vasculitis, and nephritis.

Freeman TM. Clinical practice. Hypersensitivity to Hymenoptera stings. N Engl J Med 351:1978–1984, 2004.

11. What is a honeybee? Stinger? Bee-stung lips?
Honey bee: honey, dark rum, and lemon juice; stinger: cognac and white crème de menthe: bee-stung lips: light rum, honey, and heavy cream. Back to the topic.

12. What is different about a bee sting from a wasp sting?
Bees have barbed stingers that usually remain in the victim, pulling the venom sac off of the bee. Whereas the bee dies after a single sting, a wasp is capable of stinging multiple times. It is better to remove the stinger from a bee by scraping it out with a credit card rather than by pinching and plucking it with fingers or tweezers and risking the inadvertent injection of more venom. Removal of the stinger should be done as soon as possible because the venom sac continues to pulse venom after it has detached from the bee.

13. What about "killer bees"?
African honeybees (*Apris mellifera scutellata*) were introduced into Brazil in 1956 as a potential honey producer in the tropical environment. There is little difference between the Africanized bees and European bees in terms of appearance, the nature of their venom, and the amount of venom that they carry. The difference is in their aggressive behavior. Victims typically receive multiple stings during a swarming attack and, therefore, a greater venom burden. For this reason, the Africanized honeybees have been called "killer bees."

14. After a patient has survived an anaphylactic reaction to a bee sting, what should be done to prepare the patient in case he or she is stung again in the future?
The first step is avoidance of bees and wasps. It is also prudent for the patient to carry medical identification describing his or her bee sting allergy, such as a MedicAlert Bracelet. Further, he or she should also be given prescriptions for self-injection of epinephrine (the Ana-Kit or the EpiPen) and instructed in its use.

Watson WA, Litovitz TL, Rodgers GC, Jr, et al: 2002 annual report of the American Association of Poison Control Centers Toxic Exposure Surveillance System. Am J Emerg Med 21:353–421, 2003.

HELODERMA (LIZARDS)

15. **Are there any venomous lizards in the world?**
Yes, two species: the Mexican beaded lizard (*Heloderma horridum*) and the Gila monster (*Heloderma suspectum*). Both animals live in the desert areas of the southwestern United States and in Mexico. The venom of these lizards is somewhat similar to Crotaline venom, although the clinical course is typically milder. The more serious problem with these reptiles is their powerful jaws (and their tendency to hold onto their victims). They deliver their venom by chewing and dripping the venom into the lacerations created by their teeth. Their teeth also commonly break off in the wounds and become foreign bodies and a nidus for infection if not removed. The teeth, by the way, are difficult to visualize on radiographs. They envenomate in about 70% of the bites.

16. **What is a green lizard?**
Chartreuse and 151 proof rum. Off track again, I see.

CULICIDAE (MOSQUITOS)

17. **What is the major clinical significance of mosquito bites?**
There are more than 3000 species of mosquito, and they are found on every continent, except Antarctica. They are responsible for more bites than any other blood-sucking organism. They are attracted by carbon dioxide, lactic acid, body heat, and sweat. Children under age 1 year rarely show a skin reaction to the bite; however, by age 5 years almost all children react. Both immediate and delayed hypersensitivity reactions can occur. The major significance, however, is in the role of the mosquito as a disease vector: They can transmit over a half dozen forms of encephalitis, malaria, yellow fever, dengue fever, filariasis, West Nile Virus, Ross River virus, Chikungunya fever, and Rift Valley Fever. Taubes estimates that mosquito-carried diseases will cause the death of 1 out of every 17 people alive in the world today.

Taubes G: A mosquito bites back. The New York Times Magazine, August 24, 1997, pp 40–46.

MAMMALS (BATS, DOGS, CATS, FOXES, HORSES, HUMANS, RACCOONS, SKUNKS, WOODCHUCKS)

18. **How many dog and cat bites are there annually? What is the risk of infection? What is the mortality from these bites?**
The majority of pet bites that require medical attention are from dogs. Some estimate that there are as many as 4.5 million dog bites annually causing 750,000 to seek medical attention. The

annual incidence of cat bites is probably in excess of 400,000 (due to underreporting). The risk of infection from a bite is determined by multiple factors, including the location of the bite, the type of wound, the biting species, and host factors. Dog bites to the hand, for example, may have a risk of infection as high as 30%. Cat bites carry a 15–80% rate of infection (the broad spread is likely due to the determination of what constitutes the denominator). Dog attacks are fatal for about 10–20 people annually. The victims are often infants and children and usually die from exsanguinating neck injuries.

19. **Should I give prophylactic antibiotics to the victim of a dog or cat bite?**
    This is an area of some controversy. The most effective means of reducing infection potential is through meticulous wound care. In a meta-analysis, Cummings showed a number needed to treat of 14 to prevent a wound infection after a dog bite. However, if one of the studies that Cummings included had shown an abnormally high infection rate, the conclusion would have been that low-risk wounds (immunocompetent patients with nonpuncture wounds that do not involve the hand or foot, which are treated within 12 hours and show no signs of infection) do not benefit from antibiotics. High-risk wounds, however, may do better with antibiotics in addition to meticulous wound care. When choosing antibiotic(s), consider the polymicrobial nature of these infections (*Staphylococcus, Streptococcus, Pasteurella multocida,* anaerobes, etc.) and the cost of the antibiotic.

    Cummings P: Antibiotics to prevent infection in patients with dog bite wounds: A meta-analysis of randomized trials. Ann Emerg Med 23:535–540, 1994.

    Garbutt F, Jenner R: Best evidence topic report. Wound closure in animal bites. Emerg Med J 21:589–590, 2004.

20. **What is *Capnocytophaga canimorus*?**
    Capnocytophaga canimorsus (DF2) is a fastidious gram-negative rod that can cause sepsis after a dog bite. Eighty percent of the patients who become seriously ill from this infection are immunocompromised (splenectomy, hematologic malignancy, or cirrhosis). Fortunately, it is a rare infection because it carries a 25–36% mortality.

21. **What is a "fight bite"?**
    A particularly common bite wound encountered in an urban setting is that caused by another human. A "fight bite" or "clinched fist injury" (CFI) is a human bite that occurs when the fist of one opponent strikes the teeth of a second opponent. This usually involves the knuckles of the dominant hand. The importance of this injury is that the laceration can involve the extensor tendon and its bursa, the superficial and deep fascia, and the joint capsule. These structures are contaminated with oral flora at the time of injury and are notorious for becoming infected. There are at least 42 species of bacteria in human saliva. The most frequently cultured organism from fight bites is *Streptococcus,* followed by *Staphylococcus aureus* (usually penicillin resistant); 31% of these wound infections are due to gram-negative organisms, and 43% are due to mixed gram-negative and gram-positive organisms. Up to 29% of these infections may be due to a facultatively anaerobic gram-negative rod, *Eikenella corrodens*. This organism is typically resistant to the semisynthetic penicillins, clindamycin, and the first-generation cephalosporins. However, it is usually sensitive to penicillin and ampicillin. These wounds should be meticulously cared for, with special attention given to thorough exploration and irrigation. Consider the polymicrobial nature of these infections when choosing antibiotics.

    Managing bites from humans and other mammals. Drug Ther Bull Sep 42:67–71, 2004.

22. **What is the origin of the phrase "the hair of the dog that bit you"?**
    It is a very, very old expression, probably arising from the Roman belief that *similia similibus curantur* ("like cures like"). To treat the victim of a dog bite, one would obtain samples of its hair and either burn the hair and apply it to the wound or use the hair in creating a poultice for the wound. It was thought that this would speed wound healing and recovery from rabies. By extension, another drink or two after a drinking binge would be the cure for a hangover.

23. **What types of bites are a risk for the transmission of rabies?**
Rabies is a disease caused by an RNA rhabdovirus transmitted by inoculation with infectious saliva. It is prevalent in parts of Latin America, Asia, Africa, South America, Europe, the Middle East, India, and Southeast Asia. Hawaii, England, Australia, Japan, and parts of the Caribbean are rabies free. The virus primarily affects the central nervous system and is almost always fatal. In the United States, animal bites from skunks, raccoons, bats, foxes, and woodchucks should be considered a risk. Exposures from livestock, rodents, and lagomorphs should be considered individually but rarely require postexposure prophylaxis. Consult your state health department for local recommendations.

24. **What does postexposure prophylaxis for rabies consist of?**
Postexposure prophylaxis means trying to prevent the disease before it becomes manifest after a high-risk exposure. It begins with a thorough cleansing of the wound. After cleansing, 20 IU/kg of human rabies immunoglobulin is administered (50% injected in and around the wound, if possible, and 50% given intramuscularly in the gluteal). Human diploid cell vaccine (1.0 mL) is injected into the deltoid muscle (or the anterolateral thigh in young children) on days 0, 3, 7, 14, and 28. Tip: Do not administer the rabies vaccine and the rabies immunoglobulin in the same site.

MARINE FAUNA (JELLYFISH, SHARK, VENOMOUS FISH)

25. **How do I treat jellyfish or other coelenterate stings?**
Jellyfish envenomate by injecting small harpoon-shaped spines from their nematocysts into their prey. The discharge is triggered by either physical or chemical stimulation. Frequently, "undischarged" nematocysts within the jellyfish tentacles remain in contact with the victim's skin. The concern, of course, is that the undischarged nematocysts may be stimulated to release additional venom into the victim. It is well established that acetic acid (vinegar) inhibits nematocyst discharge in *Chironex fleckeri* stings. However, acetic acid has no effect on cysts that have already discharged. Further, inhibition of nematocyst discharge is probably species specific. Effective inhibitors in one species may trigger nematocyst discharge in another. Acetic acid has been demonstrated to inhibit nematocyst discharge in all of the species of medically important Australian jellyfish.

If vinegar is not available, acidic drinks (soft drinks and fruit juices) may be tried. Although popular in folklore, urine has not been proven to inhibit nematocyst discharge and may stimulate nematocyst discharge.

Immersion of the affected extremity in hot water may be of some benefit (after acetic acid decontamination). The nematocysts that remain in the skin can be removed by applying shaving cream, talc, baking soda, or flour and by shaving the area. The same treatment can be used for the stings from sea anemones or fire coral. There is an Australian box jellyfish (*Chironex flecker*) antivenin available. The recommended dosage for the antivenom is one to three ampules.

26. **Name some venomous fish, and state what their venoms have in common. How can that feature of their venom be used in treatment?**
Stingray, scorpion fish, stonefish, catfish (freshwater catfish, sea catfish, coral catfish), oldwife fish, lionfish, zebrafish, butterfly cod, spiny dogfish, rabbit fish, ratfish, stargazer fish, surgeon fish, toadfish, weaver fish, bullrout, sculpin, and stinging sharks all have heat-labile toxins (heating destroys the toxin). Barbs and spines may remain embedded in the wound and should be promptly removed. The venoms can be rendered nontoxic by placing the affected extremity of the victim (usually the foot) into hot water (45°C) for 90 minutes.

27. **What else do I need to know about treatment of venomous fish wounds?**
   There is a stonefish antivenom available. It is a hyperimmune Fab2 horse serum preparation.
   There are three places in the United States that stock it: Sea World San Diego, Sea World Ohio,
   and the Steinhardt Aquarium in San Francisco.

   Lyon RM: Stonefish poisoning. Wilderness Environ Med 15:284–288, 2004.

28. **How many people are killed by sharks worldwide annually?**
   About 10–25. In contrast, approximately 100 million sharks are killed by people annually. In
   many oceans and with many species, overfishing to the point of extinction is a real possibility.

29. **How do you make a shark bite?**
   Try swimming by yourself in shark-infested waters at dusk through schools of bait fish, disguised
   as a seal, and dragging a bleeding, captured fish. That ought to do it. Alternatively, stay on the
   beach, mix dark rum, orange juice, sour mix, and grenadine (tall glass, ice, umbrella).

CROTALINAE, ELAPIDAE (RATTLESNAKES, COPPERHEADS, WATER MOCCASINS, CORAL SNAKES)

30. **What is a "dry" snakebite?**
   Sorry, no recipe. A dry snakebite is a bite in which no venom was introduced. About 20–25% of
   all bites from rattlesnakes in the United States do not result in envenomation. Coral snakes,
   lacking fangs, envenomate by "chewing" the skin; thus, as many as 50% of their bites are dry.
   Quick observations helpful in determining whether rattlesnake envenomation has taken place
   include the presence of fang marks that ooze nonclotting blood with surrounding ecchymosis
   and severe burning pain. These signs combined with microhematuria are characteristic of
   severe envenomation and a poor prognosis. In coral snake envenomation, there may be few
   signs at the bite site, and systemic signs may be delayed for as long as 12 hours. The
   earliest signs and symptoms to develop tend to be nausea, vomiting, headache, abdominal
   pain, diaphoresis, and pallor. Coagulopathy is not a feature of coral snake envenomation.

31. **True or false: Snakebites are uncommon but are highly lethal.**
   True and false. In the United States, snakebites are uncommon, and mortality is rare. In their
   2003 report, the AAPCC documented 6889 snakebites (venomous and nonvenomous) out of
   94,247 bites and envenomations that they tracked. In 2003, there were two deaths attributed to
   snakebites in the United States (one from a rattlesnake, one from a poisonous exotic snake).
   Moderate or major sequelae were seen in 1694 and 178 cases, respectively. The most common of
   these were from rattlesnakes (35%); the next most common were from copperheads (26.8%).

32. **List some of the epidemiologic characteristics of snakebites in the United States.**
   - 90% occur from April to October.
   - 50% occur between the hours of 2 P.M. and 9 P.M.
   - Male-to-female victim ratio is 9:1.
   - 50% of victims are age 18–28 years.
   - 80% of bites are on the fingers or hand; 15% involve the foot or ankle.
   - Ethanol intoxication is a common risk factor for the victim (especially when "pet" snakes are
     involved).

33. **List the clinical signs of crotaline (pit viper) envenomation.**
   - Rapid onset of slow spreading edema (80%)
   - Pain out of proportion to the puncture (72%)

- Weakness (65%)
- Light-headedness (52%)
- Nausea (48%)
- Erythema at the bite site (53%)
- Bleeding diathesis (52%)
- Lymphangitis, hypotension, shock, diaphoresis, chills (58%)
- Paresthesias, taste changes, fasciculations (33%)

34. What is "CroFab"? When should it be administered?

CroFab (Crotalidae Polyvalent Immune Fab by Altana, Inc) is an antivenin produced from the pooled serum of sheep immunized with one of four crotaline snake venoms, then digested with papain to produce antibody fragments (Fab and Fc). The more immunogenic Fc portion of the antibody is eliminated during purification. The four individual monospecific Fab preparations are combined to form the final antivenin product. It is provided as lyophilized powders and must reconstituted (this takes 30–40 minutes). Initial control (defined as cessation of progression of all components of envenomation including local effects, systemic effects, and coagulopathy) is obtained by the administration of 3–12 vials. After control has been established, additional two-vial doses are infused at 6, 12, and 18 hours. Since the FDA approval of CroFab, Wyeth has ceased manufacture of Polyvalent Crotalidae Antivenin (although some institutions may have supplies that have not yet been used).

Probably because of the relatively small molecule size and consequent renal clearing, the effective half-life of CroFab may be insufficient for one-dose treatment of crotaline envenomation. Scheduled retreatment is recommended.

Dart RC, McNally J: Efficacy, safety, and use of snake antivenoms in the United States. Ann Emerg Med 37:181–188, 2001.

35. Can a crotaline bite cause a compartment syndrome?

It can, but it is unlikely. In most cases, venom is deposited in the subcutaneous tissue, not in fascial compartments. Compartment syndrome cannot be diagnosed reliably in an envenomated patient without directly measuring compartment pressures because the signs and symptoms of compartment syndrome (paresthesias, decreased pulses, and pain on motion) are similar to signs and symptoms of envenomation. The only way to determine whether compartment syndrome has developed is to measure the intracompartmental pressure. Because treatment with antivenin may improve compartment pressure, if the pressure is found to be elevated initially, one should monitor the compartment pressure while administering antivenin and perform fasciotomy only when pressures remain persistently elevated above 30–40 mmHg.

One exception is the envenomated finger. A tense, blue or pale envenomated finger with absent or poor capillary refill may be treated by digit dermotomy on clinical grounds alone. To make the dermotomy, incise the skin (only) longitudinally, on the medial or lateral aspect of the digit from the web to the midportion of the distal phalanx. A digit dermotomy should not be used routinely in all finger bites; it is not appropriate for prophylactic treatment to prevent a digital compartment syndrome.

36. What is the importance of the coloring of coral snakes, and what are the active components of its venom?

This small, thin, brightly colored snake is venomous; however, the king snake, which is nonvenomous, has similar but not identical coloration. Remember:

"Red on yellow, kill a fellow" (coral snake).

"Red on black, venom lack" (harmless snake).

This rhyme helps only with the identification of North American snakes. Coral snake venom contains a neurotoxin that irreversibly binds to presynaptic nerve terminals and blocks acetylcholine receptors. It may take weeks or months to regenerate the receptors.

The clinical effects are slurred speech, ptosis, dilated pupils, dysphagia, and myalgias. Death results from progressive paralysis and respiratory failure. There is virtually no local tissue toxicity.

37. **How is coral snake envenomation treated?**

Neostigmine (2.5 mg every 30–60 minutes) and equine antivenin (Wyeth). Four to six vials of the coral snake antivenin are recommended for envenomations from the eastern coral snake or the Texas coral snake; envenomations from the western coral snake need not be treated with antivenin.

38. **What treatments have been advocated for rattlesnake bites that are now considered to be ineffective or harmful?**

Incising the wound and attempting to extract the poison by oral suction (cut and suck), electric shock to denature the toxin proteins, carbolic acid, strychnine, enemas, urine, cauterization, prophylactic antibiotics, ice packs (cryotherapy), and arterial tourniquets are probably ineffective or harmful. In the early 1900s, whiskey was advocated as an antidote (see W.C. Fields's advice at the beginning of the chapter).

39. **What nonantivenin treatments do make sense?**

The use of constriction bands, splints, and venom removal with **the Extractor** (a mechanical suction device that produces about 1 atm of negative pressure and may remove 30% of the injected venom if used within 3 minutes of the bite) are controversial, with proponents and opponents.

A constriction band (broad and flat band as opposed to a ropelike tourniquet) can be applied to exert a pressure great enough to occlude superficial veins and lymphatic channels (typically >20 mmHg) but loose enough to admit one or two fingers. It has been shown in experimental models to delay the systemic absorption of venom and may have use in cases with prolonged transport time.

A competing technique originating in Australia is the pressure-immobilization method. By firmly wrapping the bitten extremity with an elastic bandage (for pressures 40–70 mmHg) and splinting the entire extremity, the onset of significant systemic toxicity may be delayed until the patient can be treated in a facility where antivenin therapy is available. Theoretically, however, trapping the venom in the bitten extremity may worsen local necrosis. Releasing the pressure could allow a bolus of venom to be released into the systemic circulation. The relative merits of the constriction band versus the pressure-immobilization technique have not been directly compared.

In an animal model, the time to death after injection of venom can be prolonged, and the median lethal dose of venom can be increased, simply by immobilizing all four limbs (including the unbitten extremity). This technique also has not been studied clinically.

Nonsteroidal anti-inflammatory drugs may compound a crotaline venom-induced thrombocytopenic bleeding diathesis and probably should be avoided.

40. **What about some of the more exotic snakes (at least exotic by North American standards)?**

In 2003, the AAPCC reported 2732 cases of exposure to exotic snakes (poisonous, nonpoisonous, and "unknown if poisonous"). There was 1 death reported; 9 patients had life-threatening morbidity, and 52 had moderate morbidity. There is an Antivenom Index that is sent to all of the Poison Control Centers in the United States. It includes a catalog of all of the antivenins stocked by North American zoos and aquariums. Possession of exotic venomous snakes may be restricted by law, and these cases should be reported to the authorities.

WEBSITES

1. The Venom-List Mailing List/Listserv: groups.yahoo.com/group/venomlist/

2. American Association of Poison Control Centers: www.aapcc.org/

3. Snake Bite Antivenom—Resources and Producers: globalcrisis.info/latestantivenom.htm

BIBLIOGRAPHY

1. Auerbach PS (ed): Wilderness Medicine, 4th ed. St. Louis, Mosby, 2001.

2. Cummings P: Antibiotics to prevent infection in patients with dog bite wounds: A meta-analysis of randomized trials. Ann Emerg Med 23:535–540, 1994.

3. Dart RC, McNally J: Efficacy, safety, and use of snake antivenoms in the United States. Ann Emerg Med 37:181–188, 2001.

4. Dart RC, Waeckerle JF: Introduction: Advances in the management of snakebite symposium. Ann Emerg Med 37:166–167, 2001.

5. Foex B, Wallis L: Best evidence topic report. Scorpion envenomation: Does antivenom reduce serum venom concentrations? Emerg Med J 22:195–197, 2005.

6. Freeman TM: Clinical practice. Hypersensitivity to hymenoptera stings. N Engl J Med 351:1978–1984, 2004.

7. Frundle TC: Management of spider bites. Air Med J 23(4):24–26, 2004.

8. Garbutt F, Jenner R: Best evidence topic report. Wound closure in animal bites. Emerg Med J 21:589–590, 2004.

9. Hall EL: Role of surgical intervention in the management of crotaline snake envenomation. Ann Emerg Med 37:175–180, 2001.

10. Lyon RM: Stonefish poisoning. Wilderness Environ Med 15:284–288, 2004.

11. Managing bites from humans and other mammals: Drug Ther Bull 42(9):67–71, 2004.

12. Saucier JR: Arachnid envenomation. Emerg Med Clin North Am 22:405–422, ix, 2004.

13. Steen CJ, Janniger CK, Schutzer SE, et al: Insect sting reactions to bees, wasps, and ants. Int J Dermatol 44(2):91–94, 2005.

14. Swanson DL, Vetter RS: Bites of brown recluse spiders and suspected necrotic arachnidism. N Engl J Med 352:700–707, 2005.

15. Taubes G: A mosquito bites back. In The New York Times Magazine, August 24, 1997, pp 40–46.

16. Watson WA, Litovitz TL, Rodgers GC, Jr, et al: 2002 annual report of the American Association of Poison Control Centers Toxic Exposure Surveillance System. Am J Emerg Med 21:353–421, 2003.

CHAPTER 76

SMOKE INHALATION

Richard E. Wolfe, MD

1. **What is the principal cause of death in fire victims?**
   Smoke inhalation.

2. **Does smoke cause thermal injury to the lungs?**
   Not usually. Air has such a low heat capacity that it rarely produces lower airway damage. The upper respiratory tract generally cools hot air before it reaches the vocal cords. Steam, however, has 4000 times the heat-carrying capacity of air and causes severe upper airway burns with fatal glottic edema as well as bronchial mucosal destruction and alveolar hemorrhage.

3. **Why is smoke so lethal?**
   Carbon dioxide and carbon monoxide, the major components of smoke, are responsible for a drop in the concentration of ambient oxygen from 22% to 5–10%. Carbon monoxide and, more rarely, hydrogen cyanide block the uptake and use of oxygen, leading to severe tissue cellular hypoxemia. Depending on the fuel, temperature, and rate of heating, smoke contains a wide variety of toxins. Soot may act as a vehicle in transporting these toxic gases to the lower respiratory tract, where they dissolve to form acids and alkali. Removal of the soot is impaired by action of certain of these toxins on respiratory cilia, leading to severe, delayed pneumonia.

4. **What are the earliest clinical manifestations of acute inhalation injury following smoke exposure?**
   Inflamed nares, cough, sputum production, and hoarseness are the first signs of injury. This is because the nasopharynx and larynx are exposed to the highest concentration of inhaled toxins leading to the most severe chemical burns. Furthermore, the proximal airway is usually the only part of the airway subjected to thermal burns. However, even when injured, nasopharyngeal and laryngeal edema may be delayed. Furthermore, rapid progression to complete airway obstruction may occur in patients with mild symptoms. For this reason, close observation followed by early airway management is often necessary to ensure patient safety.

5. **Name the four clinical stages of smoke inhalation.**
   - **Stage 1:** Acute respiratory distress occurs 1–12 hours postinjury and is due to bronchospasm, laryngeal edema, and bronchorrhea.
   - **Stage 2:** Noncardiogenic pulmonary edema (adult respiratory distress syndrome) occurs 6–72 hours postinjury secondary to increased capillary permeability.
   - **Stage 3:** Strangulation occurs 60–120 hours postinjury from cervical eschar formation in patients with circumferential neck burns.
   - **Stage 4:** Onset of pneumonia 72 hours after injury, usually from *Staphylococcus aureus*, *Pseudomonas aeruginosa*, or gram-negative organisms.

6. **How should smoke inhalation victims be managed in the field?**
   All victims should be placed on a 100% nonrebreather mask, even if they are asymptomatic. Oxygen dramatically accelerates the washout of carbon monoxide, shortening the half-life from 4 hours at room air to about 90 minutes. Endotracheal intubation is indicated for patients in respiratory distress. When intubated, the patient should be suctioned aggressively to remove

inhaled soot. Patients with a loss of consciousness or altered mental status should be transported to a facility capable of providing hyperbaric oxygen (HBO) therapy.

7. **Why is HBO therapy theoretically beneficial in smoke inhalation?**
   - HBO therapy provides increased oxygen to poorly functioning mitochondrial enzymes inhibited by carbon monoxide and cyanide.
   - HBO therapy at 3 atm decreases the half-life of carbon monoxide to 23 minutes.
   - HBO therapy has been shown to reduce smoke-induced pulmonary edema.
   - At a cellular level, HBO therapy decreases the formation of intercellular adhesion molecule-I on the endothelial membrane, which prevents neutrophils from infiltrating the central nervous system and causing a damaging inflammatory reaction and permanent neurologic sequelae.

8. **What should I ask about the fire?**
   Ask if the patient was trapped in a closed space because significant inhalation injury would not occur in an open area. Try to determine what material was burning. The fuel is of primary importance in determining the composition of smoke and the risk to the patient.

9. **Name some fuels and the materials from which they derive.**
   - **Hydrogen cyanide:** combustion of wool, silk, nylons, and polyurethanes found commonly in furniture and paper
   - **Aldehydes, acrolein:** wood, cotton, paper, and plastic materials
   - **Hydrogen chloride, phosgene:** pyrolysis of chlorinated polymers; polyvinyl chloride (wire insulation materials); chlorinated acrylics; and wall, floor, and furniture coverings
   - **Oxides of nitrogen:** nitrocellulose film
   - **Sulfur dioxide, hydrogen sulfide:** rubber

   Cohen MA: Inhalation of products of combustion. Ann Emerg Med 12:628–631, 1983.

10. **How do I make the diagnosis of smoke inhalation injury?**
    Bronchoscopy is needed to confirm the presence of inhalation injury. Soot deposition in the airway, extensive edema, mucosal erythema, hemorrhage, and ulceration confirm that smoke inhalation has occurred. The initial bronchoscopy may be relatively normal because hyperemia and edema formation may take some time to evolve. A normal proximal airway does not rule out more distal injury.

11. **How should asymptomatic patients be managed?**
    Observe the patient for a few hours first. If still asymptomatic, provide comprehensive discharge instructions on when to return. Although the physical examination cannot reliably rule out complications such as delayed noncardiogenic pulmonary edema or pneumonia, ancillary studies and emergency department (ED) or in-hospital observation are not cost effective. The patient should be instructed to return to the ED if shortness of breath, chest pain, or fever occurs.

12. **If the patient's pulse oximetry is normal, would arterial blood gas analysis yield additional information?**
    In the presence of carboxyhemoglobin (CO), pulse oximetry may yield a falsely elevated reading. Arterial blood gases are of limited use and may be helpful only if the oxygen saturation is measured directly and not derived from the PaO_2 measurement. Although an increased alveolar-arterial gradient may correlate with smoke inhalation injury, it does not predict the severity of injury. Arterial blood gases are most useful in determining hypoventilation (increased PCO_2) and the presence of a metabolic or respiratory acidosis.

13. **Should I get a chest radiograph on all patients with a history of smoke inhalation?**
    No. A chest radiograph offers little benefit in the ED. Chest radiographs are normal immediately after smoke inhalation injury, and abnormalities appear only on a delayed basis. A chest

radiograph is not indicated in asymptomatic patients, and in most instances, it is useful only as a baseline in symptomatic patients.

14. **Can I use the standard burn formula for intravenous fluids if smoke inhalation is present?**
Patients with cutaneous and inhalation injuries pose a difficult problem because their fluid requirements are usually greater, but because of leaky capillaries, they are much more likely to develop membrane permeable pulmonary edema. Intravenous fluids must be guided by regular clinical reevaluation (breath sounds, oxygen saturation, urinary output, vital signs) rather than by formulas. Swan-Ganz monitoring may be required.

15. **Is HBO therapy the only available therapy for cyanide poisoning?**
No. All EDs should stock the Lilly cyanide antidote kit. Hydroxycobalamin (vitamin B_{12}) reduces cyanide concentrations and is available in Europe, although it has not yet been approved for use in the United States.

16. **How does the Lilly cyanide antidote kit work?**
Cyanide binds to the ferric ions, blocking the mitochondrial cytochrome oxidase pathway and cellular respiration. The cyanide antidote kit acts in two ways to limit this: (1) nitrites generate methemoglobin, creating heme-ferric ions to compete with cyanide with mitochondrial ferric ions, and (2) sulfur transferase (rhodanase) binds cyanide molecules to sulfur-forming thiocyanate, which is nontoxic and eliminated in the urine. Thiosulfate accelerates this process by increasing available sulfur molecules. (See Fig. 76-1.)

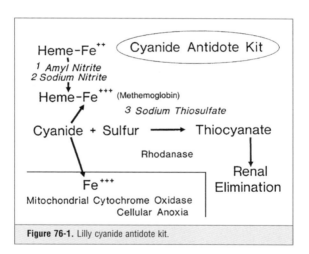

Figure 76-1. Lilly cyanide antidote kit.

17. **When should I use the cyanide antidote kit?**
Symptomatic patients can have carbon monoxide or cyanide toxicity. Inducing methemoglobinemia with amyl nitrite capsules and sodium nitrite in patients with high CO levels must be avoided until the patient is in the HBO chamber. Until then, if measured oxygen saturation is low, use the sodium thiosulfate portion of the kit. High lactate levels can help distinguish cyanide from CO because elevations in serum lactate correlate well with cyanide toxicity. This can provide an indication for administration of sodium nitrite when HBO therapy is unavailable.

KEY POINTS: SMOKE INHALATION

1. Obtain CO level and treat with O_2 any patient who has inhaled smoke in an enclosed space.

2. Consider cyanide poisoning when patient inhaled smoke from burning furniture fabric (wool, silk, or polyurethanes).

18. **How do I administer the cyanide antidote kit?**
    Amyl nitrite **inhalers** are used in patients without intravenous access. These can be used every 3–4 minutes but are less effective than intravenous sodium nitrite. If a patient is apneic, break one of the amyl nitrite inhalants inside the resuscitation bag. When an intravenous line is established, the full amount of a 10-mL ampule or 5–10 mg/kg of sodium nitrite should be administered intravenously over 4 minutes. This is followed by 12.5 g of intravenous thiosulfate.

CONTROVERSY

19. **Isn't the early respiratory failure seen in inhalation victims worsened by aggressive crystalloid resuscitation?**
    Respiratory failure from interstitial fluid accumulation is a rare event. When it occurs, it is caused by capillary leakage due to inflammation of pulmonary tissue. The amount of crystalloid used during resuscitation does not increase the risk or the severity of the resultant pulmonary edema. Fluids should not be withheld in a patient with severe cutaneous and respiratory burns.

    Holm C, Tegeler J, Mayr M: Effect of crystalloid resuscitation and inhalation injury on extravascular lung water: Clinical implications. Chest 121:1956–1962, 2002.

BIBLIOGRAPHY

1. Blinn DL, Slater H, Goldfarb W: Inhalation injury with burns: A lethal combination. J Emerg Med 6:471–473, 1988.
2. Hampson N: Hyperbaric Oxygen Therapy Committee: Hyperbaric oxygen therapy. 1999 Committee report. Kensington, MD: Undersea and Hyperbaric Medical Society, 1999.
3. Kirk MA, Gerace R, Kulig KW: Cyanide and methemoglobin kinetics in smoke inhalation victims treated with the cyanide antidote kit. Ann Emerg Med 22:1413–1418, 1993.
4. Miller K, Chang A: Acute inhalation injury. Emerg Med Clin North Am 21:573–577, 2003.
5. Murphy SM, Murray D, Smith S, Orr DJ: Burns caused by steam inhalation for respiratory tract infections in children. BMJ 328:757, 2004.
6. Ramzy PI, Barret JP, Herndon DN: Thermal injury. Crit Care Clin 15:333–352, 1999.
7. Stewart RJ, Mason SW, Taira MT, et al: Effect of radical scavengers and hyperbaric oxygen on smoke-induced pulmonary edema. Undersea Hyperb Med 21:21–30, 1994.
8. Zerbe NF, Wagner BK: Use of vitamin B12 in the treatment and prevention of nitroprusside-induced cyanide toxicity. Crit Care Med 21:465–467, 1993.

CHAPTER 77

WEAPONS OF MASS DESTRUCTION

Carl J. Bonnett, MD, and Peter T. Pons, MD

1. **Why do I need to be familiar with terrorism and weapons of mass destruction (WMD)?**

   Emergency physicians (EPs) play an integral role in the planning, preparation, and response to both natural disasters and terrorist attacks. The emergency department (ED) will be on the receiving end of any large-scale incident, and EPs will find themselves looked on as subject matter experts.

2. **What do I need to know about terrorism?**

   In the past, there was a sense that terrorists used attacks to gain publicity but possibly had some reluctance to kill too many people for fear of alienating their support base. Experts now believe that a shift has occurred and that terrorists of the 21st century are looking for maximum body counts.

   First Annual Report to The President and The Congress of the Advisory Panel to assess domestic response capabilities for terrorism involving weapons of mass destruction, aka The Gilmore Report of 1999, available at www.rand.org/nsrd/terrpanel/terror.pdf

   Hoffman, B: Inside Terrorism. Columbia University Press, New York, 1998.

3. **Describe the levels of personal protective equipment (PPE).**

   - **Level A:** Required for exposure to areas of chemical release (**hot zones**), if air concentrations exceed those that are immediately dangerous to life of health. This level includes a self-contained breathing apparatus and fully encapsulated suits that are resistant to liquid and vapor penetration.
   - **Level B:** Required for exposures that pose a potential inhalation danger. This suit is less protective than the level A suit, but when used with a self-contained breathing apparatus or a supplied air respirator, it provides adequate vapor and liquid protection.
   - **Level C:** Required when the contaminant is identified and an air-purifying respirator is appropriate for the agent involved. This level includes clothing protective for liquid and vapor and an ambient air-purifying respirator. This is the level of protection necessary for hospital personnel involved in decontamination.

4. **I thought we have hazardous materials (HAZMAT) teams to deal with this kind of thing. Aren't nuclear, biologic, and chemical (NBC) attacks basically the same thing?**

   On one level, NBC attacks are quite similar to conventional HAZMAT incidents. They both have a dangerous material that is released with the requisite need for containment, decontamination, and evacuation of injured and exposed persons. A terrorist attack, however, would probably occur in an area of high population density (subway, sporting event, etc.) and by design contaminate many people and create mass hysteria. Thus, in these kinds of attacks it will be much harder to control patient flow than traditional HAZMAT incidents, and they will certainly garner a much larger public reaction.

A biologic release will have almost no resemblance to a traditional HAZMAT event because the time of release of the agent may be days before patients present with symptoms. The exception to this is if a known substance is discovered or announced (i.e., anthrax spores).

Maniscalco PM, Christen HT: Understanding Terrorism and Managing the Consequences. Upper Saddle River, NJ, Prentice Hall, 2002.

5. What else is unique about terrorist attacks?

If a chemical truck rolls over on the highway, it is serious and unfortunate but usually "what you see is what you get." Terrorists may very well use a *diverting attack* to draw emergency medical services (EMS) resources away and then launch a larger attack against their main objective. Alternatively, they may launch a primary attack and then have a *secondary device* to target emergency responders.

Terrorist attacks are also always crime scenes and will require the coordination of multiple local, state, and federal agencies. Additionally, plans must be made to interact with and control the media, as they will draw significant attention.

Maniscalco PM, Christen HT: Understanding Terrorism and Managing the Consequences. Upper Saddle River, NJ, Prentice Hall, 2002.

6. What makes a good chemical or biologic weapon (in a terrorist's mind)?

It must be highly lethal or toxic. It must be easy to disperse over large areas and relatively stable in the environment. Additionally, it must be relatively easy to produce from readily available precursor materials. Terrorists would also like the agent to be able to be loaded into delivery systems without putting themselves at risk. Finally, the agent must be able to withstand the energy transfer during delivery (i.e., if it is loaded onto an explosive munition.)

Public health response to biological and chemical weapons: WHO guidance. 2004. Available at www.who. int/csr/delibepidemics/biochemguide/en/

RADIATION

7. What are the basic physics I need to know?

Atoms consist of a nucleus of protons and neutrons (except for hydrogen, which has no neutrons) surrounded by electrons. A given element may exist in the form of different **isotopes,** which have different numbers of neutrons. Some of these isotopes may emit particles and/or electromagnetic energy and are considered **radioisotopes.** Protection from these particles or energy is afforded by *shielding, distance,* and *decreased time of exposure.*

Mettler FA, Voelz GL: Major radiation exposure—What to expect and how to respond. N Engl J Med 346;1554–1561, 2002.

8. Review the different units of radiation.
See Table 77-1.

9. Describe the different types of radiation and their shielding requirements.
See Table 77-2.

10. What are the types of radiation injury?
See Table 77-3.

11. What are the different types of attacks?
See Table 77-4.

TABLE 77-1. DIFFERENT UNITS OF RADIATION

Radiation absorbed dose (rad)	Measure of the energy deposited into a mass of tissue by radiation
	Being replaced by the International System unit the gray (Gy)
Gray (Gy)	100 rad = 1 Gy
	1 Gy = 1 Joule/kilogram
Radiation equivalent, man (rem)	Different types of radiation have different effects on the body. Multiply by a quality factor (QF) to adjust appropriately
	Gamma radiation by definition has a QF of 1.
	1 Gy of pure gamma radiation = 1 rem
Sievert (Sv)	International unit of radiation equivalence
	1 Sv = 100 rem

FM 8-7 NATO Handbook on the Medical Aspects of NBC Defensive Operations AMedP-(B). Available at www.fas.org/nuke/guide/usa/doctrine/dod/fm8-9/toc.htm

12. **Describe the three acute radiation syndromes (ARS).**
   - **Bone marrow syndrome (also known as hematopoietic syndrome):** Occurs with a 0.7–10 Gy (70–1000 rad) exposure. Damage occurs to stem cells in the bone marrow, causing a drop in all cell lines. Patients present with anorexia, fever, and malaise. Patients receiving less than 6 Gy should survive, but it may take months to 2 years to recover. Death, if it occurs, is primarily caused by infection and bleeding.
   - **Gastrointestinal (GI) syndrome:** Occurs with 10–100 Gy (1000–10,000 rads) exposure. Patients present with severe nausea, vomiting, cramps, diarrhea, and anorexia. In the latent phase, stem cells and GI tract cells are dying. Death will occur within 2 weeks due to severe infection, electrolyte imbalance, and dehydration. The LD_{100} (dose that will kill 100% of exposed patients) is approximately 10 Gy (1000 rads).
   - **Central nervous system (CNS):** >50 Gy (5000 rads). Patients present with all the symptoms described above plus confusion, seizures, or coma. There is no recovery, and most patients will die within 3 days of exposure.

   Centers for Disease Control and Prevention: Acute radiation syndrome fact sheet for physicians. Available at www.bt.cdc.gov/radiation/arsphysicianfactsheet.asp

13. **What are the four stages of ARS?**
   - **Prodromal stage:** Patients experience nausea, vomiting, and possibly diarrhea depending on the dose. Symptoms can occur minutes to days after exposure and may last episodically from minutes to several days.
   - **Latent stage:** The initial symptoms resolve, and the patient may look and feel healthy for hours to possibly a few weeks.
   - **Manifest illness stage:** Symptoms will appear depending on the specific syndromes. They can last hours to months.
   - **Recovery or death:** The patients who do not recover will likely die within several months of the exposure. Recovery may take anywhere from several weeks up to 2 years.

   Medical Management of Radiologic Casualties Handbook, Armed Forces Radiobiology Research Institute, 1999. Available at www.afrri.usuhs.mil/www/outreach/pdf/radiologicalhandbooksp99-2.pdf

TABLE 77-2.	DIFFERENT TYPES OF RADIATION AND SHIELDING REQUIREMENTS	
Radiation	Description	Shielding
Alpha particles	Consist of two neutrons and two protons that have been ejected from the nucleus of a radioactive atom	Stopped by paper
	A doubly charged particle that loses its energy quickly in matter	
	Generally only dangerous if inhaled or swallowed	
Beta particles	High-energy electrons that are emitted from a nucleus along with an antineutrino	Interact less with target material
	Much smaller than alpha particles and have only one charge	Require plastic, glass or thin metal
	Like alpha particles, they can cause damage if swallowed or inhaled.	Some levels of PPE
	May also cause cellular damage to unprotected skin	
	Largely found in fallout radiation	
Gamma	Not particles but rather *uncharged* pulses of very high-energy electromagnetic radiation	Concrete, earth, or dense metal such as lead
	No mass or charge and only lose their energy when they collide with the electron shell of target atoms	
	Easily pass through the human body	
	Potential to cause significant cellular damage	
Neutrons	Uncharged particles emitted during nuclear detonation; not a fallout hazard	Thick concrete or significant amount of earth
	About the same mass as a proton but no charge	
	Because of this lack of charge, they interact directly with the nucleus of target atom instead of its electrons.	
	Do not react well with material so can travel large distances	
	Can cause previously stable atoms to become radioactive	

PPE = personal protective equipment.
Medical Management of Radiologic Casualties Handbook, Armed Forces Radiobiology Research Institute, 1999. Available at www.afrri.usuhs.mil/www/outreach/pdf/radiologicalhandbooksp99-2.pdf

TABLE 77-3. DIFFERENT TYPES OF RADIATION INJURY

Irradiation	Electromagnetic radiation such as gamma rays pass through an object. If that object is a person, then significant cellular damage may take place. That person is not considered radioactive and is not a threat to medical personnel.
Contamination	Particulate radiation (alpha, beta, or neutrons) is deposited on, swallowed by, or inhaled by the patient. After appropriate PPE, rescuers may provide stabilizing treatment, as the contamination is not an immediate life threat.
Incorporation	Radioactive material is ingested, inhaled, or absorbed. This allows the material to cause ongoing damage.

PPE = personal protective equipment.
Markovchick VJ: Radiation injuries. In Marx JA, Hockberger RS (eds): Rosen's Emergency Medicine: Concepts and Clinical Practice, 5th ed. St. Louis, Mosby, 2002, pp 1066–1074.

TABLE 77-4. DIFFERENT TYPES OF RADIATION ATTACKS

Nuclear detonation	If a government or terrorist group could find a way to deliver or smuggle a conventional nuclear weapon into the country, this would obviously cause a catastrophic incident. There is debate as to the existence and location of "suitcase bombs" that hypothetically could be sneaked into the United States.
Environmental release	A highly radioactive material could be set out in a public place or dispersed into the food or water supply. The actual amount of injury would be limited, but the fear this would generate makes this a useful terror tactic.
Radiation dispersal device (dirty bomb)	"Dirty bombs" are conventional explosives with radioactive material attached to them. The resulting explosion disperses the material over an area proportional to the power of the explosion. The majority of destruction will come from the explosion itself. Again, this is a terror weapon as well as an incredible nuisance. The radioactive contamination will cause fear as well as a real decontamination nightmare.
Nuclear reactor	Hypothetically, a direct attack on a nuclear reactor could cause a meltdown and subsequent release of highly radioactive material into the atmosphere.

Emergency Preparedness and Response: Radiation Emergencies Frequently Asked Questions, Centers for Disease Control. Available at www.bt.cdc.gov/radiation/emergencyfaq.asp

14. **These numbers are hurting my brain. What is the bottom line?**
    - 50% of patients who receive 3.5 Gy will be dead in 30 days without treatment.
    - An exposure of less than 1 Gy rarely leads to ARS.
    - Casualties who receive more than 8 Gy will likely die.
    - Vomiting less than 1 hour after exposure indicates a severe exposure (> 4–6 Gy) and a high likelihood of dying.
    - Nausea, vomiting, and diarrhea within 4 hours of exposure suggest a high but potentially treatable exposure.

    Koenig KL, Goans RE, Hatchett RJ, et al: Medical treatment of radiological casualties: Current concepts. Ann Emerg Med 45:643–652, 2005.

15. **Why is the absolute lymphocyte count helpful?**
    See Table 77-5.

TABLE 77-5. ROLE OF THE ABSOLUTE LYMPHOCYTE COUNT		
Minimal Lymphocyte Count Within 48 hours of Exposure	**Estimated Absorbed Dose (Gy)**	**Prognosis**
1000–3000	0–0.5	Likely no injury
1000–1500	1–2	Significant but good prognosis
500–1000	2–4	Severe, may survive
100–500	4–8	Very severe, likely die
<100	>8	Will likely die

Koenig KL, Goans RE, Hatchett RJ, et al: Medical treatment of radiological casualties: Current concepts. Ann Emerg Med 45:643–652, 2005.

16. **Why are survivalists stockpiling potassium iodine (KI) tablets?**
    An attack on or an accident at a nuclear reactor may release a cloud of radioactive iodine into the atmosphere. The principle behind taking KI tablets is to saturate the thyroid with nonradioactive iodine before one is exposed to radioactive iodine. It is only protective against radioactive iodine and not other forms of radiation. In theory, government officials should alert the public that a release contains radioactive iodine and that KI tablets are indicated. Many areas near nuclear reactors have stockpiles of KI tablets, but some people choose to have their own.

    Potassium Iodine: U.S. Food and Drug Administration. Available at www.fda.gov/cder/guidance/4825fnl.htm

17. **What other treatment options do I have?**
    Aggressive supportive care is the cornerstone of therapy. Victims of radiation exposure should be treated as immunocompromised patients with close attention paid to supporting the hematopoietic system. Other treatments include KI, diethylenetriaminepentaacetate (DTPA), Prussian blue, and Neupogen. Full coverage of these agents is beyond the scope of this chapter, but there is an excellent overview of weapons of mass destruction in general and these treatments in particular on the Centers for Disease Control and Prevention (CDC) Web site.

    Emergency Preparedness and Response: Radiation Emergencies. Centers for Disease Control. Available at www.bt.cdc.gov/radiation

CHEMICAL AGENTS

18. **List the general characteristics used to describe chemical weapons.**
    - **Volatility** describes the tendency of a liquid to evaporate into a gas. Most chemical weapons are liquids at normal atmospheric pressures and temperatures and are dispersed as fine liquid droplets after detonation. The more volatile chemicals, such as phosgene and cyanide, will evaporate into a gas quickly. Less volatile agents, such as the nerve agent VX and sulfur mustard, will remain liquid. Also, all agents except hydrogen cyanide are heavier than air and will concentrate in low lying places.
    - **Persistence** relates inversely to volatility. Persistent chemicals will remain on objects and patients longer, creating the potential for ongoing exposure and contamination. The military categorizes agents as persistent or nonpersistent based on their ability to vaporize in less than or greater than 24 hours. VX, for instance, can persist 30–80 days if conditions are right.
    - **Toxicity** is the ability of an agent to cause harm to a person. The usual measurement is the concentration-time product (Ct). This is the product of the concentration in the air times the time a patient is exposed. One can go further and look at the LCt_{50}, which is the Ct of a vapor or aerosol that will kill 50% of those exposed to the agent.
    - **Latency** is the delay between a patient being exposed to an agent and the manifestation of signs and symptoms. With some agents, the cellular damage occurs very quickly, but the evidence of that damage may be delayed significantly. Health care providers must be acutely aware of this principle because victims who do not show any clinical signs or symptoms may still be exposed and need to be decontaminated.

    Public health response to biological and chemical weapons: WHO guidance. 2004. Available at www.who.int/csr/delibepidemics/biochemguide/en/

19. **What are the different classes of chemical weapons?**
    See Table 77-6.

TABLE 77-6. CLASSES OF CHEMICAL WEAPONS			
Class	Description	Signs and Symptoms	Examples and Designation
Blister agents/ vesicants	Damages cellular components and creates blisters on dermal and mucosal surfaces minutes to hours later	Dyspnea, dermal irritation and pain, vesicles, conjunctivitis, possibly severe respiratory compromise	Lewisite (L) Nitrogen mustard Phosgene oxime Sulfur mustard
Blood agents	Absorbed into the bloodstream and interferes with aerobic metabolism	Dyspnea, chest pain, anxiety, flushed skin	Arsine (SA) Carbon monoxide Cyanogen chloride (CK) Hydrogen cyanide Potassium cyanide (KCN) Sodium cyanide (NaCN) Sodium monofluoroacetate (compound 1080)

Continued

TABLE 77-6.   CLASSES OF CHEMICAL WEAPONS—CONT'D

Class	Description	Signs and Symptoms	Examples and Designation
Caustics	Directly burn and irritate mucous membranes, skin and eyes	Burning and severe irritation, pulmonary irritation if inhaled	Hydrofluoric acid
Choking/ pulmonary agents	Irritate the lining of the lungs and throat, causing edema of the mucous membranes	Coughing, dyspnea, dysphagia, chest pain, eye irritation, burning sensation in throat	Ammonia Bromine (Br) Chlorine (Cl) Hydrogen chloride Phosgene (CG) Sulfuryl fluoride
Incapacitating agents	Cause altered mental status and affect victim's ability to think clearly	Altered mental status, anticholinergic syndrome (BZ), opioid toxidrome	3-quinuclidinyl benzilate (BZ) Fentanyl (aerosolized)
Nerve agents	Inhibit acetylcholinesterase thereby interfering with nerve transmission	Cholinergic toxidrome. Salivation, lacrimation, paralysis	Sarin (GB) Soman (GD) Tabun (GA) VX
Riot control/ tear gas	Very irritating but nonlethal agents used for crowd control and riot suppression		Bromobenzylcyanide (CA) Chloroacetophenone (CN) Chlorobenzylidenemalono-nitrile (CS) Chloropicrin (PS) Dibenzoxazepine (CR)
Vomiting agents	Ocular, nasal, and respiratory tract irritation; GI upset and vomiting	Vomiting starting minutes to hours after exposure	Adamsite (DM)

GI = gastrointestinal.
Emergency Preparedness and Response: Chemical Emergencies, Centers for Disease Control.
Available at www.bt.cdc.gov/chemical

20. **Give me a little more detail about the pathophysiology and clinical symptoms caused by nerve agents.**
    - **Pathophysiology:** All nerve agents block the enzyme acetylcholinesterase. This causes a buildup of the neurotransmitter acetylcholine (ACH) at postsynaptic junctions. This causes overstimulation of muscarinic and nicotinic receptors in the parasympathetic nervous system (PNS) and CNS. Stimulation of muscarinic receptors causes activity of exocrine glands (e.g., salivation, bronchorrhea). Stimulation of the nicotinic receptors is responsible for muscle fasciculations, flaccid paralysis, hypertension, and tachycardia.
    - **Symptoms:** This creates a cholinergic toxidrome that can be remembered by the **SLUDGE** mnemonic. Patients may exhibit some combination of **S**alivation, **L**acrimation, **U**rination, **D**efecation, **G**astrointestinal symptoms, and **E**mesis. CNS effects can cause seizures, coma, and apnea. Survivors may have psychologic changes lasting for weeks.

21. **How do I treat a patient with nerve agent toxicity?**
    Treatment is based on a three-pronged approach. Atropine is given to counteract the muscarinic effects, thereby drying up secretions and improving ventilation. Pralidoxime chloride (2-PAM) reverses the nicotinic effects of nerve agents, thereby reversing paralysis. When nerve agents combine with ACH, a process called "aging" takes place during which a permanent covalent bond is formed and the enzyme is permanently deactivated. To be effective, 2-PAM must be administered before this happens. This time ranges from 2 minutes for Soman (GD) to 48 hours for VX. Finally, seizures are treated with diazepam.

    Schultz, CH, Koenig KL: Weapons of mass destruction. In Marx JA, Hockberger RS (eds): Rosen's Emergency Medicine: Concepts and Clinical Practice, 5th ed. St. Louis, Mosby, 2002, pp 2641–2648.
    World Health Organization: Public health response to biological and chemical weapons: WHO guidance, 2004. Annex 1: Chemical Weapons. Available at www.who.int/csr/delibepidemics/annex1.pdf

22. **Just how deadly are nerve agents?**
    The lethal dose of VX, which will kill half of exposed victims (LD_{50}) is 10 mg (skin exposure) on a 70-kg man. To give you a frame of reference, this means that a drop of VX that is large enough to cover two columns on the Lincoln Memorial on the back of a U.S. penny is enough to kill half of exposed victims who have this placed on exposed skin.

    Newmark J: Nerve agents. Neurol Clin 23:623–641, 2005.

BIOLOGIC AGENTS

23. **What is bioterrorism? Is it a new phenomenon?**
    It is the intentional release of infectious viruses, infectious bacteria, or naturally derived toxins with the intent to cause incapacitation or death. Biologic warfare has been around for centuries.

    Jacobs MK: The history of biologic warfare and bioterrorism. Dermatol Clin 22:231–246, 2004.

24. **Have biologic agents ever been used by terrorists?**
    The answer is absolutely "yes." Several mailings of anthrax spores were sent through the U.S. mail in the fall of 2001. This caused 22 infections (11 cutaneous and 11 inhalational) and 5 deaths. Additionally, 750 people in Oregon became sick after eating at salad bars in four different restaurants, which had been intentionally laced with *Salmonella* by the Bagwan Sri Rajneesh sect.

    Inglesby TV, O'Toole T, Henderson DA, et al: Anthrax as a biological weapon: Updated recommendations for management. JAMA 287:2236–2252, 2002.
    Maniscalco PM, Christen HT: Understanding Terrorism and Managing the Consequences, Upper Saddle River, NJ, Prentice Hall, 2002.

25. **Doesn't it take lots of government funding and fancy equipment to make biologic agents?**

    To a point yes, but this is much less true than it is for chemical and nuclear weapons. There is a saying that "if you can make beer you can make bugs." It is not too difficult for a motivated terrorist to make a biologic weapon. The U.S. military has seized documents in Afghanistan suggesting that Al Qaeda has done research on a variety of WMD, including biologic weapons.

    Gostin LO, Sapsin JW, Teret SP, et al: The model state emergency health powers act: Planning for and response to bioterrorism and naturally occurring infectious diseases. JAMA 288:622–628.

    Maniscalco PM, Christen HT: Understanding Terrorism and Managing the Consequences, Upper Saddle River, NJ, Prentice Hall, 2002.

26. **Is there much difference between biologic attacks and the others we have talked about?**

    In many ways, biologic attacks are the most frightening. First of all, it may not be apparent that an attack has even happened until days later when symptoms arise. Even then, it may take awhile for clinicians to see a pattern and realize an attack occurred. By that time, the persons who were initially exposed may have traveled to different parts of the country or the world. If one is dealing with an agent that has a high person-to-person transmission potential, this could also cause a significant epidemic, not to mention panic and hysteria.

    Macintyre AG, Christopher GW, Eitzen E, et al: Weapons of mass destruction events with contaminated casualties: Effective planning for health care facilities. JAMA 282:242–249, 2000.

    Maniscalco PM, Christen HT: Understanding Terrorism and Managing the Consequences. Upper Saddle River, NJ, Prentice Hall, 2002.

27. **How does the CDC categorize the different biologic agents?**

    In 1999 the CDC divided up the various infectious agents into three categories (A, B, and C) according to each organism's ability to have the greatest negative impact on the public's health and potentially overwhelm public health resources (Table 77-7).

    Centers for Disease Control and Prevention: Biological and Chemical Terrorism: Strategic Plan for Preparedness and Response. Recommendations of the CDC Strategic Planning Workgroup. MMWR 49(No. RR-4):[inclusive page numbers], 2004. Available at www.cdc.gov/mmwr/PDF/rr/rr4904.pdf

28. **Describe the general characteristics used to describe biologic agents.**
    See Table 77-8.

29. **Give me a rundown on anthrax.**

    Anthrax is caused by *Bacillus anthracis,* which is an aerobic, gram-positive, spore-forming, nonmotile organism. The spores are very hardy and can exist in the environment for decades. The disease can occur as an *inhalational, gastrointestinal,* and *cutaneous* form. It was historically transmitted from livestock such as sheep. Now anthrax has been prepared and used as a weapon that is aerosolized and distributed deliberately. After the anthrax spores are inhaled, they are taken up by macrophages in the lung and taken to mediastinal lymph nodes, where they transform into vegetative cells. Once the bacteria start replicating, they produce toxins that cause edema, hemorrhage, and necrosis.

    Inglesby TV, O'Toole T, Henderson DA, et al: Anthrax as a biological weapon: Updated recommendations for management. JAMA 287:2236–2252, 2002.

30. **What are the signs and symptoms?**

    Inhalational anthrax begins with nonspecific presentation. Of 10 patients presenting with inhalational anthrax in the 2001 attacks, all had fever, chills, malaise, and fatigue. Most developed some degree of cough, chest discomfort, and dyspnea. All of them had some chest x-ray abnormality, including widened mediastinum, pleural effusions, air bronchograms, necrotizing

TABLE 77-7. CDC CATEGORIZATION OF BIOLOGIC AGENTS

Category Definitions

Category A Diseases/Agents

The U.S. public health system and primary health care providers must be prepared to address various biologic agents, including pathogens that are rarely seen in the United States. High-priority agents include organisms that pose a risk to national security because they can be easily disseminated or transmitted from person to person, result in high mortality rates and have the potential for major public health impact, might cause public panic and social disruption, and require special action for public health preparedness.

Category A

Anthrax (*Bacillus anthracis*)

Botulism (*Clostridium botulinum toxin*)

Plague (*Yersinia pestis*)

Smallpox (*Variola major*)

Tularemia (*Francisella tularensis*)

Viral hemorrhagic fevers (filoviruses [e.g., Ebola, Marburg] and arenaviruses [e.g., Lassa, Machupo])

Category B Diseases/Agents

Second highest priority agents include those that are moderately easy to disseminate, result in moderate morbidity rates and low mortality rates, and require specific enhancements of CDC's diagnostic capacity and enhanced disease surveillance.

Category B

Brucellosis (*Brucella* species)

Epsilon toxin of *Clostridium perfringens*

Food safety threats (e.g., *Salmonella* species, *Escherichia coli* O157:H7, *Shigella*)

Glanders (*Burkholderia mallei*)

Melioidosis (*Burkholderia pseudomallei*)

Psittacosis (*Chlamydia psittaci*)

Q fever (*Coxiella burnetii*)

Ricin toxin from *Ricinus communis* (castor beans)

Staphylococcal enterotoxin B

Typhus fever (*Rickettsia prowazekii*)

Viral encephalitis (alphaviruses [e.g., Venezuelan equine encephalitis, eastern equine encephalitis, western equine encephalitis])

Water safety threats (e.g., *Vibrio cholerae*, *Cryptosporidium parvum*)

Continued

TABLE 77-7.	CDC CATEGORIZATION OF BIOLOGIC AGENTS—CONT'D	
Category C Diseases/Agents	Category C
Third highest priority agents include emerging pathogens that could be engineered for mass dissemination in the future because of availability, ease of production and dissemination, and potential for high morbidity and mortality rates and major health impact.	Emerging infectious diseases such as Nipah virus and hantavirus

CDC = Centers for Disease Control and Prevention.

TABLE 77-8.	GENERAL CHARACTERISTICS OF BIOLOGIC AGENTS
Infectivity	The ability of an agent to enter, multiply, and survive in a host
	ID_{50} is the dose that would infect 50% of an exposed population.
Virulence	The relative severity of the disease
	Different strains of the same agent can cause varying severities of disease.
Incubation period	Time between exposure and onset of symptoms
Lethality	The ability of an agent to cause death
Contagiousness	Measured by the number of secondary cases occurring after exposure to the primary case
Mechanisms of transmission	Manner by which the disease is transmitted (i.e., respiratory, blood borne, vector born, food contamination)

Public health response to biological and chemical weapons: WHO guidance (2004). Available at: www.who.int/csr/delibepidemics/biochemguide/en/

pneumonic lesions, or consolidations. Any nonspecific febrile illness with pulmonary symptoms and an abnormal chest x-ray in previously healthy patients should raise the suspicion for anthrax.

Inglesby TV, O'Toole T, Henderson DA, et al: Anthrax as a biological weapon: Updated recommendations for management. JAMA 287:2236–2252, 2002.

31. **How do I treat it?**
In general, ciprofloxacin and doxycycline are the mainstays. Because the spores can last quite a long time and germinate at any time, current recommendations are to treat for 60 days.

Inglesby TV, O'Toole T, Henderson DA, et al: Anthrax as a biological weapon: Updated recommendations for management. JAMA 287:2236–2252, 2002.

32. **What else should I do if I'm serious about learning about biologic weapons?**

Read the series of articles entitled *Medical and Public Health Management Following the Use of a Biological Weapon: Consensus Statements of the Working Group on Civilian Biodefense,* which were published in the Journal of the American Medical Association (JAMA). They are available free on the JAMA Web site and are an excellent source of information.

- **Anthrax:** jama.ama-assn.org/cgi/reprint/287/17/2236.pdf
- **Botulism:** jama.ama-assn.org/cgi/reprint/285/8/1059.pdf
- **Hemorrhagic fevers:** jama.ama-assn.org/cgi/reprint/287/18/2391.pdf
- **Plague:** jama.ama-assn.org/cgi/reprint/283/17/2281.pdf
- **Smallpox:** jama.ama-assn.org/cgi/reprint/281/22/2127.pdf
- **Tularemia:** jama.ama-assn.org/cgi/reprint/285/21/2763.pdf

33. **How do I protect myself while taking care of these patients?**

As always, universal precautions are a must. Table 77-9 highlights transmission and isolation issues.

TABLE 77-9. TRANSMISSION AND ISOLATION ISSUES WITH BIOLOGIC AGENTS

Illness	Weaponized Vector	Person to Person?	Isolation Required?
Anthrax	Aerosolized particles	No	No
Botulism	Aerosol or food	No	No
Hemorrhagic fevers	Aerosolized particles	Yes	Yes
Plague	Aerosolized particles	Yes (pneumonic form)	Yes
Smallpox	Aerosolized particles	Yes	Yes
Tularemia	Aerosol or water	Likely not	No

Shannon M: Management of infectious agents of bioterrorism. Clin Pediatr Emerg Med 5:63–71, 2004.

KEY POINTS: WEAPONS OF MASS DESTRUCTION

1. The ideal terrorist weapon is cheap, is easy to manufacture, is easy to disseminate, and will produce large numbers of casualties.

2. The most likely radiologic incident will be a radiologic dispersal device that involves using a conventional explosive to disperse some radioactive material.

3. A chemical agent attack will generally be recognized by having a large number of casualties presenting with similar symptoms in a short period of time in a relatively small geographic area.

4. In the event of a biologic agent attack, all patients should be considered to be infectious until a definitive diagnosis of a nontransmissible agent in confirmed.

34. **How will I know if a biologic attack has occurred?**

As stated previously, this may be very difficult. Terrorists may not announce an attack because they would like for the disease to spread as far as possible or have the largest number of persons unknowingly exposed that they can. Dr. Paul Rega published a list of "covert assault clues" that clinicians can use to look for possible biologic attacks:

- Severe manifestations of disease in previously healthy people
- Greater than normal numbers of patients with fever, respiratory, and/or GI complaints
- Multiple patients with similar complaints from a common location
- An endemic disease that occurs during an unusual time of year
- An unusual number of rapidly fatal cases
- A greater number of sick or dead animals
- Rapidly rising and falling epidemic curve
- Larger number of patients with severe pneumonia, sepsis, sepsis with coagulopathy, fever with rash, or diplopia with progressive weakness

Burkle FM: Mass casualty management of a large-scale bioterrorist event: An epidemiological approach that shapes triage decisions. Emerg Med Clin North Am 20:409–436, 2002.

Rega P: Bio-terry: A stat manual to identify and treat diseases of biological terrorism. Maumee, Ohio, Mascap, Inc, 2000, pp 1–4.

35. **What if I suspect an attack has occurred?**

Every hospital should have a plan in place that EPs should be familiar with. If there is a suspicion of a biologic weapon (BW) release, state and local public health officials as well as the CDC and Federal Bureau of Investigation should be notified as soon as possible.

EXPLOSIVES

36. **Aren't conventional explosives pretty "old school?"**

NBC weapons are very frightening but are difficult to acquire, transport, and disperse in such a way as to create large numbers of casualties. Many more people have died as a result of conventional explosives. For example, there were 518 injuries and 168 deaths after Timothy McVeigh detonated a fuel oil and fertilizer bomb in Oklahoma City in 1995. In addition, the Madrid train bombing of March 11, 2004, the 1995 al Qaeda attacks on U.S. embassies in Tanzania and Kenya, and the multiple suicide bombings in Israel demonstrate that conventional explosives are still very much a part of the terrorist's arsenal.

Depalma RG, Burris DG, Champion HR, et al: Blast injuries. N Engl J Med 352:13, 2005.

Hoffman B: Inside Terrorism. Columbia University Press, New York, 1998.

37. **Describe the four effects of a conventional explosion.**

- **Primary** or **direct** effects are due to the direct effect of the pressure wave. This can result in tympanic membrane (TM) rupture, pulmonary barotrauma with air embolization, and rupture of hollow organs.
- **Secondary** effects include penetrating trauma from flying debris or fragments that are built into the explosive device and designed to inflict more damage on victims.
- **Tertiary** effects are caused by structural collapse or the result of persons being thrown by the blast wind. This also includes crush injuries and blunt injury from large flying objects.
- **Quaternary** effects include burns, exposure to toxic chemicals, and asphyxia.

Centers for Disease Control: Explosions and blast injuries: A primer for clinicians. Available at www.bt.cdc.gov/masstrauma/pdf/explosions-blast-injuries.pdf

Depalma RG, Burris DG, Champion HR, et al: Blast injuries. N Engl J Med 352:13, 2005.

38. Give me a quick screening method to triage victims of blast injury.

Otoscopic examination of the TM is a quick (but not foolproof) way to asses the severity of blast injury. The TM can be ruptured by an increase in atmospheric pressure as low as 5 psi above normal. If there is no TM rupture, then the chance of hollow organ injury is significantly lower. It is not zero, however. It was found that in 17 critically injured patients after the Madrid train bombing, 13 had ruptured TMs, but 4 did not. Obviously, if other symptoms such as shortness of breath are present, one must suspect other injuries.

Depalma RG, Burris DG, Champion HR, et al: Blast injuries. N Engl J Med 352:13, 2005.

39. What is "blast lung?"

It is pulmonary barotrauma after an explosion. The shearing forces exerted on the lungs during an explosion can cause pulmonary hemorrhage, pneumothorax, and pulmonary air embolism. Any patient with ruptured TMs should receive a chest x-ray and be observed for at least 8 hours.

Depalma RG, Burris DG, Champion HR, et al: Blast injuries. N Engl J Med 352:13, 2005.

DECONTAMINATION

40. What do I need to know about decontamination?

With both radiologic and chemical exposures, decontamination is critical, both for the individual patient and to prevent cross-contamination of other patients, health care workers, and facilities. The timing is different, however. Chemical decontamination is an emergency and very time critical, whereas radiation contamination is not.

41. How do I decontaminate victims of chemical exposure?

First, rescuers must use the appropriate level of PPE. Then victims must be completely disrobed but in a fashion that protects their modesty if possible. If possible, decontamination should occur in the prehospital setting before they arrive at the ED. However, as was discovered in the Tokyo subway attacks, hospitals also need to have either prebuilt or easily assembled decontamination shower facilities for patients. Washing with copious amounts of soap and water should be effective in getting surface contamination off.

U.S. Army Medical Research Institute of Chemical Defense (USAMRICD): Medical Management of Chemical casualties handbook, 3rd ed, 2000. Available at www.gmha.org/bioterrorism/usamricd/Yellow_Book_2000.pdf

42. Is there anything that will neutralize these agents?

Traditionally, it was taught to use a 0.5% hypochlorite (household bleach) solution because it inactivates biologic agents (except mycotoxins) and chemical agents. Some authors question this because it takes 15–20 minutes of contact time and can damage skin that has already been injured. Copious irrigation with water is always a safe bet.

Macintyre AG, Christopher GW, Eitzen E, et al: Weapons of mass destruction events with contaminated casualties. JAMA 283:242–249. Available at jama.ama-assn.org/cgi/reprint/283/2/242.pdf.

43. What if they are contaminated with radioactive material?

From a personal protection standpoint, once the patients are out of the hazardous environment, using level D (scrubs, masks, gloves, eye protection, and shoe coverings) is adequate. Personnel should also be issued a dosimeter to measure radiation exposure. There are two components to the decontamination process.

- **Gross decontamination** involves removing all of the patient's clothing and bagging it for appropriate disposal. The patients should be rinsed off head to toe with copious amounts of water. Care should be taken so that the water flushes material away from the eyes, nose, and mouth. This process is estimated to remove ~95% of contamination.

- **Secondary decontamination** is a much more methodical process to fully ensure that a patient is decontaminated. This should be performed with the hospital's radiation safety officer and by using radiation detection equipment. Eyes, ears, mucous membranes, and wounds should be swabbed, and the swabs should be analyzed for radioactivity. Additionally, these same areas should be copiously irrigated. The patient's eyes should be anesthetized and copiously irrigated. The ears should be checked for perforated TMs and irrigated copiously if intact. Dentures should be removed and the mouth rinsed copiously without swallowing the rinse water. Wounds should also be irrigated and covered with waterproof dressings to avoid run-off contamination from irrigating other areas.

Medical Management of Radiologic Casualties Handbook. Armed Forces Radiobiology Research Institute, 1999. Available at www.afrri.usuhs.mil/www/outreach/pdf/radiologicalhandbooksp99–2.pdf

Weingart SD, Maltz BR: CBRNE—Nuclear and Radiologic Decontamination. Available at www.emedicine.com/emerg/topic941.htm

CHAPTER 78

CARDIOVASCULAR TOXICOLOGY

Jody J. Rogers, MD, and Kennon Heard, MD

1. **What effects do different poisons have on the heart rate, blood pressure, and QRS duration?**

    A list of the presenting signs of common cardiovascular poisons is shown in Table 78-1.

TABLE 78-1. CARDIOVASCULAR EFFECTS OF DIFFERENT POISONS

Bradycardia with hypertension

- Phenylpropanolamine: Causes a reflex bradycardia because of its vasoconstrictive and hypertensive effects
- Alpha$_2$ agonists (clonidine): Usually patients progress to bradycardia and hypotension by the time they reach the hospital.

Bradycardia with hypotension and narrow-complex QRS

- Alpha$_2$ agonists (clonidine): Inhibit the release of norepinephrine in the central nervous system, resulting in vasodilation, bradycardia, and somnolence
- Beta blockers (BBs) without sodium channel effects (see later)
- Calcium channel blockers (CCBs) (see later)
- Cardiac glycosides (see later)
- Sedative-hypnotics, opiates, and barbiturates decrease CNS sympathetic outflow.
- Organophosphates and carbamates by increasing vagal tone (tachycardia also possible from stimulation of sympathetic ganglionic neurons)
- Lidocaine, tocainide (class 1b antiarrhythmics)

Bradycardia with hypotension and wide-complex QRS

- BBs with sodium channel effects (propranolol, acebutolol, metoprolol)
- CCBs (severe toxicity causes ventricular escape rhythms)
- Cardiac glycosides (severe toxicity causes ventricular escape rhythms)
- Propafenone and flecainide (class 1c antiarrhythmics that cause sodium channel blockade): Initially, patients bradycardic with wide QRS, due to decreased cardiac conduction, that may degenerate into ventricular tachycardia
- Quinidine, procainamide, and disopyramide (class 1a antiarrhythmics that cause sodium channel blockade, prolonged QRS and QT intervals): Patients may present with bradycardia, due to decreased cardiac conduction that may degenerate into ventricular tachycardia.
- Hyperkalemia from cardiac glycosides, BBs, and potassium-sparing diuretics

---

Continued

TABLE 78-1. CARDIOVASCULAR EFFECTS OF DIFFERENT POISONS—CONT'D

Tachycardia with hypertension

- Sympathomimetics (amphetamines, cocaine, LSD, marijuana, ephedrine, pseudoephedrine) by directly stimulating the sympathetic nervous system
- Anticholinergics: Due to decrease in vagal tone and agitation from delirium
- Monoamine oxidase inhibitors: Inhibit the breakdown of catecholamines in central nervous system synapses

Tachycardia with hypotension and narrow-complex QRS

- Angiotensin-converting enzyme inhibitors: Due to vasodilation and reflex tachycardia
- Alpha$_1$ antagonists (prazosin, terazosin, doxazosin): Cause vasodilation and reflex tachycardia
- Phenothiazines: Due to alpha$_1$-antagonism causing vasodilation and reflex tachycardia
- Diuretics: Cause tachycardia and hypotension secondary to dehydration
- Nitrates: Cause vasodilation and reflex tachycardia
- Theophylline and caffeine: Due to stimulation of the sympathetic nervous system

Tachycardia with hypotension and wide-complex QRS

- Tricyclic antidepressants have effects on sodium channels causing widening of the QRS complex. (In severe toxicity, this can lead to hypotension despite tachycardia from anticholinergic effects.)
- Cocaine: Sodium channel effects that late in the course override the ability to maintain blood pressure from tachycardia and vasoconstriction

CNS = central nervous system; LSD = lysergic acid diethylamide.

---

2. **What drugs cause cardiovascular toxicity by blocking cardiac sodium channels?**
    Many drugs bind to sodium channels when studied in vitro; however, some of these drugs rarely show cardiac effects or show these effects only in massive overdose. The major clinical manifestations of sodium channel blockade are prolongation of the QRS duration and ventricular arrhythmias.
    - **Drugs with primary toxic effects on sodium channel** include quinidine, flecainide, mexiletine, disopyramide, and procainamide.
    - **Drugs with sodium channel effects and other serious effects** include tricyclic antidepressants, propranolol, cocaine, chloroquine, propafenone, and thioridazine. Patients poisoned with these agents often present with other symptoms, but it is common to see prolonged QRS duration or arrhythmias as a toxic effect.
    - **Drugs with sodium channel effects that are seen only in massive ingestions** include diphenhydramine, dimenhydrinate, carbamazepine, lidocaine, and norpropoxyphene (a metabolite of propoxyphene). Patients poisoned with these agents present with other symptoms but should be observed and treated if prolonged QRS duration or arrhythmias develop.

3. **What is the antidote for drugs that cause sodium channel blockade?**
    Sodium bicarbonate (1–2 mEq/kg as a bolus) is used for the treatment of arrhythmias or prolongation of the QRS duration (>120 msec) that occurs after the ingestion of any of these

agents. If the QRS duration does not narrow after administration of sodium bicarbonate, a second bolus should be given. Hyperventilation should be initiated to induce a serum pH of 7.5–7.55. In addition to bicarbonate, patients with cardiovascular toxicity also likely require fluids and vasopressors for hypotension, benzodiazepines for seizures, and endotracheal intubation for altered mental status.

Wax PM: Sodium bicarbonate. In Goldfrank LR, Flomenbaum NE, Lewin NA, et al (eds): Goldfrank's Toxicologic Emergencies, 7th ed. New York, McGraw-Hill, 2002, pp 519–525.

4. **How do patients with a calcium channel blocker (CCB) overdose present?**
CCBs decrease calcium influx into cardiac tissue and vascular smooth muscle. The heart depends on calcium for automaticity, conduction through the atrioventricular node, and contractility. Vascular smooth muscle requires calcium to maintain tone. Patients with CCB overdose present with hypotension (owing to decreased contractility and decreased vascular tone) and initial tachycardia that often progresses to bradycardia and atrioventricular blocks. If hypotension is significant, patients may have altered mental status, organ ischemia, and acidosis.

Kerns W, Kline J, Ford MD: Beta blocker and calcium channel blocker toxicity. Emerg Med Clin North Am 12:365–390, 1994.

5. **Describe the treatment for CCB overdose.**
Begin treatment with the ABCs (airway, breathing, circulation). Gastric decontamination can proceed after the airway is adequately protected. Hypotension is treated initially with fluid boluses (i.e., 2 L NS), and symptomatic bradycardia is treated with atropine or pacing. Calcium is usually the next step in treatment for toxicity. The dose is 1–2 gm of calcium chloride intravenously and may be repeated every 10 minutes three to four times. Occasionally, an infusion of calcium may be needed. Inotropic agents, such as dopamine or norepinephrine, sometimes at high doses, are used next. Glucagon (5–10 mg IV push, then if improvement is noted start a drip at 5–10 mg/h) or high-dose insulin (1–2 units/kg bolus, then 1–2 units/h with supplemental glucose) is the next line of therapy. Heroic measures, such as extracorporeal membrane oxygenation, intraaortic balloon pump, and cardiopulmonary bypass, may be used in severe refractory cases.

Kerns W, Kline J, Ford MD: Beta blocker and calcium channel blocker toxicity. Emerg Med Clin North Am 12:365–390, 1994.
Yuan TH, Kerns WP, Thomaszewski CA, et al: Insulin-glucose as adjunctive therapy for sever calcium channel antagonist poisoning. J Toxicol Clin Toxicol 37:463–474, 1999.

6. **How do patients with beta blocker (BB) overdose present?**
BBs compete with endogenous catecholamines for receptor sites; this blunts the normal adrenergic response, leading to bradycardia, atrioventricular blocks, and hypotension from decreased contractility. Patients suffering from BB toxicity present similarly to patients with CCB overdose. There can be a few differences, however, depending on which BB is involved. Some BBs, such as propranolol, are lipid soluble. This allows entry into the central nervous system, leading to seizures and altered mental status unrelated to blood pressure. Some BBs (propranolol, acebutolol, alprenolol, oxprenolol) antagonize sodium channels, leading to a widened QRS. Sotalol also blocks potassium channels, causing a prolonged QT interval and torsades de pointes.

Kerns W, Kline J, Ford MD: Beta blocker and calcium channel blocker toxicity. Emerg Med Clin North Am 12:365–390, 1994.

7. **Describe the treatment for BB toxicity.**
Treatment is similar to that for CCB overdose. Glucagon is the drug of choice for treatment after fluids, vasopressors, and atropine. The dose of glucagon is the same as for CCB overdose. High-dose insulin therapy may be beneficial as well. Calcium has not been well studied for

treatment of BB overdose. Seizures unrelated to hypotension should be treated with benzodiazepines; sodium bicarbonate is used for QRS widening. Refractory sympathetic bradycardia should be treated with external cardiac pacing.

Kerns W, Kline J, Ford MD: Beta blocker and calcium channel blocker toxicity. Emerg Med Clin North Am 12:365–390, 1994.

8. **Describe the manifestations of acute and chronic digoxin poisoning.**
   Acute digoxin toxicity occurs after accidental or intentional ingestion of a supratherapeutic amount of digoxin-containing products. A dose of more than 1 mg in a child and more than 3 mg in an adult is potentially toxic. Patients with acute digoxin toxicity often develop gastrointestinal symptoms, such as nausea or vomiting. The most common cardiac effects are bradycardia and heart block. After acute digoxin ingestion, blockade of the cellular sodium/potassium exchange pump leads to systemic hyperkalemia. Severe hyperkalemia (serum level > 5.5 mEq/L) is associated with a mortality of greater than 90% if untreated.

   Chronic digoxin toxicity occurs when the dose or clearance of digoxin changes in a patient who is receiving digoxin therapy. Initiation of quinidine, amiodarone, spironolactone, or verapamil may change the steady-state clearance of digoxin and result in toxicity. Decreased clearance of digoxin may occur when patients develop renal insufficiency. Symptoms of chronic digoxin toxicity are often subtle and nonspecific, including confusion, anorexia, vomiting, visual changes, and abdominal pain. The patient is often bradycardic with varying degrees of heart block. Patients may develop premature atrial and ventricular contractions, supraventricular tachycardia, ventricular tachycardia, or ventricular fibrillation. In contrast to acute digoxin toxicity, serum potassium is often normal or depressed, unless the patient has hyperkalemia from renal insufficiency.

   Antman EM, Wenger TL, Butler VP: Treatment of 150 cases of life threatening digitalis intoxication with digoxin specific Fab antibody fragments: Final report of a multi-center study. Circulation 81:1744–1752, 1990.
   Lewin NA: Cardiac glycosides. In Goldfrank LR, Flomenbaum NE, Lewin NA, et al (eds): Goldfrank's Toxicologic Emergencies, 7th ed. New York, McGraw-Hill, 2002, pp 724–839.

9. **What are the indications for digoxin immune antibody fragments (Fab)?**
   The most common indications are symptomatic bradycardia, complete heart block, ventricular tachycardia, or ventricular fibrillation. Often, digoxin immune Fab must be administered to critically ill patients without laboratory confirmation of elevated digoxin levels. Fab should be administered to patients who present after an acute ingestion with hyperkalemia or hemodynamically significant dysrhythmias. The indications for Fab therapy for patients with chronic digoxin toxicity are not well defined. Therapy should be considered for patients with hemodynamically significant bradycardia, multifocal ventricular ectopy, and ventricular dysrhythmias. Because serum digoxin levels correlate poorly with symptoms, there is no serum digoxin level that is considered an absolute indication for digoxin Fab.

   Antman EM, Wenger TL, Butler VP: Treatment of 150 cases of life threatening digitalis intoxication with digoxin specific Fab antibody fragments: Final report of a multi-center study. Circulation 81:1744–1752, 1990.
   Lewin NA: Cardiac glycosides. In Goldfrank LR, Flomenbaum NE, Lewin NA, et al (eds): Goldfrank's Toxicologic Emergencies, 7th ed. New York, McGraw-Hill, 2002, pp 724–839.

10. **How is digoxin Fab dosed?**
    Digoxin Fab may be dosed in one of several ways, depending on the information available to the clinician:
    1. If the patient is critically ill, 10–20 vials should be given empirically.
    2. If the amount ingested is known, the following formula should be used: Dose ingested (mg) $\times$ 0.48 $=$ number of vials.

3. If the steady-state serum level is known, the following formula should be used: Serum digoxin level (ng/mL) × patient wt (kg)/100 = number of vials. (This normally results in a patient with chronic toxicity receiving one to three vials.)

Antman EM, Wenger TL, Butler VP: Treatment of 150 cases of life threatening digitalis intoxication with digoxin specific Fab antibody fragments: Final report of a multi-center study. Circulation 81:1744–1752, 1990.

Lewin NA: Cardiac glycosides. In Goldfrank LR, Flomenbaum NE, Lewin NA, et al (eds): Goldfrank's Toxicologic Emergencies, 7th ed. New York, McGraw-Hill, 2002, pp 724–839.

KEY POINTS: CARDIOVASCULAR TOXICOLOGY

1. The most common cause of ventricular dysrhythmias from poisoning is sodium channel blockade.

2. There is no single proven successful treatment for CCB and BB overdose, and severe ingestions often require multiple interventions.

3. Some BBs have sodium channel (i.e., propranolol) or potassium channel (i.e., sotalol) blocking effects.

4. Acute and chronic digoxin poisoning results in different clinical manifestations.

5. There is no serum digoxin level that is considered an absolute indication for digoxin immune Fab.

Acknowledgment

We would like to thank Christopher DeWitt, who authored this chapter in the previous edition and contributed substantially to this edition.

PELVIC INFLAMMATORY DISEASE

Alexander T. Trott, MD

CHAPTER 79

1. What is pelvic inflammatory disease (PID)?

An acute clinical syndrome caused by the spread of microorganisms from the vagina and cervix to reproductive organs. The organisms are most commonly sexually transmitted. PID can involve endometrium (endometritis), fallopian tubes (acute salpingitis), ovaries (oophoritis), and surrounding pelvic peritoneum (peritonitis). Any structure can be involved, either alone or in combination. Perihepatitis (Fitz-Hugh-Curtis syndrome) and tubo-ovarian abscess (TOA) can be considered within the spectrum of acute PID.

Banikarim C, Chacko MR: Pelvic inflammatory disease in adolescents. Adolesc Med Clin 15:273–285, 2004.

2. Who is at risk for PID?

Sexually active women, between the ages of 15 and 19, who use no method of contraception, are at highest risk. The risk is increased significantly if there have been recent encounters with multiple partners. Natural barriers to infection with sexually transmitted disease (STD) organisms are reduced during menses and by douching. Women in lower socioeconomic groups are at greatest risk, but the disease strikes at all levels of society. Of note is that the average age for patients admitted for PID is 32 years and TOA is more common in the older age group. Although oral contraceptives are associated with a higher rate of chlamydial infection of the cervix, oral contraceptives lower the risk and the severity of disease if it does occur. The intrauterine device increases the risk for PID. Operative procedures such as dilation and curettage, hysterosalpingography, and legal abortion may increase the risk of PID.

Sorbye IK, Jerve F, Staff AC: Reduction in hospitalized women with PID disease in Oslo over the past decade. Acta Obstet Gynecol Scand 84:290–296, 2005.

3. What are the microbiologic causes?

A complex interplay between multiple organisms exists in the setting of PID. *Chlamydia trachomatis* and *Neisseria gonorrhoeae* are the most common organisms found, with 30% of cases having both organisms present. Facultative aerobes, such as *Escherichia coli,* group B streptococcus, and *Haemophilus influenzae,* and anaerobes may be recovered as well. Other implicated organisms include *Mycoplasma hominis* and *Ureaplasma urealyticum.*

Grio R, Latino MA, Leotta E, et al: Sexually transmitted diseases and PID. Minerva Ginecol 56:141–147, 2004.

4. Can patients have more than one STD?

The presence of one STD does not preclude another. Patients with PID can have syphilis or may be infected with human immunodeficiency virus (HIV). All patients being evaluated for an STD should have a serologic test for syphilis. Testing for HIV should be considered. Vaginitis, a mild vaginal infection caused by *Candida, Trichomonas,* or *Gardnerella,* may be associated with PID. Women who have vaginal discharge or itching require testing for chlamydial infection and gonorrhea, and a microscopic examination of vaginal secretions for the common causes of vaginitis should be ordered.

Swygard H, Sena AC, Hobbs MM, et al: Trichomoniasis: Clinical manifestations, diagnosis and management. Sex Transm Infect 80:91–95, 2004.

5. **Describe the signs and symptoms of PID.**
    The signs and symptoms of PID can vary widely and range from subtle and mild to severe. Lower abdominal pain is the most common symptom of PID. It may or may not be accompanied by other symptoms such as vaginal discharge, abnormal uterine bleeding, or dysuria. Severe pain and vomiting indicate a more serious case. Physical exam may range from mild cervical motion tenderness to overt pelvic peritoneal signs accompanied by fever. An abnormal vaginal discharge is usually present. Because cases are often mild and subtle, the examiner should maintain a high index of suspicion, especially in patients with pelvic-related symptoms that do not have other explanations.

    Simms I, Warburton F, Westrom L: Diagnosis of pelvic inflammatory disease: Time to rethink. Sex Transm Infect 79:491–494, 2003.

6. **What other diseases should be considered?**
    Of all patients admitted to the hospital for PID, 25% are found to have other conditions. The most important of these conditions are ectopic pregnancy and acute appendicitis. Ruptured corpus luteum cysts, pelvic endometriosis, ovarian torsion, and pelvic adhesion are included in the differential diagnosis. In a few patients, the cause of pelvic pain is never diagnosed, despite extensive testing.

7. **Which diagnostic tests should be performed?**
    - A β-human chorionic gonadotropin pregnancy test is recommended.
    - If the pregnancy test is positive, an ultrasound is necessary to diagnose or rule out an ectopic pregnancy.
    - An ultrasound should be done on patients being considered for admission.
    - A urinalysis may reveal a urinary tract infection as a possible cause of the patient's symptoms or a coexistent infection. Because a clean-catch urine can easily be contaminated with vaginal secretions, a catheter-obtained specimen is recommended to ensure diagnostic accuracy.
    - A white blood cell count can help to indicate the severity of infection.
    - Whenever a TOA is suspected, ultrasound is recommended.
    - Cultures for *C. trachomatis* and *N. gonorrhoeae* are obtained in all patients with PID.
    - Short of laparoscopy, there is no reliable test to exclude PID.

8. **What are the consequences of PID, particularly if it is unrecognized or untreated?**
    All of the serious consequences of PID result from tubal inflammation and scarring. Acutely, PID can progress to TOA that may require surgical intervention. Ectopic pregnancy, the most serious consequence, is two to seven times more likely to occur in women with prior PID. Tubal factor infertility (TFI) is another serious sequela and is directly proportional to the number of pelvic infections and severity of infection. One of the main reasons to maintain a low index of suspicion for PID is *C. trachomatis*. Chlamydial salpingitis is often clinically mild yet can seriously damage the tubes. One of the most troublesome sequelae of PID is chronic abdominal pain, which eventually may require a hysterectomy.

    Mardh PA: Tubal factor infertility, with special regard to chlamydial salpingitis. Curr Opin Infect Dis 17:49–52, 2004.

9. **Who should be treated?**
    The older, more strict criteria for diagnosis have led to significant undertreatment of the disease. For this reason, the CDC in 2002, has re-evaluated and changed its minimum criteria and stated, "Empiric treatment of PID should be initiated in sexually active young women and other women at risk for STDs if the following minimal criteria can be met and no other cause for illness can be identified: uterine/adnexal tenderness or cervical motion tenderness."

Patients with unexplained abnormal uterine bleeding, dyspareunia, and vaginal discharge should also be considered for empiric PID treatment.

Centers for Disease Control and Prevention: Sexually transmitted diseases treatment guidelines 2002. Available at www.cdc.gov/mmwr/preview/mmwrhtm/rr5106a1.htm

10. **Who should be hospitalized?**
The main reasons to hospitalize a patient with PID are to protect future fertility and to treat moderate-to-serious disease. Most authorities agree that young, nulligravida women, regardless of infection severity, require hospitalization for the first episode. The Centers for Disease Control's Guidelines for Hospital Admission are as follows:
- Uncertain diagnosis (appendicitis cannot be ruled out)
- Suspicion of pelvic abscess
- Pregnancy
- Severe illness (high fever, peritoneal signs, vomiting)
- Adolescent patient
- Failure of outpatient therapy
- Presence of HIV infection

11. **Summarize the recommended antibiotic regimens for PID treatment.**
See Table 79-1.

TABLE 79-1. OUTPATIENT TREATMENT OF PID

Regimen A

Ofloxacin, 400 mg PO b.i.d. for 14 days

or

Levofloxacin 500 mg PO daily for 14 days

with or without

Metronidazole, 500 mg PO b.i.d. for 14 days

Regimen B

One of following: (1) ceftriaxone, 250 mg IM once; (2) cefoxitin, 2 gm IM, plus probenecid, 1 gm PO in a single dose concurrently once; *or* (3) other parenteral third-generation cephalosporin (e.g., ceftizoxime or cefotaxime)

plus

Doxycycline, 100 mg PO b.i.d. for 14 d *with or without* metronidazole 500 mg PO b.i.d. for 14 days

Parenteral regimen A

Cefotetan, 2 gm IV q 12 h; *or* cefoxitin, 2 gm IV q 6 h

plus

Doxycycline, 100 mg IV or PO q 12 h

Note: Because of pain associated with infusion, doxycycline should be given orally when possible, even when patient is hospitalized. Oral and intravenous administration of doxycycline provide similar bioavailability. If intravenous administration is necessary, lidocaine or another short-acting local anesthetic, heparin, or steroids with a steel needle or extension of the infusion time may reduce infusion complications. Parenteral therapy may be discontinued 24 hours after a patient improves clinically, and oral therapy with

Continued

TABLE 79-1. OUTPATIENT TREATMENT OF PID—CONT'D

doxycycline (100 mg b.i.d.) should continue for 14 days. When tubo-ovarian abscess is present, clindamycin or metronidazole may be used with doxycycline for continued therapy rather than doxycycline alone because it provides more effective anaerobic coverage.

Parenteral regimen B

Clindamycin, 900 mg IV q 8 h

plus

Gentamicin, loading dose IV or IM (2 mg/kg body weight), followed by a maintenance dose (1.5 mg/kg) q 8 h. Single daily dosing may be substituted.

Note: Although use of one daily dose of gentamicin has not been evaluated for the treatment of PID, it is efficacious in analogous situations. Parenteral therapy may be discontinued 24 hours after a patient improves clinically, and continuing oral therapy should consist of doxycycline, 100 mg PO b.i.d., or clindamycin, 450 mg PO q.i.d., to complete 14 days of therapy. When tubo-ovarian abscess is present, clindamycin may be used for continued therapy rather than doxycycline because clindamycin provides more effective anaerobic coverage.

b.i.d. = twice a day, IM = intramuscular, IV = intravenous, PID = pelvic inflammatory disease, PO = per os, q.i.d. = four times a day.
Adapted from Centers for Disease Control and Prevention: Sexually transmitted diseases treatment guidelines. MMWR 51(RR–6)50, 2002

12. **Does the presence of an intrauterine pregnancy effectively rule out PID?**
A common misconception is that PID cannot occur in a pregnant woman but it can occur, most commonly in the first trimester in primigravidas. Infection can take place concurrently with fertilization or throughout the first trimester, after which the uterine cavity is obliterated by the pregnancy. Although PID can occur under these conditions, it is uncommon.

Heinonen PK, Leinonen M: Fecundity and morbidity following acute PID treated with doxycycline and metronidazole. Arch Gynecol Obstet 268:284–288, 2003.

13. **Does a history of tubal ligation preclude the diagnosis of PID?**
Bilateral tubal ligation (BTL) does not preclude PID. Salpingitis following BTL occurs, on average, more than a year after the procedure. Histologically, inflammation occurs both proximal and distal to the occlusion site. TOAs have been reported as well, up to 20 years following ligation.

Levgur M, Duvivier R: PID after tubal sterilization: A review. Obstet Gynecol Surv 55:41–50, 2000.

14. **What is the appropriate follow-up for patients with PID?**
Patients treated as outpatients need close follow-up. Response to treatment should be assessed within 48–72 hours. The patient can return to the emergency department (ED), see a primary care provider, or be evaluated by a gynecologist. For reliable patients, a phone contact can suffice. For all patients, a test of cure by repeat examination and cervical cultures is recommended 2–4 weeks after the initial intervention.

KEY POINTS: PELVIC INFLAMMATORY DISEASE

1. PID can be subtle and mild but can cause extensive tubal damage.

2. Tubo-ovarian abscess is more likely to occur in older age groups.

3. Pelvic ultrasound should be done on any patient with PID being considered for admission.

4. Abnormal uterine bleeding may be the only sign of PID in some patients.

5. Neither pregnancy nor tubal ligation precludes a diagnosis of PID.

15. **Summarize the principles of management of acute PID.**
    - Rule out pregnancy.
    - Treat early and with broad-spectrum antibiotics.
    - Advise patient that her sexual partner is at risk and may need to be treated as well.
    - Maintain a low index of suspicion for the diagnosis of PID.

CHAPTER 80

SEXUAL ASSAULT

Kim M. Feldhaus, MD

1. What is the definition of sexual assault?

Definitions vary from state to state, but sexual assault generally refers to any genital, anal, oral, or manual penetration of the victim's body by way of force and without the victim's consent. Individuals who have an impaired mental function due to alcohol, drugs, sleep, or unconsciousness are unable to give consent by definition. The more traditional term "rape" is defined as forced vaginal, anal, or oral intercourse; force includes both psychological coercion and physical force. This definition of sexual assault includes attempted rapes, male and female victims, and heterosexual and homosexual rape.

Rape Abuse and Incest National Network Statistics: What is sexual assault. Available at www.rainn.org/definition.html

2. How common is sexual assault?

Every 2½ minutes, somewhere in the United States, someone is sexually assaulted. Over recent years, an average of 223,280 victims of rape, attempted rape, or sexual assault reported to law enforcement. However, research indicates that only 40% of sexual assaults are reported to law enforcement. Approximately 18% of American women have experienced a completed or attempted rape at some point in their life, and 3% of American men report a completed or attempted rape during their lifetime. Of women who report being raped, 54% were younger than the age of 18 years when they were victimized. Rape in America has been termed a "tragedy of youth." Women who are sexually assaulted as children and adolescents are at greater risk of being sexually assaulted as an adult. Although most victims of sexual assault are women, men can be assaulted by other men, and occasionally women perpetrate sexual assaults against other women or men. The vast majority of sexual assaults (80%) are perpetrated by someone whom the victim knows.

National Crime Victimization Survey 2003, Bureau of Justice Statistics, US Department of Justice, Washington DC. NCJ 207811. Available at www.ojp.usdoj.gov/bjs/pub/pdf/cv03.pdf

RAINN Statistics, Rape, Abuse, and Incest National Network (RAINN): Calculations based on US Department of Justice National Crime Victimization Survey 2003. Available at www.rainn.org/90seconds.html

RAINN Statistics, Rape Abuse and Incest National Network (RAINN): Facts about sexual assault. Available at www.rainn.org/statistics.html

3. Rape is a legal term, and usually law enforcement is requesting evidence be gathered. What role does a medical provider have in these cases?

The emergency department (ED) is the most common place for a sexual assault victim to present for acute medical care *and* forensic evidence gathering. Thirty-two percent of women older than 18 years who are sexually assaulted report being injured in the assault, and 36% sought some type of medical treatment. Always remember that the physician's primary responsibility is to provide for the patient's physical and psychological well-being first; then, if the patient consents, to provide police with corroborative forensic evidence. Victims should be encouraged to undergo an evidentiary examination as soon as possible because critical evidence may be lost if this exam is delayed. The victim may later choose not to proceed through the criminal justice system, because collection of forensic evidence does not commit him or her to seek prosecution. A comprehensive ED sexual assault protocol that addresses medical care and the evidentiary examination is necessary for optimal patient care.

Tjaden P, Thoennes N: Prevalence, incidence, and consequences of violence against women: Findings from the National Violence Against Women Survey. National Institute of Justice and Centers for Disease Control, November 1998, NCJ 172837. Available at ncjrs.org/pdffiles/172837.pdf

4. What information should be elicited in the patient history?

- Information regarding the patient's general health, medications, and allergies should be obtained along with a complete gynecologic history, including birth control usage, date and time of last consensual intercourse, last menstrual period, and history of recent gynecologic symptoms before the assault.
- A directed history of the assault includes the date, time, and location of the assault; information concerning the assailants; and the type and details of the sexual acts, including type of force or threats used. The history must be obtained in a private setting; law enforcement personnel should not be present.

Patel M, Minshall L: Management of sexual assault. Emerg Med Clin North Am 19:817–831, 2001.

5. Of what should the physical examination consist?

Rape is a crime of violence and control, not a crime of passion. The purpose of the physical examination is to detect injuries requiring treatment and to record and gather forensic evidence for prosecution. A complete head-to-toe medical examination should be done, regardless of whether law enforcement has requested a forensic exam and regardless of whether the patient has consented to a forensic exam. *General body trauma* occurs more frequently than genital trauma. Injuries may include abrasions and bruises on the arms, head and neck, signs of restraint (such as rope burns or mouth injuries), broken teeth, fractured nose or jaw from being punched or slapped, muscle soreness, or stiffness from restraint in positions allowing sexual penetration. The gynecologic examination should include a thorough search for contusions, abrasions, lacerations, bleeding, or tenderness. A Wood's lamp fluoresces most semen stains, and toluidine blue dye reveals minor traumatic genital tears. A colposcopic examination may identify cervical injuries. A careful rectal examination should be done in cases of rectal penetration, and if blood is present, anoscopy or sigmoidoscopy should be done to identify internal injuries.

Feldhaus KM: Female and male sexual assault. In Tintinalli JE, Kellen GB, Stapcznski JS (eds): Emergency Medicine: A Comprehensive Study Guide, 6th ed. New York, McGraw-Hill, 2004, pp 1851–1854.
Patel M, Minshall L: Management of sexual assault. Emerg Med Clin North Am 19:817–831, 2001.
Riggs N, Houry D, Long G, et al: Analysis of 1.076 cases of sexual assault. Ann Emerg Med 35:358–362, 2000.

6. What evidence should be gathered as part of the forensic examination?

The forensic evidence may be divided into four categories: control samples from the victim, evidence which might identify the assailant, evidence or proof of recent sexual contact, and evidence or proof of force or coercion (Table 80-1).

7. What laboratory studies are indicated?

A urine or serum pregnancy test should be done to rule out a preexisting pregnancy; if a preexisting pregnancy is present, the patient should be reassured that this pregnancy was not the result of the assault. The routine collection of gonorrhea or chlamydial cultures is debatable. A preexisting infection is present in approximately 5% of assault victims (the same as the general population); identification of these patients allows for treatment of their regular partners. If the victim does not receive prophylactic antibiotics in the ED, chlamydial and gonorrhea cultures should be repeated or performed in 2 weeks. Compliance with medical follow-up is historically poor, however. From a medicolegal perspective, positive cultures indicating

TABLE 80-1. FORENSIC EVIDENCE KIT CONTENTS

Control samples from victim
- Head hair samples
- Saliva sample
- Blood sample
- Pubic hair samples

Samples to identify assailant
- Skin swabbing for assailant's saliva
- Fingernail scrapings or clipping (from victim)
- Pubic hair combing
- Trace evidence (such as stray hair, bits of clothing)

Evidence for proof of recent sexual contact:
- Oral, vaginal, and/or anal swabs for semen
- Wet mounts of oral, vaginal, and/or anal swabs for sperm
- Skin swabbing for semen
- Any tampons, if present

Evidence for proof of force or coercion:
- Documentation of injuries found on exam
- Fingernail scrapings or clippings
- Urine or blood for toxicologic testing
- All clothing

Compiled from Patel M, Minshall L: Management of sexual assault. Emerg Med Clin North Am 19:817–831, 2001; and Feldhaus KM: Female and male sexual assault: In Tintinalli JE, Kellen GB, Stapcznski JS (eds): Emergency Medicine: A Comprehensive Study Guide, 6th ed. New York, McGraw-Hill, 2004, pp 1851–1854.

preexisting sexually transmitted diseases (STDs) have been used by defense attorneys as evidence of the victim's sexual promiscuity.

Centers for Disease Control and Prevention: Sexually transmitted diseases treatment guidelines 2002. MMWR 51(No. RR–6), 2002. Available at www.cdc.gov/std/treatment/TOC2002TG.htm

8. **What about blood alcohol levels and tests for drug use?**
In general, routine drug screens and routine alcohol levels are not recommended; proof of intoxication or drug use may be used against the victim in a court of law. However, if the tests are medically indicated and will influence your treatment (such as a patient with an unexplained altered mental status, or unexplained tachycardia), then laboratory testing may be indicated.

9. **What historical features might indicate a drug-facilitated rape?**
A history of a period of amnesia or a history of being out drinking and then suddenly feeling "very intoxicated" should raise concerns about a drug facilitated sexual assault (DFSA). Sometimes the patient simply relates a history of waking up naked, unsure of what occurred, with genital or pelvic soreness. In these situations, urine should be obtained for drug testing. This testing should be done by law enforcement to preserve chain of evidence, and victims should be informed that any previous volitional, recreational drug use (such as cocaine or marijuana) may also be revealed in the toxicologic screening. The urine sample should be

refrigerated after receipt by law enforcement to preserve the detection of drugs of abuse. Conviction of a DFSA increases the legal penalties significantly.

Anglin D, Spears KL, Hutson HR: Flunitrazepam and its involvement in date or acquaintance rape. Acad Emerg Med 4:323–326, 1997.

10. **What are the most common STDs that may be contracted as a result of a sexual assault?**

Sexual assault victims are at risk of contracting chlamydial infection, gonorrhea, bacterial vaginosis, hepatitis B, and human immunodeficiency virus (HIV). The risks of contracting a new chlamydial, gonorrheal, or bacterial vaginosis infection as the result of sexual assault are hard to estimate; risk varies according to geographical area and type of assault. In general, the risk of contracting chlamydial infection or gonorrhea is 4–17%, and the risk of contracting bacterial vaginosis is slightly higher. Hepatitis B is efficiently transmitted via sexual contact, and postexposure immunization is recommended.

Patel M, Minshall L: Management of sexual assault. Emerg Med Clin North Am 19:817–831, 2001.

11. **Is empirical antibiotic treatment of sexual assault victims indicated? How about vaccinations?**

Because of historically poor follow-up rates by sexual assault victims, along with the significant risk of contracting a new STD, prophylaxis should be offered to all victims. Effective regimens include ceftriaxone, 125 mg intramuscularly in a single dose; cefixime, 400 mg orally in a single dose; or ciprofloxacin, 500 mg orally in a single dose, for gonorrhea coverage. Patients also should be given azithromycin, 1 gm orally in a single dose, or doxycycline, 100 mg orally twice a day for 7–10 days, for chlamydial prophylaxis. The Centers for Disease Control and Prevention (CDC) also recommends a single 2-gm oral metronidazole dose to treat *Trichomonas* and bacterial vaginosis. Pregnant patients should receive ceftriaxone 125 mg intramuscular (IM) in a single dose (avoid quinolones and tetracyclines) for gonorrhea coverage, as well as erythromycin base 500 mg four times a day (q.i.d.) for 7 days or amoxicillin 500 mg three times a day (t.i.d.) for 7 days to cover *Chlamydia*. Contracting bacterial vaginosis during pregnancy carries a risk of premature rupture of membranes, preterm labor, and chorioamnionitis; pregnant women should be encouraged to follow up with gynecology and receive treatment if they develop bacterial vaginosis. The CDC also recommends that hepatitis B vaccine be administered at the time of the initial examination if victims have not been previously vaccinated. Follow-up doses of vaccine should be administered 1–2 and 4–6 months after the first dose.

Centers for Disease Control and Prevention: Sexually transmitted diseases treatment guidelines 2002. MMWR 1(No. RR–6), 2002 Available at www.cdc.gov/std/treatment/TOC2002TG.htm

12. **What is the risk of pregnancy after sexual assault?**

Although the risk of pregnancy after an isolated sexual encounter during nonfertile periods of the menstrual cycle is thought to be less than 1%, it is significantly higher at midcycle. Approximately 5% of all sexual assault victims become pregnant as a result of the assault. The presence of a preexisting pregnancy must be identified in the ED.

Resnick HS, Holmes MM, Kilpatrick DG, et al: Predictors of post-rape medical care in a national sample of women. Am J Prev Med 19:214–219, 2000.

13. **What are the current options for pregnancy prophylaxis?**

When a preexisting pregnancy has been ruled out, postcoital preparations can be used to prevent pregnancy by inhibiting or disrupting ovulation or inhibiting fertilization or implantation. Emergency contraception is not effective once implantation has occurred, and it will not disrupt an existing pregnancy. These preparations may be taken up to 5 days after sexual contact, but because their effectiveness decreases over time, ideally they should be taken within 72 hours. There are two Food and Drug Administration (FDA)–approved oral products for postcoital emergency contraception. Preven is a combination of ethinyl estradiol and levonorgestrel. Plan B contains only levonorgestrel. Common side effects include nausea, vomiting, and vaginal spotting. The latest research shows that taking both tablets of Plan B at one time (total of 150 μg levonorgestrel) is as effective as separating the two tablets by 12 hours. The failure rate with Plan B is less than 2%. If a dedicated emergency contraceptive product is not available, a levonorgestrel-containing oral contraceptive pill, such as Ovral, may be used (traditionally dosed as two tablets of Ovral now, two in 12 hours).

Cheng L, Gulmezoglu AM, Oel CJ, et al: Interventions for emergency contraception. Cochrane Database Syst Rev 3:CD001324, 2004.

Feldhaus KM: Female and male sexual assault. In Tintinalli JE, Kellen GB, Stapcznski JS (eds): Emergency Medicine: A Comprehensive Study Guide, 6th ed. New York, McGraw-Hill, 2004, pp 1851–1854.

14. What are the special characteristics of male sexual assault?

The male sexual assault victim should be treated similarly to a female victim. Special attention should be paid to the mouth, genitals, anus, and rectum. Men represent approximately 5% of reported sexual assault victims.

15. Discuss the special characteristics of pediatric sexual assault.

In pediatric sexual assault, the assailant is often known to the victim, and there is often a history of repetitive assaults. In addition to documenting signs of acute trauma, the physician should look for signs of recurrent abuse, such as healed hymenal tears, a large vaginal opening, vaginal discharge, or relaxed rectal sphincter tone. The gynecologic examination should take into account the nature of the assault and the age of the child. In the evaluation of a small child in whom a speculum examination is indicated, a nasal speculum may be used in place of a vaginal speculum. Sometimes the vaginal or rectal examination must be done under general anesthesia because of the emotional state of the child. The child should be protected from further abuse by admission to the hospital or by immediate referral to the appropriate social service agency.

16. Should pediatric patients be given prophylactic antibiotics?

Prophylactic antibiotics are not generally indicated when sexual abuse of children is suspected. The baseline infection rate in children is significantly lower than in adults, and the presence of a STD in a child is strong evidence that abuse has occurred. It is important to document the presence of the infection before treatment. In the child, chlamydial and gonorrhea cultures should be obtained from the vagina instead of the cervix.

Centers for Disease Control and Prevention: Sexually transmitted diseases treatment guidelines 2002. MMWR 51(No. RR–6), 2002. Available at www.cdc.gov/std/treatment/TOC2002TG.htm

17. State the important aspects of follow-up care for any victim of sexual assault.

Follow-up medical care should ensure that any physical injuries have healed properly, adequate pregnancy prophylaxis has been administered, STDs have been treated properly, and the victim has accessed supportive counseling. Provision of written aftercare instructions and information on community resources is essential.

18. What types of emotional trauma might sexual assault victims experience?

The development of a posttraumatic stress disorder, manifested by sleep disturbances, feelings of guilt, memory impairment, and detachment from the world and others may occur in the days to weeks following the assault. Long-term psychological sequelae in the form of rape trauma syndrome also may occur. Many communities have rape crisis centers with social workers and volunteers who are trained to provide counseling for sexual assault survivors. Sexual assault response teams have been organized in other areas to provide a coordinated approach to the sexual assault victim, including emotional support after the event. Physicians should be aware of the availability of such services so that they can recommend them to their patients.

National Center for Injury Prevention and Control: Sexual violence fact sheet. Centers for Disease Control. Available at www.cdc.gov/ncipc/factsheets/svfacts.htm

19. My patient is terrified of contracting HIV after her sexual assault. What do I do now?

Provide nonoccupational postexposure prophylaxis (nPEP).

20. What is nPEP?

nPEP refers to the provision of postexposure antiretroviral therapies for individuals who are exposed to potentially infected blood or bodily fluids from sexual contact, from injection drug use, or in other nonoccupational settings (i.e., non health care, sanitation, public safety, or laboratory employment settings).

Antiretroviral postexposure prophylaxis after sexual, injection-drug use, or other nonoccupational exposure to HIV in the United States. MMWR 54(RR02);1–20, 2005.

Recommendations from the U.S. Department of Health and Human Services. Available at www.cdc.gov/mmwr/preview/mmwrhtml/rr5402a1.htm

21. What is the risk of acquiring HIV after a sexual assault?

The estimated risk is dependent on the HIV status of the assailant, the type of sexual contact, and the amount of mucosal trauma involved. The HIV status of the source should be considered—is the assailant known to be HIV positive? Is the assailant known to be from a group with a high prevalence rate of HIV (i.e., injection drug users, commercial sex workers, or homosexual or bisexual men)? Studies in prison populations reveal that HIV infection rates are higher in male sexual assailants than in the general male population (1% versus 0.3%). In most cases of sexual assault, the HIV status of the assailant will not be known. Genital trauma, bleeding, and inflammation associated with sexual assault increase the risk of HIV transmission. In general, receptive anal intercourse carries a risk of seroconversion of 50 per 10,000 exposures. In comparison, a percutaneous needle stick from an infected source carries a 30 per 10,000 risk of contracting HIV. The risk of contracting HIV following receptive penile-vaginal intercourse is 10 per 10,000.

Antiretroviral postexposure prophylaxis after sexual, injection-drug use, or other nonoccupational exposure to HIV in the United States. MMWR 54(RR02);1–20, 2005.

Recommendations from the U.S. Department of Health and Human Services. Available at www.cdc.gov/mmwr/preview/mmwrhtml/rr5402a1.htm

22. How exactly do I provide nPEP for my patient?

Baseline HIV testing should be performed on the victim, preferably with an FDA-approved rapid-test kit (results available within 1 hour). nPEP should be begun within 72 hours after exposure—the sooner the better. If more than 72 hours have lapsed since the assault, the risks of antiretroviral therapies may outweigh the benefit. No evidence indicates that any specific antiretroviral medication or combination of medications is optimal for use as nPEP. Based on the degree of experience with certain agents, there are preferred regimens. Preferred regimens include non-nucleoside reverse transcriptase inhibitor (NNRTI)-based therapies and protease inhibitor (PI)–based therapies. Preferred NNRTI regimes include efavirenz (Sustiva) *plus* lamivudine (Epivir, 3TC) or emtricitabine *plus* zidovudine or tenofovir. PI regimens include lopinavir/ritonavir (coformulated in one tablet as Kaletra) *plus* zidovudine (AZT, Retrovir) *plus* either lamivudine or emtricitabine. Efavirenz should be avoided in pregnant women and women of child-bearing potential. Regardless of the regimen chosen, the exposed person should be counseled about the potential associated side effects and adverse events that require immediate medical attention. The use of medications to treat symptoms (e.g., antiemetics or antimotility agents) might improve medication compliance. A 3–5 day starter pack is recommended with a follow-up visit scheduled to review the results of HIV testing (if a rapid test was not used), review baseline laboratory data, discuss medication side effects, and change therapies if needed. A full 28-day course of medications should be provided at that time.

Antiretroviral postexposure prophylaxis after sexual, injection-drug use, or other nonoccupational exposure to HIV in the United States MMWR 54(RR02);1–20, 2005.

Recommendations from the U.S. Department of Health and Human Services. Available at www.cdc.gov/mmwr/preview/mmwrhtml/rr5402a1.htm

KEY POINTS: CARE OF THE SEXUAL ASSAULT VICTIM

1. First and foremost, care for the victim's medical and emotional needs.

2. Collection of forensic evidence is requested by law enforcement and may not be performed without the victim's consent.

3. All victims should be offered prophylactic antibiotics for sexually transmitted diseases.

4. Women of child-bearing age should be informed about emergency contraception; if it is not offered to the victim at the hospital, a referral should be made so the patient may receive it in a timely manner.

5. Written referral to community resources for post-assault counseling is critical.

CHAPTER 81

SPONTANEOUS ABORTION, ECTOPIC PREGNANCY, AND THIRD-TRIMESTER BLEEDING

Dane M. Chapman, MD, PhD

1. What is spontaneous abortion or miscarriage?

Termination of pregnancy before achieving fetal weight or maturity compatible with survival—less than 20–22 weeks' gestation or 500 g or less fetal weight.

Goddijn M, Leschot NJ: Genetic aspects of miscarriage. Baillieres Best Pract Res Clin Obstet Gynaecol 14:855, 2000.

2. State the incidence and timing of spontaneous miscarriage.

Ten to 20% of clinically recognized pregnancies less than 20 weeks miscarry; 80% of these occur in the first 12 weeks of gestation. Approximately 70% of all spontaneous abortions occur before pregnancy is clinically detected.

Wilcox, AJ, Weinberg, CR, O'Connor, JF, et al: Incidence of early loss of pregnancy. N Engl J Med 319:189, 1988.

KEY POINTS: MOST COMMON CAUSES OF SPONTANEOUS ABORTIONS

1. First 4–8 weeks of gestation: Abnormal development of the zygote with chromosomal abnormalities in 50–60% of spontaneous abortions

2. Later in the first trimester:
   - Isolated chromosomal abnormalities
   - Maternal factors (insufficient progesterone support, alcohol use, cocaine use, tobacco use, nonsteroidal anti-inflammatory drug, or caffeine use)
   - Structural uterine abnormalities that lead to hemorrhage into the decidua basalis with subsequent necrotic changes in the area of implantation (The ovum becomes partially or completely detached, acts as a foreign body in the uterus, stimulates contractions, and results in expulsion of uterine contents.)

---

3. What are the five stages (types) of miscarriage?

- Any pregnant patient with vaginal bleeding in the first half of pregnancy and a closed internal os is said to have a **threatened abortion.** Crampy abdominal pain or back pain may be present.
- If the internal os is open on examination, this is an **inevitable abortion.**
- Patients with products of conception present in the cervical os or the vaginal canal are described as having an **incomplete abortion,** whereas **complete abortions** occur after all products of conception have been passed. Pain and bleeding cease after a complete abortion.

- In a **missed abortion,** the conceptus dies but is not passed, with retention of products of conception in utero for 4–8 weeks or more, at which time the uterine size decreases and symptoms of pregnancy regress, usually spontaneously.

4. **Describe the sonographic findings in a healthy pregnancy.**
There is a distinct, well-formed gestational ring, with central echoes indicating a fetal pole that should be present by 5–6 weeks. A sac with no central echoes from an embryo or fetus implies, but does not prove, death of the conceptus. An ovum with no visible fetus in the sac may be a blighted ovum due to a degenerated or absent embryo. Serial sonograms are important to follow the progression or lack of fetal growth.

Deaton JL, Honore GM, Huffman CS, Bauguess P: Early transvaginal ultrasound following an accurately dated pregnancy: The importance of finding a yolk sac or fetal heart motion. Hum Reprod 12:2820, 1997.

5. **What are important questions to consider during exmination and treatment of spontaneous abortion?**
   - Is the patient hemodynamically stable?
   - Is there abdominal tenderness or rebound (indicating a possible ectopic pregnancy [EP])?
   - Are products of conception visible in the cervical os or vaginal canal (an incomplete abortion)?
   - Is the cervical os open (an inevitable abortion) or closed?

Nadukhovskaya L, Dart R: Emergency management of the nonviable intrauterine pregnancy. Am J Emerg Med 19:495–500, 2001.

6. **What are the earliest symptoms of a miscarriage?**
Bleeding or spotting is usually first, followed by crampy abdominal pain.

7. **What is the treatment of threatened or incomplete abortion?**
   1. Identify an intrauterine pregnancy (IUP) by ultrasound, if not previously documented, to rule out an EP.
   2. Restrict sexual intercourse and strenuous physical exercise.
   3. Follow serial quantitative human chorionic gonadotropin (hCG) tests. If levels decrease, prognosis is poor.
   4. If bleeding persists, obtain hematocrit and hemoglobin tests.
   5. If bleeding is perfuse, causing hypotension, uterine evacuation is necessary.
   6. If bleeding continues once fetus has been delivered, consider methargen or oxytocin.
   7. If an incomplete abortion, dilation and evacuation or dilation and curettage with local cervical anesthesia and procedural sedation is required. If there is tissue protruding from the os on pelvic examination, removal can be attempted by gentle traction with ring forceps, which in most instances decreases the amount of uterine hemorrhage.

8. **What is the prognosis for patients with threatened abortion?**
Patients with bleeding and a closed internal os have a risk of miscarriage estimated at 35–50%, although the fetal loss rate is probably higher in emergency department (ED) populations. If fetal cardiac activity is shown on ultrasound, risk of subsequent miscarriage is much lower. There is no treatment regimen that influences the course of a threatened abortion. Expectant management for women in early pregnancy failure can be as effective as medical or surgical management if the fetus is less than 13 weeks of gestation and the mother has stable vital signs and no fever. Successful spontaneous abortion occurs in 91% of women with incomplete miscarriages and 26% with missed abortions.

Luise C, Jermy K, May C, et al: Outcome of expectant management of spontaneous first trimester miscarriage: Observational study. BMJ 324:873, 2002.
Shelley JM, Healy D, Grover S: A randomized trial of surgical, medical and expectant management of first trimester spontaneous miscarriage. Aust N Z J Obstet Gynaecol 45:122, 2005.

9. **What is a septic abortion?**

   A spontaneous abortion complicated by endometritis, parametritis, or peritonitis.

10. **What are the signs and symptoms of a septic abortion?**
    - Malodorous discharge from the cervix or vagina
    - Pelvic and abdominal pain
    - Fever
    - Uterine tenderness
    - Hyperthermia, which may be an indication of endotoxic shock

11. **Do diagnostic radiographs cause spontaneous abortion?**

    No. Diagnostic radiographs (< 10 rads) place a pregnant woman at little or no increased risk for miscarriage, although there is a risk for the development of fetal chromosomal abnormalities. Therapeutic radiation and antineoplastic agents *do* increase the incidence of spontaneous abortion.

12. **What factors are associated with spontaneous abortion and/or fetal abonormalities?**
    - Cigarette, alcohol (at high-exposure range), or cocaine use
    - Progesterone-containing, but not copper-containing, intrauterine devices increase the risk of spontaneous abortion. (Oral contraceptives taken either before or during pregnancy have not been associated with spontaneous abortion.)
    - Environmental chemicals (anesthetic agents, arsenic, aniline, benzene, ethylene oxide, formaldehyde, lead)
    - Accutane (isotretinoin) (Do *not* use in pregnant women or in women planning to become pregnant.)
    - Caffeine consumption during pregnancy
    - Nonsteroidal anti-inflammatory drug use during conception
    - Increased risk with increased maternal parity and increased maternal and paternal age (The frequency increases from 12% in women younger than age 20–26 to 40% in women age 40.)
    - Conception within 3 months after a live birth
    - Systemic disease of the mother (e.g., diabetes mellitus, cancer, hypothyroidism, or hyperthyroidism)
    - Laparotomy: The closer the surgery to the pelvic organs, the greater the risk of spontaneous abortion
    - Increased life stress: May increase the risk of spontaneous abortions in women greater than 11 weeks' gestation, implying an increased risk of miscarriage of chromosomally normal fetuses
    - Uterine defects including acquired leiomyomas where the location is more important than the size and submucous fibroids are more dangerous; and developmental abnormalities including müllerian duct malformation or fusion and a septate, bicornate, or unicornate uterus

    Boyles SH, Ness RB, Grisso JA, et al: Life event stress and the association with spontaneous abortion in gravid women at an urban emergency department. Health Psychol 19:510–514, 2000.

    Cnattingius S, Signorello LB, Anneren G, et al: Caffeine intake and the risk of fist-trimester spontaneous abortion. N Engl J Med 343:1839, 2000.

    Li DK, Liu L, Odouli R: Exposure to non-steroidal anti-inflammatory drugs during pregnancy and risk of miscarriage: Population based cohort study. BMJ 327:368, 2003.

    Nybo Andersen AM, Wohlfahrt J, Christens P, et al: Maternal age and fetal loss population based register linkage study. BMJ 320:1708–1712, 2000.

13. **Is trauma a major factor associated with spontaneous abortion?**

    No. Fetuses are well protected by maternal structures and amniotic fluid from minor falls or blows, but penetrating trauma such as a gunshot wound or stab wound is dangerous to the fetus.

14. **Is exposure to spermicide before or after conception deleterious to a pregnancy?**
No.

15. **Define cervical incompetence.**
Cervical incompetence is the painless dilation of the cervix during the second trimester, followed by spontaneous rupture of membranes, with subsequent expulsion of uterine contents.

16. **Name the drug used to prevent Rh immunization.**
Rh immunoglobulin or RhoGAM. Any pregnant woman who is experiencing vaginal bleeding must have an Rh (rhesus) type checked; if she is Rh negative and less than 12 weeks' gestation, she should receive a mini-dose of RhoGAM, 50 μg. If she is greater than 12 weeks' gestation, the full dose of RhoGAM, 300 μg, should be given.

Grant J, Hysolp M: Underutilization of Rh prophylaxis in the emergency department: A retrospective survey. Ann Emerg Med 21:181–183, 1992.

17. **What follow-up instructions should be given to a patient with a threatened abortion?**
Careful instructions are given to return if she has a significant increase in pain, bleeding, or signs of hemodynamic instability, such as syncopal episodes. The patient should be instructed to bring any tissue she passes in with her to the ED or her primary care physician (PCP). Arrangements to repeat quantitative hCG measurements should be made. Patients with a history of recurrent miscarriages should be referred to a specialist for further testing.

18. **What about the emotional aspects of an early miscarriage?**
Miscarriage is associated with a significant amount of psychological stress and grieving. Important therapeutic messages include informing the patient that early miscarriages are common and that miscarriages are usually due to chromosomal abnormalities and not to the patient's own actions.

Zaccardi R, Abbott J, Koziol-McLain J: Loss and grief reactions after spontaneous miscarriage in the emergency department. Ann Emerg Med 22:799–804, 1992.

19. **What is an ectopic pregnancy?**
An ectopic pregnancy (EP) is a pregnancy in which implantation of the gestational sac occurs outside of the uterus. In most cases, the pregnancy is located in the fallopian tubes, but EPs can occur in the interstitial or cornual portion of the uterus (2%), intra-abdominally (1.5%), on the ovary (0.1%), or within the cervix (0.1%). EP occurs in approximately 1 in 60 pregnancies in the United States; the risk is higher in older women and minorities. EP is still the leading cause of pregnancy-related first-trimester maternal deaths. Most ED series report that about 7% of first-trimester patients presenting to EDs have an EP diagnosed. Typically, patients with EP will present with abdominal pain, amenorrhea, or vaginal bleeding. However, more than 50% of women with EP are asymptomatic before tubal rupture and do not have a risk factor for EP.

Alsuleiman SA, Grimes EM: Ectopic pregnancy: A review of 147 cases. J Reprod Med 27:101, 1982.
Fylsra DL: Tubal pregnancy: A review of current diagnosis and treatment. Obstet Gynecol Surv 53:320, 1998.
Stovall TG, Kellerman AL, Ling FW, Buster JE: Emergency department diagnosis of ectopic pregnancy. Ann Emerg Med 19:1098, 1990.

20. **What are common risk factors for EP?**
- Pelvic inflammatory disease, which can be seen histologically in 50% of patients with EP
- Prior EP
- Tubal ligation
- Intrauterine device use

- Pelvic surgery
- Infertility and fertilization procedures (New technology, such as artificial fertilization, ovulation stimulation, and surgical procedures that result in salvage of potentially abnormal fallopian tubes, also may contribute to the increased incidence.)
- Risk of heterotopic (combined intrauterine and ectopic) pregnancy: Cited as 1 in 30,000 pregnancies, but more recent estimates put the risk at closer to 1 in 4000 (The risk in infertility patients with pregnancy stimulation or embryo transfer procedures may be much higher.)
- Risk of EP low in women with painless vaginal bleeding during the first trimester (but occasionally women with EP present this way initially)
  Odds ratios are given in Table 81-1.

TABLE 81-1. ODDS RATIOS FOR RISK FACTORS FOR ECTOPIC PREGNANCY

Degree of Risk	Risk Factors
High (odds ratios = 2.4–25)	Previous ectopic pregnancy
	Previous tubal surgery
	Tubal pathology
	In utero DES exposure
Moderate (odds ratios = 2.1–21)	Previous genital infections
	Infertility
	Multiple sexual partners
Low (odds ratios = 0.9–3.8)	Previous pelvic/abdominal surgery
	Smoking
	Vaginal douching
	Early age of intercourse (<18 years)

DES = diethylstilbestrol.
Adapted from data in Ankum WM, Mol BWJ, Van Der Veen F, Bossuyt PMM: Risk factors for ectopic pregnancy—a meta-analysis. Fertil Steril 65:1093, 1996.

21. **How reliable are routine serum and urine pregnancy tests in a patient with EP?**
Sensitive serum or urine pregnancy tests are almost always positive in EP. β-hCG is secreted from the time of implantation and is detectable about 7–8 days after implantation of the fertilized ovum. Qualitative pregnancy tests positive at a level of 10–50 mIU/mL are positive in 99% of patients with EP. Home pregnancy tests and less sensitive tests with higher thresholds may be falsely negative. Serum and urine tests provide similar accuracy for qualitative testing if their thresholds are similar.

22. **What clinical signs and symptoms useful to increase suspicion of an EP?**
The classic picture of EP is of vaginal bleeding, pelvic or abdominal pain, prior missed menses, and an adnexal mass. This picture is neither sensitive nor specific. Missed menses occur in only 85% of EP patients. Vaginal bleeding and pain may occur only later, when the growing EP begins to fail or overstretch its abnormal implantation site. Adnexal masses are palpated in only 50% of patients, even under anesthesia; they may represent the corpus luteum of the pregnancy rather than the ectopic gestation itself. Patients at high risk for EP are those with first-trimester

pregnancy and either pelvic pain or risk factors for EP. Peritoneal signs, severe pain on pelvic examination, and cervical motion tenderness also increase suspicion of EP. There is, however, no constellation of historical factors or findings that confirms or excludes EP with sufficient reliability to avoid ancillary studies discussed subsequently.

Abbott JT, Emmans L, Lowenstein SR: Ectopic pregnancy: Ten common pitfalls in diagnosis. Am J Emerg Med 8:515–522, 1990.

Dart RG, Kaplan B, Varaklis K: Predictive value of history and physical examination in patients with suspected ectopic pregnancy. Ann Emerg Med 33:283–290, 1999.

23. What are the incidence and risk factors for tubal rupture?

The overall rate of tubal rupture is 18% and does not affect subsequent IUP. Risk factors include the following:

- Never having used contraception
- History of tubal damage and infertility
- Induction of ovulation
- High level of β-hCG (at least 10,000 IU/L, when the EP was suspected to have ruptured)

Job-Spira N, Fernandez H, Bouyer J, et al: Ruptured tubal ectopic pregnancy: Risk factors and reproductive outcome of a population-based study in France. Am J Obstet Gynecol 180:938, 1999.

24. Why are corpus luteum cysts frequently confused with EPs?

The corpus luteum of the ovary, originating from the graafian follicle, supports the pregnancy with secretion of hCG and progesterone during the first 6–7 weeks of gestation and may become cystic, growing to 5 cm in diameter or more. Cyst rupture can occur in the first trimester, presenting as a patient in early pregnancy with sudden pain, unilateral peritoneal findings, adnexal tenderness, and perhaps a mass.

25. What is the most efficient way to diagnose or exclude EP in the ED?

Ultrasound evaluation of early pregnancy is the best first ancillary study. Of patients, 50–75% have a definitive diagnosis of either IUP or EP (less commonly) from imaging. Normal IUPs can be seen by transvaginal sonography by about 5.5 weeks' gestation. EPs occasionally can be seen, but the more common finding is an empty uterus. In 25–50% of patients seen in the first trimester for vaginal bleeding or pain, ultrasound is indeterminant. The risk of EP can be defined further by obtaining a quantitative hCG level if the ultrasound is inconclusive. IUP, if present, should be detected on ultrasound when the hCG concentration is greater than 2000 IU/L.

Paul M, Schaff E, Nichols M: The roles of clinical assessment, human chorionic gonadotropin assays, and ultrasonography in medical abortion practice. Am J Obstet Gynecol 183:S34, 2000.

26. What is the role of quantitative hCG? Should it be a *stat* test in every patient with possible EP?

Levels of hCG double every 2–3 days during the first 7–8 weeks of normal pregnancies. Because many women do not know the date of their last menstrual period, quantitative levels may be useful to estimate gestational age and correlate with expected sonographic findings (see earlier). With hCG greater than 2000 mIU/mL, a healthy IUP should be visible by transvaginal sonography. Failure to double normally during the first 7 weeks indicates the pregnancy is failing—either within the uterus or at an ectopic site. EP is likely if the ultrasound is indeterminant and the quantitative hCG is greater than 2000 mIU/mL or is rising on serial measurements (usually done at 48-hour intervals). A rapidly falling hCG level (less than half of the original in 48 hours) is unlikely to be an EP, whereas slowly falling levels are consistent with EP. A failed pregnancy is likely to be ectopic if dilation and curettage fails to detect villi or if no products of conception are found at the time of miscarriage. The most efficient method of diagnosing EP is to measure the hCG level only if the ultrasound is indeterminant. An alternative algorithm that is almost as efficient employs an initial hCG level and an ultrasound when the hCG level is greater than 2000 mIU/mL.

Hajenius PJ, Engelsbel S, Ankum WM, et al: Serum human chorionic gonadotropin measurement in the diagnosis of ectopic pregnancy when transvaginal sonography is inconclusive. Fertil Steril 70:972–981, 1998.

27. **Does every patient with bleeding or pain in the first trimester require ultrasound before discharge from the ED?**
Urgent sonography is for patients with acute pain, significant risk factors, or unreliable follow-up. Most patients can be managed with the possibility that they could be harboring an EP. They should get an urgent ultrasound within 1–2 days; daytime sonographic studies frequently are more complete and accurate. All first-trimester complaints are treated as *rule out EP* until an IUP is shown on ultrasound. These patients can be scheduled for a follow-up outpatient ultrasound, but they should be instructed to return immediately to their PCP or the ED if they have increasing pain or vaginal bleeding.

Garcia CR, Barnhart KT: Diagnosing ectopic pregnancy: Decision analysis comparing six strategies. Obstet Gynecol 97:464–470, 2001.

28. **What are the ultrasound findings in patients with suspected EP?**
See Table 81-2.

TABLE 81-2. ULTRASOUND FINDINGS IN PATIENTS WITH SUSPECTED EP	
Diagnostic of IUP	**Indeterminate**
Double gestational sac	Empty uterus
Intrauterine fetal pole or yolk sac	Nonspecific fluid collections
Intrauterine fetal heart activity	Echogenic material
Diagnostic of EP	Abnormal sac
Ectopic fetal heart activity or	Single gestational sac
Ectopic fetal pole	
Suggestive of EP	
Moderate or large cul-de-sac fluid without IUP	
Adnexal mass* without IUP	

EP = ectopic pregnancy, IUP = intrauterine pregnancy.
*Complex mass most suggestive of EP but cyst also can be seen with EP.
Modified from Dart RG: Role of pelvic ultrasonography in evaluation of symptomatic first trimester pregnancy. Ann Emerg Med 33:310–320, 1999.

29. **What patients with EPs can be discharged from the ED?**
Women who are unstable with significant pain or signs of significant blood loss require admission. ED or inpatient observation may be useful in stable patients with worrisome symptoms, risk factors, or expected poor compliance to facilitate rapid sonography, quantitative hCG interpretation, or specialist consultation. Stable patients with indeterminant ultrasound results (*rule out EP*) or known but relatively asymptomatic EPs may be followed on an outpatient basis. Conservative outpatient treatment modalities for EP are becoming more common. Expectant management or chemotherapy for women with few symptoms and low hormonal levels should be directed by the patient's obstetrician. The role of the ED physician is to consider the diagnosis, make every effort to exclude or make the diagnosis of EP expeditiously, make the

patient aware of the differential diagnosis and signs that should be of concern to her, and ensure access to close follow-up care for this potentially serious problem.

30. Which EPs should be treated medically with methotrexate?

Methotrexate, a folic acid antagonist that inhibits DNA synthesis and cell reproduction, is a chemical poison for the rapidly growing cells of pregnancy and has replaced surgery for many patients with small EPs (usually without fetal heart tones, < 3 cm diameter, or hCG level < 5000 mIU/mL IRP [International Reference Preparation] without signs of significant peritoneal bleeding). It should only be ordered by an obstetrician/gynecologist. Failure rates of about 10% are seen, so the patient still must be followed closely. Patients commonly have significant pain and may have peritoneal findings several days after treatment with methotrexate. Abnormal vital signs, a decreasing hematocrit, or diffuse peritoneal signs are indications that rupture of the EP may have occurred. The gynecologist administering methotrexate should always be involved in assessment of these patients. Medical treatment is often less expensive than laparoscopic surgery. Single-dose methotrexate is effective in 85% of patients.

Barnhart KT, Gosman G, Asnby R, Sammel M: The medical management of ectopic pregnancy: A meta-analysis comparing "single-dose" and "multidose" regimens. Obstet Gynecol 101:778, 2003.

Morlock RJ, Lafata JE, Eisenstein D: Cost-effectiveness of single-dose methotrexate compared with laparoscopic treatment of ectopic pregnancy. Obstet Gynecol 95:407, 2000.

KEY POINTS: CANDIDATES FOR MEDICAL TREATMENT WITH METHOTREXATE ✔

1. An asymptomatic ectopic pregnancy

2. The ability and willingness to comply with post-treatment monitoring

3. Serum β-hCG concentration less than 5000 mIU/mL before treatment

4. Tubal size less than 3 cm and no fetal cardiac activity on ultrasonographic examination

31. Name the sources and causes of third-trimester vaginal bleeding.

The sources are the vagina, cervix, and uterus. In the following list, life-threatening causes are indicated by an asterisk:

- Placenta previa: 0.3–0.5% of live births*
- Placental abruption: 0.8–1.2% of pregnancies (15–20% present without vaginal bleeding)*
- Uterine rupture: 0.05% of pregnancies*
- Marginal sinus rupture
- Bloody show
- Local trauma
- Cervical polyps and lesions

McKennett M, Fullerton JT: Vaginal bleeding in pregnancy. Am Fam Physician 51:639–646, 1995.

32. What is placenta previa? How is it diagnosed?

Placenta previa occurs when the placenta implants on or near the cervical os. Total coverage of the cervical os by placenta is called **complete placenta previa,** whereas subtotal coverage is called **partial placenta previa. Marginal placenta previa** occurs when the margin of the placenta approaches but does not cover any of the cervical os. Placenta previa is dangerous, as vaginal penetration or manipulation of the placenta during a pelvic examination may rupture blood vessels and cause massive hemorrhage, which in turn may cause maternal or fetal demise. Placenta previa is diagnosed by color flow Doppler ultrasound, which is 82% sensitive and 91–96% specific in diagnosing placenta previa. Placenta previa frequently is diagnosed early in pregnancy and followed with serial ultrasound studies until delivery. Occasionally, gravid women present with vaginal bleeding and an undiagnosed placental abnormality. If vaginal bleeding occurs, it is generally painless and bright red in color. Palpation of the fetus is not difficult. Fetal heart tones are heard, and there is no coagulopathy.

Chou MM, Ho ES, Lee YH: Prenatal diagnosis of placenta previa accreta by transabdominal color Doppler ultrasound. Ultrasound Obstet Gynecol 15:28–35, 2000.

33. How is placenta previa treated?

If the diagnosis is considered, call for an immediate obstetric consultation. Do not perform a pelvic examination unless you are in the operating room or delivery suite with an experienced obstetrician because life-threatening bleeding may occur if the placenta is inadvertently manipulated. Place the patient on her left side in the recumbent position. In patients who are hemodynamically stable with small amounts of bleeding, start an intravenous line, and admit the patient for ultrasound, serial maternal vital signs, and fetal monitoring. In selected cases, delivery is delayed to optimize fetal development. If serious vaginal bleeding occurs, start two large-bore intravenous lines, administer oxygen, monitor fetal heart tones, and admit the patient for delivery.

Crane S, Chun B, Acker D: Treatment of obstetrical hemorrhagic emergencies. Curr Opin Obstet Gynecol 5:675–682, 1993.

34. What is placental abruption (abruptio placentae)? Why is it dangerous?

The premature separation of the placenta from its insertion on the uterine wall where a large amount of blood may collect between the placenta and the uterine wall, causing maternal shock and fetal demise. Abruption occurs spontaneously or after mild, moderate, or severe trauma. The uterus is firm or hard, and the patient reports severe abdominal pain. Hypotension may occur, and vaginal bleeding occurs in about 80% of patients. If vaginal bleeding does occur, the blood is dark red. This presentation is in contrast to the painless, bright red bleeding of placenta previa. The presence of additional blood in the uterus makes palpating the fetus and measuring fetal heart tones difficult. Coagulopathy may occur. Placental abruption is diagnosed by ultrasound.

35. Describe the treatment of placental abruption.

Start two large-bore intravenous lines, and administer oxygen. Monitor fetal heart tones and the mother's vital signs frequently. If possible, place on a fetal monitor. Obtain coagulation studies to diagnose coagulopathy (prothrombin time [PT], partial thromboplastin time [PTT], fibrinogen, and fibrin splint products). If the mother and fetus are stable, arrange an immediate ultrasound. Take unstable patients directly to the operating room or delivery suite for delivery.

36. What is uterine rupture? Why is it dangerous?

A grave complication of late pregnancy in which the uterus ruptures, usually during contractions. It can produce massive, life-threatening intra-abdominal hemorrhage. Maternal mortality is 8%, and fetal mortality is about 50%. Uterine rupture presents sudden abdominal pain and shock late in pregnancy associated with uterine contractions. There is scant vaginal bleeding, and the abdomen is extremely tender.

37. What is the treatment of uterine rupture?

Start two large-bore intravenous lines, and administer oxygen with immediate transfer to the operating room or delivery suite for laparotomy and hysterectomy. Ultrasound may be necessary in selected cases to distinguish uterine rupture from placental abruption.

38. **Describe the non-life-threatening causes of third-trimester vaginal bleeding.**
Bloody show is a pink mucous discharge caused by cervical changes that precedes labor by several hours to a week. The cervix is prone to hemorrhage during late pregnancy, and local trauma from vaginal penetration, including intercourse, may cause bleeding. Cervical erosions or preexisting polyps produce limited bleeding. Marginal sinus rupture is a premature separation of the placenta limited to the placental margin.

Acknowledgments

I express appreciation to the previous authors, Kim M. Feldhaus, Jean T. Abbott, and John M. Howell, for their contributions to previous edition chapters that were combined and updated to form this chapter and to Angela B. Chapman for her help in preparing the manuscript.

CHAPTER 82

PREECLAMPSIA AND ECLAMPSIA

Jennie A. Buchanan, MD

1. **What is preeclampsia?**

   Preeclampsia is a syndrome that occurs after 20 weeks of gestation. It is associated with hypertension, proteinuria, edema, visual disturbances, headache, and epigastric or right upper quadrant pain.

2. **Define the criteria for the diagnosis of preeclampsia.**
   - Blood pressure of 140 mmHg systolic or higher and 90 mmHg diastolic or higher, which occurs after 20 weeks of gestation in a woman with normal blood pressure previously
   - Proteinuria, defined as a urinary excretion of 0.3 gm protein or higher in a 24-hour period

3. **What are the criteria for the diagnosis of severe preeclampsia?**
   - Blood pressure > 160/110 mmHg
   - Proteinuria (5 g/L in 24 hours)
   - Oliguria (< 400 mL in 24 hours)
   - Visual or cerebral disturbances
   - Pulmonary edema or cyanosis
   - Epigastric or right upper quadrant pain
   - Impaired liver function tests
   - Fetal growth restriction
   - Thrombocytopenia

   Sibai BM: Hypertension. In Gabbe SG, Niebyl JR, Simpson JL (eds): Obstetrics: Normal and Problem Pregnancies, 4th ed. Philadelphia, Churchill Livingstone, 2002, pp 945–1004.

4. **Is every hypertensive woman considered preeclamptic?**

   No. Hypertension during pregnancy can be categorized into four different categories:
   - Preeclampsia/eclampsia
   - Chronic hypertension
   - Chronic hypertension with preeclampsia
   - Gestational hypertension

   Chronic hypertension precedes pregnancy. Chronic hypertension superimposed with preeclampsia poses greater risk for mother and fetus than either condition alone. The majority of cases of gestational hypertension occur after 37 weeks of gestation, and the diagnosis is often suspected until a more specific diagnosis can be assigned.

5. **What causes preeclampsia?**

   The etiology of preeclampsia is unknown. Many theories have been proposed but are currently unproven. Research has focused on the incomplete degree of trophoblastic invasion by the placenta often associated with preeclampsia. The hypoperfused placenta releases toxic mediators, which result in organ hypoperfusion and damage.

6. **Who is at risk for preeclampsia?**

   Preeclampsia is primarily a disease of first pregnancies. Risk factors include family history, obesity, multifetal gestation, preeclampsia in prior pregnancy, poor outcome in prior pregnancy, chronic hypertension, renal disease, insulin-dependent diabetes, thrombophilias, vascular and connective tissue disorders, African-American race, age older than 35 years, smoking, elevated cholesterol, and lower socioeconomic status.

Bhattacharya S, Campbell DM: The incidence of severe complications of preeclampsia. Hypertens Pregnancy 24:181–190, 2005.

7. What is the incidence of preeclampsia?
Between 5% and 8%.

Cunningham FG, Gant NF, Leveno KJ, et al: Hypertensive disorders in pregnancy. In: Williams Obstetrics, 21st ed. New York, McGraw-Hill, 2001, pp 567–618.

8. State the laboratory tests used to predict who will develop preeclampsia/eclampsia.
- Hemoglobin and hematocrit: Hemoconcentration supports the diagnosis, but values may be lower if hemolysis is present.
- Platelet count: Thrombocytopenia is associated with preeclampsia.
- Creatinine level: Abnormal or increasing levels in association with oliguria are often associated with the syndrome.
- Uric acid: Increased levels suggest the diagnosis.
- Serum transaminase levels: Suggest liver involvement
- Albumin, lactic acid dehydrogenase, blood smear, and coagulation profile: Indicate extent of endothelial leak, presence of hemolysis, and coagulopathy

9. What new lab value may be helpful in discerning who will develop preeclampsia?
Brain natriuretic peptide.

Kale A, Kale E, Yalinkaya A, et al: The comparison of amino-terminal probrain natriuretic peptide levels in preeclampsia and normotensive pregnancy. J Perinat Med 33:121–124, 2005.

10. How should blood pressure be treated in preeclampsia?
Antihypertensive medications should be utilized when diastolic blood pressure is 105–110 mmHg or higher. Medications used to control blood pressure include the following:
- Hydralazine, 5–10 mg doses intravenously every 15–20 minutes until desired response is reached
- Labetalol, 20 mg intravenous bolus dose followed by 40 mg if not effective within 10 minutes; then 80 mg every 10 minutes with a maximum dose of 220 mg

Nifedipine and sodium nitroprusside can also be utilized (follow fetus for cyanide toxicity if nitroprusside is utilized). Diuretics and angiotensin-converting enzyme inhibitors are contraindicated.

Cunningham FG, Gant NF, Leveno KJ, et al: Hypertensive disorders in pregnancy. In: Williams Obstetrics, 21st ed. New York, McGraw-Hill, 2001, pp 567–618.

11. What is the optimal treatment for preeclampsia?
For mild preeclampsia, deliver if the patient is at term. If the patient is premature, hospitalize and check labs, urine, serial blood pressures, start magnesium sulfate when in labor or at time of induction. In severe disease, start magnesium; monitor labs, pulmonary status, and urine; keep blood pressure between 90–105 mHg with hydralazine or labetalol; deliver or consider cesarean for primigravida, unfavorable cervix, and gestational age less than 32 weeks.

12. What are the current prophylaxis and treatment of eclamptic seizures?
Prophylaxis should be utilized in all patients during labor, delivery, and 24 hours postpartum. Magnesium sulfate is still the drug of choice in the United States, although controversy still

exists. The loading dose is 4–6 gm of magnesium sulfate in a 10% solution infused slowly over 5–10 minutes. Maintenance dose is 2–3 gm per hour with magnesium levels checked every 6 hours.

13. **How does magnesium toxicity present?**
Magnesium toxicity presents initially with loss of patellar reflexes (8–12 mg/dL), feeling of warmth with flushing, somnolence, slurred speech, muscular paralysis, respiratory difficulty, and finally cardiac arrest (30–35 mg/dL). If the patient becomes toxic, calcium gluconate 10 mL of a 10% solution can be utilized intravenously.

Abbot J, Houry D: Acute complications of pregnancy. In: Rosen's Emergency Medicine Concepts and Clinical Practice, 5th ed. St. Louis, Mosby, 2002, pp 2413–2433.

KEY POINTS: PREECLAMPSIA AND ECLAMPSIA

1. Preeclampsia and eclampsia can present postpartum.

2. Magnesium sulfate is the treatment for eclampsia.

3. Be alert if a woman presents with elevated blood pressure in the second or third trimester.

14. **What is the best mode of delivery for a preeclamptic woman?**
In mild preeclampsia, a vaginal term delivery is recommended. There are no randomized clinical trials that have evaluated vaginal verses cesarean delivery in severe preeclampsia or eclampsia. The decision to undergo a cesarean should based on the individual patient.

Walker JJ: Pre-eclampsia. Lancet 356:1260–1265, 2000.

15. **What is eclampsia?**
Eclampsia is defined as the presence of new-onset grand mal seizures in a woman with preeclampsia.

16. **How is eclampsia treated?**
   - ABCs should be addressed, immediately. Often an oral airway is needed.
   - Administer oxygen.
   - Place lines, monitor fetus and mother, urine output (Swan Ganz catheter can be placed).
   - Administer magnesium sulfate.
   - Consider diazepam (Valium), 10 mg IV push, if patient seizes a second time.
   - Emergent delivery is the definitive treatment.

17. **Does a patient have to be pregnant to become preeclamptic/eclamptic?**
No. Preeclamptic symptoms can worsen after delivery, and postpartum preeclampsia and eclampsia are well-described phenomena. Symptoms usually develop in the first 24–48 hours after delivery but may not occur until weeks post delivery.

18. **What is HELLP syndrome?**
HELLP syndrome is described in conjunction with severe preeclampsia:
   - **H** = Hemolysis
   - **EL** = Elevated Liver enzymes
   - **LP** = Low Platelets
   Patients present with epigastric or right upper quadrant pain, nausea, vomiting, and nonspecific viral prodrome. Patients with HELLP do not often present with severe hypertension or proteinuria.

19. **Who is at risk for HELLP syndrome?**
    Caucasian patients and preeclamptic patients who have been managed conservatively are at risk for HELLP.

20. **What is an acute life-threatening complication of HELLP syndrome?**
    HELLP is associated with placental abruption, renal failure, and subcapsular hepatic hematoma ruptured or unruptured. Patients with hepatic rupture present with shock, shoulder pain, ascites, and pleural effusion. Fetal mortality ranges from 7.7–60%, and maternal mortality ranges from 0–24%.

    Sibai BM: Hypertension. In Gabbe SG, Niebyl JR, Simpson JL (eds): Obstetrics: Normal and Problem Pregnancies, 4th ed. Philadelphia, Churchill Livingstone, 2002, pp 945–1004.

21. **Name the most frequent cause of maternal death in preeclampsia/eclampsia.**
    Central nervous system disorders, including microinfarctions, cerebral edema, subarachnoid hemorrhage, cortical and subcortical hemorrhages, and large intracerebral hematomas.

22. **What are the fetal risks in a preeclamptic/eclamptic pregnancy?**
    Because of impaired uteroplacental blood flow and placental infarction, the fetus is at risk for intrauterine growth restriction, oligohydramnios, placental abruption, and nonreassuring fetal status during antepartum monitoring.

    Sibai BM: Hypertension. In Gabbe SG, Niebyl JR, Simpson JL (eds): Obstetrics: Normal and Problem Pregnancies, 4th ed. Philadelphia, Churchill Livingstone, 2002, pp 945–1004.

23. **Can preeclampsia be prevented?**
    Recent studies have focused attention on low-dose aspirin, calcium, and antioxidant therapy to prevent preeclampsia. Aspirin has shown little benefit, and studies have failed to prove the benefit of calcium. Vitamin C and E therapy has shown some promise in preventing preeclampsia; however, these studies need to be confirmed by randomized trials.

    American College of Obstetricians and Gynecologists: Diagnosis and management of preeclampsia and eclampsia. ACOG Practice Bulletin No. 33. Obstet Gynecol 99:159–167, 2002.

Acknowledgment

I gratefully acknowledge the contributions of Robert S. Van Hare, MD, author of this chapter in the previous edition.

CHAPTER 83

CHILDBIRTH

Richard O. Jones, MD

1. I'm an emergency medical (EM) physician. Why should I learn about childbirth?
The unplanned delivery of babies in the Emergency Department (ED) is a fact of life. The main objective is always a healthy baby and mother. Involvement of obstetrics and pediatrics is appropriate as soon as it is evident that a delivery is going to occur in the ED. *Labor and delivery* is a natural process, which usually proceeds to its conclusion without difficulty. In most cases, little intervention is required on the part of the health care provider. Most mistakes in the care of the mother and baby are made as the result of lack of preparation and planning.

2. When a pregnant patient is brought to the ED, what factors should direct treatment?
After the mother is evaluated and stabilized, the baby can be evaluated. If your hospital has obstetric coverage, notify the on-call obstetrician as soon as possible.

3. What do I need to do to stabilize a pregnant patient brought into the ED?
After vital signs and the chief complaint are obtained, the next step should probably be to establish intravenous (IV) access, especially if the patient appears to be in labor or is having vaginal bleeding or leakage of fluid from her vagina.

4. What information do I need to care properly for the pregnant patient?
Important information to obtain is the patient's due date and the number of deliveries she has had. Next, find out if she feels the baby moving and if she is having contractions, vaginal bleeding, or leakage of fluid from the vagina. Then inquire about problems with the pregnancy and current medications. Once that information is obtained, find out where she is getting her prenatal care and the name of her doctor or midwife.

5. How are the baby and pregnancy evaluated?
Fetal heart tones should be obtained as soon as the mother is stabilized. A normal fetal heart rate is between 110–160 bpm. Next, the fundal height (the distance in centimeters from the symphysis pubis to the top of the pregnant uterus) should be measured to give a rough estimate of gestational age. For example, a fundal height of 32 cm would indicate a gestational age of roughly 30–34 weeks. An ultrasound, if available, can provide much more information. External fetal monitoring can identify the pattern of the fetal heart rate and the mother's contraction pattern.

6. What is false labor?
False labor is characterized by contractions without cervical change. This is a common occurrence.

7. When can the diagnosis of true labor be made?
When the patient is having effacement (thinning) and dilation of the cervix with contractions.

8. How can I ascertain uterine contractions?
By palpating the uterus. The uterus will become more firm and "ball" up when contracting. Contractions may last from 30–90 seconds and may occur as frequently as 1 minute apart.

9. **How long does labor usually last?**
   In primigravidas, labor lasts an average of 10 hours but can last as long as 26 hours. In multiparas, this time may be shortened to less than 7 hours, but can last as long as 20 hours.

10. **What is the most important sign of the progress of labor?**
    Progressive dilation of the cervix.

11. **How do you check cervical dilation?**
    Under sterile conditions, a digital pelvic examination is performed. The diameter of the cervical opening in front of the baby's head is estimated in centimeters. The measurements vary from closed up to 10 cm. Practice is required for accuracy.

12. **Describe a normal labor process.**
    Labor is usually divided into three parts: first stage, second stage, and third stage.

13. **Define the first stage of labor.**
    The first stage starts when contractions begin and lasts until the cervix is completely dilated to 10 cm. During this stage, the cervix thins out (effaces) and dilates in response to the uterine contractions. The first stage is divided into latent phase, active phase, and deceleration phase. The latent phase can last 20 hours (average 6.5 hours) in a primigravida and 14 hours (average 5 hours) in a multigravida. During the active phase, the most rapid dilation of the cervix takes place. The contractions are much stronger and more painful than in the latent phase. This phase usually lasts no longer than 5 hours in a primigravida and 3 hours in a multigravida. The deceleration phase takes place in the last hour or so before the cervix is completely dilated at 10 cm. During this phase, dilation slows, and the head begins to descend down the birth canal.

14. **Define the second stage of labor.**
    This stage begins when the cervix is completely dilated and ends when the baby is delivered. The patient may be allowed to push when the cervix is completely dilated. This shortens the second stage. Even if the patient does not push, the uterine contractions will cause delivery. The second stage can last 2 hours in a primigravida and usually is much shorter in a multigravida.

15. **Define the third stage of labor.**
    The third stage begins after the baby is delivered and ends when the placenta is delivered. The third stage usually does not last more than 30 minutes.

16. **If the evaluation shows the patient is in labor but is not very dilated, can she be taken to the labor and delivery suite?**
    If delivery is not imminent, taking the patient to Labor and Delivery is the best option. If the patient is well along in labor and delivery is imminent, you should prepare for delivery in the ED. Make sure an emergency delivery pack is available.

17. **What should be in an emergency delivery pack?**
    The contents of an emergency delivery pack may vary from ED to ED. At a minimum, each pack should contain:
    - A bulb syringe to clear the baby's nose and mouth
    - Sterile gloves [in various sizes] for the delivering health care provider
    - Sterile towels to dry off baby and a baby blanket to keep the baby warm
    - Four Kelly clamps for clamping the umbilical cord or vaginal or perineal bleeders
    - Mayo scissors to cut the umbilical cord
    - Two-ring forceps
    - Three packs of 4 × 4 sponges
    - Container for placenta

18. **How can I determine if a delivery is imminent?**

    This can be difficult. Some patients will not appear to be in any distress 1 minute, and there is a baby in the bed the next minute. If delivery is imminent, most patients will feel the urge to push or bear down in response to the pressure of the baby as it moves down the birth canal. The patient may say, "The baby is coming," or "I have to have a bowel movement." She may be visibly bearing down or pushing with contractions. If examination of the patient reveals the cervix is 6 cm or more dilated, delivery may occur before or during transport to Labor and Delivery.

19. **What do I do when I have a laboring pregnant patient in the ED and the baby can be seen distending the mother's perineum?**

    After making sure the obstetrician and pediatrician have been called, get ready for the delivery. Wearing sterile gloves, apply gentle pressure against the presenting part to prevent sudden expulsion and to allow gradual stretching of the perineum.

20. **Should I put traction on the baby to help the delivery?**

    In most cases, the mother will push the baby out without help. Pulling on the baby may interrupt the normal delivery process unless you are experienced with deliveries. The best way to assist with the delivery is to use your hands to help control and guide the delivery of the baby. The baby may deliver very quickly, so keep a good grip. Be sure to note the time of delivery.

KEY POINTS: CHILDBIRTH IN THE EMERGENCY DEPARTMENT

1. Labor and delivery is a natural process, which usually proceeds to its conclusion without difficulty. In most cases, minimal intervention is required on the part of the health care provider.

2. When evaluating a pregnant patient in the ED, stabilization and resuscitation of the mother will result in optimal prognosis of the baby.

3. During delivery, the health care provider should not attempt to speed up the process by manipulating the baby. In most cases, it is unnecessary to do more than attempt to guide and control the process.

21. **If the umbilical cord is wrapped around the neck during a delivery, what should I do?**

    If the cord is wrapped around the neck, it should be pulled gently over the head, if possible, so that it does not tighten as the baby is being born. If the cord is too tight to lift over the head, carefully apply two clamps to the cord and cut the cord between the clamps. Then the cord can be unwound from around the neck and the baby delivered.

22. **What do I do now that the baby is delivered?**

    Holding the baby head down, suction the nose and mouth with a bulb syringe. Most babies can cough out the amniotic fluid without help, as long as they are held head down. "Spanking" the baby is unnecessary. Then apply two clamps to the umbilical cord (at least several centimeters from the baby's abdomen), and cut the cord between the clamps. Next, to prevent the baby from becoming too cold as a result of evaporation of amniotic fluid on the skin, the baby should be dried and kept warm. After drying, the baby can be placed on the mother's abdomen for skin-to-skin contact, which provides warmth. See Chapter 66 if the baby is having problems after delivery and no pediatrician is available.

23. **She has not delivered the placenta. What should I do now?**
There is no hurry to deliver the placenta unless there is heavy bleeding. If there is heavy bleeding, have the mother try to push out the placenta. Do not pull on the cord. Gently but firmly massaging the uterus through the mother's lower abdominal wall above the pubic bone may help control blood loss and may help deliver the placenta. If the placenta delivers spontaneously, massage the uterus gently but firmly to keep it contracted into a firm "ball." As long as the uterus stays firmly contracted, bleeding should be minimal.

24. **How much bleeding is normal with a delivery?**
Usually a delivering mother will lose 200–300 mL of blood with a delivery. Up to 500 mL is considered within the normal range.

25. **The placenta is out, but there was a tear in the perineum that is bleeding. What do I do?**
As with any laceration, applying pressure usually stems the bleeding until the obstetrician arrives. If the delay is too long, clamp the bleeding site with a Kelly clamp. If that is unsuccessful or the clamp cannot be left in place, give local anesthetic and suture the laceration with interrupted sutures to control the bleeding. Transfer the patient and placenta to your Labor and Delivery unit, when stable.

26. **Where can I read more about pregnancies and deliveries?**
There are several excellent obstetric textbooks available. One of the most popular is *Obstetrics*, edited by Dr. Steve Gabbe, published by Churchill Livingstone.

BIBLIOGRAPHY

1. Cunningham FG, Gant NF, Leveno KJ, et al: Williams Obstetrics, ed 21. New York, McGraw-Hill, 2001.
2. Gabbe S, Niebyl JR, Simpson JL: Obstetrics: Normal and Problem Pregnancies, ed 4. New York, Churchill-Livingstone, 2002.

MULTIPLE TRAUMA

Peter Rosen, MD

CHAPTER 84

1. **What is multiple trauma?**
   Significant injury to more than one major body system or organ.

2. **Can severity of injury be determined at the scene?**
   Not accurately because many younger patients have great cardiovascular reserves and do not demonstrate evidence of injuries that may be serious until they decompensate. A variety of different trauma scales and scoring devices have been developed to quantify the extent of injury. These devices are imperfect, however, and to maintain an acceptable safety margin, systems need to **overtriage** potential multiple-trauma victims. Transport to a trauma center should be based on the mechanism of injury, underlying disease, physiologic parameters such as alterations in vital signs and neurologic status, and the presence of obvious multiple organ system injury.

3. **Define mechanism of injury.**
   Mechanism of injury refers to the events and conditions that lead to visible and occult traumatic injuries. Significant mechanism of injury is associated with a higher likelihood of multiple trauma. Less obvious mechanism is of greater concern with increasing age or preexisting disease. A 70-year-old patient with ankylosing spondylitis is much less able to tolerate blunt trauma to the spinal column and pelvis than is a healthy younger person.

4. **Give examples of significant mechanisms of injury.**
   Blunt trauma
   - Automobile crashes: Fatality at the scene or in the same vehicle, passenger ejection, vehicle rollover, significant interior damage
   - Automobile-pedestrian accidents: High speed, damage to exterior of vehicle
   - Falls: Greater than one story (12–15 feet)
   Penetrating trauma
   - Gunshot wounds to head, neck, or torso
   - Stab wounds to neck or torso

5. **List the first steps in managing multiple trauma in the emergency department (ED).**
   - Activate the trauma resuscitation team.
   - Designate a trauma captain and call for O-negative blood if indicated by prehospital course and vital signs.
   - Transfer the patient from the ambulance stretcher or other conveyance to the ED resuscitation bed using spinal injury precautions if indicated.
   - Quickly obtain a history, including the mechanism of injury, field treatment, and response to this field treatment.
   - Obtain vital signs while the patient is being undressed.
   - Assess the ABCs and intervene as necessary.
   - Draw blood for type, crossmatching, and baseline laboratory testing.

6. How should the patient be undressed?

Because immobilization is necessary until the spine can be cleared, all movement should be avoided. To obtain complete visualization rapidly while protecting the spine, simply cut the clothes away. Keep in mind that one of the purposes of clothing removal is to rid the patient of objects that can cause further damage to the patient or injury to the health care providers, such as shards of broken glass, bits of metal, or weapons.

7. What are the ABCs (and D) of trauma?

- A = Airway
- B = Breathing
- C = Circulation
- D = Disability

8. Discuss assessment of the airway.

Airway patency is evaluated by listening for vocalizations, asking for the patient's name, and looking in the patient's mouth for signs of obstruction (blood, emesis, or foreign debris). The trauma captain must determine if the patient needs active airway management and verify that supplemental oxygen is being administered continuously to all patients who do not require immediate intubation.

Mandatory indications for airway management in trauma include the following:

- Massive facial injuries
- Head injury with Glasgow Coma Scale (GCS) less than 8
- Penetrating injury to the cranial vault
- Missile penetrating injury to the neck
- Blunt injury to the neck with expanding hematoma or alteration of the voice
- Multisystem trauma with persistent shock

Relative indications for airway management in trauma include the following:

- Upper airway obstruction from any cause
- Any patient with injuries impairing ventilation
- Flail chest with increasing respiratory rate or deteriorating oxygenation
- Any patient with one or more rib fractures who is going to need a ventilator or a general anesthetic
- Patients with bilateral pneumothorax
- Bilateral missile penetrating injuries of the thorax
- Patients with severe hypovolemic shock
- Patients with recurrent hemothorax or who do not respond to tube thoracostomy

9. How is breathing assessed?

Ventilation is assessed by observing for symmetric rise and fall of the chest and by listening for bilateral breath sounds over the anterior chest and axillae. The chest should be palpated gently for subcutaneous air and bony crepitus. Oxygen saturation should be monitored continuously. The trauma captain determines whether or not tube thoracostomies or ventilatory support is needed immediately.

10. How is circulation assessed?

Circulatory function is assessed by noting the patient's mental status; skin color and character (cool and clammy versus warm and dry); vital signs; and presence or absence of radial, femoral, and carotid pulses. Continuous cardiac monitoring should be started. Prehospital vascular access and type and amount of volume infused are assessed. The trauma captain determines whether additional vascular access or volume of crystalloid is needed and whether blood should be administered. A FAST ultrasound examination should be performed on any patient with torso trauma to detect free fluid (blood) in the abdomen or perineum. See Chapter 5.

11. How is disability assessed?

The patient's neurologic status should be assessed (level of consciousness and gross motor function). An initial ED GCS rating should be ascertained, and this should be compared with the prehospital GCS. With any alteration of consciousness, it is useful to perform a rectal examination to determine anal sphincter tone.

12. What type of intravenous access should be established in a patient with major trauma?

At least two large-bore (16G) intravenous catheters should be placed. Forearm or antecubital veins are the preferred sites for initial access. Although subclavian and internal jugular catheters allow central venous pressure monitoring, they rarely provide access for high-volume intravenous infusions unless a Cordis introducer is left in place. These routes should be used only if no other access exists, and catheters should be placed on the ipsilateral side of the chest trauma unless a subclavian vascular injury is suspected. Femoral lines and saphenous cutdowns are indicated in patients with a dropping blood pressure because large-volume infusions will be needed quickly. Central line placement is aided by use of an ultrasound probe. This will also make femoral line insertion safer.

13. Where should cutdowns be performed?

The ankle. The distal saphenous vein can be found between the anterior tibialis tendon and the medial malleolus.

KEY POINTS: MULTIPLE TRAUMA

1. Trauma care is a team sport involving prehospital providers and emergency physicians and surgical staff.

2. All trauma patients should be completely undressed and examined.

3. All trauma victims must be assessed for occult bleeding in the cranial vault, chest, and abdomen.

4. When indicated by mechanism of injury, symptoms, or signs, spinal precautions must be maintained until the spine is cleared.

---

14. What parameters should be monitored in multiple trauma victims?

Vital signs, neurologic status, cardiac rhythm, oxygen saturation, and, if possible, central venous pressure and urinary output. Hypothermia adversely affects outcome, and core temperature can drop rapidly when the patient is disrobed and receives large quantities of cold intravenous fluid. Tachypnea is a sensitive sign of hypoxia and acidosis and should be measured accurately rather than estimated. Neurologic status, skin color and character, and urinary output over time should be monitored.

15. When should blood be administered?

O-negative (universal donor) blood should be reserved for patients who are in arrest from hypovolemic shock. If 50 mL/kg of crystalloid is infused rapidly and there is no significant improvement in the patient's circulatory status, type-specific noncrossmatched blood should be administered if available. Otherwise, use type O initially. (For more details, see Chapter 4.)

16. Are laboratory tests useful?

No, although all major trauma victims should have a clot blood tube sent for type and crossmatch. Baseline values of hematocrit and serum amylase (or preferably lipase) may be useful in detecting occult injuries and preexisting anemia. Urinalysis should be done to detect hematuria. Many trauma centers obtain an extensive trauma panel, which may be useful if the patient requires surgery or has underlying disease. No laboratory test defines injury however, and the trauma panel is of little use in determining initial management, disposition, or need for surgery. Common initial lab tests in multiple trauma include the following:

- Complete blood cell count
- Type and crossmatch
- Electrolytes
- Urinalysis
- Blood urea nitrogen, creatinine
- Blood alcohol as indicated
- Glucose
- Toxicology as indicated
- Prothrombin and partial thromboplastin times
- Amylase, lipase

17. What is the secondary survey?

The complete physical examination performed after the ABCs have been assessed and stabilized. This survey includes assessment of the chest, abdomen, pelvis, back, and extremities. A repeat neurologic examination and rectal examination also should be done. The purpose of the rectal examination is to determine if there is gross blood in the rectum, if there is adequate sphincter tone and sensation, and if the prostate gland is in a normal position.

18. Which radiologic studies need to be obtained immediately?

When the patient is stabilized, portable radiographs of the lateral cervical spine, chest, and pelvis should be obtained. In gunshot wounds, portable films in two planes may be needed to determine the location of the bullet. If the mechanism of injury is an ejection or a fall, a cross-table lumbar spine film should be added to the initial series.

19. How do I prioritize diagnostic tests?

Prioritization is based on potential life threats. After external hemorrhage is controlled, diagnosing intraperitoneal hemorrhage takes precedence. Unless an indication for immediate laparotomy is present, the patient should undergo diagnostic peritoneal lavage, abdominal computed tomography (CT) scan, or abdominal ultrasound to assess the intraperitoneal cavity. After these procedures, attention should be focused on ruling out correctable intracranial hemorrhage, such as a subdural or an epidural hematoma. Based on the mechanism of injury and the initial course, other specialized studies to evaluate the aorta and the retroperitoneum should be done. If the patient has a bleeding diathesis (e.g., hemophilia) or is on an anticoagulant, even minor head injury mandates a CT scan.

20. How are fluids managed in pediatric trauma?

Start with a bolus of 20 mL/kg of normal saline (NS) or lactated Ringer's (LR). This can be repeated until up to 50 mL/kg has been reached. At this point, start packed red blood cells at 10 mL/kg.

21. What is the significance of blunt abdominal trauma in the pregnant woman?

- During the first trimester, the fetus is well protected, and the best treatment for the fetus is to protect the mother from hypovolemic shock.
- In the second trimester, the fetus is more vulnerable and must be monitored for signs of placental abruption.
- In the third trimester, the fetus is the most vulnerable, and even minor trauma necessitates fetal monitoring for several hours. If the signs of abruption occur, emergency caesarian section must be performed.

BIBLIOGRAPHY

1. Feliciano DV, Moore EE, Mattox KL (eds): Trauma, 3rd ed. Stamford, CT, Appleton & Lange, 1996.

2. Gin-Shaw S, Jorden RC: Approach to the multiple trauma patient. In Marx JA, Hockberger RS, Walls RM (eds): Rosen's Emergency Medicine: Concepts Clinical Practice, 5th ed. St. Louis, Mosby, 2002, pp 242–256.

3. Greenfield LJ, Mulholland MW, Oldham KT, et al (eds): Surgery: Scientific Principles and Practice, 2nd ed. Philadelphia, Lippincott-Raven, 1997.

4. Rosen P, Legome E: General principles of trauma. In Wolfson AB, Hendey GW, Hendry PL, et al (eds): Harwood-Nuss' Clinical Practice of Emergency Medicine, 4th ed. Philadelphia, Lippincott Williams & Wilkins, 2005, pp 890–899.

CHAPTER 85

MAXILLOFACIAL TRAUMA

Carlo L. Rosen, MD

1. **What are the facial bones?**
   The facial bones are the frontal, temporal, nasal, ethmoid, lacrimal, palatine, sphenoid, zygoma, maxilla, and mandible.

2. **What is the initial approach to a patient with maxillofacial trauma?**
   The initial management of patients with facial trauma should follow the ABCs (airway, breathing, circulation) of trauma resuscitation. The airway is the primary concern and can be challenging in these patients. Significant facial trauma may cause swelling or distortion of the airway as a result of bleeding, loose teeth, or fractures. In patients with mandibular fractures, the tongue loses its support and can occlude the airway. Early endotracheal intubation should be considered in patients with significant midface or mandibular trauma, especially if they exhibit any signs of airway distress. Standard methods of intubation, such as rapid-sequence intubation, should be attempted first. However, airway distortion resulting from facial trauma sometimes necessitates a cricothyrotomy. All patients with facial and head trauma should be assumed to have a cervical spine injury. In-line cervical spine stabilization should be used during intubation. The incidence of cervical spine injuries in patients with facial trauma is 1–4%.

   Ellis E, Scott K: Assessment of patients with facial fractures. Emerg Med Clin North Am 18:411–448, 2000.

3. **Which procedure is contraindicated in patients with maxillofacial trauma?**
   Nasogastric tube placement should not be performed because of the risk of intracranial placement through a fracture in the cribriform plate. The small size and flexibility of the nasogastric tube allow it to be misdirected through a fracture into the brain. There is also a theoretical concern about placing a nasotracheal tube through the cribriform plate into the brain. However, an endotracheal tube is larger and more rigid than a nasogastric tube. The literature suggests that the risk of intracranial placement of a nasotracheal tube is low.

   Rosen CL, Wolfe RE, Chew S, et al: Blind nasotracheal intubation in the presence of facial trauma. J Emerg Med 15:141–145, 1997.

4. **What is a blow-out fracture? What is the entrapment syndrome?**
   A blow-out fracture is a fracture of the orbital floor that results from a direct blow to the orbit. Increased intraorbital pressure causes rupture of the floor of the orbit. The entrapment syndrome is binocular diplopia and paralysis of upward gaze that results from entrapment of the inferior rectus muscle in the orbital wall defect. Diplopia is noted by having the patient follow and count fingers on upward gaze. Other physical findings include infraorbital anesthesia and enophthalmos (posterior displacement of the globe into the orbit). Patients may have tenderness or step-offs at the infraorbital rim or subcutaneous emphysema secondary to a fracture into the maxillary sinus. Ophthalmologic evaluation for associated orbital trauma (globe rupture, hyphema, retinal tear or detachment, blindness), despite an initially normal visual acuity and funduscopic examination, should be considered.

KEY POINTS: CLINICAL SIGNS OF ORBITAL FRACTURES

1. Eyelid edema

2. Enophthalmos

3. Proptosis

4. Limitation of upward gaze

5. Diplopia

6. Infraorbital anesthesia

7. Subcutaneous emphysema

5. What are Le Fort fractures?

The Le Fort classification is used to describe maxillary fractures (Fig. 85-1). Midface fractures are diagnosed by grasping the upper alveolar ridge and noting which part of the midface moves. Le Fort I, a transverse fracture just above the teeth at the level of the nasal fossa, allows movement of the alveolar ridge and hard palate. Le Fort II, a pyramid fracture with its apex just above the bridge of the nose and extending laterally and inferiorly through the infraorbital rims,

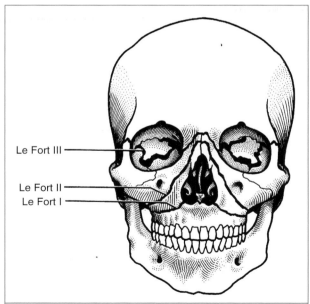

Figure 85-1. Le Fort classification of facial fractures. Le Fort I: palatofacial disjunction. Le Fort II: pyramidal disjunction. Le Fort III: craniofacial disjunction.
(From Cantrill SV: Face. In Marx JA, Hockberger RS, Walls RM, et al [eds]: Rosen's Emergency Medicine Concepts and Clinical Practice, 5th ed. St. Louis, Mosby, 2002, Fig. 35-8, p 325.)

allows movement of the maxilla, nose, and infraorbital rims. Le Fort III, the most serious of the Le Fort fractures, represents complete craniofacial disruption and involves fractures of the zygoma, infraorbital rims, and maxilla. It is rare for these fracture types to occur in isolation; they usually occur in combination (one type on one side of the face and another on the other side).

KEY POINTS: RADIOGRAPHIC SIGNS OF ORBITAL BLOW-OUT FRACTURES

1. "Hanging teardop sign": Oribital fat herniating into the maxillary sinus
2. Air-fluid levels in the maxillary sinus

6. **When are nasal radiographs indicated?**
   Almost never. Nasal fractures typically are a clinical diagnosis without the need for routine radiographs. Physical examination may reveal swelling, angulation, bony crepitus, deformity, pain on palpation, epistaxis, and periorbital ecchymosis. Nasal radiographs are neither sensitive nor specific for fractures. The results do not alter management.

7. **What is a septal hematoma? Why is it important?**
   All patients with nasal trauma and suspicion of a nasal fracture require inspection of the nasal septum for a septal hematoma. This is a collection of blood between the mucoperichondrium and the cartilage of the septum. It appears as a grape-like swelling over the nasal septum. If left undrained, it may result in septal abscess, necrosis of the nasal cartilage, and permanent deformity. If a septal hematoma is identified, incision and drainage is indicated in the emergency department (ED), followed by nasal packing, anti-staphylococcal antibiotics (prophylaxis for toxic shock syndrome), and prompt referral.

8. **When should a consultation be obtained for a nasal fracture?**
   Most nasal fractures do not require immediate reduction unless there is significant deformity and malalignment. After anesthetizing the nose with lidocaine or tetracaine-soaked gauze or pledgets, early reduction of an angulated fracture is performed by exerting firm, quick pressure toward the midline with both thumbs. Patients should be referred to a maxillofacial or plastic surgeon for follow-up in 4–7 days. Immediate consultation is suggested for nasal fractures with associated facial fractures, cerebrospinal fluid rhinorrhea, and sustained epistaxis.

9. **How is a frontal sinus fracture diagnosed?**
   Frontal sinus fracture should be suspected in any patient with a severe blow to the forehead. The clinical signs include supraorbital nerve anesthesia, anosmia, cerebrospinal fluid rhinorrhea, subconjunctival hematoma, crepitus, and tenderness to palpation. The preferred diagnostic modality is computed tomography (CT) to determine if there is involvement of the anterior or posterior walls of the sinus or intracranial hemorrhage.

10. **How are frontal sinus fractures treated?**
    After surgical consultation, patients with nondisplaced anterior wall fractures may be discharged on prophylactic antibiotics, with instructions to avoid Valsalva maneuvers and to follow up in 1 week with the surgical consultant. Patients with displaced anterior wall and sinus floor fractures require surgical consultation, admission, and antibiotic therapy. Patients with posterior wall fractures require antibiotics and immediate neurosurgical consultation.

11. **What are the classic zygoma fractures?**

The zygoma is the third most commonly fractured facial bone (after the nose and mandible). Zygoma fractures are classified into three basic types:

1. **Arch:** The bone may be fractured in one or two places and may be nondisplaced or displaced medially. Pain and trismus are caused by bony arch fragments abutting the coronoid process of the mandible. Because the masseter muscle originates on the zygoma, any movement causes further arch disruption. The fracture is diagnosed by the plain radiograph bucket-handle view (submentovertex).

2. **Tripod:** This is the most serious type of zygoma fracture and involves the infraorbital rim, the zygomaticofrontal suture, and the zygomaticotemporal suture. Clinical signs include deformity (flatness of the cheek), infraorbital nerve hypesthesia, inferior rectus muscle entrapment, and diplopia on upward gaze. Although these fractures may be detected on plain radiographs (Waters and Caldwell views), CT is necessary to better define the extent of the fracture. For these fractures, admission and consultation with a maxillofacial surgeon are required.

3. **Body:** Fracture of the body of the zygoma, which involves the clinical signs and symptoms of the tripod fracture, results from severe force and leads to exaggerated malar depression.

12. **What is the tongue blade test?**

Patients with mandible fractures have mandibular tenderness and deformity, sublingual hematoma, and malocclusion on physical examination. The jaw appears asymmetric, with deviation toward the side of the fracture. The tongue blade test is performed by asking the patient to bite down on a tongue depressor. The tongue blade should be twisted by the examiner. If there is no fracture, the patient should be able to break the blade. In the presence of a mandible fracture, the patient opens his or her mouth and the tongue blade remains intact.

MacLaughlin J, Colucciello S: Maxillofacial injuries. In Wolfson AB, Hendey GW, Hendry PL, et al (eds): Harwood-Nuss' Clinical Practice of Emergency Medicine, 4th ed. Philadelphia, Lippincott Williams & Wilkins, 2005, pp 928–937.

13. **Which imaging studies should be ordered to diagnose a mandible fracture?**

If available, the Panorex view is the most useful view for detecting mandible fractures. It provides a 180-degree view of the mandible and can detect fractures in all regions of the mandible, including symphyseal fractures that can be missed with the other views. Mandible fractures are the second most common facial fracture. Multiple fractures are common ($>50\%$) because of the ring structure of the bone. Always check for a second fracture. The standard mandible series includes the posteroanterior view (for detecting fractures of the angle and body of the mandible), lateral oblique views (for detection of rami fractures), and the Townes view (anteroposterior view that projects the rami and condyles). A condylar fracture may be missed by plain radiographs. If this fracture is suspected and the plain radiographs are negative, facial CT is indicated.

Druelinger L, Guenther M, Marchand EG: Radiographic evaluation of the facial complex. Emerg Med Clin North Am 18:393–410, 2000.

14. **What are the most commonly fractured areas of the mandible?**

The most commonly fractured areas are the body, the condyle, and the angle of the mandible.

Isenhour JL, Colucciello SA: Maxillofacial trauma. In Ferrera PC, Colucciello SA, Marx JA, et al (eds): Trauma Management, An Emergency Medicine Approach. St. Louis, Mosby, 2001, pp 180–196.

15. **What is the mechanism for a temporomandibular joint dislocation? How is it treated?**

Temporomandibular joint dislocation can result from blunt trauma to the mandible, but it also can occur after a seizure or with yawning. Patients with a temporomandibular joint dislocation present with jaw deviation away from the side of the dislocation if it is a unilateral dislocation or with the mandible pushed forward if it is a bilateral dislocation. After conscious sedation with a benzodiazepine for masseter muscle relaxation and a narcotic for pain relief, the emergency physician should place gauze-wrapped thumbs on the posterior molars. The mandible is then pushed downward and posterior.

16. **When is a CT scan indicated in the evaluation of maxillofacial trauma?**
In patients with a history of facial trauma but with minimal physical findings consistent with fractures or an equivocal examination, plain radiography can be used as a screening test. The standard plain film series of the face includes a Waters (occipitomental) view, Caldwell (occipitofrontal) view, submentovertex view, and lateral view. The Waters view visualizes the orbital rim, infraorbital floor, maxilla, and maxillary sinuses and is useful as an initial examination in patients with suspected orbital floor fractures. Performance of this view requires that the cervical spine be clear because the patient is in the prone position. Fluid in the maxillary sinus is indirect evidence of fracture. The Caldwell view allows visualization of the superior orbital rim and the frontal sinuses. The lateral view shows the anterior wall of the frontal sinus and the anterior and posterior walls of the maxillary sinus.

In patients with physical findings that are highly suggestive of facial fractures (tenderness, step-offs, crepitus, or evidence of entrapment), some authors recommend proceeding directly to CT. This allows appropriate surgical planning. High-resolution, thin-cut CT scanning is the preferred modality for the elucidation of bony and soft tissue destruction inherent in maxillofacial trauma. This is the preferred test in any patient with suspected tripod, orbital, or midface fractures. In patients with suspected orbital fractures, CT scan with coronal and axial sections should be ordered (2- to 3-mm cuts).

Druelinger L, Guenther M, Marchand EG: Radiographic evaluation of the facial complex. Emerg Med Clin North Am 18:393–410, 2000.

17. **How do I recognize an injury to Stenson's duct?**
Stenson's (parotid) duct arises from the parotid gland and courses from the level of the external auditory canal (superficial) through the buccinator muscle to open at the level of the upper second molar (Fig. 85-2). Any laceration at this level may involve the parotid gland, parotid duct, or buccal branch of the facial nerve. Laceration of the parotid system is recognized by a flow of saliva from the wound or bloody drainage from the duct orifice. Careful exploration reveals whether the flow is from the parotid gland or duct. The buccal branch of the facial nerve travels in close proximity to Stenson's duct; injury leads to drooping of the upper lip, which indicates a possible parotid duct injury. To assess for parotid duct patency, the parotid gland should be milked to see if saliva is expressed from the intraoral opening of the parotid duct. Damage to the duct requires repair over a stent and plastic surgical consultation.

Cantrill SV: Face. In Marx JA, Hockberger RS, Walls RM, et al (eds): Rosen's Emergency Medicine Concepts and Clinical Practice, 5th ed. St. Louis, Mosby, 2002, pp 314–329.

18. **When should closure of a facial laceration be deferred?**
Closure of facial lacerations in the ED depends on the severity of facial and systemic injuries. Complex lacerations in patients needing operative intervention should be cleansed with normal saline, covered with dampened gauze, and deferred for intraoperative closure. Closure of the highly vascular tissues of the face may be delayed for up to 24 hours. Wounds involving the facial nerve, lacrimal duct, parotid duct, and avulsions should be referred on presentation to the appropriate surgeon for definitive care.

19. **How do I control persistent hemorrhage from a facial laceration?**
First, inject with 1% lidocaine with epinephrine. If hemorrhage continues and discrete arterial or venous bleeders can be visualized, they can be ligated with absorbable suture. If hemorrhage is from muscle, pack with gauze followed by external pressure.

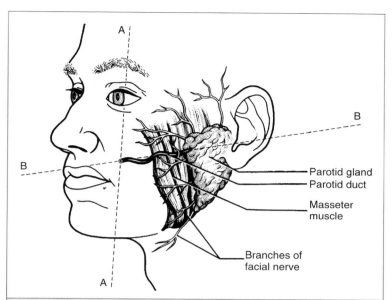

Figure 85-2. Parotid gland and parotid duct with nearby branches of the facial nerve. Line B demonstrates approximate course of parotid duct from parotid gland, entering mouth at junction of lines A and B.
(From Cantrill SV: Face. In Marx JA, Hockberger RS, Walls RM, et al [eds]: Rosen's Emergency Medicine Concepts and Clinical Practice, 5th ed. St. Louis, Mosby, 2002, Fig. 35-6, p 323.)

20. How is the ear anesthetized?

A subcutaneous circumferential injection of plain lidocaine should be placed at the base of the pinna. Lacerations in the external auditory require topical anesthesia with 4% lidocaine or local injection.

CHAPTER 86

CERVICAL SPINE AND SPINAL CORD TRAUMA

Michael J. Klevens, MD, and Robert M. McNamara, MD

1. **What is the annual incidence of spinal cord injury (SCI)?**
   Forty cases per million population in the United States. In other words, 11,000 new cases each year!

2. **Name the most common causes of SCI.**
   - Vehicular crashes (50.4%)
   - Falls (23.8%)
   - Violence, primarily gunshot wounds (11.2%)
   - Sports (9.0%)
   - Other (5.6%)

3. **What are the most common levels of injury?**
   The most frequent level of injury is C5, followed by C4, C6, T12, C7, and L1. Overall about half are cervical injuries.

4. **In patients discharged from the hospital with neurologic impairment, what percentage has paraplegia and what percentage has tetraplegia (quadriplegia)?**
   - Incomplete tetraplegia (34.3%)
   - Complete paraplegia (25.1%)
   - Complete tetraplegia (22.1%),
   - Incomplete paraplegia (17.5%)

   One percent has complete recovery by discharge. An injury to one of the eight cervical vertebrae can cause tetraplegia. Persons with paraplegia have injuries to the thoracic, lumbar, or sacral regions.

5. **If most spinal injuries do not cause neurologic injury, why do I care?**
   The management of any spinal injury is important because improper care can result in permanent neurologic injury. It is important to have an index of suspicion for injury and proper immobilization and handling of the patient. It is imperative to have good-quality radiographs, because inadequate studies and interpretation errors can lead to permanent injury.

6. **What is the financial impact of a SCI?**
   The health care and living costs can vary greatly, depending on what severity of injury was sustained and the age of the individual at time of injury. The estimated yearly costs can range from $14,000 to $122,000. This does not include the first year costs, which range from $200,000 to $683,000. The lifetime costs can range from $435,000 to $2.7 million.

7. **What is the average age of the person who sustains a SCI?**
   SCI is devastating in that it primarily affects young healthy adults. Since 2000, the average age at injury is 38.0 years. The predominant age range is between 16 and 30. An overwhelming percentage of injuries are suffered by males.

8. **Name the causes of reduced life expectancy in SCI patients.**
   Pneumonia, pulmonary emboli, and sepsis.

9. **Are there any underlying conditions That could precipitate or heighten the chance of a SCI?**

   Less force is required to cause fractures in the elderly. Rheumatoid arthritis can lead to subluxation problems at C1 and C2. Normal development of the odontoid may not occur in a Down's syndrome patient. Osteoporosis and metastatic cancer may lead to a vertebral fracture with insignificant trauma.

10. **How do I immobilize the potential spinal injury patent?**

    When any spinal injury is suspected, the entire spine should be immobilized with a long board. The cervical spine is immobilized with a hard collar. There are several different types of stiff cervical collars, such as the Philadelphia or Ambu brand collars. The emergency medical service (EMS) stabilization may also include the forehead taped to the board and accessory towel, sandbag, or other bolsters to prevent further neck movement. The sandbag and tape method without a rigid collar support should not be used.

11. **How should one approach the patient with potential spinal injury?**

    There are several mnemonics for the initial stabilization of any trauma patient. ATLS teaches the **ABCDE** mnemonic:
    - **A** = **A**irway
    - **B** = **B**reathing
    - **C** = **C**irculation
    - **D** = **D**isability
    - **E** = **E**xposure

      According to another mnemonic, a proper history is **A MUST**:
    - **A** = **A**ltered mental state. Check for drugs or alcohol.
    - **M** = **M**echanism. Does the potential for injury exist?
    - **U** = **U**nderlying conditions. Are high risk factors for fractures present?
    - **S** = **S**ymptoms. Is pain, paresthesia, or neurologic compromise part of the picture?
    - **T** = **T**iming. When did the symptoms begin in relation to the event?

12. **What should be assessed on physical examination?**

    There are two key areas: the spine itself and the neurologic examination. The spine is palpated to assess for tenderness, deformity/step-off, and muscle spasm. It is important to understand that the examiner feels only the posterior elements of the vertebrae; therefore, a fracture may be present despite a lack of tenderness. The neurologic examination should include motor function, sensory function, some aspect of posterior column function (position and vibration), and a rectal examination. In an unconscious patient, the only clues may be poor rectal tone, priapism, absence of deep tendon reflexes, or diaphragmatic breathing.

13. **What is neurogenic shock? How is it treated?**

    Neurogenic shock is a syndrome with loss of neurologic function and accompanying autonomic tone. This is usually exhibited by flaccid paralysis with loss of reflexes and loss of urinary and rectal tone. Accompanying this are bradycardia, hypotension, hypothermia, and ileus. The diagnosis of neurogenic shock should only be made after all other forms of shock have been eliminated. Hypotension is usually successfully treated with rapid infusion of crystalloid. If intravenous fluids are not adequate to maintain organ perfusion, the use of dopamine or Neo-Synephrine may be beneficial. Bradycardia can be treated with atropine or dopamine. In refractory bradycardia, a pacemaker may be required. In most cases of neurogenic shock, hypotension resolves within 24–48 hours.

14. **What are the general principles of emergency treatment in the patient with spinal cord trauma?**
First, do no harm. As stated previously, that means proper immobilization and coordinated movement of the patient, when absolutely necessary. A higher level of cervical injury results in a more devastating injury to the patient. Any patient with an injury above C5 probably should be intubated because the phrenic nerve roots, which supply the diaphragm, emerge from C3 to C5. Rapid-sequence intubation (RSI) oral-tracheal intubation with manual in-line C-spine stabilization has been proven to be the safest way to intubate these patients. Early gastric and bladder decompression are also indicated. Overhydration should be avoided so as to not cause pulmonary edema. The absence of pain below the level of injury can mask other injuries. The patient with neurologic deficit faces a difficult hospital stay, and the emergency department (ED) should use full sterile precautions for any procedure such as urinary catheters or central venous access when possible.

15. **How do I determine which patients need spine radiographs?**
There are two validated decision rules available to the emergency physician. One is the National Emergency X-Radiography Utilization Study (NEXUS) decision rule. The other is the Canadian C-Spine Rule (CCR). Both have been shown to reduce the number of radiographs necessary to identify important cervical C-spine injury.

16. **What are the NEXUS criteria?**
   - No midline cervical tenderness
   - No focal neurologic deficit
   - Normal alertness
   - No intoxication
   - No painful distracting injury

   If patients meet the criteria, there is a high likelihood that they have a low probability of injury and that cervical radiography is not needed. In this large multicenter study, the overall rate of missed cervical spine injuries was less than 1 in 4000 patients. Note that there are specific definitions of the previous five criteria that must be reviewed when applying the NEXUS criteria.

17. **What is the CCR?**
The CCR asks three questions:
   - Is there any high-risk factor that mandates radiography (i.e., age > 65, severe mechanism, or focal neurologic signs)?
   - Can the patient be assessed safely for range of motion (simple mechanism, sitting position in the ED, ambulatory at any time, delayed onset of neck pain, or absence of midline cervical spine tenderness)?
   - Can the patient actively rotate the neck 45 degrees to the left and the right?

   This study had a sensitivity of 100% and a specificity of 42.5% for identifying clinically important C-spine injuries. Again, one needs to review the rule completely before applying it to patients.

18. **Can these decision rules be applied to children?**
It is difficult to validate the NEXUS or CCR in children because there has been a paucity of studies in this population. Additionally, some of the criteria in the CCR and NEXUS are difficult to verify in toddlers and children because of their inherent immaturity and unpredictability.

19. **Which type of radiographs should be obtained?**
The standard three-view of the C-spine is an anteroposterior (AP), lateral, and open-mouth (odontoid). During the initial evaluation, a cross-table lateral radiograph should be taken because the patient doesn't have to move. It is extremely important that C-spine precautions not be discontinued based solely on the cross-table lateral. Some studies have reported that up to

18% of cervical spine injuries are missed with the cross-table lateral radiograph alone. The most commonly missed injuries are at C1-C2, followed by the lower C6-C7-T1 junction.

20. **How do I interpret the lateral cervical spine radiograph?**
    The first rule is to make sure that the radiograph is technically adequate and that the top of T1 is visible on the film. Next, follow the mnemonic **ABCS:**
    - **A** = **A**lignment. Check for a smooth line at the anterior and posterior aspect of the vertebral bodies and the spinolaminar line from C1 to T1 (Fig. 86-1).
    - **B** = **B**ones. Check each vertebral body to ensure that the anterior and posterior heights are similar (> 3 mm difference suggests fracture); follow the vertebrae out to the laminae and spinous process. Look carefully at the upper and lower cervical segments where fractures are likely to be missed. Examine the ring of C2, which can show a fracture through the upper portion of the vertebral body of C2.
    - **C** = **C**artilage. Check the intervertebral joint spaces and the facet joints.
    - **S** = **S**oft tissue spaces. Look for prevertebral swelling, especially at the C2-C3 area (> 5 mm) and check the predental space (Fig. 86-2), which should be less than 3 mm in adults and less than 5 mm in children. From C4 to C7 the soft tissue thickness should not be greater than 22 mm.

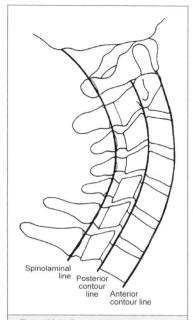

Spinolaminal line Posterior contour line Anterior contour line

Figure 86-1. Curve of alignment.

21. **What are the indications for flexion-extension views of the cervical spine?**
    Based on the NEXUS study, flexion-extension imaging is unnecessary in the acute evaluation of patients with blunt trauma. A computed tomography (CT) or magnetic resonance imaging (MRI) would give more information in the presence of specific clinical concerns for ligamentous damage or fracture not diagnosed on plain films.

22. **When would a CT or MRI be ordered?**
    Routine indications are when plain radiographs are inconclusive or difficult to interpret and you have suspicion of spinal injury. A CT is good for detection of bony injury and to identify surgical conditions such as hematoma or disk fragments within the spinal canal. With the advent of rapid helical scanning, many centers are increasing their use of the CT scan in place of plain radiographs, especially if the patient has an indication for a head CT. A CT

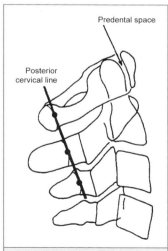

Predental space

Posterior cervical line

Figure 86-2. Posterior cervical line and predental space.

scan is also needed for the clearance of the cervical spine in comatose or obtunded patient. In a study of patients with traumatic brain injury, 5.4% of the patients had C1 or C2 fractures, and 4% had occipital condyle fractures that were not visualized on the three-view radiography series. An MRI is useful to identify injury to the spinal cord itself in the face of neurologic deficit. The MRI can show areas of contusion and edema within the spinal space. An MRI can also detect rupture of intervertebral disks and ligamentous injury. The MRI is not as good as CT for the identification of vertebral fractures.

23. What is SCIWORA?

It is spinal cord injury without radiographic abnormalities. Children are more susceptible to SCIWORA because of the greater elasticity of their cervical structures. This leads to transient spinal column subluxation and stretching of the spinal cord. These pediatric patients may have a brief episode of upper extremity weakness or paresthesias with delayed development of neurologic deficits that appear hours to days later.

KEY POINTS: SPINAL CORD TRAUMA

1. It is important to have an index of suspicion for injury and ensure proper immobilization and handling of the patient.

2. Use clinical decision rules such as NEXUS or Canadian C-spine rule to minimize cervical spine radiographs.

3. The use of steroids in blunt spinal cord trauma is not standard of care.

4. Special populations, such as pediatric and geriatric, need a more thorough work-up than the normal adult.

5. The three-view cervical spine series is mandatory in evaluations if you are getting radiographs, whereas the flexion-extension view is not needed in the acute setting.

---

24. Describe the Jefferson, Hangman, Clay Shoveler's, and Chance fractures.

- **Jefferson fracture** is a burst fracture of the ring of C1 that occurs from axial loading.
- **Hangman's fracture** is a disruption of the posterior arch of C2.
- **Clay-Shoveler's fracture** is a fracture of the spinous process that is classically caused by forceful cervical extension.
- **Chance fracture** is a vertebral fracture, usually in the lumbar segment, involving the posterior spinous process, pedicles, and vertebral body. It is caused by the flexion forces on the spinal column. This is associated with the use of lap belts.

25. Describe the incomplete cord syndromes or injuries.

- **Anterior cord syndrome** results in loss of function in the anterior two thirds of the spinal cord from damage to the corticospinal and spinothalamic pathways. Findings include loss of voluntary motor function and pain and temperature sensation below the level of the injury, with preservation of the posterior column functions of position and function. The key issue is the potential reversibility of this lesion if a compressing hematoma or disk fragment can be removed. This condition requires immediate neurosurgical evaluation.
- **Central cord syndrome** results from injury to the central portion of the spinal cord. Because more proximal innervation is placed centrally within the cord, this lesion results in greater involvement of the upper extremities than of the lower extremities. Bowel or bladder

control usually is preserved. The mechanism of injury is hyperextension of a cervical spine with a cord space narrowed by congenital variation, degenerative spurring, or hypertrophic ligaments. This syndrome can occur without actual fracture or ligamentous disruption.

- **Brown-Séquard syndrome** is a hemisection of the spinal cord, usually from penetrating trauma. Contralateral sensation of pain and temperature is lost, and motor and posterior column functions are absent on the side of the injury.
- **Cauda equina syndrome** is an injury to the lumbar, sacral, and coccygeal nerve roots causing a peripheral nerve injury. There can be motor and sensory loss in the lower extremities, bowel and bladder dysfunction, and loss of pain sensation at the perineum (saddle anesthesia).

26. **What is the significance of sacral sparing and spinal shock?**
Sacral sparing refers to the preservation of any function of the sacral roots, such as toe movement or perianal sensation. If sacral sparing is present, the chance of functional neurologic recovery is good. Spinal shock is a temporary concussive-like condition in which cord-mediated reflexes, such as the anal wink, are absent. Spinal shock also may result in bradycardia and hypotension. The extent of cord injury—and prognosis—cannot be determined until these reflexes return.

27. **What can physicians do to prevent spinal injuries?**
Get involved in injury prevention and education. Due to the predominance of vehicle crashes causing SCIs, one can work to reduce driving under the influence of alcohol and drugs. Further, the use of safety belts should be emphasized at discharge in every ED visit, regardless of the reason the person came in for treatment. Diving and sporting injuries can be reduced by proper public education and coaching.

CONTROVERSY

28. **What is the status of steroids in spinal cord trauma?**
This has been a very controversial topic. In 1975 the first National Acute Spinal Cord Injury Study (NASCIS) was established. This was followed by NASCIS 2 and NASCIS 3, which was completed in 1998. The dosage of methylprednisolone was an initial bolus of 30 mg/kg intravenously over 15 minutes, followed 45 minutes later by a continuous infusion of 5.4 mg/kg/h for 23 hours. This was given within 3 hours of injury. When the therapy was initiated 3–8 hours after injury, patients were maintained on an infusion for 47 hours. Initial support for the use of steroids was encouraging, but multiple reviews of the NASCIS study and other literature have shown that there is insufficient evidence to support the use of corticosteroids in the treatment of patients with acute SCI. Many believe that there were study design, data presentation, interpretation, and analysis flaws in the NASCIS study. Further, a recent Level I study showed that patients treated with methylprednisolone had a higher incidence of complications such as gastrointestinal (GI) bleed and respiratory complications. Unfortunately, the overwhelming desire for any improvement has made steroid therapy a de facto standard of care at many institutions. This conflicts with recent position statements by the American Academy of Emergency Medicine, Canadian Association of Emergency Physicians, American Academy of Neurological Surgeons, and the Congress of Neurological Surgeons. In conclusion, the use of steroids is an option but is certainly not a standard of care. Other promising but not proven therapies include ganglioside GM-1, opiate receptor antagonists, calcium channel antagonists, and glutamate receptor antagonists.

WEBSITES

1. American Academy of Emergency Medicine: www.aaem.org/positionstatements/steroidsinacuteinjury.shtml

2. Canadian Association of Emergency Physicians: www.caep.ca/002.policies/002–01.guidelines/steriods-acute-spinal.htm

3. Eastern Association For The Surgery of Trauma: www.east.org

4. National Spinal Cord Injury Statistical Center: www.spinalcord.uab.edu

BIBLIOGRAPHY

1. American College of Surgeons: Advanced Trauma Life Support, 6th ed. Chicago, 1997.

2. Bracken MB: Steroids for acute spinal cord injury. Cochrane Database Syst Rev Issue 2, Art. No.: CD001046, DOI:10.1002/14651858.CD001046, 2002.

3. Bracken MB, Shepard MJ, Holford TR, et al: Administration of methylprednisolone for 24 or 48 hours or tirilazad mesylate for 48 hours in the treatment of acute spinal cord injury: Results of the third national acute spinal cord injury randomized controlled trial. JAMA 227:1597–1604, 1997.

4. Congress of Neurological Surgeons: Cervical spine immobilization before admission to the hospital. Neurosurgery 50(3 Suppl):S7–17, 2002.

5. Congress of Neurological Surgeons: Pharmacological therapy after acute cervical spinal cord injury. Neurosurgery 50(3 Suppl):S63–72, 2002.

6. Davis JW, Phreaner DL, et al: The etiology of missed cervical spine injuries. J Trauma Injury Infect Cri Care 34:342–346, 1993.

7. Dickinson G, Stiell IG, Schull M, et al: Retrospective application of the NEXUS low-risk criteria for cervical spine radiography in Canadian emergency departments. Ann Emerg Med 43:507–514, 2004.

8. Dreyer SJ, Boden SD: Natural history of rheumatoid arthritis of the cervical spine. Clin Orthop Rel Res 366:98–106, 1999.

9. Geiderman JM: General principles of orthopedic injuries. In Marx JA, Hockberger RS, Walls RM(eds): Rosen's Emergency Medicine, 5th ed. St. Louis, Mosby, 2002, p 468.

10. Hockberger RS, Kirshenbaum KJ: Spine. In Marx JA, Hockberger RS, Walls RM(eds): Rosen's Emergency Medicine, 5th ed. St. Louis, Mosby, 2002, p 350.

11. Knopp R: Comparing NEXUS and Canadian C-spine decision rules for determining the need for cervical spine radiography. Ann Emerg Med 43:518–520, 2004.

12. Link TM, Schuierer G, Hufendiek A, et al: Substantial head trauma: Value of routine CT examination of the cervicocranium. Radiology 196:741–754, 1995.

13. Masuda K, Iwasaki M, Seichi, et al: Cervical myelopathy in an adult due to atlantoaxial subluxation associated with Down syndrome: a case study. J Orthop Sci 8:227–231, 2003.

14. Mower WR, Hoffman J: Comparison of the Canadian C-spine rule and NEXUS decision instrument in evaluating blunt trauma patients for cervical spine injury. Ann Emerg Med 43:515–517, 2004.

15. National Spinal Cord Injury Statistical Center, University of Alabama at Birmingham, 2004 Annual Statistical Report, June 2004, p 119.

16. Nesathurai S: Steroids and spinal cord injury: revisiting the NASCIS 2 and NASCIS 3 trials. J Trauma 45:1088–1093, 1998.

17. Perron AD, Huff JS: Spinal cord disorders. In Marx JA, Hockberger RS, Walls RM(eds): Rosen's Emergency Medicine, 5th ed. St. Louis, Mosby, 2002, pp 1497–1505.

18. Pollack CV Jr, Hendey GW, Martin DR, et al: Use of flexion-extension radiographs of the cervical spine in blunt trauma. Ann Emerg Med 28:8–11, 2001.

19. Pollard ME, Apple DF: Factors associated with improved neurological outcomes in patients with incomplete tetraplegia. Spine 28:33–39, 2003.

20. Ruoff, B, West OC: The cervical spine. In Schwartz DT, Reisdorff E (eds): Emergency Radiology. St. Louis, McGraw-Hill, 2000, pp 269–318.

21. Spencer MT, Bazarian JJ: Are corticosteroids effective in traumatic spinal cord injury. Ann Emerg Med 41:410–413, 2003.

22. Stiell IG, Clement CM, McKnight D, et al: The Canadian c-spine rule versus the NEXUS low-risk criteria in patients with trauma. N Engl J Med 349:2510–2518, 2003.

23. Stiell IG, Wells GA, Vandemheen KL, et al: The Canadian c-spine rule for radiography in alert and stable trauma patients. JAMA 286:1841–1848, 2001.

24. Sweeney TA, Marx JA: Blunt neck injury. Emerg Med Clin North Am 11:71–79, 1993.

25. Viccellio P, Simon H, Pressman BD, et al: A prospective multicenter study of cervical spine injury in children. Pediatrics 108:E20, 2001.

26. Wagner R, Jagoda A: Spinal cord syndromes. Emerg Med Clin North Am 15:699, 1997.

27. Yealy DM, Auble TE: Choosing between clinical prediction rules. N Engl J Med 349:2553–2554, 2003.

CHAPTER 87

HEAD TRAUMA
Edward Newton, MD

1. **What is the scope of head injury in the United States?**

   There are more than 1.5 million emergency department (ED) visits and approximately 70,000 deaths as a result of head injury every year in the United States. Although the incidence of severe head injury is decreasing, most likely owing to the preventive benefits of helmets and seat belts and air bags in automobiles, head trauma remains the most lethal traumatic injury and accounts for a large proportion of patients with permanent disability. The peak incidence of head injury is in the 15- to 24-year-old age group, with males affected twice as often as females. The spectrum of head injury includes relatively minor problems, such as lacerations and scalp contusions, and major, often lethal, intracranial trauma. Distinguishing between minor and potentially lethal head injuries while using diagnostic resources appropriately is one of the most difficult tasks facing the emergency physician.

2. **What groups of patients are at particular risk from head trauma?**

   Because assessment of mental status is such an integral part of the evaluation of head-injured patients, patients who are unable to communicate because they are preverbal (e.g., infants), intoxicated, mentally impaired, aphasic, or they have a language barrier pose a special challenge. When such communication barriers are present, there should be a lower threshold for obtaining a computed tomography (CT) scan.

   Certain age groups are at higher risk for intracranial injury:
   - **Infants** are at higher risk because of their relatively large head size and compressibility of the skull. Infants also are at high risk for nonaccidental trauma (e.g., **shaken baby syndrome**), in which case an accurate history may be unavailable or deliberately withheld. If the cranial sutures and fontanelles are not closed, the cranium can expand as a result of intracranial bleeding. Infants can bleed sufficiently intracranially to produce hemorrhagic shock, whereas in older children and adults, another source of bleeding is inevitably responsible for shock.
   - The **elderly** also are at higher risk of intracranial injury, particularly subdural hematoma (SDH). Cerebral atrophy results in stretching of bridging veins from the dura to the brain parenchyma, making these veins vulnerable to tearing from deceleration forces.
   - **Chronic alcoholics** are at risk because of their greater frequency of head trauma, cerebral atrophy, and coagulopathy. Patients who are taking anticoagulants or antiplatelet agents or who have intrinsic **bleeding diatheses** bleed more actively than patients with normal coagulation and have higher mortality from brain injury.

   Cheung DS, Kharasch M: Evaluation of the patient with closed head trauma: An evidence based approach. Emerg Med Clin North Am 17:9–23, 1999.

KEY POINTS: PATIENTS AT HIGH RISK FOR HEAD INJURY

1. Very young and very old patients

2. Chronic alcoholics

3. Patients with coagulopathy

3. What is a cerebral concussion?

Sudden, transient loss of central neurologic function secondary to trauma. It is characterized by loss of consciousness, transient amnesia, confusion, disorientation, or visual changes, without any gross cerebral abnormalities.

4. What is the postconcussive syndrome?

Although the patient may have a completely normal neurologic examination after a concussion, there are common sequelae from this type of injury. Patients frequently report migraine-type headaches, dizziness, inability to concentrate, and irritability. Although in 90% of cases these symptoms resolve within 2 weeks, they may persist for up to 1 year. Treatment is supportive, and the long-term prognosis is good. A phenomenon known as the **second impact syndrome** is recognized in which a second head trauma during a vulnerable period after a concussion results in severe and often fatal diffuse cerebral edema. Consequently, athletes should be held out of contact sports until all postconcussive symptoms have resolved.

5. How do you detect cerebrospinal fluid (CSF) leaks caused by basilar skull fractures?

A patient with signs of basilar skull fracture (raccoon eyes, hemotympanum, or Battle's sign) with clear drainage from the nose or ear canal should be suspected of having a CSF leak. Analysis of the glucose content of the drainage by glucometer or laboratory analysis may distinguish CSF (containing 60% of serum glucose levels) from nasal mucus (glucose not present). In cases in which blood is mixed with CSF, applying a drop of the fluid to filter paper reveals CSF in a target shape with blood at the center and pink-tinged CSF forming an outer ring. Bedside tests are neither specific nor sensitive for detecting CSF leaks.

6. How are CSF leaks treated?

CSF leaks through tears in the dura generally are managed conservatively. The use of prophylactic antibiotics is controversial because they have not been shown to reduce significantly the incidence of meningitis and may select for antibiotic-resistant bacteria. Patients must be followed closely until the dural tear heals because of the risk of meningitis. Dural tears that fail to close spontaneously over 2–3 weeks usually require operative repair.

7. How does a patient with epidural hematoma present?

Epidural hematoma occurs in 5–10% of severe head injuries. In the classic pattern, a patient who loses consciousness from the initial concussion, gradually recovers over a few minutes, and enters a lucid interval wherein he or she is relatively asymptomatic and has a normal neurologic examination. During this interval, accumulation of arterial blood in the epidural space, usually from a lacerated middle meningeal artery, eventually causes compression and shift of brain across the midline. This process is accompanied by a second reduction in the level of consciousness and the pupillary and motor signs of herniation. This classic pattern occurs in only about 30% of cases, however. Many patients who remain unconscious after the initial impact or in minor hemorrhages may not develop increased intracranial pressure (ICP) at all. The characteristic CT scan appearance of an epidural hematoma is a hyperdense lenticular collection of blood that indents adjacent brain parenchyma and does not extend beyond cranial sutures where the dura is attached.

8. **How does an SDH present?**

SDH may be acute, subacute (6–14 days), or chronic (>14 days after trauma).

- **Acute SDH** is associated with a high incidence of underlying brain injury. The presentation varies with the severity of the underlying injury, but patients commonly present with a diminished level of consciousness, headache, and focal neurologic deficits corresponding to the area of brain injury. If sufficient bleeding occurs, ICP increases, and herniation may occur. The characteristic appearance of an acute SDH on CT scan is a collection of hyperdense blood in a crescent-shaped pattern conforming to the convexity of the hemisphere and often extending past cranial sutures. At times, the injury causes a minimal amount of bleeding, and the patient does not immediately seek medical care. The SDH undergoes lysis over a period of several days and eventually organizes into an encapsulated mass.
- **Subacute** or **chronic SDH** is a difficult clinical diagnosis because the symptoms are vague and common (e.g., persistent headache, difficulty concentrating, lethargy), and the trauma may have been forgotten. Even the CT scan diagnosis is difficult because subacute SDH becomes isodense and indistinguishable from surrounding brain unless special CT techniques are used. Chronic SDH appears as an encapsulated lucent collection of fluid in the same position as the acute type.

9. **What is axonal shear injury?**

Axonal shear injury occurs during abrupt deceleration because white and gray matter have different densities and different rates of deceleration. This produces a shearing force that may tear axons at the white-gray interface, resulting in coma or other severe neurologic derangements. The CT scan may appear completely normal or show only small petechial hemorrhages. Magnetic resonance imaging (MRI) of the brain is a more sensitive tool in detecting these injuries but is currently impractical in the acute phase.

10. **What is brain herniation?**

Herniation is caused by increased ICP. Because the cranium is a rigid structure, pressure varies with the volume of its contents. Approximately 10% of intracranial volume is blood; another 10% is CSF, and the remainder is brain parenchyma and intracellular fluid. An increase in any of these compartments by blood, tumor, or edema causes a predictable response. Initially, CSF is forced into the spinal canal, and the ventricles and cisterns collapse. When this has occurred, ICP rises steeply, and the brain parenchyma shifts away from the accumulating blood and herniates through one of several spaces, eventually causing death by compressing the brain stem.

11. **List the four types of herniation syndrome.**

- Uncal herniation
- Central herniation
- Cingulate herniation
- Posterior fossa cingulation

12. **Describe uncal herniation syndrome.**

The uncus is the most medial portion of the hemisphere and is often the first structure to shift below the tentorium that separates the hemispheres from the midbrain. As the uncus is forced medially and downward, the ipsilateral third cranial nerve is compressed, producing pupillary dilation, ptosis, and oculomotor paresis. As herniation progresses, the ipsilateral cerebral peduncle and pyramidal tract are compressed, resulting in contralateral hemiplegia.

In approximately 10% of cases, the hemiparesis occurs on the same side as the brain lesion, making this a less reliable finding for localizing the injury. Further progression results in brain stem compression with respiratory and cardiac arrest. Transtentorial herniation of this type is the most common variety.

13. What is central herniation syndrome?

Occasionally, hematomas located at the vertex or frontal lobes cause simultaneous downward herniation of both hemispheres through the tentorium. Clinical findings are similar to uncal herniation, except that bilateral motor weakness occurs.

14. How does cingulate herniation occur?

Rarely, the cingulate gyrus is forced medially beneath the falx by an expanding lateral hematoma, causing compression of the ventricles and impairing cerebral blood flow.

15. Explain posterior fossa herniation.

Bleeding or edema in the posterior fossa can result in herniation of the cerebellar tonsils either upward through the tentorium or downward through the foramen magnum. In the latter case, coma and fatal brain stem dysfunction may occur rapidly and with little warning.

16. What is the ED treatment for increased ICP?

1. **Maintain adequate cerebral perfusion pressure.** Although there is often misguided reluctance to hydrate vigorously patients with concomitant head and systemic injuries, cerebral perfusion must be maintained for resuscitation to be successful. Hypotension must be avoided, and often laparotomy to correct intraabdominal bleeding must take precedence over neurosurgical intervention to maintain cerebral perfusion.

2. **Avoid secondary injuries to the central nervous system.** After brain trauma, there is a cascade of secondary neuronal metabolic injuries that are detrimental to recovery of neurologic function. At present, few interventions have proved effective in limiting these changes. Certain other treatable conditions either increase the metabolic demands of the brain or decrease cerebral perfusion and worsen the prognosis unless they are corrected. The **5 Hs (hypotension, hypoxia, hypercarbia, hypoglycemia,** and **hyperthermia)** and **seizures** are conditions that should be avoided or corrected in the ED. Anticonvulsant prophylaxis with diphenylhydantoin is indicated particularly for penetrating injuries and depressed skull fractures. Raising the head of the bed while maintaining spinal precautions may decrease ICP slightly but also decreases cerebral perfusion pressure. Coagulopathies should be corrected with fresh frozen plasma, and platelet transfusion should be considered in patients who have recently taken aspirin or other antiplatelet drugs.

3. **Hyperventilation.** Carbon dioxide is one of the main determinants of cerebrovascular tone. High levels produce cerebral vasodilation; low levels cause vasoconstriction. Hyperventilation to a PCO_2 level of 25 mmHg decreases blood flow to the brain by 50%, which decreases the vascular compartment of the brain, "buying some time" for definitive surgical interventions. When blood flow to the brain decreases, delivery of oxygen and glucose also decreases, resulting in ischemic injury and worse edema. The optimal level of hypocarbia is uncertain at present, but most clinicians recommend mild hyperventilation, with a PCO_2 level of 30–35 mmHg as the goal. To accomplish this degree of hypocarbia, it is necessary to intubate the patient with rapid-sequence intubation and mechanically ventilate with settings determined by arterial blood gases to maintain the PCO_2 between 30 and 35 mmHg. The indication for implementing hyperventilation is increased ICP resulting in clinical signs of focal neurologic deficit (i.e., herniation). Hyperventilation is not used prophylactically but is reserved for patients with elevated ICP and clinical deterioration.

4. **Diuresis.** The use of an osmotic diuretic, such as mannitol, 0.5–1.0 g/kg intravenously over 15 minutes, or a loop diuretic, such as furosemide, 0.5–1.0 mg/kg intravenously, is effective

in reducing brain edema. Infusion of mannitol creates an osmotic gradient between the intravascular space and the extracellular fluid, drawing fluid from the extracellular fluid and reducing brain water content and ICP. Mannitol is filtered by the kidneys, producing systemic dehydration. Clinical experience and animal studies seem to support the concomitant administration of osmotic diuretics and volume resuscitation in patients with hypovolemic shock.

5. **Ventriculostomy.** Although generally an intensive care unit (ICU) technique, removal of CSF through a ventriculostomy is occasionally implemented in the ED and is perhaps the most effective way of rapidly lowering ICP.

6. **Barbiturates.** Conscious patients who are paralyzed for intubation also must be sedated. A short-acting barbiturate such as thiopental is the ideal agent for this purpose because it lowers ICP, prevents seizures, and decreases cerebral metabolism. Such agents cannot be used in a hypotensive patient, however. In these cases, a reversible agent, such as morphine, 0.1 mg/kg; lorazepam, 0.01 mg/kg; or midazolam, 1 mg/kg/h, is preferred because adverse effects on blood pressure and cardiac output can be reversed by specific antagonists. Etomidate, 0.2 mg/kg, is a short-acting agent that decreases ICP without adversely affecting cardiac output, cerebral perfusion pressure, and systemic blood pressure. Fentanyl, 3–5 µg/kg, causes a slight increase in ICP and is not the preferred agent for sedation of a head-injured patient.

7. **Hypertonic saline.** Various concentrations of hypertonic saline ranging from 3% to 7.5% have been used to simultaneously decrease brain edema, maintain cerebral perfusion pressure, and restore systemic volume. It has been shown to be at least as effective as mannitol in treating elevated ICP. Patients receiving hypertonic saline will develop significant hypernatremia and hyperosmolarity. These abnormalities should be allowed to correct themselves gradually over a period of several days.

Chestnut RM: Management of brain and spinal injuries. Crit Care Clin North Am 20:25–55, 2004.

Guha A: Management of traumatic brain injury: Some current evidence and applications. Postgrad Med J 80:481–488, 2004.

Rosner MJ, Rosner SD, Johnson AH: Cerebral perfusion pressure: Management protocol and clinical results. J Neurosurg 83:949–961, 1995.

Stochetti N, Maas AI, Chieregato A, et al: Hyperventilation in head injury: A review. Chest 127:1812–1817, 2005.

Wade CE, Grady JJ, Kramer GC, et al: Individual patient cohort analysis of the efficacy of hypertonic saline/dextran in patients with traumatic brain injury and hypotension. J Trauma 42(Suppl 5):S61–S65, 1997.

Walls RM: Rapid sequence intubation in head trauma. Ann Emerg Med 22:1008–1013, 1993.

KEY POINTS: TREATMENT OF HEAD INJURY

1. Maintain cerebral perfusion and avoid hypotension.

2. Maintain oxygenation.

3. Secure airway using rapid-sequence intubation (RSI) if the Glasgow Coma Scale (GCS) is less than 8.

4. Seizure prophylaxis with diphenylhydantoin (15 mg/kg IV).

5. Hyperventilate to $pCO_2 = 30$–35 mmHg only if patient has elevated ICP and is clinically deteriorating.

6. Diuresis using either mannitol or hypertonic saline.

7. Correct coagulopathy.

17. **Does hypothermia have a role in the ED treatment of increased ICP?**

Some evidence suggested that reducing core body temperature to 32–34°C might be protective for the injured brain. Recent prospective studies have not demonstrated a benefit, and routine induction of hypothermia is not recommended. Fever should be treated aggressively, however, and patients who arrive in the ED with mild hypothermia should be allowed to passively rewarm.

18. **If a patient has a normal CT scan after head trauma, is it completely safe to discharge him or her home?**

Nothing is completely safe. There are well-documented instances of delayed epidural and subdural bleeding many hours after injury. Consequently, although it is generally safe to discharge such patients, head injury instructions should be given to responsible family members, and the patient should be instructed to return immediately if symptoms worsen. If the patient is socially isolated or unreliable, a judgment has to be made regarding the seriousness of the mechanism of injury and the risk of discharge. Intoxicated patients should be kept under observation until their mental status can be evaluated properly.

af Geijerstam JL, Britton M: Mild head injury: Reliability of early computed tomographic findings in triage for admission Emerg Med J 22:103–107, 2005.

19. **Because CT scan is available, is there any role for plain skull films?**

The usefulness of plain radiographs of the skull has been far outstripped by more informative imaging modalities such as CT and MRI. Skull films still have certain indications in evaluation of the following:

- Penetrating trauma (gunshot wounds)
- Suspected depressed skull fracture
- Suspected basilar skull fracture
- As part of the skeletal survey for suspected child abuse
- In patients with prior craniotomies or shunts

CHAPTER 88

TRAUMATIC OPHTHALMOLOGIC EMERGENCIES

Harold Thomas, MD

1. **Name the two most time-critical emergencies in ophthalmology.**
   Central retinal artery occlusion and chemical burns to the eyes.

2. **What is the treatment for a chemical burn of the eye?**
   Immediate copious irrigation of the eyes (for at least 20 minutes). Irrigation should be initiated before transport to the emergency department (ED).

3. **How do you know when you have irrigated the eye enough?**
   Nitrazine paper can be used to ensure that the pH has been corrected to normal. This usually requires at least 3 L of normal saline in each eye and continuous irrigation for 20 minutes. Alkalis, which cause the most damaging burns, tend to adhere to the tissue of the eye and are difficult to remove completely with irrigation. After irrigation, emergent ophthalmologic consultation is indicated.

4. **What is the significance of pain from an eye injury that is not relieved with topical anesthesia?**
   Complete symptomatic relief with topical anesthesia indicates a superficial injury involving only the cornea. If a patient still has significant pain after application of anesthetic drops, a deeper injury (often traumatic iritis) must be suspected, even in the presence of an obvious superficial injury.

5. **List nine potential injuries that must be considered in a patient sustaining a blunt injury to the eye.**
   - Blow-out fracture of the floor of the orbit
   - Corneal abrasion
   - Anterior hyphema
   - Lens dislocation
   - Traumatic mydriasis
   - Vitreous hemorrhage
   - Retinal detachment
   - Traumatic iritis
   - Ruptured globe (rare after blunt injuries)

6. **What is the most common eye injury seen in the ED?**
   Corneal abrasion with or without a superficial foreign body.

7. **How is corneal abrasion diagnosed?**
   The anesthetized eye can be stained with fluorescein and illuminated by an ultraviolet or Wood's lamp; corneal defects fluoresce bright yellow-orange. Visual acuity should be checked, and the eye should be inspected, with particular emphasis on the anterior chamber to look for an anterior hyphema.

8. **What is the treatment for a corneal abrasion?**
   Because this injury is extremely painful, narcotic analgesics are indicated. **Never dispense topical anesthesia from the ED.** One frequently overlooked aspect of therapy is the instillation

of a cycloplegic, usually cyclopentolate (Cyclogyl), to relieve the ciliary spasm that commonly accompanies this injury. Patients also need evaluation for tetanus prophylaxis. Most should receive topical antibiotics, drops, or ointment.

9. **What is the role of an eye patch in treatment of corneal abrasions?**
   A pressure patch previously was considered the most important aspect of management of a corneal abrasion. Patches were thought to increase comfort and hasten healing. It is now known that not only are eye patches uncomfortable but also they do not increase healing and may promote infection. They do *not* prevent the involved eye from moving and should not be used for most superficial corneal abrasions. If you do use a patch, be sure to instruct the patient not to drive because depth perception depends on binocular vision.

   Campanile TM, St Clalir DA, Benaim M: The evaluation of eye patching in the treatment or traumatic corneal epithelial defects. J Emerg Med 15:769–774, 1997.

10. **How does a corneal abrasion from a contact lens differ from other causes of corneal trauma?**
    Corneal abrasions secondary to overuse of contact lenses are much more likely to have a bacterial process involved, often *Pseudomonas*. These patients should receive topical antibiotics effective against *Pseudomonas* organisms (tobramycin or gentamicin) and should never be patched. If the emergency physician is unable to do a slit-lamp examination, early ophthalmologic referral to rule out ulcerative keratitis (corneal ulcer) is indicated.

    Schein OD: Contact lens abrasions and the nonophthalmologist. Ann J Emerg Med 11:606–608, 1993.

11. **What is the most common location of an ocular foreign body?**
    Foreign bodies often are lodged just beneath the upper eyelid along the palpebral conjunctiva. The eyelid needs to be everted with a cotton swab to examine this area adequately. Conjunctival foreign bodies should be suspected when many vertical linear streaks are noted on the cornea with fluorescein examination.

12. **What is the proper treatment for a corneal foreign body?**
    First, topical anesthesia is applied, usually proparacaine. Nonembedded foreign bodies should be removed with a sterile, moist cotton swab. Embedded foreign bodies are removed with a 27G needle or an eye spud. Most metallic foreign bodies leave a residual rust ring that should be removed in approximately 24 hours, after the cornea has softened.

13. **What is an anterior hyphema?**
    A collection of blood in the anterior chamber of the eye; it is seen as a layering of cells that pool along the bottom of the eye when the patient is sitting upright. When the patient is lying down, a hyphema is not recognized easily; it may appear as a diffuse haziness of the anterior chamber. Small hyphemas, termed **microhyphemas,** may be identified only with a slit lamp.

14. **How is an anterior hyphema treated?**
    The standard in the past was to admit all patients for bed rest; today the dominant tendency is toward outpatient management. The patient should be kept upright, the eye patched, and ophthalmologic consultation initiated, at least by phone. Complications include rebleeding, glaucoma formation (particularly in patients with sickle-cell trait), and corneal staining.

15. **What physical findings lead to the suspicion of a blow-out fracture?**
    Classic findings with a blow-out fracture (fracture of the inferior orbital wall with herniation of the global contents into the maxillary sinus) are (1) decreased sensation over the inferior orbital rim, extending to the edge of the nose and ipsilateral upper lip, secondary to compromise of the inferior orbital nerve; (2) enophthalmos, or a sunken appearance of the eye, which may be

masked by edema; and (3) paralysis or limitation of upward gaze (manifested as diplopia), resulting from entrapment of the inferior rectus muscle.

KEY POINTS: OPHTHALMOLOGIC EMERGENCIES

1. Preservation of vision in a chemical burn is directly related from time of exposure to time initiating irrigation; do not wait for the patient to arrive at the hospital.

2. Never patch a patient with an eye injury related to contact lens; a patch provides a perfect environment for bacterial proliferation. These patients should be treated with aminoglycoside ointment.

3. Diplopia on upward gaze is the hallmark of a blow-out fracture of the orbital floor.

16. **What is traumatic mydriasis?**
An efferent pupillary defect manifested by a dilated (in most instances irregular) pupil that does not react to direct or consensual light, usually as a result of minor trauma to the eye. Because such a patient is at risk for other more serious eye injuries, a careful eye examination is mandatory. The possibility of uncal herniation secondary to intracranial injury should be considered if level of consciousness is decreased in the presence of a perfectly round, nonreactive, unilateral, dilated pupil. If level of consciousness is unaltered, this is most likely an isolated ocular injury.

17. **Why is a history of hammering metal on metal important in a patient presenting with an eye complaint?**
Often a small, high-velocity fragment penetrates the globe with minimal or no physical findings. This injury, which can cause inflammation weeks later, is diagnosed with soft tissue radiographs of the orbit or a computed tomography (CT) scan of the globe.

18. **Which eyelid lacerations should be repaired by an ophthalmologist or plastic surgeon?**
    - Those involving the lid margin or gray line
    - Those involving the tear duct mechanism along the lower eyelid
    - Those involving the tarsal plate or levator muscle

19. **When should penetration of the globe be suspected?**
The pupil is usually misshapen, pointing in the direction of the penetration. The globe may appear soft because of decreased intraocular pressure. Intraocular pressure should not be tested if a penetrating injury is suspected because the pressure promotes extrusion of aqueous humor.

20. **What is the significance of a subscleral (subconjunctival) hemorrhage?**
Subscleral hemorrhages are usually benign and often occur spontaneously with complete resolution over 2–3 weeks. When associated with trauma, other potentially more serious eye injuries should be suspected and ruled out.

21. **List traumatic ophthalmologic injuries that require immediate ophthalmologic consultation.**
    - Chemical burns of the eye
    - Orbital hemorrhage with increased intraocular pressure

- Perforation of the globe or cornea
- Lacerations involving the lid margin, tarsal plate, or tear duct
- Lens dislocation

22. **Name two ophthalmologic injuries that require urgent ophthalmologic consultation (within 12–24 hours).**
Anterior hyphema and blow-out fracture.

23. **What is solar keratitis?**
Also known as **flash burns** or **snow blindness,** solar keratitis is a corneal injury secondary to overexposure to ultraviolet light. Diagnosis is made with fluorescein staining, which shows multiple punctate lesions of the cornea. Treatment consists of resting the eyes with adequate narcotic analgesia. Spontaneous resolution can be expected in 12–24 hours.

24. **What is the significance of a retro-orbital hematoma?**
Bleeding behind the globe (retro-orbital hematoma) can lead to elevated orbital pressure, which can be greater than the perfusion pressure of the retina and result in ischemia. Treatment is a lateral canthotomy, which releases the canthus that holds the eye in its socket. This allows for proptosis of the globe, which (temporarily) relieves the elevated retro-orbital pressure, preserving blood flow to the retina.

McInnes G, Howes D: Lateral canthotomy and cantholysis: A simple, vision-saving procedure. Can J Emerg Med 4:54, 2002.

25. **What is the cause of a dilated pupil that fails to constrict with topical pilocarpine?**
A dilated pupil that fails to constrict with topical miotic agents is due to topical application of a mydriatic agent often because of rubbing the eye after application of a scopolamine patch (for motion sickness).

CHAPTER 89

NECK TRAUMA

Jeffrey J. Schaider, MD

1. **Why is neck trauma a complicated topic?**

   The lack of bony protection makes the anterior neck especially vulnerable to severe, life-threatening injuries. The exposed anatomic structure of the neck, which contains many vital structures of the vascular, airway, and gastrointestinal systems, provides a fertile ground for debate and myriad opinions about modality of treatment.

2. **What are the most urgent concerns in the initial management of neck trauma?**

   Airway and **hemorrhage control.** Airway management comes before anything else discussed in this chapter. Early endotracheal intubation is indicated for any patient with existing or potential airway compromise. Delay in airway management increases the difficulty of intubation because of swelling and compression of the anatomic structures. Bleeding should be controlled with pressure rather than with blind clamping. The wound should be examined to determine whether it has violated the platysma. Injudicious probing of the wound may be dangerous, however, because a vascular structure that has ceased to bleed may resume with disastrous consequences when its tamponade is released.

3. **What is the preferred method to secure the airway?**

   Rapid-sequence induction with oral tracheal intubation should be the initial airway approach in patients with none to minimal distortion of their airway. Patients with airway distortion with anticipated difficult bag-valve-mask ventilation should have their airway managed with local airway anesthesia or sedative-assisted oral tracheal intubation. The preferred sedative medications include versed and fentanyl because they are reversible or ketamine because it does not depress spontaneous respirations. Although the risks of blind nasal tracheal intubation include breaking away clots and damaging a distorted airway, a recent study from Denver found that blind nasal tracheal intubation had a 90% success rate in the prehospital phase. Surgical airway via cricothyrotomy should be employed if endotracheal intubation is unsuccessful. Tracheostomy is preferred over cricothyrotomy if there is severe damage to the larynx and cricoid cartilage.

   Schaider JJ, Bailitz J: Neck trauma: Don't put your neck on the line. Emerg Med Pract 5:1–23, 2003.
   Weitzel N, Kendall JL, Pons P: Blind nasotracheal intubation for patients with penetrating neck trauma. J Trauma 56:1097–1101, 2004.

4. **What common findings indicate significant neck injury?**

   - Injuries involving the **vascular system** result in hematomas, bleeding, pulse deficit, shock, and neurologic deficit secondary to arterial interruption.
   - **Laryngeal trauma** causes voice alteration, airway compromise, subcutaneous emphysema, crepitus, and hemoptysis.
   - Signs and symptoms of **esophageal disruption** include pain and tenderness in the neck, resistance of the neck to passive motion, crepitus, dysphagia, and bleeding from the mouth or nasogastric tube. The diagnosis of esophageal disruption is difficult because of injuries to other overlying structures. Ancillary testing must be used to assist in the diagnosis of these injuries.

     For more details, see Table 89-1.

TABLE 89-1. SIGNS AND SYMPTOMS OF SYSTEM INJURIES

Vascular	Aerodigestive
Hematoma	Respiratory distress
Hemorrhage	Stridor
Neurologic deficit	Cyanosis
Pulse deficit	Hemoptysis
Horner's syndrome (carotid injury)	Tracheal deviation
Hypovolemic shock	Subcutaneous emphysema
Vascular bruit or thrill	Pneumothorax
Altered sensorium	Sucking wound
Harsh, machinery-like precordial murmur	Dysphonia, aphonia, hoarseness
(air embolism)	Dysphagia
	Odynophagia

5. **What are the signs and symptoms of blunt carotid artery trauma?**
Of patients with blunt carotid trauma, 25–50% have no external signs of trauma. Delayed neurologic signs are the rule rather than the exception; only 10% of patients have symptoms of transient ischemic attacks or strokes within 1 hour of injury. Most patients develop symptoms within the first 24 hours, but 17% develop symptoms days or weeks after injury. Carotid artery injuries may present with a hematoma of the lateral neck, bruit over carotid circulation, Horner's syndrome, transient ischemic attack, aphasia, or hemiparesis. The clinical manifestations of vertebral artery injury include ataxia, vertigo, nystagmus, hemiparesis, dysarthria, and diplopia.

6. **Name the main controversy regarding management of penetrating neck trauma.**
The management of penetrating neck trauma that violates the platysma. In the 1990s, physicians and surgeons changed from a mandatory exploration policy for penetrating neck wounds to a selective management approach.

7. **What is mandatory exploration for penetrating neck wounds?**
All patients who have wounds that penetrate the platysma muscle in the neck are explored surgically to determine the presence or absence of injury to the deeper structures in the neck. Some ancillary diagnostic testing (angiography, esophagography, esophagoscopy, laryngoscopy) may be done preoperatively, depending on the location of the wound and the stability of the patient.

8. **What are the advantages and disadvantages of mandatory exploration for penetrating neck wounds?**
During the 1940s, mandatory exploration was instituted for all penetrating wounds that violate the platysma. This policy reduced mortality significantly and remained the only mode of therapy until the mid-1970s. Proponents of mandatory exploration warn of the catastrophic complications from delayed treatment and missed injuries. Neck exploration is relatively simple, and a negative exploration has low morbidity and mortality. However, because the negative exploration rate (no injuries found at surgery) is 50%, the cost of the operation and the added length of hospital stay are unwarranted. Many of these operations could be avoided with the selective approach to neck exploration.

KEY POINTS: EARLY AIRWAY MANAGEMENT FOR NECK INJURIES

1. Manage airway early before airway distortion occurs.
2. Use oral tracheal intubation with rapid-sequence intubation (RSI) as initial airway management option.
3. Do not paralyze patients with significant airway distortion who cannot be ventilated.
4. Tracheostomy may be necessary as rescue airway if there is a hematoma over or damage to cricoid cartilage.

9. **Describe the theory behind the selective surgical management of penetrating neck wounds.**
   With the improved sensitivity and specificity of ancillary diagnostic testing (angiography, carotid duplex scanning, computed tomography [CT], esophagography, esophagoscopy, laryngoscopy), a nonoperative approach to a select group of patients, based on physical examination and results of ancillary tests, is safe. The selective approach has reduced the negative exploration rate from 50% to 30%.

10. **What are the three anatomic zones of the neck?**
    - **Zone I** is the area below the cricoid cartilage.
    - **Zone II** extends from the cricoid cartilage to the angle of the mandible.
    - **Zone III** extends from the angle of the mandible to the base of the skull.
    Figure 89-1 illustrates the zones of the neck.

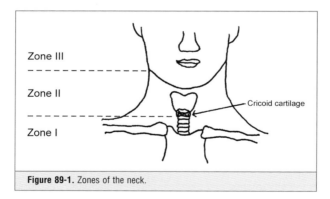

Figure 89-1. Zones of the neck.

11. **Why is the neck divided into three zones?**
    The location of the injury plays a major role in assessing the need for angiography:
    - All **zone I** injuries require angiography to determine the integrity of the thoracic outlet vessels. In stable but symptomatic patients needing surgery, angiography should be done preoperatively because positive findings necessitate a thoracotomy before neck exploration.
    - The familiar anatomy of **zone II,** coupled with relative ease of surgical exposure, minimizes the need for angiography in symptomatic patients undergoing surgery.

Some clinicians observe asymptomatic patients with penetrating injuries without angiography. Others perform angiography, carotid duplex scanning, or helical CT on asymptomatic patients to detect occult injuries and involvement of vertebral vessels before observation.

- The management of **zone III** injuries is controversial because of the complex anatomy of the area and the difficulty in obtaining adequate exposure. Most clinicians agree that for asymptomatic patients not undergoing surgery, angiography is necessary to assess the status of the internal carotid artery and the intracerebral circulation. For symptomatic patients, preoperative angiography is helpful because high internal carotid artery injuries are difficult to visualize at operation and may require carotid artery ligation and concomitant extracranial-intracranial bypass.

Demetriades D, Theodorou D, Cornwell E, et al: Evaluation of penetrating injuries of the neck: Prospective study of 223 patients. World J Surg 21:47–48, 1997.

Knaut AL, Kendall JL: Penetrating neck trauma. In Wolfson AB, Hendey GW, Hendry PL, Linden CH, Rosen CL, Schaider JJ (eds): Clinical Practice of Emergency Medicine, 4th ed. Philadelphia, Lippincott, Williams & Wilkins, 2005, pp 956–962.

12. **Can carotid duplex scanning or helical CT angiography (HCTA) replace angiography for detection of vascular injuries in penetrating neck injuries?**
With experienced operators, carotid duplex scanning approaches 100% sensitivity for excluding zone II and III vascular injuries in stable, asymptomatic patients with penetrating neck injuries. Because carotid duplex scanning has a lower specificity (85–95%), positive carotid duplex scanning should be followed by carotid angiography before making a decision regarding surgical intervention. In recent studies using multidetector helical CT scanners, HCTA had sensitivities of 90–100%, a specificity of 100%, a positive predictive value of 100%, and a negative predictive value of 98% in detecting carotid artery injuries. The limitations and pitfalls of the HCTA include artifacts produced by the shoulders of large patients or by bullet fragments and other metallic foreign bodies. Streak artifacts can simulate an intimal tear. In cases with inadequate studies or doubtful HCTA results, the study should be considered nondiagnostic, and the patients must undergo conventional angiography. Helical CT angiographic examinations have only a 1.1% reported incidence of nondiagnostic results.

Fry WR, Dort JA, Smith RS, et al: Duplex scanning replaces arteriography and operative exploration in the diagnosis of potential cervical vascular injury. Am J Surg 168:693–695, 1994.

LeBlang SD, Nunez DB: Noninvasive imaging of cervical vascular injuries. Am J Roentgenol 175:1269–1278, 2002.

Montalvo BM, LeBlang SD, Nunez DB Jr, et al: Color Doppler sonography in penetrating injuries of the neck. Am J Neuroradiol 17:943–951, 1996.

Múnera F, Cohn S, Rivas LA: Penetrating Injuries of the neck: Use of helical computed tomographic angiography. J Trauma 58:413–418, 2005.

Múnera F, Soto JA, Palacio D, et al: Diagnosis of arterial injuries caused by penetrating trauma to the neck: Comparison of helical CT angiography and conventional angiography. Radiology 216:356–362, 2000.

13. **What diagnostic testing is preferred in detection of blunt vascular injuries?**
- Blunt vascular injuries were found in 27% of high-risk patients screened for blunt vascular injury (combination of injury mechanism [cervical hyperextension or hyperflexion, direct cervical blow, near-hanging] and injury pattern [carotid canal, midface, and cervical spine fracture]). **Angiography** is the study of choice in acutely injured and symptomatic patients. Of lesions, 90% occur at the bifurcation of carotids or higher. Four-vessel angiography is recommended because multiple vessel injuries occur in 40–80%.
- The diagnostic accuracy of **HCTA** has not been studied extensively in blunt trauma. In a small study comparing CT angiography with conventional angiography, CT angiography had a sensitivity of 85% and specificity of 71%. CT angiography has been shown to decrease significantly the time to diagnose the injury.

- **Color flow Doppler ultrasound** provides rapid identification and quantification of arterial dissection, but it is unable to assess distal upper extracranial and intracranial internal carotid artery and is operator dependent. With an experienced operator, ultrasound can be used as a screening test in lower-risk patients.
- **Magnetic resonance (MR) angiography** accurately detects carotid and vertebral artery injuries with a sensitivity and specificity greater than 95% for carotid artery dissection. It is ideal for follow-up or for stable patients; MR angiography is difficult to perform in an acutely injured unstable patient.

Biffl WL, Moore EE: Identifying the asymptomatic patient with blunt carotid arterial injury. J Trauma 47:1163–1164, 1999.

Ullman E: Blunt neck trauma. In Wolfson AB, Hendey GW, Hendry PL, Linden CH, Rosen CL Schaider JJ (eds): Clinical Practice of Emergency Medicine, 4th ed. Philadelphia, Lippincott, Williams Wilkens, 2005, pp 953–956.

14. **Which diagnostic studies are important in suspected laryngeal injuries?**
    - Soft tissue cervical **radiographs** may show a fractured larynx, subcutaneous air, or prevertebral air.
    - **CT** accurately identifies the location and extent of laryngeal fractures. CT should be done when the diagnosis of a laryngeal fracture is still suspected despite a negative examination of the endolarynx or when flexible laryngoscopy cannot be done (e.g., intubated patient).
    - Flexible **laryngoscopy** provides valuable information regarding the integrity of the cartilaginous framework and the function of the vocal cords.

15. **Are diagnostic studies necessary in suspected esophageal injuries?**
    Yes. Soft tissue cervical radiographs may show subcutaneous emphysema or an increased prevertebral shadow. Chest radiograph findings include pleural effusion, pneumothorax, mediastinal air, and mediastinal widening. Esophageal contrast studies should be done initially with radiopaque contrast medium (Gastrografin); if negative, studies should be repeated with barium to increase diagnostic yield. Radiographic imaging is difficult because of the high false-negative rate. Esophagography has a 30–50% false-negative rate and should be followed by esophagoscopy in patients with suspected esophageal injury. Rigid endoscopy is more sensitive than flexible endoscopy. No one study can exclude esophageal perforation; a combination of physical signs, plain and contrast radiographs, and esophagoscopy should be used to make the diagnosis. Isolated esophageal injuries after blunt injury are extremely rare.

CHAPTER 90

CHEST TRAUMA

Justin C. Chang, MD, and Robert C. Jorden, MD

1. **How should the patient with chest trauma be approached?**
   One must immediately identify actual or potential life threats based on the clinical evaluation. This evaluation consists of the standard inspection, auscultation, and palpation.
   - **Inspection.** Completely undress the patient and visually inspect the entire chest, which necessitates rolling over a supine patient. Look for a flail chest (paradoxical movement of the chest wall) and sucking chest wounds. Identify the exact location, number, and type (i.e., penetrating or blunt) of wounds.
   - **Auscultation.** Listen for diminished or absent breath sounds and bowel sounds in the chest. The former indicate a pneumothorax if the subcutaneous emphysema is located over the ribs or a pneumomediastinum if the location is supraclavicular. Bony crepitus indicates a rib or sternal fracture with the potential for intrathoracic injury.
   - **Palpation.** It is important to palpate the chest wall gently at first to detect subcutaneous emphysema and bony crepitus. The former indicates a major blow to the chest with rib fractures and the potential for underlying organ damage (e.g., pulmonary contusion), and the latter, depending on location, indicates pneumothorax or pneumomediastinum.

2. **What is a flail chest?**
   A flail chest occurs when a segment of the chest wall becomes unattached from the rest of the chest. It occurs in one of three settings:
   - Two or more ribs are broken in two or more places.
   - More than one rib is fractured in association with costal cartilage disarticulation.
   - The costal cartilages on both sides of the sternum are disarticulated, resulting in a sternal or central flail segment. The significance of a flail chest lies in the tremendous force that caused it and the near certainty of associated intrathoracic injuries.

3. **What is the treatment for flail chest?**
   The condition of the underlying lung generally dictates the treatment. Underlying pulmonary contusion and resultant hypoxemia indicate the need for intervention. In general, a flail chest should be treated supportively; if the patient is doing well and tolerating the flail (i.e., blood gases do not show hypoxemia or hypercarbia), only supplemental oxygen is indicated. If the patient is in respiratory distress either clinically or as indicated by blood gas analysis or oxygen saturation measurements, intubation and positive-pressure ventilation should be initiated. Positive-pressure ventilation results in uniform expansion of the chest from within and stabilizes the flail segment.

4. **What are the radiographic findings of a tension pneumothorax?**
   There should not be any because this diagnosis should be made on clinical grounds, and treatment should be undertaken before a radiograph is obtained. If a radiograph is obtained, a hyperlucent, overexpanded hemithorax with an evident pneumothorax and a mediastinal shift to the opposite side would be observed.

5. **What are the clinical signs of a tension pneumothorax?**
   Respiratory distress, an overexpanded hemithorax, hyperresonance to percussion, absent or markedly diminished breath sounds, tracheal shift away from the pneumothorax (the trachea

must be palpated above the sternal notch; it is not appreciated on inspection), tachycardia, jugular venous distention, subcutaneous emphysema, and hypotension. In addition, in patients who are intubated and are being bag ventilated, increasing resistance to ventilation (requiring more manual pressure to insufflate air into the lungs) is often the earliest sign of tension pneumothorax. The most reliable and easiest to appreciate signs of tension pneumothorax are absent breath sounds, hypotension, tachycardia, and, if no hypovolemia is present, jugular venous distention or elevated central venous pressure (CVP).

6. **Why does tension pneumothorax cause hypotension?**
   The mediastinal shift compromises vena caval blood return to the heart. The severely altered preload results in reduced stroke volume, reduced cardiac output, and hypotension.

7. **What is the treatment for a tension pneumothorax?**
   Immediate reduction in the intrapleural pressure on the affected side is mandatory! For patients in extremis, the best way to accomplish this is also the quickest: placement of a 14G over-the-needle catheter over the fourth or fifth rib in the midaxillary line, followed by aspiration with a 50-mL syringe. After vital signs improve, the procedure should be followed immediately by **tube thoracostomy,** which is the definitive treatment. For patients who are stable, aspiration need not precede insertion of a chest tube.

8. **What are the radiologic findings of pulmonary contusion?**
   Characteristic findings on chest radiographs consist of solitary or multiple patchy, ill-defined areas that may be either localized or diffuse resulting from blood and secretions accumulating in the alveoli and interstitial spaces of the lung. Although often visible within 1–2 hours following blunt chest trauma injury, these findings sometimes may not appear until several hours after injury.

9. **What is the signficance of a sternal fracture?**
   Sternal fractures are often associated with more serious injuries to the underlying great vessels and myocardium and necessitate further evaluation. Sternal fractures are often missed on initial anteroposterior chest radiographs, and are best viewed on lateral chest films, or by computed tomography (CT) scan.

10. **What significant history should be obtained if the patient was involved in a motor vehicle accident?**
    - What was the nature of the accident (rollover, head-on collision)?
    - Was the patient wearing a seat belt? If so, what type?
    - Did the air bag deploy?
    - Was the steering wheel or windshield broken?
    - Was there substantial vehicular damage?
    - Was there intrusion into the passenger space?

    When a frontal deceleration mechanism is operative, one should consider not only chest wall injuries and pulmonary contusion but also two other specific entities—myocardial contusion and aortic rupture.

11. **How is myocardial contusion diagnosed and treated?**
    Unfortunately, there is no gold standard for the diagnosis of myocardial contusion short of autopsy. Many modalities have been used in the attempt, including electrocardiogram (ECG), echocardiography, cardiac enzyme analysis, and radionucleotide scanning. Because a contusion rarely causes serious dysrhythmias or compromises cardiac output, there is a trend away from aggressive monitoring of patients based on mechanism only. Instead, most recommend using ECG and clinical assessment as a screening device. A normal ECG in the absence of hemodynamic instability precludes the need for extended monitoring and probably effectively

rules out a clinically significant contusion. Treatment is symptomatic, with dysrhythmia control and measures to optimize cardiac output.

Fildes JJ, Betlej TM, Manglano R, et al: Limiting cardiac evaluation in patients with suspected myocardial contusion. Am Surg 61:832–835, 1995.

12. **What is the most common ECG finding in patients with myocardial contusion?**
Sinus tachycardia with nonspecific ST-T wave changes, although any ECG abnormality can be seen. An abnormal ECG or unexplained hypotension in the proper clinical setting may merit further diagnostic evaluation and admission.

13. **How can anyone survive a ruptured aorta?**
Approximately 85–90% of patients with aortic rupture die, and they do so before medical aid reaches them. The 10–15% who survive do so because not all three layers of the aorta are ruptured; the adventitia remains intact and temporarily contains the hemorrhage. Left untreated, this injury usually results in complete rupture and exsanguination, usually in hours to days, but this may be delayed for years in the form of a pseudoaneurysm rupture.

14. **What is the mechanism of a traumatic aortic tear?**
The thoracic aorta is particularly susceptible to acceleration-deceleration shearing forces because the arch is less mobile than the heart and the aorta distal to the ligamentum arteriosum. Frontal or transverse deceleration causes shearing forces at the points of fixation, with the most common site for disruption being just distal to the left subclavian artery. Vertical acceleration-deceleration injuries such as falls may result in a tear of the ascending aorta with coronary artery compromise or acute pericardial tamponade.

15. **Describe the first steps in diagnosing aortic rupture.**
Traditionally, the initial screening for aortic rupture includes obtaining the mechanism of injury and a standard upright chest radiograph. The finding of an abnormal-appearing or widened mediastinal silhouette usually triggers additional workup for these patients. Other suggestive radiographic findings include deviation of the nasogastric tube to the right, an apical cap, left pleural effusion, loss of the aortic window or the left pleural stripe, and depression of the left mainstem bronchus. A supine chest radiograph can have a falsely widened mediastinum, and aortic rupture can be present even with a normal-appearing chest radiograph. If clinical suspicion is strong enough based on mechanism or clinical findings, further evaluation of the aorta by helical chest CT or aortography is warranted.

Fabian TC, Richardson JD, Croce MA, et al: Prospective study of blunt aortic injury: Multicenter trial of the American Association for the Surgery of Trauma. J Trauma Inj Infect Crit Care 47:374–383, 1997.

16. **Should aortography or helical CT be used in diagnosing aortic rupture?**
Classically, aortography has been considered the gold standard for diagnosing this condition. It is a relatively safe procedure with high sensitivity and specificity. It is also an invasive, costly, and time-consuming procedure, however, which may not be available at all institutions or during off hours.

The introduction of helical CT technology has resulted in CT becoming the preferred method of diagnosis. It is more widely available, quicker, and accessible 24 hours a day, and many trauma patients often require a trip to the CT scanner for other reasons. Large, prospective studies have shown helical CT to have 100% sensitivity and 100% negative predictive value for diagnosing traumatic aortic injury. Patients with negative scans effectively require no further evaluation. Helical CT also can diagnose subtle intimal injuries sometimes missed by aortography. The major drawback with helical CT is its lower specificity compared with aortography. Nevertheless, used as a screening test, helical CT has dramatically reduced the number of unnecessary aortograms performed. A dynamic helical CT scan of the chest is acceptable as an initial screening test for traumatic aortic dissection because a completely normal CT scan effectively rules out aortic injury.

Dyer DS, Moore EE, Ilke DN, et al: Thoracic aortic injury: How predictive is mechanism and is chest computed tomography a reliable screening tool? A prospective study of 1,561 patients. J Trauma 48:673–683, 2000.

Fabian TC, Davis KA, Gavant ML, et al: Prospective study of blunt aortic injury: Helical CT is diagnostic and antihypertensive therapy reduces rupture. Ann Surg 227:666–677, 1998.

17. **How is penetrating chest trauma managed?**
   Multiple diagnostic and therapeutic approaches exist, depending on the location of the chest wound and the nature of the wounding implement.

18. **What is the significance of the location of the wound?**
   Wound location dictates the clinical approach by virtue of the organs at risk. From a functional standpoint, wounds are categorized as central, peripheral, thoracoabdominal, and those in adjacent areas (abdomen and neck). Anatomically speaking, central wounds are located anteriorly (bordered by the midclavicular lines, the clavicles superiorly, and the costal margins inferiorly). All other wounds are considered peripheral; they are either lateral (bordered by the midclavicular lines, the posterior axillary lines, the axilla, and the costal margins) or posterior (bordered by the posterior axillary lines, the shoulders, and the costal margins).
   Thoracoabdominal wounds are those in the inferior positions of all three anatomic areas. The inferior portions are defined by the nipple line anteriorly, the sixth rib laterally, and the tip of the scapulas posteriorly. Any wound below these landmarks is considered thoracoabdominal.

19. **How are penetrating wounds of the central region managed?**
   Patients who are grossly unstable require transfer to an operating room for an emergent thoracotomy with no emergency department (ED) workup. Stable patients should be monitored closely while a diagnostic workup (consisting of aortography, an esophagogram with or without esophagoscopy, and possibly bronchoscopy) is done. If the workup is negative, observation for 24–48 hours is appropriate; if positive, surgical intervention is needed. A helical CT scan of the chest can be extremely useful to determine the presence and location of mediastinal hemorrhage. If the hemorrhage is periaortic or direct signs of aortic injury are seen, the patient should proceed to aortography or possibly directly to the operating room.

20. **What trauma victims can potentially benefit from ED thoracotomy (EDT) ?**
   Victims of blunt trauma with documented asystole, or who require >5–10 minutes of prehospital cardiopulmonary resuscitation (CPR) and arrive to the ED with no signs of life (pupillary response, respiration, or motor activity) are generally regarded as being unsalvageable. Because survival is essentially 0% for this population, EDT is considered futile care.
   Victims of penetrating trauma who arrest in the field but arrive with <15 minutes of prehospital CPR are potentially salvageable and candidates for EDT. The population that appears to benefit the most from EDT are those victims of penetrating chest trauma who arrest immediately on, or after, their arrival to the ED. Immediate release of a pericardial tamponade or temporary repair of a cardiac laceration can be life saving.

Powell DW, Moore EE, Cothren CC, et al: Is emergency department resuscitative thoracotomy futile care for the critically injured patient requiring prehospital cardiopulmonary resuscitation? J Am Coll Surg 199:211–215, 2004.

21. **When should pericardial tamponade be suspected?**
   Acute pericardial tamponade is a clinical condition that results from the accumulation of blood and clots in the pericardial space. When pericardial pressure exceeds cardiac filling pressure, shock and ultimately death rapidly ensue. It should be suspected in any patient with a

penetrating wound of the chest (particularly in the central area) who develops hypotension, tachycardia, and elevated CVP after tension pneumothorax has been treated or ruled out. The quickest and most accurate means of diagnosing a pericardial effusion is bedside ultrasonography.

Plummer D, Brunette D, Asinger R, et al: Emergency department echocardiography improves outcome in penetrating cardiac injury. Ann Emerg Med 21:709–712, 1992.

KEY POINTS: CONTRAINDICATIONS FOR ED THORACOTOMY

1. Blunt traumatic arrest with documented asystole

2. Blunt traumatic arrest with prehospital CPR > 5 minutes and no signs of life

3. Penetrating traumatic arrest with CPR > 15 minutes and no signs of life

4. Penetrating traumatic arrest and asystole without the possibility of cardiac tamponade

KEY POINTS: CLINICAL FINDINGS OF PERICARDIAL TAMPONADE

1. Hypotension

2. Tachycardia

3. Elevated central venous pressure or jugular venous distension

4. Remember these are also seen in tension pneumothorax!

22. **How is acute pericardial tamponade treated?**
The proper course of action in a grossly unstable patient is **pericardiocentesis,** preferably ultrasound-guided, followed by immediate transfer to the operating room. If vital signs are lost in the ED, an immediate thoracotomy is indicated. Patients with less severe hypotension, or in situations in which an operating room is not immediately available, may benefit from placement of a pericardial catheter to allow for repeat aspirations until arrangements can be made for transfer for more definitive therapy.

23. **Should all patients with a stab wound of the chest be admitted to the hospital?**
Patients with peripheral wounds not in the thoracoabdominal area who are stable and have an initial chest radiograph that is normal usually do not require admission. They should be observed in the ED and have a repeat upright chest radiograph and hematocrit done in 4–6 hours. If repeat studies are normal, the patient may be discharged.

24. **Are peripheral gunshot wounds that cross the mediastinum handled differently?**
Determining missile trajectory based on entry wound and final resting position or exit wound is not always accurate. Nevertheless, if the estimated trajectory does traverse the mediastinum, these patients require a more thorough diagnostic evaluation while they are observed as inpatients. They should undergo the same work-up as patients who have sustained a penetrating injury of the central chest.

25. How are thoracoabdominal wounds managed?

By virtue of their low chest location, such wounds risk injury to the infradiaphragmatic, intraperitoneal, and retroperitoneal organs. There is no clear consensus on how to manage these patients. Some recommend observation alone, basing surgical intervention on positive physical findings. Others use diagnostic peritoneal lavage with lowered red blood cell criteria ($>$ 5000 or 10,000 red cells as opposed to the usual 50,000–100,000). Others use laparoscopy as a more definitive but more difficult and time-consuming means of evaluation. Posterior thoracoabdominal wounds are particularly difficult to evaluate because retroperitoneal injuries are predominant, and they are undetected by peritoneal lavage. Occult colon injuries can also be easily missed. Observation with a variable diagnostic work-up is recommended. Some merely observe, whereas others recommend adding an intravenous pyelogram, diagnostic peritoneal lavage, abdominal CT scan, the addition of contrast-enhanced enemas to CT scans, or varying combinations of these alternatives.

Merlotti GJ, Dillon BC, Lange DA: Peritoneal lavage in penetrating thoraco-abdominal trauma. J Trauma 28:17–23, 1988.

Phillips T, Sclafani SJ, Goldstein A: Use of the contrast-enhanced CT enema in the management of penetrating trauma to the flank and back. J Trauma 26:593–601, 1986.

CHAPTER 91

ABDOMINAL TRAUMA

S. Jason Moore, PA, MS, and Ernest E. Moore, MD

1. **Discuss the key aspects of the history and physical examination in the initial evaluation of abdominal trauma.**
   The history is important in establishing the tempo, sequence, and extent of early diagnostic efforts. Glean as much relevant information as possible from the prehospital providers while they are in the emergency department (ED). They were at the scene and can paint you a picture of what transpired. The primary survey is the initial search and correction of life-threatening injuries and is followed by a comprehensive examination of the patient, the secondary survey. Always consider lower thoracic and upper abdominal trauma as a unit and anticipate both thoracic and abdominal injuries. Abdominal tenderness and guarding are common with significant injury, whereas rebound tenderness and rigidity are relatively infrequent. Most importantly, 20–40% of patients with serious intra-abdominal injury in the context of multisystem trauma may be asymptomatic.

2. **What are some of the biomechanical differences between blunt and penetrating trauma?**
   - **Blunt trauma** results from a combination of crushing, stretching, and shearing forces. The magnitude of these forces is proportional to the mass of the object, rate of change in velocity (acceleration and deceleration), direction of impact, and elasticity of the tissues. Injury results when the sum of these forces exceeds the cohesive strength and mobility of the tissues involved.
   - **Penetrating injuries** result from the dissipation of energy and tissue disruption along the path of the offending projectile. Typically, injuries result in localized tears or contusions of involved organs. The magnitude of injury depends on the kinetic energy imparted by the penetrating object and the trajectory. Gunshot wounds can produce extensive tissue damage $(KE = MV^2)$.

3. **What are the common injury patterns produced by blunt abdominal trauma?**
   Blunt injuries usually represent energy transfer to underlying visceral and vascular structures in the anatomic region sustaining the direct impact and can be compounded by crushing against the rigid vertebral column. Specific examples are as follows:

Direct Impact	Resultant Injuries
Right lower rib fractures	Liver, gallbladder
Left lower rib fractures	Spleen, left kidney
Mid-epigastric contusion	Duodenum, pancreas, small bowel mesentery
Lumbar transverse process fracture	Kidney, ureter
Anterior pelvic fracture	Bladder, urethra

4. **What are the most commonly injured organs as a result of blunt abdominal trauma?**
   - Spleen (40–55%)
   - Liver (35–45%)
   - Small bowel (5–10%)

5. **What diagnostic tools are most helpful for the evaluation of blunt abdominal trauma?**
   - Ultrasound (US)
   - Diagnostic peritoneal lavage (DPL)
   - Computed tomography

6. **Which is the initial test of choice?**
   The Focused Assessment with Sonography for Trauma (FAST) exam is currently the initial test of choice in the evaluation of potential blunt abdominal trauma. It is noninvasive, portable, and easily repeatable, allowing for serial exams. It is reasonably sensitive (86–98%) for the detection of significant free intraperitoneal fluid and provides screening for the pleural and pericardial spaces. The major disadvantages are as follows:
   - It does not identify or quantitate specific organ injury well.
   - It does not identify the precise site and magnitude of bleeding.
   - It does not accurately evaluate hollow viscous injury or the retroperitoneum.

7. **Explain the role of DPL.**
   DPL is a rapid, extremely sensitive (98–100%) technique for detecting intraperitoneal hemorrhage and is relatively effective in detecting hollow viscus injury. In a hemodynamically stable patient, DPL is a valid modality for determining the source of computed tomography (CT)-visualized abdominal free fluid without solid organ injury. Disadvantages include the following:
   - Lack of organ specificity
   - Inability to evaluate the retroperitoneum
   - Morbidity of an invasive procedure
   Contraindications include morbid obesity, multiple previous abdominal surgeries, and portal hypertension (risk of variceal perforation).

8. **What is role of CT?**
   CT has an important role as a noninvasive diagnostic adjunct in the early evaluation of suspected abdominal and pelvic injuries. In addition to excellent sensitivity (93–98%) for intraperitoneal hemorrhage, CT adds injury specificity and shows the magnitude of solid-organ injury, allowing for controlled nonoperative management. The CT is especially suited for the following scenarios:
   - Any patient whose mechanism of injury or physical examination is suggestive of blunt abdominal trauma or retroperitoneal injuries
   - Hemodynamically stable patients with localized abdominal signs but without signs of peritonitis
   - Stable patients whose US and DPL are equivocal or difficult to perform
   - Patients whose serial physical examinations are unreliable or untenable due to altered mental status (e.g., head injury, intoxication)
   Disadvantages include the following:
   - Need for intravenous contrast
   - Logistical issues involving transport from the ED
   - CT not reliable for early detection of either pancreatic fractures or hollow viscous injuries (The presence of free fluid alone does not mandate immediate operative exploration because the incidence of gastrointestinal [GI] perforation is low.)

9. **How are DPL results interpreted following blunt abdominal trauma?**
   DPL is considered positive if greater than 10 mL of free blood is aspirated. Otherwise, 1 L of warmed 0.0% sodium chloride is infused (15 mL/kg in children). If the clinical condition permits, the patient is rolled from side to side to enhance intraperitoneal sampling. The saline bag is lowered to the floor for the return of lavage fluid by siphonage. A minimal recovery of 75% of lavage effluent is required for the test to be considered valid. The fluid is analyzed for red blood cell (RBC) and white blood cell (WBC) counts, lavage amylase, alkaline phosphatase, and bilirubin. The criteria for a positive DPL are outlined in Table 91-1.

TABLE 91-1. CRITERIA FOR POSITIVE DPL AFTER ABDOMINAL TRAUMA		
Index	**Positive**	**Equivocal**
Aspirate		
Blood	>10 mL	
Fluid	Enteric contents	
Lavage		
RBCs	>100,000/mm^3	>20,000/mm^3
WBCs	>	>500/mm^3
Enzymes	Amylase >20 IU/L *and* alkaline phosphatase >3 IU	Amylase >20 IU/L *or* alkaline phosphatase >3 IU
Bilirubin	Greater than serum level	

DPL = diagnostic peritoneal lavage, RBCs = red blood cells, WBCs = white blood cells.

10. **Describe the management priorities for blunt abdominal trauma.**
    The initial management consists of a through history of events (paramedics and family), fluid resuscitation for any sign of hypovolemia, systematic physical examination, and directed laboratory and diagnostic studies as dictated by the physiologic status of the patient. The preferable initial screening test is the bedside US. If intraperitoneal fluid is identified, the patient's hemodynamic status determines whether to proceed to laparotomy or CT for scanning. For stable patients with equivocal US or signs of peritoneal irritation, CT scanning is appropriate. Hemodynamically stable, alert patients with a negative US and laboratory tests are followed with serial physical examinations and US.

11. **What are the most commonly injured organs in penetrating abdominal trauma?**
    - Stab wounds: Liver (40%), small bowel (30%), diaphragm (20%), and colon (15%)
    - Gunshot wounds: Small bowel (50%), colon (40%), liver (30%), and vascular structures (25%)

12. **List the common patterns of injury associated with penetrating abdominal wounds.**
    See Table 91-2.

TABLE 91-2. COMMON PATTERNS OF INJURY ASSOCIATED WITH PENETRATING ABDOMINAL WOUNDS

Region	Likely Injury	Frequently Associated Injuries
Right upper quadrant	Liver	Diaphragm, gallbladder, right colon
Left upper quadrant	Spleen	Stomach, pancreas (tail), left kidney, diaphragm
Mid-epigastric	Stomach	Pancreas (body), abdominal aorta
	Duodenum	Inferior vena cava
	Portal vein	Hepatic artery, common bile duct
	Superior mesenteric artery	Pancreas (neck), left renal vein, abdominal artery
Pelvis	Iliac artery	Iliac vein, bladder, rectum

13. **Which diagnostic tests are most useful for the initial evaluation for penetrating abdominal wounds?**
    The management of penetrating abdominal wounds is dichotomous:
    - **Gunshot wounds** that violate the peritoneum warrant mandatory laparotomy.
    - **Stab wounds** can be managed selectively.

    Only two thirds of stab wounds to the anterior abdomen penetrate the peritoneal cavity, and only half of those entering the peritoneum produce injuries requiring laparotomy. Consequently, the first diagnostic question is whether the stab wound traverses the peritoneum. Local wound exploration, done under local anesthetic in the ED, answers this question reliably. Patients with an unequivocally negative wound exploration can be discharged. If peritoneal violation has occurred, the next question is whether significant intra-abdominal injury is involved. DPL has proved to be exceedingly useful in the decision for laparotomy in this scenario. In a hemodynamically stable patient in whom peritoneal integrity is indeterminate, laparoscopy may be used to ascertain violation of the peritoneum.

14. **Describe the management priorities for penetrating abdominal trauma.**
    A thorough history of relevant events is essential, along with crystalloid infusion for signs of hypovolemia. Hemodynamic instability, obvious evisceration, peritoneal signs, and intraperitoneal fluid shown by US (unless suspected ascites secondary to cirrhosis) are indications for immediate laparotomy. The diagnostic studies are guided by anticipated trajectory. The management of a stable patient with an abdominal stab wound is local wound exploration followed by DPL or observation if fascial penetration is identified. Gunshot wounds that traverse the peritoneum mandate immediate laparotomy. Radiopaque markers placed on the entrance and exit wounds with anteroposterior and lateral abdominal films are important to map the bullet path. When the wound is in proximity to the thorax, a chest radiograph must be obtained to ensure the bullet has not entered the chest.

15. **What are the absolute indications for laparotomy following blunt or penetrating abdominal trauma?**
    Peritonitis and hemodynamic instability are absolute indications, regardless of injury mechanism.

16. **What is the "seat belt mark" sign? What is its significance?**
The seat belt mark sign is an ecchymotic imprint of the seatbelt on the anterior chest or abdomen of a restrained patient from a motor vehicle collision. It is indicative of rapid deceleration and is associated with a 20% incidence of intra-abdominal injuries. Once the seat belt mark is identified, a CT is the diagnostic test of choice to exclude hollow organ injuries.

KEY POINTS: ABDOMINAL TRAUMA

1. Any patient who exhibits hemodynamic instability or signs of peritonitis following abdominal trauma requires emergent laparotomy.

2. In a lucid patient with blunt abdominal trauma, your clinical examination is the best guide for your selection of diagnostic tests.

3. A negative abdominal ultrasound does not reliably exclude significant intraperitoneal injury.

4. Observing a trauma patient is an active process, which means serial physical examinations and repeat abdominal ultrasonography.

17. **What are the unique concerns in a pregnant patient with abdominal trauma?**
The prevailing rule when managing a pregnant trauma patient is that optimal care of the mother ensures the best outcome for the fetus. Pregnancy alters the susceptibility to blunt injury and the physiologic response to injury. The gravid uterus occupies the pelvis and lower abdomen and is vulnerable to a variety of insults from direct blows or seat belt injuries. These insults result in a spectrum of injuries from minor soft tissue contusions to uterine wall disruption, placental abruption, potential exsanguinations, and fetal loss. The significance of relatively minor injuries mandates an aggressive posture in the early evaluation of pregnant patients. US and DPL (open technique) are used routinely; the gravid uterus is evaluated simultaneously with US and noninvasive fetal monitoring. Hemodynamic instability, uterine rupture, placental abruption, or fetal distress indicates the need for emergent abdominal exploration and uterine evacuation with the rare possibility of hysterectomy. (See Chapter 93.)

18. **What are the specific concerns in the child with abdominal trauma?**
Pediatric trauma provides unique challenges because of patient size and different injury patterns. The elasticity of the child's lower rib cage and the relatively large size of the abdominal cavity increase susceptibility to intra-abdominal injury. Blunt injuries commonly are minor, with modest liver or splenic fractures that are self-limited. Pancreatic fractures and intestinal perforation are infrequent in children. Despite the enthusiasm for nonoperative management, an aggressive operative policy is warranted in the context of pediatric multisystem trauma because of the child's limited physiologic reserve. Although grossly positive DPLs in hemodynamically stable children can be elucidated further by CT scan to verify solid-organ injury amenable to expectant care, abdominal exploration is undertaken promptly for hemodynamic instability, need for ongoing blood transfusions, or DPLs positive by enzymes. (See Chapter 94.)

BIBLIOGRAPHY

1. American College of Surgeons Committee on Trauma: Advanced Trauma Life Support Manual, 7th ed. Chicago, American College of Surgeons, 2004.

2. Alexander K, Simons R, Torreggiani W et al: Intraabdominal free fluid without solid organ injury in blunt abdominal trauma: An indication for laparotomy. J Trauma 52:1134–1140, 2002.

3. Allen T, Mueller M, Bonk T et al: Computed tomographic screening without oral contrast solution for blunt bowel and mesenteric injuries in abdominal trauma. J Trauma 56:314–322, 2004.

4. Branney SW, Moore EE, Cantril SV et al: Ultrasound based key clinical pathway reduces the use of hospital resources for the evaluation of blunt abdominal trauma. J Trauma 42:1086–1090, 1997.

5. Burch JM, Franciose RJ, Moore EE: Trauma. In Schwart SI (ed): Principles of Surgery, 7th ed. New York, McGraw-Hill, 1998, pp 155–221.

6. Chiu W, Shanmuganathan K, Mirvis S et al: Determining the need for laparotomy in penetrating torso trauma: A prospective study using triple-contrast enhanced abdominopelvic computed tomography. J Trauma 51:860–869, 2001.

7. Demetriades D: Indications for laparotomy. In Moore EE, Feliciano DV, Matttox KL(eds): Trauma, 5th ed. New York, McGraw Hill, 2002, pp 593–612.

8. Dror S, McKenney M, Cohn S et al: A prospective evaluation of ultrasonography for the diagnosis of penetrating torso injury. J Trauma 56:953–959, 2004.

9. Fakhry S, Watts D, Daley B et al: Current diagnostic approaches lack sensitivity in the diagnosis of perforation blunt small bowel injury (SBI): Findings from a large multiinstitutional trail. J Trauma 54:295–306, 2003.

10. Henneman PL, Marx JA, Moore EE et al: Diagnostic peritoneal lavage: Accuracy in predicting necessary laparotomy following blunt and penetrating trauma. J Trauma 30:1345–1355, 1990.

11. Livingston D, Laery R, Passannate M et al: Free fluid on abdominal computed tomography without solid organ injury after blunt abdominal injury does not mandate celiotomy. Am J Surg 182:6–9, 2001.

12. Malhotra AK, Fabian TC, Katsis SB et al: Blunt bowel and mesenteric injuries: The role of screening computed tomography. J Trauma 48:991–999, 2000.

13. McCarter FD, Luchette FA, Malloy M et al: Institutional and individual learning curves for focused abdominal ultrasound for trauma. Ann Surg 231:689–700, 2000.

14. Omert L, Salyer D, Dunham M et al: Implications of the "contrast blush" finding on computed tomographic scan of the spleen in trauma. J Trauma 51:272–278, 2001.

15. Oschsner MG, Knudson MM, Pachter HL et al: Significance of minimal or no intraperitoneal fluid visible on CT scan associated with blunt liver and splenic injuries. J Trauma 49:505–514, 2000.

16. Peizman AB, Heil B, Rivera L et al: Blunt splenic injury in adults: Multi-institutional study. J Trauma 49:177–194, 2000.

17. Stassen NA, Lukan JK, Carillo EH et al: Abdominal seat belt marks in the era of focused abdominal sonography for trauma. Arch Surg 137:718–723, 2002.

18. Wong Y, Wang L, See L et al: Contrast material extravasation on contrast-enhanced helical computed tomographic scan of blunt abdominal trauma: Its significance on the choice, time, and outcome of treatment. J Trauma 54:164–170, 2003.

CHAPTER 92

PELVIC FRACTURES AND GENITOURINARY TRAUMA

Sarrah Goodwin, MD, and Walter L. Biffl, MD

1. Why are pelvic fractures so deadly?

Pelvic fractures can lead to life-threatening hemorrhage. Sources of bleeding include the pelvic bones themselves, surrounding soft tissue, and the extensive arterial and venous networks running through the pelvic ring. The considerable force required to fracture the pelvis typically results in significant associated injuries in up to 90% of patients. Collectively, these factors account for high rates of morbidity and mortality.

Scalea TM, Burgess AR: Pelvic fractures. In Moore EE, Feliciano DV, Mattox KL (eds): Trauma, 5th ed. New York, McGraw-Hill, 2004, pp 779–807.

2. What is the approach to the patient with a pelvic fracture?

The evaluation begins with the primary survey (the ABCs) and resuscitation. Unstable patients with pelvic fractures require a multispecialty approach, with the fundamental objectives of (1) control of hemorrhage, (2) reversal of shock, (3) identification of associated injuries, and (4) prioritization of treatment based on threat to life. Life-threatening associated injuries are evaluated and treated simultaneously with systematic assessment of the pelvic fractures. Because these patients may require coordinated interventions by multiple specialties, the immediate presence of the attending trauma surgeon, attending orthopedic surgeon, and interventional radiologist in the emergency department (ED) is warranted. (See Fig. 92-1.)

Biffl WL, Smith WR, Moore EE, et al: Evolution of a multidisciplinary clinical pathway for the management of unstable patients with pelvic fractures. Ann Surg 233:843–850, 2001.

KEY POINTS: APPROACH TO PATIENTS WITH A PELVIC FRACTURE

1. Control of hemorrhage

2. Reversal of shock

3. Identification of associated injuries

4. Prioritization of treatment based on threat to life

---

3. How do you examine the patient with a pelvic fracture?

Very carefully! The physical examination directed at the pelvis includes gentle manual compression of the bony pelvis and inspection of the perineum, rectum, and vagina for ecchymosis, ongoing bleeding, and open wounds. An unstable pelvic fracture is NOT a "teaching case"—every manipulation leads to further hemorrhage, as bony edges disrupt clot and lacerate tissue and blood vessels. Plain anteroposterior radiography of the pelvis is a priority in patients with suspected fracture. Hemodynamically stable patients may be evaluated further with

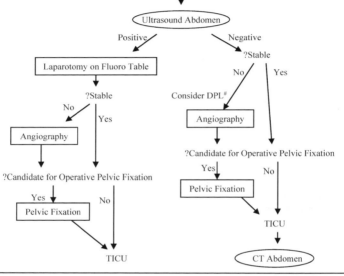

Pelvic Fracture Clinical Pathway

Hemodynamically Unstable Patient with Biomechanically Unstable Pelvic Fracture

Immediate Notification: Attending Trauma and Orthopaedic Surgeon, Blood Bank, Interventional Radiology
Resuscitate with 2 Liters Crystalloid
Wrap Pelvis with Sheet, Tape Knees and Ankles, Consider External Fixation Device
Place CVP Line
Transfuse PRBCs and FFP 1:1; 5 U PLTs for each 5 U PRBCs
Rule Out Thoracic Source (Portable Chest X-Ray)

Ultrasound Abdomen

DPL may be warranted in the setting of refractory shock

Figure 92-1. Management of patients with a pelvic fracture. CVP = central venous pressure, PRBCs = packed red blood cells, FFP = fresh frozen plasma, PLTs = platelets, DPL = diagnostic peritoneal lavage, TICU = trauma intensive care unit.

additional views (e.g., inlet/outlet) or computed tomography (CT), but this should not interfere with resuscitation or necessary interventions.

Scalea TM, Burgess AR: Pelvic fractures. In Moore EE, Feliciano DV, Mattox KL (eds): Trauma, 5th ed. New York, McGraw-Hill, 2004, pp 779–807.

4. How are pelvic fractures classified?
The Tile classification, based on pelvic stability, is useful for reconstructive planning:
- Tile A: Rotationally and vertically stable
- Tile B: Rotationally unstable, vertically stable
- Tile C: Rotationally and vertically unstable
A commonly used scheme is that of Young and Burgess, which is based on injury mechanism and is more helpful in assessing the risk of hemorrhage:
Anteroposterior compression (APC)
- APC I: Pubic symphyseal diastasis < 2.5 cm, no significant posterior ring injury
- APC II: Pubic symphyseal diastasis > 2.5 cm, tearing of anterior sacral ligaments

- APC III: Complete disruption of pubic symphysis and posterior ligament complexes
Lateral compression (LC)
- LC I: Posterior compression of sacroiliac (SI) joint without ligament disruption
- LC II: Posterior SI ligament rupture, sacral crush injury
- LC III: LC II, with APC injury to contralateral pelvis
Vertical shear injuries consist of displaced fractures of the anterior rami and posterior columns, including SI dislocation.

Tile M: Acute pelvic fractures. I: Causation and classification. J Am Acad Orthop Surg 4:143–160, 1996.
Young JWR, Burgess AR, Brumback RJ, et al: Pelvic fractures: Value of plain radiography in early assessment and management. Radiology 160:445–451, 1986.

5. **What are the sources of bleeding from major pelvic fractures?**
The most frequent source is of venous origin, but arterial bleeding can lead quickly to hemodynamic compromise. Massive bleeding is often associated with vertical shear or APC fractures. The internal iliac arterial system (in particular, the superior gluteal artery bridging the SI joint) may be affected by SI disruption. Significant blood loss can occur from vesicular branches of the pudendal artery in association with pubic diastasis and anterior fractures. Injury to the veins in the superior gluteal and pudendal distributions and the lumbosacral venous plexus also contributes significantly to retroperitoneal and pelvic hemorrhage. LC fractures are not usually associated with major blood loss because they result in compression of local vasculature.

Scalea TM, Burgess AR: Pelvic fractures. In Moore EE, Feliciano DV, Mattox KL (eds): Trauma, 5th ed. New York, McGraw-Hill, 2004, pp 799–807.

6. **Name three goals of mechanical pelvic stabilization.**
- Reduce pelvic volume.
- Promote tamponade of bleeding bone and vessels.
- Prevent further fracture motion.

Scalea TM, Burgess AR: Pelvic fractures. In Moore EE, Feliciano DV, Mattox KL (eds): Trauma, 5th ed. New York, McGraw-Hill, 2004, pp 799–807.

7. **Discuss four methods of pelvic stabilization.**
- **Wrapping the pelvis with a sheet and binding the knees and ankles with tape.** This intervention should be performed immediately on discovery of an unstable pelvic fracture, particularly before patient transport. Prolonged use may result in extremity or abdominal compartment syndrome.
- **Anterior external fixation.** This is becoming the standard intervention for acute pelvic stabilization. It is most effective with the anteroposterior open-book fracture. More complex fractures such as vertical shear injury may also benefit from early stabilization, but fixation is not as complete because of the instability of the posterior column.
- **Pelvic C-clamp.** This intervention is more effective than a standard anterior frame in stabilizing the posterior pelvis.
- **Pneumatic antishock garment (PASG).** Use is controversial, particularly in prehospital care in urban areas with short transport times. Given the efficacy of pelvic wrapping, there is little role for the PASG today.

Mohany K, Musso D, Powell JN, et al: Emergent management of pelvic ring injuries: An update. Can J Surg 48:49–56, 2005.

8. **When should patients with pelvic trauma undergo laparotomy?**
The risk of active intraperitoneal visceral bleeding is 20–30% in association with pelvic fracture. Ultrasound should be utilized during initial evaluation of unstable patients to exclude

hemoperitoneum. If ultrasound is not available, diagnostic peritoneal lavage (DPL) should be done at the supraumbilical ring to avoid dissecting pelvic hematoma. Ultrasound showing overt intraperitoneal fluid, or a grossly positive DPL, should prompt immediate laparotomy. In the patient with a normal ultrasound or DPL positive by red blood cell count only, the pelvic bleeding should be managed first. In this case, the key decision is whether to employ skeletal fixation alone, or selective arterial embolization; prompt consultation of orthopedic and interventional radiology specialists is imperative. (See Fig. 92-1.)

Scalea TM, Burgess AR: Pelvic fractures. In Moore EE, Feliciano DV, Mattox KL (eds): Trauma, 5th ed. New York, McGraw-Hill, 2004, pp 779–807.

9. **How frequently are rectal injuries associated with pelvic injuries? How are they managed?**
Approximately 5% of major pelvic fractures are associated with rectal injuries. These complex injuries result in a high mortality rate secondary to septic complications. Current management principles consist of fecal diversion, presacral drainage, and perineal debridement as needed. Although some studies have shown that presacral drainage may be unnecessary, these were based on small patient samples.

Burch JM, Feliciano DV, Mattox KL: Colostomy and drainage for civilian rectal injuries: Is that all? Ann Surg 209:600–611, 1989.
Gonzalez RP, Falimirski ME, Holevar MR: The role of presacral drainage in the management of penetrating rectal injuries. J Trauma 45:656–661, 1998.

10. **What are the major causes of death following pelvic trauma?**
The mortality associated with unstable pelvic fractures is 30–50%. Early mortality results from uncontrolled hemorrhage, refractory shock, or associated multisystem injuries. Delayed mortality is most frequently the result of septic complications or multiple organ failure and may be up to 50% in the subset of patients with open pelvic fractures.

Scalea TM, Burgess AR: Pelvic fractures. In Moore EE, Feliciano DV, Mattox KL (eds): Trauma, 5th ed. New York, McGraw-Hill, 2004, pp 779–807.

11. **What types of injuries are associated with genitourinary trauma?**
Pelvic fracture can cause posterior (above the urogenital diaphragm) urethral tears or bladder trauma, whereas perineal straddle injury is more likely to cause anterior urethral tear. Fractures of the lower ribs, lower thoracic, or lumbar vertebrae are often associated with renal or ureteral injuries.

Coburn M: Genitourinary trauma. In Moore EE, Feliciano DV, Mattox KL (eds): Trauma, 5th ed. New York, McGraw-Hill, 2004, pp 809–849.

12. **What is considered a true genitourinary emergency?**
Most genitourinary trauma is not life threatening and can be addressed after stabilization of the patient, including necessary operative control of significant hemorrhage and contamination. However, renal pedicle injury can lead to uncontrolled hemorrhage or renal ischemia. The kidneys are not fixed and move to a limited degree on the vascular pedicle. Complete severance of this pedicle can lead to exsanguination, whereas lesser injury to the renal vessels can cause thrombosis and subsequent ischemia. This is typically seen with deceleration injury. Early diagnosis and surgical intervention are crucial for salvage of the affected kidney.

Schneider RE: Genitourinary trauma. In Rosen P, Barkin RM (eds): Emergency Medicine: Concepts Clinical Practice, 4th ed. St. Louis, Mosby, 1998, pp 582–601.

KEY POINTS: UROLOGIC TRAUMA

1. Renal injury is the most frequent urologic trauma.

2. Renal pedicle injury can lead to uncontrolled hemorrhage or ischemia.

3. Clinical signs of kidney damage may include flank ecchymosis, lateral abdominal tenderness or mass, hematuria, or fracture of lumbar posterior ribs or lumbar vertebrae.

4. Gross hematuria or persistent microhematuria warrant evaluation.

5. Urologic injury may be present in the absence of hematuria.

13. **What four clinical signs may indicate injury to the kidney?**
    - Flank ecchymosis
    - Lateral abdominal tenderness or mass
    - Hematuria
    - Fracture of lumbar posterior ribs or lumbar vertebrae

    Coburn M: Genitourinary trauma. In Moore EE, Feliciano DV, Mattox KL (eds): Trauma, 5th ed. New York, McGraw-Hill, 2004, pp 809–849.

14. **What is the general management strategy for renal injury?**
    Nonoperative management is appropriate in the large majority of patients because injuries will heal spontaneously. Surgery is indicated for hemodynamic instability, ongoing bleeding, or urinary extravasation. However, minimally invasive techniques, such as angioembolization for hemorrhage and stenting for urinary extravasation, may allow renal salvage.

    Coburn M: Genitourinary trauma. In Moore EE, Feliciano DV, Mattox KL (eds): Trauma, 5th ed. New York, McGraw-Hill, 2004, pp 809–849.

15. **What diagnostic tools can be used to evaluate renal trauma?**
    CT is the preferred modality for the evaluation of blunt abdominal trauma. It allows for comprehensive evaluation of all intra-abdominal structures. Helical CT has increased sensitivity for ureteral injury. Intravenous pyelography (IVP) is less sensitive and does not allow for evaluation of nonurologic injuries. However, it may still be used in cases of suspected renal or ureteral injury when CT is unavailable, or if urologic imaging is required in the operating room. Renal angiography may be indicated in the presence of a suspected vascular injury, although it has also largely been replaced by CT. Magnetic resonance imaging (MRI) has imaging capabilities similar to CT but is far more expensive, time consuming, and not as readily available. MRI may be useful in stable patients with contrast allergies.

    Smith JK, Kenney PJ: Imaging of renal trauma. Radiol Clin North Am 41:1019–1035, 2003.

16. **When should ureteral trauma be suspected?**
    In the presence of penetrating injuries in proximity to the ureter. These are the least common of the genitourinary injuries. Hematuria may be absent when the ureter is completely transected. Ureteral injuries can be detected by CT or IVP and should be managed operatively.

    Schneider RE: Genitourinary trauma. In Rosen P, Barkin RM (eds): Emergency Medicine: Concepts Clinical Practice, 4th ed. St. Louis, Mosby, 1998, pp 582–601.

17. **What are the associated clinical findings with bladder injury?**
    Traumatic bladder rupture is an uncommon injury secondary to the protected location of the bladder within the pelvis. This injury most often occurs in conjunction with pelvic fracture but

can also be seen with lower abdominal compression due to lap belt or steering wheel injuries. Gross hematuria is present in greater that 95% of patients.

Iverson AJ, Morey AF: Radiographic evaluation of suspected bladder rupture following blunt trauma: Critical review. World J Surg 25:1588–1591, 2001.

18. **How should bladder injury be evaluated?**
The two main diagnostic modalities for evaluation of bladder injury are CT cystography and conventional retrograde cystography. The accuracy of either method depends on adequate distention of the bladder. Bladder imaging is mandatory in the setting of gross hematuria with pelvic fracture. Relative indications include gross hematuria without pelvic fracture and pelvic fracture with microhematuria. Penetrating trauma in the vicinity of the bladder should be evaluated with a cystogram regardless of the presence of hematuria.

Coburn M: Genitourinary trauma. In Moore EE, Feliciano DV, Mattox KL (eds): Trauma, 5th ed. New York, McGraw-Hill, 2004, pp 809–849.

19. **When should urethral injury be suspected?**
Blood is visualized at the urethral meatus in 80–90% of patients with urethral injury. Other signs of urethral injury are penile, scrotal, or perineal hematomas or a high-riding prostate on rectal examination. If urethral injury is suspected, insertion of Foley catheter should be deferred until retrograde urethrogram can be performed. The ED management of complete urethral disruption is transcutaneous suprapubic cystostomy.

Coburn M: Genitourinary trauma. In Moore EE, Feliciano DV, Mattox KL (eds): Trauma, 5th ed. New York, McGraw-Hill, 2004, pp 809–849.

20. **How is a retrograde urethrogram performed?**
The urethrogram is obtained using a 12 Fr urinary catheter secured in the meatal fossa by inflating the balloon to approximately 3 mL. Alternatively, a catheter-tipped syringe may be used. Standard water-soluble contrast material (25–30 mL) is injected under gentle pressure as the anteroposterior and oblique views are taken.

Coburn M: Genitourinary trauma. In Moore EE, Feliciano DV, Mattox KL (eds): Trauma, 5th ed. New York, McGraw-Hill, 2004, pp 809–849.

21. **What is the diagnostic approach to asymptomatic microhematuria in the patient with blunt trauma?**
Asymptomatic microscopic hematuria is not a good predictor of genitourinary tract injury. The amount of blood in the urine does not correlate with severity of injury. The relatively low incidence of positive studies requiring surgery does not justify an extensive radiographic evaluation. Close follow-up of these patients and repeat urinalyses are recommended, with additional studies only if the hematuria persists. Controversy still exists regarding the evaluation of pediatric patients with asymptomatic microhematuria. Pediatric patients are more susceptible to significant renal injury with relatively benign mechanisms, and consequently many advocate imaging studies with any degree of hematuria regardless of symptoms.

Coburn M: Genitourinary trauma. In Moore EE, Feliciano DV, Mattox KL (eds): Trauma, 5th ed. New York, McGraw-Hill, 2004, pp 809–849.

22. **What is a penile fracture?**
A sudden tear in the tunica albuginea with subsequent rupture of the corpora cavernosum. It occurs only in the erect penis and usually is associated with falls or sudden unexpected moves during sexual intercourse. It has also been reported with direct blunt trauma. A sudden intense pain associated with a snapping noise and immediate detumescence usually occurs. Most authors support surgical intervention in an attempt to restore normal function and prevent angulation. Inability to urinate, bleeding from the urethral meatus, or extravasation of urine may

indicate injury to the corpora spongiosum and urethra, which occurs in approximately 20% of cases.

Schneider RE: Genitourinary trauma. In Rosen P, Barkin RM (eds): Emergency Medicine: Concepts Clinical Practice, 4th ed. St. Louis, Mosby, 1998, pp 582–601.

23. **What is the role of ultrasound in the evaluation of testicular trauma?**
Testicular injuries are most often caused by a fall or a kick to the scrotal area. Ultrasound is a valuable tool in assessing the integrity of the testicles. Adequate palpation may be prevented by hematoma formation. Ultrasound can distinguish between simple hematoma and disruption of the parenchyma. Failure to suspect and diagnose testicular rupture may result in subsequent loss of the testicle.

Schneider RE: Genitourinary trauma. In Rosen P, Barkin RM (eds): Emergency Medicine: Concepts Clinical Practice, 4th ed. St. Louis, Mosby, 1998, pp 582–601.

CHAPTER 93

TRAUMA IN PREGNANCY

Jedd Roe, MD, MBA

1. **What is the most important concept I need to remember from this chapter?**
   Fetal outcome is largely related to maternal morbidity. The best fetal resuscitation is aggressive maternal resuscitation.

2. **How common is trauma in pregnancy?**
   An estimated 6–7% of pregnancies are complicated by trauma. In blunt abdominal trauma, the usual causes are motor vehicle accidents (MVAs) (60%), falls (22%), and direct blows (17%) to the abdomen. One study showed the serious MVAs accounted for a 7% maternal mortality rate, whereas the fetal mortality rate was 15%. Of falls, 80% occur after 32 weeks of gestation.

   Shah AJ, Kilcline BA: Trauma in pregnancy. Emerg Med Clin North Am 21:615–629, 2003.

3. **Is physical or sexual abuse seen frequently in pregnant patients?**
   Yes. One large study reported a prevalence of abuse in pregnant women in urban settings of 32%. Of physically abused women, 60% reported two or more episodes of assault. Injury was more common to the head, neck, and extremities; a fourfold increase in the incidence of genital trauma was noted in this population. When pregnant patients are physically abused, there is a higher incidence of low-birth-weight infants, low maternal weight gain, maternal anemia, and drug and alcohol abuse. Homicides account for one third of maternal trauma deaths. Another study showed that three screening questions asked of emergency department (ED) pregnant patients can detect the majority of patients who are victims of partner abuse, which suggests that screening for domestic violence should be pursued with pregnant trauma patients. (See Chapter 102.)

   Feldhaus KM, Koziol-McLain J, Amsbury HL, et al: Accuracy of 3 brief screening questions for detecting partner violence in the emergency department. JAMA 277:1400–1401, 1997.

   Ikossi DG, Lazar AA, Morabito D, et al: Profiles of mothers at risk: An analysis of injury and pregnancy loss in 1,195 trauma patients. J Am Coll Surg 200:49–56, 2005.

4. **How do physiologic changes in pregnancy affect the evaluation of the trauma victim?**
   First, decreasing blood pressure and rising heart rate might indicate hypovolemic shock in a nonpregnant woman, but in pregnancy this may merely reflect physiologic changes or supine positioning. Because of increased blood volume, signs of shock may not be clinically apparent until 35% of maternal blood volume is lost. Given the markedly increased blood flow to the uterus, there is a new potential source of blood loss that requires aggressive investigation. Because physiologic changes result in a decreased maternal oxygen reserve, tissue hypoxia develops more rapidly in response to a traumatic insult.

5. **How do physiologic changes of pregnancy affect laboratory values?**
   A physiologic anemia is seen as the plasma volume rises by more than twice the amount of red blood cells. It is not unusual for one to see hematocrits of 32–34% by the third trimester. Fibrinogen levels are double those seen in other trauma patients. Disseminated intravascular coagulation (DIC) may be seen with normal fibrinogen levels. Because of hormonal stimulation

of the central respiratory drive, PCO_2 falls to 27–32 mmHg, and injury sufficient to cause a respiratory acidosis might be manifested by what ordinarily would be considered a normal PCO_2 of 40 mmHg.

6. **Are serious maternal injuries required for fetal injury to be present?**
Not always. Although in utero damage is often associated with maternal pelvic fractures, 7% of maternal cases of minor trauma have been associated with poor fetal outcome. Direct injuries to the fetus in utero are unusual, but given the size of the fetal head, when direct trauma occurs, fetal head injury is the most common injury.

El Kady D, Gilbert WM, Anderson J, et al: Trauma during pregnancy: An analysis of maternal and fetal outcomes in a large population. Am J Obstet Gynecol 190:1661–1668, 2004.

7. **Name the most common causes of fetal death.**
Maternal death, maternal shock, and placental abruption.

8. **How does placental abruption occur?**
Abruption results from the separation of a relatively inelastic placenta from an elastic uterus secondary due to a shearing, deceleration force. There may be little or no external evidence of such a mechanism. Although abruption may be present in 50% of patients with life-threatening injuries, it also exists in 2–4% of minor mechanisms. Classically, the clinical findings of abruption have included vaginal bleeding and abdominal and uterine tenderness. In many cases, fetal distress may be the only presenting sign because the reduction in placental blood flow to the fetus causes hypoxia and acidosis. DIC may occur with placental injury, and evaluation for DIC can be performed by screening with a serum fibrinogen level, with low levels stimulating the sending of a more complete DIC panel.

Shah AJ, Kilcline BA: Trauma in pregnancy. Emerg Med Clin North Am 21:615–629, 2003.

9. **How often does ultrasound detect cases of placental abruption?**
Because a large separation must be present for ultrasound to be diagnostic, it detects only about half of cases. In many instances, fetal distress is present before the clear visualization of an abruption by ultrasound. Fetal mortality from abruption is reported to be 30–68%. Usually an abruption large enough to place the fetus at risk becomes apparent within 48 hours. Detection of fetal distress mandates prompt delivery of the fetus.

10. **Are radiologic investigations harmful to the fetus?**
Fetal organs are maximally sensitive to radiation when younger than 8 weeks of gestational age. Most authorities agree that a radiation dose of less than 100 mGy carries no significant fetal risk. In general, all radiographic studies should be undertaken with appropriate fetal shielding. All **clinically indicated** studies should be done regardless of any radiation concerns. Consideration also should be given to nonradiographic alternative evaluation with ultrasound. Table 93-1 lists doses received from exposure during production of commonly ordered investigations.

11. **How should these patients be managed in the field?**
Given the reduced maternal oxygen reserve, oxygen therapy is crucial. Intravenous volume resuscitation with crystalloid should proceed as with other trauma patients. Avoid compression of the inferior vena cava by transporting the patient on her left side, or if the patient is immobilized, elevate the right side of the backboard to 15 or 20 degrees. Aside from early transport, the most important aspect of prehospital management is to notify the ED so that the appropriate obstetric consultants may participate on the trauma team.

Shah AJ, Kilcline BA: Trauma in pregnancy. Emerg Med Clin North Am 21:615–629, 2003.

TABLE 93-1. RADIATION DOSES DURING COMMONLY ORDERED INVESTIGATIONS

Examination	Estimated Dose to Uterus/Fetus (mGy)
Cervical spine series	<0.03
Extremity (one view)	<0.01
Chest posteroanterior radiograph	<0.01
Head CT	<0.05
Pelvis radiograph	22.0
Lumbar spine anteroposterior/lateral	3.5
Chest CT (helical)	0.13
Abdominal CT	26.0

CT = computed tomography.
www.perinatology.com/exposures/Physical/Xray.htm

12. **What are the priorities for ED management?**
The prehospital therapies mentioned previously should be continued. Of particular interest is the history of this pregnancy with attention directed at estimating gestational age and fetal viability. After the usual primary and secondary survey, a sterile speculum examination should be performed to evaluate for the presence of vaginal fluid, opening of the cervical os, and genital tract trauma. Continued aggressive resuscitation with warmed lactated Ringer's solution (less acidotic, more physiologic) and blood is especially important given the physiologic changes mentioned previously.

Shah AJ, Kilcline BA: Trauma in pregnancy. Emerg Med Clin North Am 21:615–629, 2003.

13. **How do I begin to evaluate the fetus?**
First, determine the size of the uterus and the presence of abdominal and uterine tenderness. Uterine size, measured in centimeters from the pubic symphysis to fundus, provides a rough estimate of gestational age and potential viability. Carefully inspect the vaginal introitus for evidence of vaginal bleeding. Next, assess for fetal distress, which may be the earliest indication of maternal hypovolemia. Abnormal fetal heart rates are greater than 160 bpm and less than 120 bpm. As soon as possible after patient arrival, continuous cardiotocographic monitoring (CTM) should be initiated to ascertain early signs of fetal distress (e.g., decreased variability of heart rate or fetal decelerations after contractions). Ultrasound should be done promptly thereafter to confirm gestational age, fetal viability, and the integrity of the placenta.

14. **Is diagnostic peritoneal lavage (DPL) safe and accurate in pregnant women?**
DPL has been reported to be safe and accurate when using an open, supraumbilical technique. Although the cell count thresholds and clinical indications for DPL are the same, ED ultrasound has become the more prevalent investigation. The physiologic changes that take place with pregnancy and the elimination of radiation exposure from abdominal computed tomography (CT) provide persuasive arguments for aggressive use of ED ultrasound as a diagnostic tool. With the exception of concern for diaphragmatic injury secondary to penetrating trauma, the need for DPL as an evaluation modality has largely been supplanted by the use of ED ultrasound (Focused Abdominal Sonogram of Trauma [FAST]) to determine rapidly the presence of intraperitoneal hemorrhage.

KEY POINTS: TRAUMA IN PREGNANCY

1. Aggressive maternal resuscitation is the best therapy for the fetus.

2. The fetus may be in acute distress with little or no maternal manifestations.

3. Ultrasound is the investigation of choice to evaluate the maternal abdomen and the fetus.

4. All clinically necessary radiologic investigations should be performed regardless of radiation concerns.

15. **What is fetomaternal hemorrhage (FMH)?**

Hemorrhage of fetal blood into the usually distinct maternal circulation. The incidence of FMH in trauma patients has been reported to be 30% (four to five times the incidence of noninjured controls). With FMH, the complications of maternal Rh sensitization, fetal anemia, and fetal death can occur. Laboratory techniques are not sensitive enough to diagnose FMH accurately. The prudent course is to give Rh immunoglobulin to all Rh-negative patients who present with the suspicion of abdominal trauma because a 300-mg dose of Rh immunoglobulin given within 72 hours of antigenic exposure prevents Rh isoimmunization. Massive transfusion (>30 mL) into the maternal circulation sometimes is seen with severe abdominal trauma. The Kleihauer-Betke (KB) test is a test that detects fetal erythrocytes in the maternal circulation, and positive KB tests have not been shown to alter management except in Rh-negative patients. However, one study showed that the incidence of positive KB tests did not differ between low-risk pregnant patients and maternal trauma patients. Given the inaccuracy of the KB test in the setting of trauma, administration of Rh immunoglobulin should proceed as described previously.

Dhanraj D, Lambers D: The incidences of positive Kleihauer-Betke test in low-risk pregnancies and maternal trauma patients. Am J Obstet Gynecol 190:1461–1463, 2004.

16. **When is cesarean section indicated?**

The first factor to be considered is the stability of the mother. If the mother has sustained serious injuries elsewhere and is critically ill, she may not be able to tolerate an additional procedure and the blood loss it would entail. Next, fetuses whose gestational age is 24 weeks or whose weight is estimated to be greater than 750 gm are predicted to have a 50% survival rate in the neonatal intensive care unit (ICU) setting and are considered viable. The most common indication for cesarean section is fetal distress. Other indications are uterine rupture and malpresentation of the fetus. Perimortem cesarean section should be done when ultrasound or uterine size suggests viability (i.e., above the umbilicus) and maternal decompensation is acute. Resuscitation should be instituted within 6 minutes, but fetal survival has occurred 15 minutes after maternal decompensation.

17. **Which pregnant patients with abdominal trauma require admission for fetal monitoring?**

Any viable (>24 weeks) fetus requires CTM. CTM is recommended even for patients without external evidence of trauma because it has been well documented that these patients are at risk from placental abruption, and CTM is sensitive for its detection. Current guidelines suggest that these patients be observed for a minimum of 4 hours with a cardiotocograph. If any abnormalities or uterine contractions are discovered, the observation should be extended 24 hours.

Shah AJ, Kilcline BA: Trauma in pregnancy. Emerg Med Clin North Am 21:615–629, 2003.

WEBSITE

www.perinatology.com/exposures/Physical/Xray.htm

BIBLIOGRAPHY

1. El Kady D, Gilbert WM, Anderson J, et al: Trauma during pregnancy: An analysis of maternal and fetal outcomes in a large population. Am J Obstet Gynecol 190:1661–1668, 2004.

2. Feldhaus KM, Koziol-McLain J, Amsbury HL, et al: Accuracy of 3 brief screening questions for detecting partner violence in the emergency department. JAMA 277:1400–1401, 1997.

3. Ikossi DG, Lazar AA, Morabito D, et al: Profiles of mothers at risk: An analysis of injury and pregnancy loss in 1,195 trauma patients. J Am Coll Surg 200:49–56, 2005.

4. Neufeld JD: Trauma in pregnancy. In Marx JA (ed): Rosen's Emergency Medicine: Concepts Clinical Practice, 5th ed. St. Louis, Mosby, 2002, pp 256–266.

CHAPTER 94

PEDIATRIC TRAUMA

Daniel S. Kim, MD, and Walter L. Biffl, MD

1. **Which children get injured? How do they do it?**
   Every year, nearly one in three children is injured, and trauma is the leading cause of mortality for children younger than 14 years. Motor vehicle crashes account for most deaths in all age groups, followed by drownings, house fires, homicides, and falls in descending order. A very common site of lethal pediatric trauma is the home. Boys are injured twice as often as girls. Falls are the most common cause of severe injury in infants and toddlers; bicycle crashes are the most common cause in children and adolescents.

   > Centers for Disease Control and Prevention: www.cdc.gov/nchs/pressroom/05facts/lifeexpectancy.htm
   > Tepas JJ III, Schinco MA: Pediatric trauma. In Moore EE, Feliciano DV, Mattox KL (eds): Trauma, 5th ed. New York, McGraw-Hill, 2004, pp 1021–1039.

2. **Aren't children just small adults?**
   No. Anatomically, three unique characteristics in children require special consideration:
   - A smaller body mass results in more force applied per unit area, with a propensity toward multiple injuries in a child.
   - A child's incompletely calcified skeleton allows internal organ damage without overlying fractures.
   - A high body surface area-to-volume ratio results in significant thermal energy loss and early hypothermia in a child.

3. **How do the ABCs differ between children and adults?**
   They don't. Airway, breathing, and circulation always take priority.

4. **Which factors affect the patency of a child's airway?**
   Craniofacial disproportion (the child's occiput is relatively large compared with the midface) results in cervical flexion when the child is lying supine. Compared with an adult, a child has a large tongue, floppy epiglottis, and increased lymphoid tissue; these factors may contribute to airway obstruction. The sniffing position (slight superior and anterior positioning of the midface) is employed to maintain a patent airway. Infants are obligate nasal breathers, so their nares should not be occluded. Oral airways should be inserted only in unconscious children because they may induce vomiting. The airway should be inserted straight, rather than upturned, then rotated downward in the oropharynx, as is often done in adults.

5. **Which factors affect endotracheal intubation of a child?**
   A child's larynx lies higher and more anterior in the neck, and the vocal cords have a more anterocaudal angle; the cords may be more difficult to visualize for intubation. The narrowest part of a child's airway is the cricoid ring, which forms a natural seal with the endotracheal tube. In adults, the narrowest portion is at the level of the vocal cords; because of the triangular shape of the larynx's cross-section at that level, a balloon is necessary to stabilize the tube in adults. Uncuffed tubes are generally used in children younger than 9 years. The size of the tube is estimated by the diameter of the child's external nares or little finger. The trachea is short, so the tube should be placed just 2–3 cm distal to the vocal cords. Nasotracheal intubation should not be attempted in children younger than 12 years.

6. **Describe rapid-sequence intubation in a child.**

See Figure 94-1.

Brown Medical School, Department of Surgery, Division of Trauma and Critical Care: Trauma Handbook, 2004, pp 28–29. Available at intra.lifespan.org/TraumaRes/

Zelicof-Paul A, Smith-Lockridge A, Schnadower D, et al: Controversies in rapid sequence intubation in children. Curr Opin Pediatr 17:355–362, 2005.

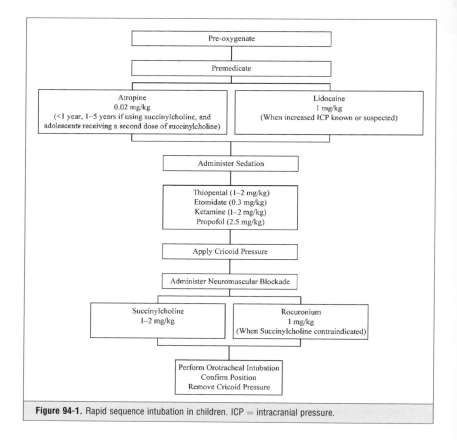

Figure 94-1. Rapid sequence intubation in children. ICP = intracranial pressure.

7. **What do I do if I cannot endotracheally intubate the patient?**

A surgical airway should be performed. If time permits, tracheostomy is the procedure of choice because of the risk of subglottic stenosis in young children who undergo cricothyroidotomy. (In an emergency, however, a cricothyroidotomy is relatively simple and life saving.) As a temporizing measure, needle cricothyroidotomy with a 14 or 16G catheter allows jet insufflation of oxygen. However, it does not provide adequate ventilation.

8. **How do I recognize shock in a pediatric patient?**

Children have an increased physiologic reserve and often maintain vitals signs in the normal range even in the presence of shock. Tachycardia and poor skin perfusion are the primary responses to hypovolemia. Other, more subtle signs include a decreased pulse pressure, mottling of the skin, cool extremities, capillary refill greater than 2 seconds, and a depressed level of consciousness. The systolic blood pressure is normally greater than 70 mmHg + twice the age in years. A 30% blood loss is required for change in vital signs. Hypotension indicates a loss of 45% of blood volume and often is accompanied by bradycardia.

9. **What are normal vital signs by age group.**
See Table 94-1.

TABLE 94-1. NORMAL VITAL SIGNS BY AGE GROUP			
Age (yr)	Heart Rate (bpm)	Blood Pressure (mmHg)	Respiratory rate (resp/min)
0–1	120	80/40	40
1–5	100	100/60	30
5–10	80	120/80	20

Adapted from O'Neill JA: The injured child. In O'Neill JA, Grosfeld JL, Fonkalsrud EW, Coran AG, Caldamone AA (eds): Principles of Pediatric Surgery, 2nd ed. St. Louis, Mosby, 2003, pp 143–149.

10. **Name the preferred sites for venous access.**
In decreasing order of preference, peripheral, intraosseous (particularly in very young children), percutaneous femoral-subclavian-external jugular-internal jugular, saphenous vein cutdown at the ankle.

11. **What are some considerations regarding an intraosseous line?**
It is most appropriate in children younger than 6 years and allows administration of virtually any fluid and blood product or drug and even allows blood draws. The preferred site is the proximal tibia below the tibial tuberosity. It should not be placed distal to a fracture and should be removed when peripheral intravenous access is secured. It may be complicated by cellulitis or osteomyelitis.

12. **What is a child's normal blood volume?**
80 mL/kg.

13. **How should I resuscitate a pediatric trauma patient?**
A 30% reduction in blood volume generally is required to manifest signs of shock. The 3:1 rule (crystalloid resuscitation-to-blood loss) applies as it does in adults. For a 20-mL/kg blood loss, 60 mL/kg should be given. Either warmed normal saline or lactated Ringer's solution can be given in boluses of 20 mL/kg. After 60 mL/kg, consideration should be given to transfusing warmed packed red blood cells (10 mL/kg). At this point, a surgeon should be involved.

14. **Why are children prone to head trauma?**
They lead with their head because it is larger in proportion to their body than that of an adult.

15. **Which kinds of head injuries do children get?**
Compared with adults, mass lesions are less common, but cerebral edema and postinjury seizures are more common. Hemorrhagic shock may occur secondary to blood loss in the subgaleal or epidural space, because of open cranial sutures and fontanels. Bulging sutures or fontanelles suggest a significant brain injury and/or cerebral edema and warrant aggressive management and neurosurgical consultation before decompensation occurs.

16. **Which children need cranial imaging after head trauma?**

Symptoms (history of loss of consciousness, vomiting, drowsiness, irritability, headache, amnesia) or signs of neurologic anomalies (scalp hematoma, depressed mental status, seizures, focal deficits) warrant a head computed tomography (CT). If the child is asymptomatic, neurologically intact, and has no scalp hematoma, no studies are required regardless of age. In a neurologically normal but mildly symptomatic older child, a CT may be done; alternatively, the child may be admitted for observation or sent home with a reliable parent. Return to the hospital and CT scan are advised for deterioration. Neurologic abnormalities, depressed skull fracture, or signs of basilar skull fracture warrant CT scanning.

Quayle KS: Minor head injury in the pediatric patient. Pediatr Clin North Am 46:1189–1199, 1999.

17. **What is SCIWORA?**

SCIWORA stands for spinal cord injury without radiographic abnormality. Plain spine radiographs are normal in two thirds of children with spinal cord injury. Therefore, in children with evidence of a spinal cord injury, normal films do not exclude injury, and a high-resolution CT should be followed by magnetic resonance imaging (MRI) and flexion-extension views. Continued immobilization and appropriate consultation are warranted if there is suspicion of spinal cord injury, particularly in the presence of neurologic deficits.

Pang D: Spinal cord injury without radiographic abnormality in children, 2 decades later. Neurosurg 55:1325–1343, 2004.

18. **How common is pseudosubluxation of the cervical spine?**

About 40% of children younger than 7 years demonstrate anterior displacement of the anterior border of C2 on C3. Approximately 20% of children up to 16 years also demonstrate pseudosubluxation. This radiographic finding can be minimized by placing the patient in a sniffing position. It can be differentiated from true subluxation by evaluating the *posterior* margin of the vertebral bodies (i.e., the anterior aspect of the spinal canal) for step-offs.

19. **How common are rib fractures in children?**

Not very. The compliant chest wall allows unimpeded transmission of energy to the underlying thoracic organs, potentially resulting in life-threatening contusions. Because of the force required to break elastic bones in young children, two thirds of children with rib fractures have associated organ injuries. A mobile mediastinum allows tension pneumothorax to develop more readily than in adults.

20. **How reliable is physical examination to exclude abdominal trauma?**

Abdominal pain and tenderness are relatively sensitive but highly nonspecific signs of intra-abdominal injuries. Decompression of the bladder and stomach, which almost invariably is distended in children who have been crying, may facilitate the examination, but some diagnostic test is generally warranted.

21. **Compare and contrast the primary diagnostic modalities for evaluating children for abdominal trauma.**

CT, diagnostic peritoneal lavage, and ultrasonography, are the primary diagnostic tests. CT is appropriate in stable patients. It is the most specific of the tests, identifying solid organ and (less accurately) hollow viscus injuries. It also evaluates the retroperitoneum. However, it is time consuming and usually requires sedation in young children. Diagnostic peritoneal lavage is better-than-95% accurate in identifying injuries, but it is invasive and too nonspecific. Because most solid organ injuries can be managed nonoperatively, the finding of a hemoperitoneum alone, without hemodynamic instability, does not warrant operative exploration. It is most useful in patients who are hemodynamically unstable or in patients whose abdomen cannot be serially evaluated, for example because they require an emergency neurosurgical or orthopedic intervention under general anesthesia. Ultrasound is simple, rapid, repeatable, and accurate in identifying hemoperitoneum. It may be used to triage unstable patients to the operating room or to rapidly exclude the abdomen as a source of significant blood loss. If equivocal, further imaging or diagnostic peritoneal lavage may be required, depending on the urgency of the situation. Growing experience with Focused Abdominal Sonography for Trauma (FAST) in children suggests that it can replace peritoneal lavage for the unexaminable patient.

Partrick DA, Bensard DD, Moore EE, et al: Ultrasound is an effective triage tool to evaluate blunt abdominal trauma in the pediatric population. J Trauma 45:57–63, 1998.

Soudack M, Epelman M, Maor R, et al: Experience with focused abdominal sonography for trauma (FAST) in 313 pediatric patients. J Clin Ultrasound 32:53–61, 2004.

Suthers SE, Albrecht R, Foley D, et al: Surgeon-directed ultrasound for trauma is a predictor of intra-abdominal injury in children. Am Surg 70:164–167, 2004.

22. What is a handlebar injury?

An injury (typically a duodenal hematoma or pancreatic injury) resulting from a bicycle handlebar—or elbow—striking the child in the right upper quadrant or epigastrium. Renal trauma is seen if the handlebar injury is off midline.

Arkovitz MD, Johnson N, Garcia VF: Pancreatic trauma in children: Mechanisms of injury. J Trauma 42:49–53, 1997.

23. What is the seat belt complex?

Ecchymosis of the abdominal wall, a flexion-distraction injury of the lumbar spine (Chance fracture), and intestinal or mesenteric injury.

Bensard DD, Beaver BL, Besner GE, Cooney DR: Small bowel injury in children after blunt abdominal trauma: Is diagnostic delay important? J Trauma 41:476–483, 1996.

24. Which burn wounds require intravenous hydration?

Greater than 10% total body surface area (BSA) in infants or 15% total BSA in older children. In addition, any child who is not tolerating adequate oral hydration (noted by poor oral intake or hourly urine output less than 0.5 mL/kg/h) and most patients with concomitant inhalation injuries should receive intravenous hydration. All children who require intravenous hydration should be treated as inpatients.

O'Neill JA: Burns. In O'Neill JA, Grosfeld JL, Fonkalsrud EW, Coran AG, Caldamone AA (eds): Principles of Pediatric Surgery, 2nd ed. St. Louis, Mosby, 2003, pp 197–204.

25. How much of a problem is nonaccidental trauma?

It is the most common cause of traumatic death in the first year of life. Of abused children, 50% who are released to those who abuse them ultimately sustain fatal nonaccidental trauma injuries. (See Chapter 64.)

BIBLIOGRAPHY

1. American College of Surgeons Committee on Trauma: Advanced Trauma Life Support for Doctors, 7th ed. Chicago, American College of Surgeons, 2004. Available at www.facs.org/trauma/atls/index.html.

CHAPTER 95

MUSCULOSKELETAL TRAUMA AND CONDITIONS OF THE EXTREMITY

Steven J. Morgan, MD, and Anand A. Parekh, MRCS (Eng)

GENERAL PRINCIPLES

1. What are the immediate treatment priorities in an open fracture?

As in any trauma patient, the immediate priorities are the ABCs: airway, breathing, and circulation. Any break in the skin near a fracture site should be assumed to communicate with the fracture until proved otherwise. After careful examination with neurologic and vascular assessment, the wound should be cleaned of gross contamination, and a sterile dressing impregnated with a 1% povidone-iodine (Betadine) solution should be applied. Direct pressure can be used for hemorrhage control. Axial realignment and splinting immobilize the bone, decreasing blood loss and protecting the soft tissue from further damage. Probing of the wound, wound cultures, extensive irrigation, and multiple examinations of the wound should be avoided, owing to the increased potential for secondary contamination and soft tissue damage. Tetanus prophylaxis and intravenous antibiotics are usually administered. A first-generation cephalosporin, with or without an aminoglycoside, is used most commonly for antibiotic prophylaxis. When open fractures occur in grossly contaminated environments, such as barnyards, penicillin is added, secondary to the increased risk of anaerobic organisms. Consult an orthopedic surgeon immediately.

Note: An open fracture is an orthopedic emergency!

2. What percentage of polytrauma patients have unrecognized fractures at the time of admission?

Of patients with multiple system injuries, up to 20% have unrecognized fractures at the time of initial assessment. In general, these do not typically involve the axial skeleton or long bones. These unrecognized injuries are located most commonly in the hands and feet. This important fact shows the need for repetitive examination of the multiply injured patient and discussions with the family of the injured party regarding the potential of unrecognized fractures.

3. What is compartment syndrome?

A condition that develops when the pressure in the confined space of the muscle compartment exceeds the filling pressure of the venules and the arterioles supplying the muscle, resulting in muscle ischemia and edema. This increases intracompartmental pressure further setting up a vicious cycle, eventually leading to necrosis of muscle and nerve tissue. Conditions or situations that cause an increase in the compartment contents or decrease the expansive nature of the compartment can result in compartment syndrome. Common causes include fracture, crush injuries, hemorrhage, postischemic swelling after repair of vascular injury, tight-fitting casts or dressings, military antishock trousers (MAST), and burns.

4. What are the signs and symptoms of acute compartment syndrome?

The classic diagnosis of acute compartment syndrome is indicated by the **5 Ps:**

- **Pain** is the earliest and most common symptom associated with compartment syndrome. It is typically more severe than what is normally expected, based on the associated cause, and is often exacerbated when the muscles of the involved compartment are put on stretch. Pain is typically ischemic in nature and often not relieved by narcotics.

- **Paresthesia** is another common finding but indicates a prolonged period of increased compartment pressures.
- **Pallor, pulselessness,** and **paralysis** are late findings, and the condition is often not reversible at that point.

There are various methods of measuring intracompartmental pressure to obtain objective evidence of compartment syndrome. The gold standard of diagnosis is a positive clinical examination combined with a plausible history. Missed or delayed diagnosis of compartment syndrome is catastrophic, warranting a high index of suspicion and early specialist consultation.

Exertional compartment syndrome is characterized by exercise induced compartmental pain and swelling that resolves with rest. Acute compartment syndrome may complicate this condition. It is therefore prudent *always* to exclude compartment syndrome in a painful limb due to uncertain etiology to avoid disastrous complications.

5. **What are the most common sites of compartment syndrome?**
   The volar compartment of the forearm and the anterior compartment of the leg. The deep posterior compartment of the leg is the site most often missed for this event. Supracondylar fractures of the humerus in children and both-bone forearm fractures are the injuries most commonly associated with this process in the upper extremity. Proximal tibial fractures are the most common cause of compartment syndrome in the leg. Compartment syndrome also is known to occur in the hands, feet, thighs, and upper arm. Fractures may or may not be present.

6. **What is the treatment of compartment syndrome?**
   Surgical release of the investing fascia of the compartment (fasciotomy) is the only effective treatment for this condition. Temporary measures that may be used to prevent compartment syndrome include elevation of the extremity to above heart level and maintenance of a normal arteriole filling pressure by maintaining a normotensive blood pressure.

7. **Describe the trauma patient who can have his or her cervical spine clinically cleared.**
   See Chapter 86.

8. **Describe the joint fluid analysis consistent with septic arthritis.**
   See Chapter 52.

9. **How do I diagnose a traumatic open joint?**
   Probing of a wound in proximity to a joint is insufficient, may increase the risk of infection, and generally should be avoided. Radiographs of the involved joint may reveal the presence of air in the joint, indicating joint violation. The definitive diagnosis is made by performing an arthrogram. Sterile saline combined with a small amount of methylene blue should be injected in the joint. A significant amount of fluid needs to be injected to distend the joint. The traumatic wound is inspected for egress of the injected fluid. The fluid should be withdrawn from the joint.

10. **When should I order radiographs? How many should I order?**
    - Radiographs should be ordered based on the physical examination findings.
    - Radiographs should include the joints above and below the perceived area of injury.
    - Two orthogonal views always should be obtained.

    Obtaining radiographs should not obstruct the resuscitation process in the multiply injured patient. In situations in which significant deformity of the limb results in vascular compromise or devitalization of the overlying skin, radiographs should be delayed, pending emergent realignment and splinting of the involved extremity.

HAND AND UPPER EXTREMITY

11. **What is the best method to control bleeding in a hand or forearm laceration?**
Direct pressure. Tourniquets are rarely necessary. The practice of blindly placing clamps into the wound is dangerous and often can damage structures in close proximity to the offending vessel, such as the median or ulnar nerve.

12. **What metacarpophalangeal joint most commonly sustains a laceration when an individual engages in "fist diplomacy"?**
The third metacarpophalangeal joint because it is the most prominent knuckle when making a fist.

13. **How much deformity can be tolerated in a metacarpal fracture?**
Rotational deformity is not tolerated well and should be corrected. Rotation in a metacarpal neck or shaft fracture causes the fingers to cross when the individual makes a fist. Flexion deformity of the fracture is the most common and best tolerated. You can accept 10, 20, 30, and 40 degrees of flexion in the index through small fingers. A greater degree of deformity is tolerated at the small finger, secondary to the increased motion at the carpometacarpal joint. The same is true for a thumb metacarpal fracture, in which 40° of angular deformity can be accepted.

14. **What bacterium is often associated with cat bites, and what is the antibiotic treatment?**
Pasteurella multocida. Penicillin G, co-amoxiclav (orally [PO]), or ampicillin/sulbactam (Unasyn) (intravenous [IV]). Use doxycycline in penicillin-allergic patients.

15. **What should be done with an amputated part that may be replanted?**
1. Remove gross contamination by irrigating with saline.
2. Wrap the part in a saline-moistened (not soaked) sterile gauze.
3. Place the wrapped part into a sealed plastic bag or container.
4. Place the bag or container into an ice water bath.
Never put the amputated part straight onto ice!

16. **List traumatic amputations that should be considered for replantation.**
- Any amputation in a child
- Multiple finger amputations
- Thumb
- Hand
- Arm
    The ultimate decision always should be deferred to a hand surgery specialist. It is usually best to defer detailed discussion of replantation with the patient or family to the consulting microvascular specialist.

17. **What is the appropriate treatment for a patient with pain in the snuffbox of the wrist and normal radiographs after a traumatic event to the wrist?**
The scaphoid is easily palpable in the anatomic snuffbox of the wrist. The snuffbox is the space between the extensor pollicis longus and the extensor pollicis brevis. Tenderness in this area is suggestive of a scaphoid fracture. The absence of fracture on the initial radiographs is common. As the necrotic bone at the fracture site is resorbed, the fracture line often becomes apparent on radiographs approximately 14 days after injury. Individuals with this condition should be immobilized in a thumb spica splint or cast and referred to an orthopedist for evaluation. For this reason, bone scans and magnetic resonance imaging (MRI) are not indicated in the acute evaluation.

18. **State the incidence and common causes of posterior shoulder dislocations.**
Incidence is 5% of shoulder dislocations. Tonic-clonic seizures, electrical shock, and direct anterior shoulder trauma are causes.

19. **What percentage of patients with first-time anterior shoulder dislocations experience a recurrent dislocation?**
Of patients aged 30 years or younger, 90% experience a recurrent dislocation. For older patients, the percentage is lower and more variable, depending on the mechanism of injury.

20. **What are the potential complications of anterior shoulder dislocation?**
The axillary nerve is at risk for injury at the time of dislocation. Careful examination of the deltoid muscle should be done to assess motor function. The axillary nerve also provides sensation to the lateral aspect of the shoulder (regimental badge area), and sensation should be checked in this area. In addition to axillary nerve injury, a rotator cuff tear can occur at the time of dislocation.

21. **How is a rotator cuff tear diagnosed?**
The patient often complains of pain with overhead activity, night pain, and pain with abduction of the arm. The patient has difficulty abducting the arm and often is unable to lift the arm above the level of the shoulder. With the shoulder in 90-degree abduction, 30-degree forward flexion, and maximal internal rotation, the patient cannot resist against downward pressure on the extremity (supraspinatus strength test). A drop test is done in the same manner with the arm simply at 90-degree abduction. The patient is not able to lower the arm **slowly** from 90-degree abduction. When these conditions exist, it is important to differentiate a rotator cuff tear from subacromial impingement (condition that irritates the rotator cuff). Inject 10 mL 1% lidocaine in the subacromial space. If the patient obtains pain relief and still cannot initiate abduction, the diagnosis of rotator cuff tear is confirmed.

22. **How is a posterior sternoclavicular dislocation diagnosed?**
Radiographs are generally unsuccessful. Computed tomography (CT) scan is the most sensitive diagnostic modality.

23. **Describe the significance of anterior versus posterior dislocation of a sternoclavicular joint.**
    - **Anterior** dislocations are not associated with major complications and are treated easily with a sling.
    - Of **posterior** sternoclavicular dislocations, 25% are associated with complications, including rupture or compression of the trachea; esophageal occlusion or rupture; lung contusion; and laceration or occlusion of the superior vena cava, subclavian vein, or artery. Reduction of posterior sternoclavicular dislocation should be done only in the operating room, with a cardiothoracic surgeon immediately available.

24. **What is the most common neurologic deficit seen with a humeral shaft fracture?**
The radial nerve may be stretched (**neurapraxia**) or rarely lacerated (**neurotmesis**). This condition typically occurs with fractures involving the distal one third of the humerus. Disability includes inability to extend the wrist and fingers at the metacarpophalangeal joints and numbness on the dorsum of the radial side of the hand. Interphalangeal extension, representing ulnar and median nerve function, is preserved. Triceps function is preserved because it is innervated by branches of the radial nerve proximal to the radial groove.

25. **What is the difference between a nightstick fracture and a Monteggia fracture?**
    - A fracture of the ulna (typically the proximal one third) with a radial head dislocation is a **Monteggia** fracture. This fracture occurs as a result of a fall on an outstretched hand with

associated valgus force on the extremity. The treatment requires internal fixation of the ulna fracture.

- A **nightstick** fracture is a fracture of the ulna resulting from a direct blow to the shaft of the ulna. There is no associated injury to the proximal radial ulnar humeral joint. In most cases, these injuries can be treated by closed means and early range of motion. Nightstick fractures with significant comminution, greater than 10 degrees of angulation or greater than 50% displacement, may be considered for operative fixation.

26. **What nerve is commonly injured in a Monteggia fracture?**
The posterior interosseous nerve lies in close proximity to the neck of the radius. When the radial head is dislocated, this nerve is often stretched, resulting in a neurapraxia and inability to extend the thumb or wrist.

LOWER EXTREMITY AND PELVIC FRACTURES

27. **Name the major complications directly related to pelvic fracture.**
Hemorrhage and urologic injuries, including bladder rupture and urethral tear.

28. **What is the mortality rate in patients with open pelvic fracture?**
Mortality has decreased from 50% in the 1980s to 10–25% due to a move toward a multidisciplinary approach and advances in critical care.

   Grotz MRW, Allami MK, Harwood P, et al: Open pelvic fractures: Epidemiology, current concepts of management outcome. Injury 2005;1:1–13. [PMID: 15589906]

29. **Discuss the major management considerations of hemorrhage in patients with pelvic fracture.**
See Chapter 92.

30. **What are the incidence and mechanism of injury in posterior hip dislocation?**
Greater than 80% are posterior and result from a force directed posteriorly to a flexed knee, as occurs when the knee strikes the dashboard in a motor vehicle accident.

31. **What are the complications of posterior hip dislocation?**
- **Sciatic nerve deficit** is found in about 10% of patients, resulting in weakness or loss of hamstring function in the thigh and all of the muscles of the leg.
- **Avascular necrosis** occurs in 10–15% of patients but increases almost to 50% if reduction is delayed beyond 12 hours.
- Even with prompt reduction, 20% of patients develop **osteoarthritis.**
- The risk of **recurrent dislocation** is increased during early rehabilitation following traction.

32. **How is posterior hip dislocation differentiated clinically from a femoral neck fracture or intertrochanteric femoral fracture?**
Both result in lower extremity shortening. In posterior hip dislocation, the hip is flexed, adducted, and internally rotated. This is often referred to as the position of modesty. With a femoral neck or intertrochanteric fracture, the lower extremity is not flexed but is shortened, abducted, and externally rotated.

33. **How much blood loss can be expected with a fracture of the femoral shaft?**
500–1500 mL.

34. How are femoral shaft fractures best stabilized in the emergency department (ED)?

Hare longitudinal traction, involving a self-contained traction unit. Most emergency providers carry these and can place them in the field or ambulance. Hare traction should not be left in place for more than 2 hours without frequent neurovascular checks because of the potential for compartment syndrome and vascular compromise. A second option is placement of a distal femoral traction pin and in-line traction connected to the bed or gurney. A proximal tibial pin may also be used provided there is no knee injury. Conventional splinting is ineffective.

35. Why do patients with hip pathology present with knee pain?

A patient with a hip problem may complain only of pain to the anterior distal thigh and medial aspect of the knee. The knee and the hip share a common innervation through the obturator nerve. Always suspect a hip problem in a patient who complains of knee pain without corresponding findings on physical examination. Careful examination of the knee and hip, with appropriate radiographs of the hip, is necessary to complete the evaluation.

36. Name the most common injury associated with traumatic hemarthrosis of the knee joint.

Anterior cruciate ligament rupture. If fat globules are noted in the joint aspiration fluid, the possibility of an associated intra-articular fracture should be pursued.

37. Name the ligament most commonly associated with an inversion ankle sprain.

Anterior talofibular ligament. The calcaneofibular ligament also can be injured in more severe sprains.

38. Describe the treatment for ankle sprains.

Ankle sprains are treated by the **RICE** protocol:

R = **R**est
I = **I**ce
C = **C**ompression
E = **E**levation

  Early protected weight bearing with crutches and an early range-of-motion program should be instituted. More severe sprains may require a short period of immobilization.

39. Discuss the Ottawa rules regarding radiographs of the ankle.

The Ottawa rules were developed from a large study done in Ottawa, Canada, which examined the necessity of routine ankle radiography in the assessment of patients with ankle injuries. It was determined that radiographs are not required when the following conditions are met:

- The examiner is experienced.
- The patient does not have significant deformity of the ankle.
- The examination is consistent with an ankle sprain.
- There is no tenderness on examination over the medial or lateral malleolus (palpate posteriorly from the tip of the malleolus to 6 cm proximally).
- The patient was able to bear weight on the injured ankle immediately after the injury or in the ED.

40. What is a locked knee? What are the most common causes?

The patient is unable to extend the knee actively or passively beyond 10- to 45-degree flexion. True locking and unlocking occur suddenly. The most common causes are a tear of the medial meniscus, a loose body or **joint mouse** (osteochondral fragment) in the knee, or a dislocated patella.

41. What injuries are associated with a calcaneal fracture?

Depending on the exact mechanism of injury and the type of calcaneal fracture, 10–50% of patients have an associated compression fracture of the lumbar or lower thoracic spine. Of calcaneal injuries, 10% are bilateral, and about 25% are associated with other lower extremity injuries; 10% can result in a compartment syndrome of the foot, requiring fasciotomy.

42. What vascular injury must be considered with a tibiofemoral knee dislocation?

Injury or compression of the popliteal artery. Cadaver studies showed that anterior dislocations tend to cause intimal flaps and occlusion, whereas posterior dislocations are more likely to cause a rupture of the popliteal artery. Injuries also occur at the trifurcation just distal to the popliteal fossa. Postreduction angiography should be considered for all patients with abnormal pulse examination or ankle-brachial index.

PEDIATRIC ORTHOPEDICS

43. What is a torus or buckle fracture?

This fracture is typically seen in the metaphysis of the radius but is not limited to this bone. **Torus** means a round swelling or protuberance. In children, the cortical bone and metaphyseal bone fail in compression (**buckling**), while the opposite cortex remains intact. The area of bone that fails in compression forms a torus. Because the opposite cortex remains intact, these fractures are stable and require splint or cast immobilization for 4 weeks.

44. What is a greenstick fracture?

Children's bones have increased elasticity. An angular force applied to a long bone of a child causes a greenstick fracture. One cortex fails in tension, while the opposite cortex bows but does not fail or fracture in compression. The fracture is similar to what occurs when one attempts to break a green branch of a tree. This fracture pattern is common in the radius and ulna. These fractures require reduction, and often the fracture must be completed to achieve an adequate reduction. Immobilization in a cast is required for 6 weeks.

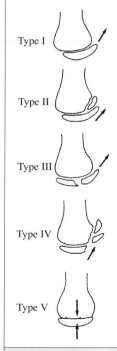

Figure 95-1. Salter-Harris classification of epiphyseal injuries.

45. What is the Salter-Harris classification? What is its clinical significance?

A method of classifying epiphyseal injuries (Fig. 95-1). Fractures involving the epiphysis may result in growth disturbance, and parents must be informed of this potential. About 80% of these injuries are Salter-Harris types I and II, both of which have a low complication rate. Salter-Harris types III, IV, and V injuries have a more variable prognosis. Displaced Salter-Harris types III and IV fractures may require open reduction to restore the normal relationship of the epiphysis and articular surface. The five types are summarized as follows:

- Type I: Fracture extends through the epiphyseal plate, resulting in displacement of the epiphysis (this may appear merely as widening of the radiolucent area representing the growth plate).
- Type II: Fracture is as above, with an additional fracture of a triangular segment of metaphysis.

- Type III: Fracture line runs from the joint surface through the epiphyseal plate and epiphysis.
- Type IV: Fracture line also occurs in type III but also passes through adjacent metaphysis.
- Type V: A crush injury of the epiphysis occurs, which may be difficult to determine by x-ray examination.

46. **Describe the vascular complications associated with pediatric supracondylar humerus fractures.**
   Displaced supracondylar humerus fractures in children have a 5% incidence of vascular compromise. The brachial artery typically is compressed or lacerated by the anteriorly displaced humeral shaft. Posterior lateral displacement of the supracondylar fracture is the fracture pattern most likely to result in vascular injury. The child with a viable hand and absent pulse should undergo prompt reduction and fracture fixation in the operating room, with re-evaluation of the vascular status after the procedure. In the patient with an absent pulse and a devascularized hand, longitudinal traction and splinting should be done in the ED in an attempt to reconstitute flow to the distal extremity. Prompt consultation with orthopedic and vascular surgeons is required.

47. **Describe the neurologic complications associated with pediatric supracondylar humerus fractures.**
   The anterior interosseous nerve (branch of the median nerve) is potentially the most commonly injured nerve. This nerve innervates the deep compartment of the forearm, which consists of the flexor digitorum profundus to the index, the pronator quadratus, and the flexor pollicis longus. The nerve can be checked by evaluating flexor pollicis longus function at the interphalangeal joint of the thumb. The radial nerve is the next most commonly injured nerve, followed by the ulnar nerve. A thorough physical examination must be done to identify these injuries, a difficult task in the small child.

KEY POINTS: MUSCULOSKELETAL TRAUMA AND CONDITIONS OF THE EXTREMITY

1. Remember the ABCs: airway, breathing, and circulation.

2. Compartment syndrome is an important diagnosis for exclusion.

3. *Never* place an amputated part directly on ice or immerse in water.

4. Multidisciplinary approach is paramount in the treatment of pelvic hemorrhage.

5. *Always* rule out infection in a child presenting with atraumatic hip pain.

6. Bleeding from a wound is best controlled with *direct* pressure.

48. **What is a nursemaid's or pulled elbow? What is its management?**
   A longitudinal pull on the outstretched arm of a 1- to 5-year-old child may result in a subluxation of the annular ligament over cartilaginous radial head. The child typically presents with pseudoparalysis of the injured extremity. Radiographs are negative for fracture or radial head dislocation. Reduction involves simultaneous supination of the forearm and flexion of the elbow. A distinct click over the radial head signifies reduction. The child often begins to use the extremity within minutes of reduction. The parent or caregiver should be educated to avoid longitudinal traction on the arm to prevent this from occurring in the future.

49. **Describe the potential implications of a humeral or femoral fracture in a small child.**
In the nonambulating child with these fractures, the suspicion of child abuse should be high. An unwitnessed event or a history that does not correspond to the injuries is another potential sign of abuse. Careful examination of the child should be done, looking specifically for skin bruises or burns, retinal hemorrhage, and evidence of previous fracture. A skeletal survey should be considered because the presence of fractures at different stages of healing is a sign of abuse. All cases of suspected abuse need to be reported to the local authority. (See Chapter 64.)

50. **What is Waddell's triad?**
The constellation of injuries in a child struck by a car:
- Femoral fracture
- Intrathoracic or intra-abdominal injury
- Head injury

51. **Which nontraumatic hip disorders cause a limp in a child?**
Septic arthritis, transient synovitis (ages 2–12 years), idiopathic avascular necrosis (boys, ages 5–9 years), slipped capital femoral epiphysis (SCFE) (boys, ages 10–16 years), Perthes' disease, and juvenile rheumatoid arthritis; all of which are uncommon. Transient synovitis is probably the most common cause of nontraumatic limp in a child but is a diagnosis of exclusion.

Symptomatic treatment is prescribed for transient synovitis, including nonsteroidal anti-inflammatory drugs and non-weight bearing or bed rest. Untreated or delayed treatment of septic arthritis can lead to irreversible and catastrophic sequelae from permanent damage and deformation of the articular cartilage. Infection in a child presenting with atraumatic hip pain must be convincingly ruled out. The white blood cell count, erythrocyte sedimentation rate, and body temperature frequently are elevated in cases of infection. If doubt persists, the gold standard is hip aspiration, usually done in the operating room. Standard anteroposterior and lateral radiographs of the hip differentiate between Perthes' disease and a slipped capital femoral epiphysis.

52. **What are the early radiographic findings of an SCFE?**
Any asymmetry of the relationship of the femoral head to the femoral neck should raise the suspicion of SCFE, even if evident on only one x-ray view. If anteroposterior and lateral radiographs are normal, frog-leg views should be obtained. Comparison of the two hips may not be helpful in discerning subtle changes because SCFE is bilateral in 20% of cases.

53. **What is the ED management of a child with injury and tenderness over an open epiphysis but a normal radiograph?**
It is best to assume the child has sustained an undeterminable fracture of the physis (Salter-Harris type I or V). Immobilize the joint in a posterior splint, and keep the child non-weight bearing if the lower extremity is involved. Parents should be notified of the possibility of this type of injury and the potential for growth disturbance. The need for prompt follow-up must be emphasized and is best arranged before discharging the child from the ED. A nondisplaced physeal fracture that becomes displaced because of lack of immobilization can have significant long-term consequences. Short-term extremity immobilization in an appropriately applied splint or cast is well tolerated. When in doubt, immobilize.

BIBLIOGRAPHY

1. Browner BD, Trafton PG, Green NE, et al (eds): Skeletal Trauma: Basic Science, Management, and Reconstruction, 3rd ed. Philadelphia, W.B. Saunders, 2002.
2. Green DP, Hotchkiss RN, Pederson WC: Green's Operative Hand Surgery, 4th ed. New York, Churchill Livingstone, 1999.

3. Lovell WW, Winter RB, Morrissy RT, Weinstein SL: Lovell and Winter's Pediatric Orthopaedics, 5th ed. Philadelphia, Lippincott Williams & Wilkins, 2001.

4. Rockwood CA, Green DP, Bucholz RW, Heckman JD: Rockwood and Green's Fractures in Adults, 5th ed. Philadelphia, Lippincott Williams & Wilkins, 2001.

5. Rockwood CA, Green DP, Bucholz RW, Heckman JD: Rockwood and Green's Fractures in Children, 5th ed. Philadelphia, Lippincott Williams & Wilkins, 2001.

CHAPTER 96

HAND INJURIES AND INFECTIONS

Michael A. Kohn, MD, MPP

1. Are hand problems important in emergency medicine?
Yes. Our hands are our interface to the mechanical world, so they are frequently injured or exposed to infection. There are 4.8 million emergency department (ED) visits per year for hand/wrist injuries. At least one of every eight injury-related ED visits is for a hand/wrist injury.

2. List the essential elements of the history.
- Age
- Dominant hand
- Occupation
- How, where, and when injury occurred
- Posture of hand when injured
- Tetanus status
- Prior injury or disability of the hand

3. List the elements of a complete hand examination.
- Initial inspection of skin and soft tissue
- Vascular examination
- Evaluation of tendon function
- Nerve examination (motor and sensory)
- Determination of joint capsule integrity
- Skeletal examination

4. What is topographical anticipation?
Looking at the skin wound and thinking about which underlying structure (vessel, tendon, nerve, bone, ligament, or joint) could be injured. Know the anatomy. Do not hesitate to consult an atlas.

5. What is the normal posture of the hand at rest?
With the wrist in slight extension, the resting fingers normally assume a "cascade," progressively more flexed from index to small. (See this by relaxing your own hand with the wrist in slight extension.) An alteration in the normal posture can lead to immediate diagnosis of major tendon and joint injuries.

6. Does dorsal swelling signify an injury or infection in the dorsum of the hand?
No. Most of the palmar lymphatics drain to lymph channels and lacunae located in the loose areolar layer on the dorsum of the hand. Always check for a palmar wound when a patient presents with dorsal swelling.

7. What is the Allen test? How is it performed?
The Allen test verifies patency of the radial and ulnar arteries as follows: Occlude radial and ulnar arteries. Have patient open and close hand five or six times. Hand should blanch. Release ulnar artery; blanching should resolve within 3–5 seconds. Repeat test, releasing radial artery instead of ulnar artery. Blanching should resolve within 3–5 seconds. The most accurate form of the Allen test uses digital blood pressures rather than return of color to monitor reperfusion.

8. **How is function of the flexor digitorum superficialis (FDS) tendon tested?**
   The FDS inserts on the middle phalanx and flexes the proximal interphalangeal (PIP) joint. The flexor digitorum profundus (FDP) inserts on the distal phalanx and flexes the PIP and the distal interphalangeal (DIP) joints. The FDS muscle-tendon units should be independent of one another, whereas the FDP tendons arise from a common muscle belly. Testing the FDS of a finger entails flexing it at the PIP joint, while stabilizing the other three fingers in full extension, thereby taking the FDP out of action as a potential flexor of the PIP joint.

9. **In which finger is the test of FDS function unreliable?**
   Because the FDP to the index finger can be independent of the other profundi, the FDS test is unreliable in the index finger. Flexion at the PIP joint may be due to the FDP, even with the other fingers stabilized in extension. Suspected index finger FDS injuries must be explored.

10. **Why is the flexor or palmar aspect of the hand called the "OR side," whereas the extensor or dorsal aspect is the "ED side"?**
    In contrast to the extensors, the flexor tendons run through delicate sheaths. Because of these sheaths, repairing flexor tendons requires more expertise and a more controlled environment in the operating room than repairing extensor tendons does.

11. **How is a partial tendon laceration diagnosed?**
    If the location of the skin laceration is suspicious, rule out an underlying partial tendon laceration by exploration and direct visualization under tourniquet hemostasis. Because a flexor tendon runs through its sheath like a piston through a cylinder, a sheath laceration implies a partial tendon laceration, which is visible only when the hand is in the same posture as when injured. A bloodless field and direct visualization of the tendon during full range of motion must occur to rule out a partial tendon laceration.

12. **How do I test the extrinsic extensor tendons?**
    The extrinsic extensors alone extend the metacarpophalangeal (MCP) joints, whereas they combine with tendons from the interossei and lumbricals to form the extensor mechanism that extends the interphalangeal joints. To test the extrinsic extensor, lay the hand, palm down, on a flat surface and ask the patient to elevate the digit.

13. **Can extensor function to a finger be intact despite complete laceration of the extensor digitorum communis (EDC) to that finger?**
    Yes. The juncturae tendinum interlink the EDC tendons at the midmetacarpal level. Even if the EDC to a finger is completely lacerated in the dorsum of the hand, extension at the MCP still may be possible because of the junctura.

14. **How do I test sensory nerve function?**
    Assess nerve function before the use of anesthesia. Test digital nerves by checking two-point discrimination on the volar pad. The two points should be 5 mm apart and aligned longitudinally.

15. **What are the sensory distributions of the median, ulnar, and radial nerves?**
    See Fig. 96-1.

16. **How is motor function of the median, ulnar, and radial nerves tested?**
    - **Median:** Abductor pollicis brevis (APB)—abducts the thumb against resistance while palpating the APB muscle belly.
    - **Ulnar:** First dorsal interosseous—abducts the index finger against resistance.
    - **Radial** (no intrinsics): Extensor pollicis longus (EPL)—extends the thumb interphalangeal joint against resistance.

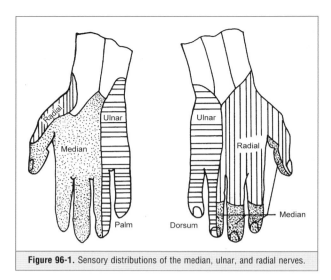

Figure 96-1. Sensory distributions of the median, ulnar, and radial nerves.

17. **Which is the most frequently dislocated carpal bone?**
The carpal bones from radial to ulnar side are as follows:
- Proximal row—scaphoid, lunate, triquetrum, pisiform
- Distal row—trapezium, trapezoid, capitate, hamate
    The **lunate** is most frequently dislocated. Its blood supply comes through the volar and dorsal ligaments from the radius. If both ligaments are ruptured, avascular necrosis results.

18. **Which is the most frequently fractured carpal bone?**
The scaphoid. Its distal blood supply increases the likelihood of avascular necrosis in the proximal segment after fracture.

19. **What is the classic sign of a scaphoid fracture?**
Snuffbox tenderness. Even without radiographic evidence of a fracture, the patient with tenderness to palpation of the anatomic snuffbox gets a thumb spica splint and must have a repeat radiograph in 2 weeks.

20. **How do I control hemorrhage from a hand injury?**
Direct pressure and elevation. This will work 99.9% of the time. Elevate and hold pressure for 10 minutes by the clock. Very rarely, an incomplete arterial laceration requires a proximal tourniquet for temporary control, followed by sensory examination, anesthesia, scrub, and exploration under good light and magnification to tie off the bleeder. **Never blindly clamp a bleeder.**

21. **Why the rule, "no blind clamping of bleeders"?**
In the hand, the arteries run in close approximation to the nerves. Blindly clamping an artery may irreparably damage the associated nerve. Also, the clamp may damage a section of vessel vital to successful reanastomosis.

22. **What should be done with an amputated digit?**
Gently clean the digit with sterile saline, wrap it in moist gauze, place it in a sterile container, and float the container in ice water. (Avoid direct contact between ice and tissue to prevent freezing.)

23. What should be done with a devascularized but still partially attached digit?
Leave part attached (preserves veins for reimplantation), gently wrap in moist gauze, and apply a bulky dressing.

24. What are the indications and contraindications for reimplantation?
- **Indications:** Multiple finger injury; thumb amputations (especially proximal to interphalangeal joint); single finger injury in children; clean amputation at hand, wrist, or distal forearm (A clean amputation at the wrist may be easier to reimplant than multiple-digit amputations.)
- **Contraindications:** Severe crush or avulsion, heavy contamination, single-finger amputations in adults, severe associated medical problems or injuries, severe multilevel injury of amputated part, willful self-amputation
  Bottom line: Give the hand surgeon the opportunity to decide.

25. Which are the most deceptive of all serious hand injuries?
High-pressure injection injuries (from paint guns, grease guns, or hydraulic lines) initially may seem innocuous, often involving just the fingertip. In the most recently published case series (from England), 6 out of 15 high-pressure injection injuries resulted in some form of amputation, and only one patient regained normal sensation, despite aggressive early surgical treatment.

Christodoulou L, Melikyan EY, Woodbridge S, Burke FD: Functional outcome of high-pressure injection injuries of the hand. J Trauma 50:717–720, 2001.

26. List Kanavel's four cardinal signs of flexor tenosynovitis.
- Slightly flexed posture of the digit
- Fusiform swelling of the digit
- Pain on passive extension
- Tenderness along the flexor tendon sheath
  Flexor tenosynovitis requires admission and surgery.

Kanavel AB: Infection of the Hand. Philadelphia, Lea & Febiger, 1925.

27. What is a paronychia? How is it treated?
A common bacterial infection involving the folds of skin that hold the fingernail in place. In the absence of visible pus, treatment should consist of warm moist compresses, elevation, and antistaphylococcal antibiotics. If pus is present, do the minimum necessary to drain and maintain drainage. This usually consists of simply elevating the eponychial fold or making a small incision. Bilateral paronychia indicates subungual pus and necessitates removal of the proximal part of the nail plate.

28. How is whitlow different from a paronychia?
Whitlow is infection of the tissue around the nail plate with herpes simplex virus (rather than bacteria). The discharge is serous and crusting rather than purulent. The patient also may have perioral cold sores. Do **not** incise and drain herpetic whitlow.

29. What is a felon? How is it treated?
A painful and potentially disabling infection of the fingertip pulp. Treatment is controversial. Some clinicians argue for immediate drainage of the tensely swollen and painful fingertip pad. Others argue that early treatment with antibiotics, elevation, and immobilization may prevent the need for surgical drainage. Even if drainage is necessary, the best method is also a matter of controversy. The full fishmouth incision has fallen out of favor, but the three-quarter fishmouth incision and the simple lateral incision are both acceptable.

30. What is a football jersey finger? How is it treated?
Rupture of the FDP occurs commonly when a football player catches his or her finger in an opponent's jersey. The tendon is avulsed from its insertion at the palmar base of the distal

phalanx, often taking a bone fragment along. Surgical repair within the next several days is indicated.

31. What is a mallet finger? How is it treated?

A mallet finger is the opposite of a football jersey finger; the insertion of the extensor tendon, rather than the flexor tendon, is avulsed from the dorsum of the distal phalanx, often pulling off a bone fragment. Appropriate treatment is to splint the DIP joint in extension (not hyperextension) for 6 weeks.

32. Describe a subungual hematoma. How is it treated?

A collection of blood under the nail plate can be painful. Classically, this occurs when a weekend carpenter strikes his or her thumb with a hammer. Relieving the pressure by nail trephination (poking a hole in the nail) will make you a hero to the patient. Use electrocautery, a red-hot paperclip, or an 18G needle (twisting it between your fingers like a drill bit). Removal of an intact nail plate is almost never indicated.

33. What is a gamekeeper's thumb? How is it diagnosed?

A torn ulnar collateral ligament of the thumb MCP joint. In 1955, the injury was reported in 24 Scottish game wardens, arising from their technique for breaking the necks of wounded rabbits. The injury is more properly called **skier's thumb** because it most commonly occurs when a skier either catches the thumb on a planted ski pole or falls while holding a pole in the outstretched hand. The injury is potentially severely disabling. Complete rupture of the ligament always requires surgery. ED treatment consists of a thumb spica splint and referral. One way to test for injury to the ulnar collateral ligament of the thumb MCP is to hand the patient a heavy can (e.g., of soda) or bottle (e.g., of hydrogen peroxide). If the injury is present, the patient will be unable to hold the object in the usual way, either supinating to balance the object in the palm or dropping it.

Cambell CS: Gamekeeper's thumb. J Bone Joint Surg 37B:148–149, 1955.

34. What is a boxer's fracture?

Fracture of the fifth (small finger) metacarpal is common in barefisted pugilists. Because the small finger metacarpal is second only to the thumb metacarpal in mobility, large angles of angulation are tolerated without functional deficit. Nevertheless, attempts to correct significant angulation of an acute boxer's fracture are warranted. Any rotational deformity must be corrected. A laceration accompanying a boxer's fracture is assumed to be a fight bite.

35. What is a fight bite?

The most notorious of all nonvenomous bite wounds is the fight bite. As the name implies, the injury occurs when the soon-to-be-patient punches his or her adversary in the teeth, lacerating the dorsum of one or more MCP joints. Other names for this injury such as **morsus humanus** or **closed fist injury** have been proposed. **Fight bite** is more compact, descriptive, and poetic. All such wounds require formal exploration, including extension of the skin laceration if necessary. They should be débrided, irrigated, dressed open (no sutures), and splinted. If the wound penetrates the extensor hood, the MCP joint requires thorough washout, and strong consideration should be given to hospitalization for intravenous (IV) antibiotics and meticulous wound care. If the wound is already infected, hospitalization is mandatory.

Perron AD, Miller MD, Brady WJ: Orthopedic pitfalls in the ED: Fight bite. Am J Emerg Med 20:114–117, 2002.

Welch C: Human bite infections of the hand. N Engl J Med 215:901, 1936.

KEY POINTS: HAND INJURIES AND INFECTIONS

1. Because scaphoid fractures are frequently radiographically occult, even without x-ray evidence of a fracture, the patient with tenderness to palpation of the anatomic snuffbox should be treated with a thumb spica splint and repeat evaluation in 1–2 weeks.

2. The most deceptive of serious hand injuries is the high-pressure injection injury sustained while testing a hydraulic paint or oil gun because, despite seeming innocuous on initial presentation, these injuries require aggressive, surgical management.

3. Any laceration over the dorsal MCP joint is suspicious for a fight bite. Fight bites require meticulous exploration and wound care. If the wound penetrates the extensor hood, thorough joint washout and IV antibiotics are required.

36. Are human bites more dangerous than other animal bites?
No. The fight bite gave human bites their reputation for being more prone to infection than other animal bites. This probably has more to do with the location of the bite and the typical delay in treatment than with the mix of organisms in the human mouth. True human bites (occlusive bites rather than fight bites) have no higher infection rates than animal bites. If humans punched animals in the teeth, these animal fight bites would have high infection rates also.

37. Name six true hand emergencies.
- Amputation or other devascularization injury
- Compartment syndrome
- Third-degree burn
- High-pressure injection injury
- Flexor tenosynovitis
- Septic joint

BIBLIOGRAPHY

1. American Society for Surgery of the Hand: The Hand: Examination and Diagnosis. Blue Book, 3rd ed. New York, Churchill Livingstone, 1990.

2. American Society for Surgery of the Hand: The Hand: Primary Care of Common Problems. Red Book, 2nd ed. New York, Churchill Livingstone, 1985.

3. Carter PR: Common Hand Injuries and Infections: A Practical Approach to Early Treatment. Philadelphia, W.B. Saunders, 1983.

4. Daniels JM II, Zook EG, Lynch JM: Hand and wrist injuries. Part II: Emergent evaluation. Am Fam Physician 69:1949–1956, 2004.

5. Lampe EW (with illustrations by F Netter): Surgical Anatomy of the Hand. Clin Symp 403, 1988.

CHAPTER 97

BURNS

Michelle Tartaglia, MD

1. **How should thermal burn patients be assessed initially in the emergency department (ED)?**

   Always start with the ABCs. Airway evaluation for inhalation injury is critical early in the patient's course. Assess respiratory status, and provide supplemental oxygen if necessary. Evaluate for circulation and hemodynamic status with vital signs, pulses, and capillary refill. The ABCs should be followed by a complete secondary survey including evaluation of burn size and depth, associated trauma, and possible cervical spine injury. As with any ED patient, past medical history, medications, allergies, and tetanus immunization status are also important. Also, it is important to speak with the emergency medical service (EMS) transport team to determine if the patient was trapped in an enclosed space or if exposure to toxic substances is a concern.

KEY POINTS: TYPES OF BURNS COMMONLY SEEN IN THE ED

1. Thermal (most common)

2. Solar (i.e., sunburn)

3. Chemical

4. Electrical

5. Radiation

2. **How do you evaluate for inhalation injury?**

   Risk factors for inhalation injury include flame burns, exposure to smoke in an enclosed space, and associated trauma. Signs of possible inhalation injury are burns around the face and mouth, soot in the nose or mouth, and carbonaceous sputum. Respiratory symptoms such as dyspnea, hoarseness, wheezing, and stridor are highly suggestive of inhalation injury. A toxicologic evaluation for carbon monoxide or cyanide should always be considered in the patient with inhalation injury. (See Chapter 76.)

3. **What about thermal burns to the airway?**

   Because of the great capacity for heat dissipation in the oropharynx and nasopharynx, thermal burns to the lower airways are uncommon except in the setting of steam inhalation. Direct thermal burns to the airway are usually limited to the upper airway and present as mucosal edema, erythema, and ulceration.

4. **What are the indications for intubation in the burn patient?**

   Early intubation is always preferred over observation. Inhalation injury can produce a rapid progression of edema that can make orotracheal intubation difficult or impossible. Any evidence of airway involvement (voice changes, stridor, wheezing, mucosal edema) or low oxygen saturation is an indication for intubation. It should also be considered in patients with severe burns to the face and neck, even if initial respiratory status is adequate.

5. **Are there any specific issues related to intubation in the burn patient?**
Again, early intubation is the key to avoiding complications of airway edema and possible "crash" intubation. Orotracheal rapid-sequence intubation (RSI) is appropriate. Fiberoptic intubation can be considered in the stable patient. Emergency cricothyrotomy may be necessary if airway edema prevents orotracheal tube placement. Remember, many RSI drugs can contribute to hypotension. Avoid complications with adequate fluid resuscitation and careful selection of RSI medications.

6. **What about succinylcholine?**
Succinylcholine is frequently reported as contraindicated in the burn patient due to changes in muscle receptors that can cause hyperkalemia. These changes take place over the first 7–10 days after the burn. This is not a concern in the acute burn patient encountered in the ED.

7. **How is the burn injury evaluated?**
Begin with a complete physical examination including the back and the perineum. Document the locations burned and the depth of the burns.
- **First-degree burns** involve only the epidermis and are erythematous and painful, without blisters. They are usually described as looking like a sunburn. These do not count toward the total body surface area (TBSA) when calculating the burn size.
- **Second-degree burns** are characterized as superficial or deep partial-thickness burns. They are painful, and their color can vary from red to mottled to pale. Blisters may be thin- or thick-walled depending on the depth of the burn. *Superficial partial-thickness burns* are erythematous and have thin-walled fluid-filled blisters. These usually heal in 2–3 weeks without scarring. *Deep partial-thickness burns* extend further into the dermis, are usually pale pink or mottled, and have thick-walled blisters. These burns will usually heal in 3–9 weeks but tend to develop hypertrophic scars—surgical treatment is usually necessary.
- **Third-degree burns** involve all layers of the dermis. The skin is firm, white, or charred, and is often described as "leathery." This represents complete tissue destruction, and surgery is necessary except in the smallest of third-degree burns.
- **Fourth-degree burns** extend to deeper tissues including subcutaneous fat, muscle, and bone. Significant débridement and reconstruction are required.

    Kao CC, Garner WL: Acute burns. Plast Reconstr Surg 105:2482–2493, 2000.

8. **What is so concerning about circumferential full-thickness burns?**
As fluid leaks from damaged tissues into adjacent soft tissues, the leather-like full-thickness burn prevents tissue expansion, thus causing compression of internal structures. Circumferential burns of the neck can lead to airway compromise. Circumferential burns of the chest can lead to respiratory insufficiency. Circumferential burns to the extremities can cause vascular compromise similar to compartment syndrome. Evaluation of pulses and Doppler signals is absolutely necessary. Signs of poor perfusion to a distal extremity are cyanosis, deep tissue pain, paresthesias, and cold skin. Escharotomy is mandatory in this setting and can be performed by the emergency physician or a surgeon.

9. **How is TBSA calculated? Why is it important?**
Estimation of the percentage of body surface area burned helps direct fluid resuscitation, determines appropriate disposition of the burn patient, and allows meaningful communication with consultants and burn units. There are several methods to estimate TBSA. The rule of nines divides the regions of the body into approximate percentages of total surface area

(Fig. 97-1). The Lund and Browder chart has similar divisions but allows for variations in infancy and childhood (Fig. 97-2). With either chart, document the areas of second- and third-degree burns on the chart and calculate a total percentage of TBSA burned.

10. **What is burn shock?**
Burn shock is a complex interaction of intravascular fluid loss and release of vasoactive substances and inflammatory mediators. Initial fluid loss is due to tissue destruction at the burn site that causes increased vascular permeability. Fluid shifts into the extravascular space and is quickly lost through the damaged skin.

11. **How do you determine appropriate fluid resuscitation in the burn patient?**
The Parkland formula is a widely used calculation to estimate the initial fluid needs of the severely burned patient (greater than 20% TBSA). The fluid requirement (of lactated Ringer's solution) is calculated for the first 24 hours. One half of this is administered over the first 8 hours. The second half is administered over the following 16 hours.

$$\text{Fluid required} = \text{body weight(kg)} \times \text{TBSA (2nd and 3rd degree)} \times 4\text{mL}$$

Remember, this is an estimate. Monitor adequacy of fluid resuscitation by following vital signs and urine output. Goal urine output is 30 mL/h in adults and 1–2 mL/kg/h in children. (Don't forget the Foley catheter.)

12. **How do you manage a patient with burns *and* trauma?**
Patients with combined burns and trauma are at greater risk for morbidity and mortality than either alone. These patients are at higher risk for inhalation injury and tend to require greater fluid resuscitation than isolated burn patients. Generally, aggressive burn resuscitation should be started, and life-threatening traumatic injuries should be treated initially. Transfer to a burn unit can be delayed until the traumatic injuries have been stabilized.

Santaniello JM, Luchette FA, Esposito TJ, et al: Ten year experience of burn, trauma, and combined burn/trauma injuries comparing outcomes. J Trauma 57:696–701, 2004.

13. **What are the criteria for referral to a burn center?**
The American Burn Association has developed a list of criteria that warrant referral to a specialized burn unit. Their Website also contains a list of verified burn centers. Referral does not always require transfer to the burn unit but may include instruction in wound treatment or plans for follow-up.

- Partial-thickness burns > 10% TBSA
- Burns that involve the face, hands, feet, genitalia, perineum, or major joints
- Third-degree burns
- Electrical burns, including lightning injury
- Chemical burns
- Inhalation injury
- Burns in patients with preexisting medical disorders that could complicate management, prolong recovery, or affect mortality
- Any patient with burns and concomitant trauma in which the burn injury poses the greatest risk of morbidity or mortality

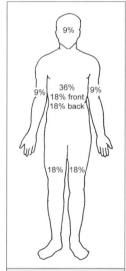

Figure 97-1.
Percentages used in determining extent of burn by "rule of nines." (From Miller RH: Textbook of Basic Emergency Medicine, 2nd ed. St. Louis, Mosby, 1980.)

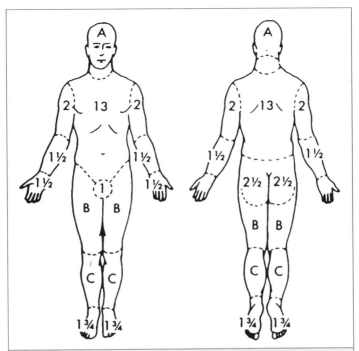

Figure 97-2. Classic Lund and Bowden chart. The best method for determining percentage of body surface burn is to mark areas of injury on a chart and then compute total percentage according to patient's age. (From Artz CP, Yarbrough DR III: Burns: Including cold, chemical, and electrical injuries. In Sabiston DC Jr [ed]: Textbook of Surgery, 11th ed. Philadelphia, W.B. Saunders, 1977.)

- Burned children in hospitals without qualified personnel or equipment for the care of children
- Burn injury in patients who will require special social, emotional, or long-term rehabilitative intervention

American Burn Association: www.ameriburn.org. Excerpted from Guidelines for the Operations of Burn Units, Resources for Optimal Care of the Injured Patient: Committee on Trauma, American College of Surgeons, 1999.

14. **Are there any burns that can be managed in the outpatient setting?**
Partial-thickness burns involving less than 10% TBSA or full-thickness burns involving less than 2% TBSA without risk of functional or cosmetic complications can usually be treated as an outpatient.

15. **How are outpatient burns treated in the ED?**
All burns should be cleaned with saline or water and a mild cleanser. Ruptured blisters should be débrided. There is controversy in the burn community over treatment of intact blisters; most sources recommend débridement of the blister or aspiration of the fluid to prevent infection of the blister fluid. Topical antibiotics such as bacitracin ointment or silver sulfadiazine should be applied liberally and covered with a nonadhesive dressing and a bulky bandage. Immobilization

may be necessary if the burn crosses a joint. The patient should follow up in 24 hours in the ED or with a physician experienced in burn care. If there are any questions concerning outpatient management, consultation with a burn center is appropriate.

16. **Is there anything special about facial burns?**
Facial burns should not be treated with silver sulfadiazine because it can cause pigmentation changes in the healing tissue. Antibiotic ointment alone, without dressings, is adequate for facial burns. Again, follow-up in 24 hours is recommended.

17. **What about pain control?**
Burns are painful, and large doses of narcotics are sometimes necessary. Intravenous (IV) narcotics can be started in the field and repeated if needed. Adequate pain control may require substantial doses of pain medications. These should only be withheld if administration is life threatening due to hemodynamic status. Also, don't forget to provide adequate oral analgesics for outpatient management. Superficial partial-thickness burns can be the most painful.

18. **Is there any role for cold water or ice in the treatment of burns?**
Initially, small burns can be cooled with saline-soaked gauze for short periods of time. Cold water applied to larger burns can result in systemic hypothermia and all the related complications. Ice should never be used, as it can cause further tissue damage.

19. **Should I check tetanus immunization status?**
Always check the status of tetanus immunization and update if needed.

20. **What are the special considerations in burn care in children?**
Children younger than 2 years have increased morbidity and mortality from burns. Consider admission even in minor burns in this age group. Do not forget the possibility of nonaccidental trauma. Ask about conditions around the home, and assess for safety. The reliability of the parents is another consideration in evaluating need for inpatient management of a pediatric burn. Do not forget that any suspicion of child abuse must be reported to child protective services.

21. **What are the special considerations in adults?**
Burn patients older than 60 years are at increased risk of morbidity and mortality from their injuries. Also, past medical history is important. Patients with human immunodeficiency virus (HIV), immune suppression (transplants, steroids), diabetes, cardiac disease, chronic obstructive pulmonary disease (COPD), or substance abuse may all require inpatient management of minor burns to monitor and treat complications of the chronic disease.

WEBSITE

American Burn Association: www.ameriburn.org

BIBLIOGRAPHY

1. Edlich RF, Bailey TL, Bill TJ: Thermal burns. In Marx JA, Hockberger RS, Walls RM, et al (eds): Rosen's Emergency Medicine Concepts and Clinical Practice, 5th ed. St. Louis, Mosby, 2002, pp 801–812.

2. Holmes JH, Heimbach DM: Burns. In Brunicardi FC, Andersen DK, Billiar TR, et al (eds): Schwartz's Principles of Surgery, 8th ed. New York, McGraw Hill, 2004, pp 189–204.

3. Schwartz LR, Balakrishnan C: Thermal burns. In Tintinalli JE, Kelen GD, Stapczynski JS (eds): Emergency Medicine: A Comprehensive Study Guide, 6th ed. New York, McGraw-Hill, 2004, pp 1220–1226.

4. Sheridan RL: Burns. Crit Care Med 30(11 suppl):S500–S514, 2002.

5. Sheridan RL: Burn care: Results of technical and organizational progress. JAMA 290:719–722, 2003.

CHAPTER 98

WOUND MANAGEMENT

Vincent J. Markovchick, MD

1. **Why is wound healing important?**
   Approximately 12 million traumatic wounds are treated in emergency departments (EDs) across the United States annually. This constitutes about 10% of all ED visits. Patients judge the competency of a physician based on their ultimate functional or cosmetic results and the development of complications.

2. **What is the difference between functional and cosmetic closure?**
   Functional closure is closure of a wound in such a fashion as to return the patient to earliest full use of the injured part. A **cosmetic repair** is one that is done so as to result in the least visible scarring.

3. **How do I remember what steps to take when repairing a wound?**
   Use the mnemonic **LACERATE:**
   - **L = Look.** Evaluate the wound to determine the most appropriate closure. Also be sure to examine thoroughly distal to the wound for movement, sensation, and pulsation.
   - **A = Anesthetize.**
   - **C = Clip and clean.** Clipping hair leads to less infection than shaving. Methodical irrigation is one of the best ways to decrease infection risk.
   - **E = Equipment.** Be prepared. Have everything needed for repair at the bedside, including laceration kit, sterile gloves, suture, and dressing.
   - **R = Repair.** Perform the repair. Devitalized tissue may need to be débrided.
   - **A = Assess results.** Reevaluate the wound when the repair is near completion to determine the need for additional sutures.
   - **T = Tetanus.** Give tetanus prophylaxis for dirty or contaminated wounds when the patient has not had a booster in 5 years or for clean wounds when the patient has not had a booster in 10 years.
   - **E = Educate.** Educate the patient on how to care for the wound, signs of infection, and the timing of suture removal.

4. **Which factors increase the visibility of scars and compromise wound healing? How are they minimized?**
   See Table 98-1 on the following page.

5. **What aspects of history should be obtained in a patient with a traumatic wound?**
   The time, setting, and mechanism of injury are essential because these features help determine whether the wound is contaminated, may contain a foreign body, or has the potential for infection. The patient's current medications and immune status (acquired immunodeficiency syndrome [AIDS], diabetes, chemotherapy), the patient's occupation, and dominant hand if a hand injury has occurred are important. The patient's tetanus immunization history and allergies (specifically regarding anesthetics, antibiotics, or latex gloves) must be obtained.

6. **What are the most important aspects of the physical examination?**
   To perform an adequate examination, it is important to be familiar with underlying anatomy, especially in the regions of the face, neck, hands, and feet. Examination of the injured site should

TABLE 98-1. MINIMIZING FACTORS THAT INCREASE VISIBILITY OF SCARS

Contributing Factors	Methods to Minimize Scarring
Direction of wound, e.g., perpendicular to lines of static and dynamic tension	Layered closure; proper direction in elective incisions of wound
Infection necessitating removal of sutures débridement, resulting in healing by secondary intention and a wide scar	Proper wound preparation; irrigation, and use of delayed closure in contaminated wounds
Wide scar secondary to tension	Layered closure; proper splinting and elevation
Suture marks	Remove all percutaneous sutures within 7 days
Uneven wound edges resulting in magnification edges and of scar by shadows	Careful, even approximation of wound top layer closure to prevent differential swelling of edges
Inversion of wound edges	Proper placement of simple sutures or use of horizontal mattress sutures
Tattooing secondary to retained dirt or foreign body	Proper wound preparation and débridement
Tissue necrosis	Use of corner sutures on flaps, splinting, and elevation of wounds with marginal circulation or venous return; excise nonviable wound edges before closure
Compromised healing secondary to hematoma	Use of properly conforming dressing and splints
Hyperpigmentation of scar or abraded skin	Use of 15 or greater SPF sunblock for 6 months
Superimposition of blood clots between healing frequent wound edges	Proper hemostasis and closure; H_2O_2 swabbing; proper application of compressive dressings
Failure to align anatomic structures properly such as vermilion border	Meticulous closure and alignment; marking or placement of alignment suture before distortion of wound edges with local anesthesia; use of field block

From Markovchick V: Suture materials and mechanical after care. Emerg Med Clin North Am 10:673–689, 1992.

begin with identification of any motor, sensory, and vascular deficits. With extremity injuries, examination can be conducted in the absence of hemorrhage by temporarily inflating a sphygmomanometer or placement of a finger tourniquet proximal to the injury. Palpation of the bones adjacent to the site of injury may detect instability or point tenderness of an underlying fracture. Direct inspection always should be performed when there is a suspicion of a tendon or joint capsule injury or presence of a foreign body.

7. **What is the most important step I can take to prevent infection?**
For all traumatic wounds, irrigation with normal saline at 8–10 psi should be done with a >18G or 19G needle and a 30-mL syringe. The optimal volume of irrigant has not been determined; however, 60 mL per centimeter of wound length has been used as a guideline. In the presence of gross contamination, copious irrigation should be done and débridement considered. Although diluted 1% povidone-iodine (Betadine) solution is not likely to cause significant tissue injury, its use has not been shown to produce a significant benefit when compared with saline. Exploration; débridement when indicated; hemostasis; and proper repair, dressing, and immobilization are essential adjuncts for proper wound management. Antibiotics have no proven prophylactic benefit in the normal host. For contaminated or dirty extensive wounds, a mechanical irrigation device should be used to remove all dirt and decrease the bacterial count. A stiff brush, such as a toothbrush or sharp debridement should be used to remove dirt that remains after irrigation.

8. **Which anesthetic agent should be used for local anesthesia?**
Selection of an appropriate anesthetic depends on many factors, including age of the patient, underlying health, prior drug reactions, wound size and location, and practice environment in the ED. Lidocaine traditionally has been the standard agent for local anesthesia in the ED; however, bupivacaine has advantages over lidocaine, related mainly to duration of anesthesia. Patients receiving bupivacaine experience significantly less discomfort during the 6-hour postinfiltration period. Also, in a busy ED, use of bupivacaine may prevent the need to reanesthetize a wound when repair has been interrupted by the arrival of a higher acuity patient.

9. **What causes the pain of local anesthetic infiltration, and how can it be prevented?**
Pain from the infiltration of lidocaine and bupivacaine is caused by distention of tissue from too-rapid injection with too large a needle directly into the dermis. Also, these agents are acidic, which causes pain. Pain from infiltration can be minimized by injecting slowly, subcutaneously, with a small, 25G or 27G needle, directly through the wound margins. Pain from infiltration can be reduced by buffering the anesthetic agent with 1 mL of sodium bicarbonate for every 10 mL of lidocaine. Bupivacaine does not lend itself to buffering because it precipitates as its pH rises. Warming of lidocaine and bupivacaine is an efficacious and inexpensive method of decreasing the pain of infiltration.

10. **What is the toxic dose of lidocaine and bupivacaine?**
Table 98-2 summarizes the maximum dose and duration of action of lidocaine, bupivacaine, and procaine, alone and in combination with epinephrine. When calculating the dose of milligrams infiltrated, 1 mL of 1% lidocaine = 10 mg of lidocaine, and 1 mL of 0.25% bupivacaine = 2.5 mg of bupivacaine. Lower maximal doses should be used for patients with

TABLE 98-2. MAXIMUM DOSE AND DURATION OF ACTION OF ANESTHETICS			
Anesthetic	Class	Maximum Dose	Duration
Lidocaine	Amide	4.5 mg/kg	1–2 h
Lidocaine with epinephrine	Amide	7 mg/kg	2–4 h
Bupivacaine	Amide	2 mg/kg	4–8 h
Bupivacaine with epinephrine	Amide	3 mg/kg	8–16 h
Procaine	Ester	7 mg/kg	15–45 min
Procaine with epinephrine	Ester	9 mg/kg	30–60 min

chronic illness, for very young or very old patients, or when infiltrating highly vascular areas or mucous mucosa.

11. **Describe the presentation of lidocaine toxicity.**
In general, toxicity should not occur unless the recommended dosing is met or exceeded. The caveat to that statement is that toxicity may take place at lower than maximal doses when infiltrating highly vascular areas or mucous membranes or in patients at the extremes of age or chronically ill patients. The main effects are on the central nervous and cardiovascular systems. Central nervous system effects present as lightheadedness, nystagmus, and sensory disturbances, including visual aura or scotoma, tinnitus, perioral tingling, or a metallic taste in the mouth. Slurred speech, disorientation, muscle twitching, and finally seizures may follow. The cardiovascular effects are manifested by hypotension, bradycardia, and prolonged electrocardiogram (ECG) intervals. In severe toxicity, the end result is coma and cardiorespiratory arrest.

12. **What can I use to anesthetize a patient who is allergic to amide and ester anesthetics?**
Subdermal diphenhydramine may be injected locally to obtain short-acting analgesia. Prepare a 0.5–1.0% solution by diluting 1 mL of 50 mg/mL diphenhydramine into 5–10 mL of saline. The anesthetic effect may take several minutes to become evident. Do not exceed a total dose of 50 mg in adults or 1 mg/kg in children. The patient may become drowsy after the injection.

13. **What are the contraindications to epinephrine as an adjunct to lidocaine and bupivacaine?**
Anesthetics with epinephrine should not be used on digits, on pinna, circumferentially around the penis, or in areas with poor or marginal blood supply, such as flap wounds of the anterior pretibial area. Epinephrine decreases resistance to infection because of its potent vasoconstrictor effect. In areas of the body such as the scalp and face, the vasoconstriction and resulting hemostasis aid in the exploration and repair of the wound and do not seem to increase wound infection.

14. **What is LET (LAT)?**
A topical anesthetic that consists of a mixture of **lidocaine** (4%), **epinephrine (adrenaline)** 1:1000, and **tetracaine** (0.5%). LET has been shown to be efficacious for wound anesthesia. It has a good margin of safety. It is now the topical agent of choice. For optimal effect it should be placed directly into the wound.

15. **What are the contraindications to LET?**
They are the same as for lidocaine or bupivacaine with epinephrine.

16. **When do I use procedural sedation?**
Procedural sedation is a pharmacologic means of lowering the level of consciousness for procedures to be performed easily with optimal results. See Chapter 65.

17. **What is a contaminated wound?**
Any wound that has a high inoculum of bacteria. Some examples are full-thickness bites; wounds of the perineum or axilla in which there is normally a high skin flora count; and wounds that are exposed to contaminated water, such as from ponds, lakes, or coral reefs.

18. **List factors that contribute to wound infection.**
- Wound age
- Presence of foreign material

- Amount of devitalized tissue
- Presence of bacterial contamination
- Advanced patient age
- Ability of the host to mount an adequate immune response

19. **Is a dirty wound the same as a contaminated wound?**
No. **Road rash,** resulting from road gravel, has a low bacterial count. In contrast, wounds that occur in a barnyard or are exposed to soil contaminated with fecal material have a high bacterial count and are contaminated.

20. **What causes tattooing?**
The retention of foreign material and incorporation of it in the dermis during the healing process. To prevent this cosmetic complication, all foreign material and dirt must be removed through proper débridement, scrubbing, and irrigation at the time of the initial patient encounter. A stiff brush, such as a toothbrush, and soap is useful to remove dirt and asphalt embedded in the dermis.

21. **How do I treat road rash?**
Anesthetize the area with viscous lidocaine and circumferential or field block anesthesia. Remove all foreign bodies with the methods described previously. Consider dressing with **silver sulfadiazine,** which greatly reduces the pain and may obviate the need the potent oral analgesics for deep, extensive, painful abrasions.

22. **When do I get an x-ray?**
Radiographs are useful to search for a foreign body or to look for an associated fracture. Obtain a radiograph if the history is suspicious for a foreign body (e.g., broken glass) and the wound penetrates muscle fascia or the entire depth of the wound cannot be visualized. In the case of some bite wounds or lip lacerations with broken or avulsed teeth, radiographs should be considered to search for teeth. With severe pain or structural instability, radiographs may reveal an underlying open fracture, which necessitates an orthopedic consultation in most cases.

23. **Which type of foreign bodies found in wounds are visible on radiographs?**
Glass, metal, and gravel. In general, glass larger than 2 mm and gravel larger than 1 mm can be seen on radiographs. Foreign bodies that are radiolucent (not visible on radiographs) include wood, plastics, and some aluminum products.

24. **What is the best method for hair removal?**
Clipping or cutting hair with scissors as opposed to shaving has been shown to result in lower wound bacterial counts and decreased rates of infection.

25. **Define the three different types of wound closure.**
- **Primary closure** is closure of wound margins with sutures, staples, glues, or adhesive tapes no longer than 24 hours after injury.
- **Delayed primary closure** is closure of a wound 3–5 days after wounding to decrease the risk of infection.
- **Secondary closure,** or healing by secondary intention, is allowing a wound to heal by granulation without mechanical approximation of the wound margins.

26. **Which wounds should be closed primarily?**
Any clean (not initially contaminated) wound if it is less than 6–8 hours old and is located anywhere on the body except for the face and scalp, which may be closed primarily up to 24 hours because of the rich vascular supply and resistance to infection.

27. **When should secondary closure be used?**
For contaminated wounds that penetrate deeply into tissue and cannot be irrigated adequately before closure. Examples of such wounds are puncture wounds of the sole of the foot or palm of the hand and stab wounds that penetrate into subcutaneous tissue and muscle.

28. **When should delayed primary closure be used?**
It should be strongly considered for all contaminated wounds that are gaping or have significant amounts of tension. It decreases the risk of infection, optimizes the cosmetic result, and accelerates the healing process.

29. **How is a wound prepared for delayed primary closure?**
The wound should be examined thoroughly, prepared, débrided, and irrigated. Hemorrhage should be controlled. A fine layer of mesh gauze should be laid in the wound; the wound should be packed open and followed closely. At 3–5 days, if there is no purulent drainage or wound-margin erythema, the wound may be closed in the same fashion as if it were being closed primarily.

30. **What is the most important step when closing a lip laceration through the vermilion border?**
Placement of the first suture at the vermilion border. Use nonabsorbable suture to close the edges of the vermilion border. Be sure to line up the edges precisely. The remainder of the lip should be closed with absorbable suture. The skin should be closed with nonabsorbable suture.

31. **When are surgical staples indicated?**
To reapproximate linear lacerations that do not involve cosmetically sensitive areas, such as the face. Two approaches are commonly employed. One approach involves two operators with one everting both wound edges with forceps while the other staples the wound together. If only one operator is available, the wound edges should be aligned and one edge everted with forceps in one hand while stapling with the other. Staples work best in wounds that are perpendicular, that is, 90 degrees to the surface, rather than with shelving angular lacerations because these tend to overlap.

32. **What is surgical glue, and how is it used?**
2-Octyl cyanoacrylate (Dermabond) is a polymer currently being used as an alternative for wound repair. Cyanoacrylate acts rapidly, polymerizing within 30 seconds at room air. It is best used for linear lacerations under low tension and may replace 5–0 or 6–0 sutures. The wound can be held together manually, and the cyanoacrylate can be painted over the wound in three to four coats to ensure adequate closure. Be careful not to apply any adhesive within the wound because this will impede healing. The adhesive sloughs off in 7–10 days. Do not use antibiotic ointment or any other type of ointment on the wound because it destroys the adhesive bond.

33. **How do I remove tissue adhesive?**
First, avoid getting tissue adhesive into undesirable areas by applying protective covering and petroleum jelly to areas surrounding the wound. Apply light coats of the adhesive and quickly wipe off excess fluid. You have about 15 seconds before the adhesive dries. If the adhesive dries on an undesirable area (e.g., eyelid glued shut), the bond may be loosened with petroleum jelly or antibiotic ointment.

34. **Summarize the advantages and disadvantages of the available techniques for wound closure.**
See Table 98-3.

TABLE 98-3. ADVANTAGES AND DISADVANTAGES OF WOUND CLOSURE TECHNIQUES

Technique	Advantages	Disadvantages
Sutures	Time-honored method	Removal required
	Meticulous closure	Anesthesia required
	Greatest tensile strength	Greatest tissue reactivity
	Lowest dehiscence rate	Slowness of application
Staples	Rapidity of application	Less meticulous closure than with sutures
	Low tissue reactivity	May interfere with CT and MRI
	Low cost	May result in uneven wound edges
Tissue adhesives	Rapidity of application	Lower tensile strength than sutures
	Patient comfort	Dehiscence over high-tension areas (joints)
	Resistance to bacterial growth	Will inhibit wound healing if placed in the wound
	No need for removal	High cost
	No risk of needle stick	
Surgical tapes	Least tissue reactivity	Lower tensile strength than sutures
	Lowest infection rates	Highest rate of dehiscence
	Rapidity of application	Cannot be used in hairy areas
	Patient comfort	Must remain dry
	Low cost	

CT = computed tomography, MRI = magnetic resonance imaging.
From Singer AJ, Hollander JE, Quinn JV: Evaluation and management of traumatic lacerations. N Engl J Med 337:1142–1148, 1997, with permission.

35. **Which sutures are used, how is the wound repaired, and when do I remove the sutures?**
See Table 98-4.

36. **How are bites treated?**
See Fig. 98-1.

37. **What should be included in all follow-up instructions?**
Instructions on local wound care, signs of infection, and time of suture removal. Antimicrobial ointment may be applied to decrease the risk of infection; however, when tissue adhesives have been used, ointments dissolve the adhesive and may cause separation of the wound. Sunlight should be avoided, and sunscreen should be used to help minimize hyperpigmentation and scarring. Inform patients that all wounds will heal with a scar, all wounds may get infected, and all wounds may have retained foreign material.

TABLE 98-4. USE OF SUTURES FOR WOUND REPAIR

Location	Suture Material	Technique of Closure and Dressing	Suture Removal
Scalp	3-0 or 4-0 nylon or polypropylene	Interrupted in galea; single tight layer in scalp; horizontal mattress if bleeding not well controlled by simple sutures	7–12 days
Pinna (ear)	6-0 nylon or 5-0 SA in perichondrium	Close perichondrium with 5-0 SA interrupted; close skin with 6-0 nylon interrupted; stint dressing	4–6 days
Eyebrow	4-0 or 5-0 SA and 6-0 nylon	Layered closure	4–5 days
Eyelid	6-0 nylon or silk	Single layer horizontal mattress	3–5 days
Lip	4-0 silk or SA (mucosa) 5-0 SA (Sq, muscle); 6-0 (skin); 4-0 SA	Three layers (mucosa, muscle, skin) if through and through, otherwise two layers	3–5 days
Oral cavity	4-0 SA	Simple interrupted or horizontal mattress; layered closure if the muscularis of the tongue is involved	7–8 days or allow to dissolve
Face	4-0 or 5-0 SA (Sq); 6-0 nylon (skin)	If full-thickness laceration, layered closure desirable	3–5 days
Neck	4-0 SA (Sq); 5-0 nylon (skin)	Two-layered closure for best cosmetic results	4–6 days
Trunk	4-0 SA (Sq, fat); 4-0 or 5-0 nylon (skin)	Single or layered closure	7–12 days
Extremity	3-0 or 4-0 SA (Sq, fat, muscle); 4-0 or 5-0 nylon (skin)	Single or layered closure is adequate, although a layered or running Sq closure may give a better cosmetic result; apply a splint if the wound is over a joint	7–14 days
Hands and feet	4-0 or 5-0 nylon	Single-layer closure only with simple or interrupted horizontal mattress suture, at least 5 mm from cut wound edges; horizontal mattress sutures should be used if there is much tension on wound edges; apply splint if wound is over a joint	7–12 days
Nailbeds	5-0 SA	Gentle, meticulous placement to obtain even edges. Replace nail under cuticle	Allow to dissolve

SA = synthetic absorbable sutures such as Vicryl and Dexon, Sq = subcutaneous.
From Markovchick V: Soft tissue injury and wound repair. In Reisdorff EJ, Roberts MR, Wiegenstein JG (eds): Pediatric Emergency Medicine. Philadelphia, W.B. Saunders, 1993, pp 899–908.

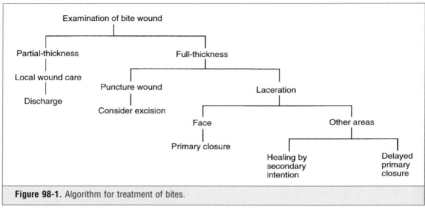

Figure 98-1. Algorithm for treatment of bites.

38. **How do I remember the direction of the lines of skin tension?**
    You don't, unless you have a photographic memory. Refer to Figs. 98-2 and 98-3.

39. **Are there any controversies in wound care?**
    The primary controversy relates to the use of prophylactic antibiotics. Their use is widespread and has developed with little scientific support. In general, the use of prophylactic antibiotics is not warranted in the normal host. Antibiotic therapy is indicated in patients with soft tissue wounds who are prone to infective endocarditis. Antibiotics may be indicated when the risk for infection is high, including wounds of the distal foot; contaminated wounds; wounds in which there has been a delay in irrigation and débridement; and wounds that contain fecal material, pus, saliva, or vaginal secretions. Prophylactic antibiotic use should never replace proper wound decontamination. To meet the "standard of care," as perceived by many, and to decrease cost to the patient, generic antibiotics should be used.

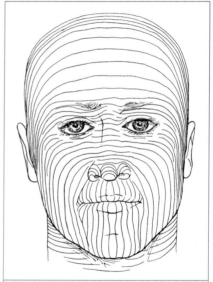

Figure 98-2. Direction of the lines of skin tension for the face. (From Marx J, Hockberger R, Well R, et al [eds]: Rosen's Emergency Medicine: Concepts and Clinical Practice, 5th ed. Philadelphia, Mosby, 2002, p 738.)

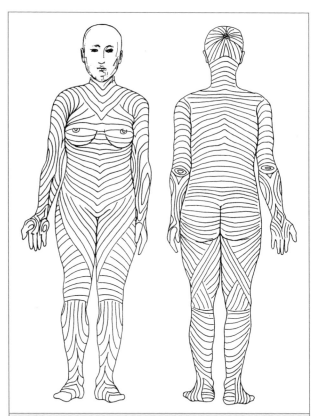

Figure 98-3. Direction of the lines of skin tension for the body. (From Marx J, Hockberger R, Well R, et al [eds]: Rosen's Emergency Medicine: Concepts and Clinical Practice, 5th ed. Philadelphia, Mosby, 2002, p 739.)

KEY POINTS: WOUND MANAGEMENT

1. Use a tourniquet, if necessary, on extremities to adequately examine and repair the wound.

2. Irrigation pressure must be at least 8 psi.

3. Wounds may be irrigated with tap water or sterile saline.

4. If soap is used, irrigation should follow.

5. A stiff brush (toothbrush) will remove ground-in dirt.

BIBLIOGRAPHY

1. Hollander JE, Singer AJ: Wound management. In Harwood-Nuss AL, Wolfson AB (eds): The Clinical Practice of Emergency Medicine, 3rd ed. Philadelphia, Lippincott Williams & Wilkins, 2005, pp 912–921.

2. Hollander JE, Singer AJ, Valentine SM, Shofer FS: Risk factors for infection in patients with traumatic lacerations. Acad Emerg Med 8:716–720, 2001.

3. Howell JM, Chishholm CD: Wound care. Emerg Med Clin North Am 15:417–425, 1997.

4. Markovchick V: Suture materials and mechanical after care. Emerg Med Clin North Am 10:673–689, 1992.

5. Markovchick V: Soft tissue injury wound repair. In Reisdorf EJ, Roberts MR, Wiegenstein JG (eds): Pediatric Emergency Medicine. Philadelphia, W.B. Saunders, 1993, pp 899–908.

6. Markovchick V: Soft tissue injuries. In Barkin R, Rosen P (eds): Emergency Pediatrics: A Guide to Ambulatory Care. Philadelphia, Mosby, 2003, pp 505–514.

7. Schilling CG, Bank DE, Borchert BA, Klatzko MD: Tetracaine, epinephrine (adrenaline), and cocaine (TAC) versus lidocaine, epinephrine, and tetracaine (LET) for anesthesia of lacerations in children. Ann Emerg Med 25:203–208, 1995.

8. Simon B, Hern HJ: Wound management principles. In Marx J, Hockberger R, Well R, et al (eds): Rosen's Emergency Medicine, 6th ed. Philadelphia, Mosby, 2006, pp 842–858.

9. Singer AJ, Hollander JE, Quinn JV: Evaluation and management of traumatic lacerations. N Engl J Med 337:1142–1148, 1997.

10. Wilson JL, Kocurek K, Doty BJ: A systematic approach to laceration repair: tricks to ensure the desired cosmetic result. Postgrad Med 107:77–88, 2000.

ACUTE PSYCHOSIS

Eugene E. Kercher, MD

CHAPTER 99

1. What is acute psychosis?

Psychosis is a dysfunction in the capacity for thought and information processing. The individual is unable to coherently perceive, retain, process, recall, or act on information in a consensually validated way. There is a decreased ability to willfully mobilize, shift, sustain, and direct attention. A major feature of the psychotic state is the failure in ranking the priority of stimuli. The ability to act on reality is unpredictable and diminished because the patient is unable to distinguish internal from external stimuli.

2. What is the difference between organic and functional psychosis?

- **Organic psychosis** refers to a reversible or nonreversible dysfunctional mental condition that can be identified as a disturbance in the anatomy, physiology, or biochemistry of the brain.
- **Functional psychosis** refers to a dysfunctional mental condition identified as schizophrenia, a major affective disorder, or other mental disorders with psychotic features.

3. What are the types of psychoses?

Classification of psychosis is found in the *Diagnostic and Statistical Manual of Mental Disorders (DSM-IV-TR)*, which is divided appropriately into functional and organic varieties. Most organically caused acute psychoses result from dementia, withdrawal states, and intoxications. Schizophrenia and the affective disorders are the major contributors to functionally caused acute psychoses.

American Psychiatric Association: Diagnostic and Statistical Manual of Mental Disorders, 4th ed, revised. Washington, DC, American Psychiatric Association, 2000, pp 297–343.

Allen M: Managing the agitated psychotic patient: A reappraisal of the evidence. J Clin Psychiatry 61:11–20, 2000.

4. List the possible causes of alcohol-related organic psychosis.

- Chronic alcoholism
- Thiamine deficiency (i.e., diet, starvation, and emesis)
- Alcohol-dependent withdrawal states
- Comorbid substance abuse
- Comorbid psychotic and mood disorder
- Alcohol idiosyncratic intoxication (pathologic intoxication)

Bresler RE, Klinger BI, Erickson BJ: Acute intoxication and substance abuse among patients presenting to a psychiatric emergency service. Gen Hospital Psychiatry 18:183, 1996.

5. Is there a brief, self-limited, and nonorganic psychosis?

Yes. Some individuals may become acutely and briefly psychotic after exposure to an extremely traumatic experience. If such a psychosis lasts for fewer than 4 weeks, it is termed a brief psychotic disorder. Precipitants of the psychosis include the death of a loved one or a life-threatening situation, such as combat or a natural disaster, or other life stressors. Patients with hysterical, borderline, and narcissistic personalities are prone to brief psychotic disorder, and some studies support a genetic vulnerability. Emotional turmoil, confusion, and extremely bizarre behavior and speech are common symptoms on presentation.

6. **How does a patient in a psychotic state typically present to the emergency department (ED)?**
Patients who are in a psychotic state may act strangely (i.e., mannerisms, posturing), dress bizarrely, respond to hallucinations, harbor false and delusional beliefs, and consistently confuse the reality of events. They are frequently impulsive and in constant danger of acting on distorted perceptions or delusional ideas resulting in unintentional injury or death. Clarity of oneself and the environment is consistently blurred. The patient is unable to discriminate the stimuli that he or she perceives. Thinking is disorganized and incoherent, as evidenced from the patient's speech. Memory is impaired in registration, retention, and recall. Orientation may be impaired, especially for time. Psychomotor behavior may be hypoactive or hyperactive. Emotions can range from apathy and depression to fear and rage.

7. **Why does the psychotic patient come to the ED?**
Psychotic patients frequently are brought to the ED by relatives or friends who no longer can safely control the patient's behavior. Frequently, a psychotic patient is brought in by police or paramedics because the psychotic condition has become potentially dangerous to self or others. Some patients come to the ED seeking refuge from their overwhelming fears.

8. **Why is it important to control psychotic behavior immediately?**
Patients who present in a psychotic state have no impulse control. They cannot distinguish internal from external stimuli and are unable to prioritize their reactions to them. Because of this dysfunction, they should always be considered a significant danger to themselves or to others.

9. **How can the potential for violent behavior be detected in the psychotic patient?**
The best way to deal with violent behavior is to prevent it. Emergency physicians should recognize patients who are obviously confused, irrational, paranoid, or excited. Emergency physicians must also develop an intuitive vigilance to detect the possibility of violence in patients who present more rationally and less floridly psychotic. Any history or comment that suggests violence should be taken seriously. The potential for violence in general is particularly high in patients who are psychotic secondary to illicit drug use.

10. **Are there behavioral controls that can be used immediately for the psychotic patient?**
Yes. Recognizing the chance of violence and physical harm, definitive steps should be taken to avoid confrontation:
- **Environmental:** Keep the environment simple and stimuli-free, and minimize staff changes.
- **Interpersonal:** Assume the role of patient advocate, and engage the patient in a calm and self-assured voice. Recognize the patient's right to privacy and dignity.

KEY POINTS: ACUTE PSYCHOSIS

1. No impulse control

2. Least restrictive restraint

3. Inadequate history

4. Organic versus functional

5. No support system

11. **What option can be exercised if the patient becomes increasingly disorganized and agitated?**
Institute a formalized and rehearsed physical restraint plan (see Chapter 101). On summons by the physician, security guards should appear at the door, so the patient can see and feel their presence. This "show of force" indicates that any display of violence will not be tolerated and often helps the patient to organize and regain control of his or her thoughts and behavior. When the patient is physically restrained, he or she should be searched thoroughly for weapons or sharp objects.

12. **Are there further methods of control if the patient continues to experience acute agitated psychotic behavior?**
Always use the least restrictive form of restraint: isolation → restraints → psychotropic medication. The gold standard medical treatment for acute agitated psychosis is still parental haloperidol plus lorazepam or diphenhydramine. There is no evidence that atypical antipsychotic medications are more efficacious or cost effective. Anxiolytic medication can be helpful in the acute presentation.

Wright P, Birkett M, David SR, et al: Double-blind, placebo-controlled comparison of intramuscular olanzapine and intramuscular haloperidol in the treatment of acute agitation in schizophrenia. Am J Psychiatry 158:1149–1151, 2001.

13. **How should priorities be set when I first encounter a psychotic patient?**
    1. Assess ABCs (airway, breathing, circulation) (if necessary).
    2. Observe (quickly assess impulse control and tendency to physically act out).
    3. Control and manage psychotic behavior (if necessary).
    4. Obtain a history (gather from everyone who has been involved with the patient).
    5. Differentiate between organic and functional causes via a formal mental status examination.
    6. Do a physical examination, to include a complete set of vital signs.
    7. Obtain laboratory (toxicologic and metabolic studies) tests as deemed appropriate and a head computed tomography (CT) scan on first psychotic breaks if not drug induced.
    8. Obtain psychiatric consultation and disposition.

14. **What are other sources of information for psychotic patients, who are usually historically unreliable?**
Because acutely psychotic patients may not be able to provide an adequate history, all available sources for obtaining information must be explored. This may include speaking to emergency medical services (EMS) personnel, family, friends, neighbors, and law enforcement officers and reviewing old medical records. A telephone conversation with caregivers and significant others can also be helpful.

15. **What historical information is important?**
    1. Onset. Did the behavior change suddenly or gradually?
    2. Longitudinal course. What was the precipitating event? Is this the first such event? What was the behavior like on previous events?
    3. Psychosocial setting. Establish some idea regarding the patient's support system.
    4. Previous psychiatric disease, that is, organic brain disease, the use or misuse of medication, history of illicit drug use.

16. **List pharmacologic agents that can cause acute psychosis.**
    - Digitalis
    - Corticosteroids
    - Isoniazid (INH)
    - Disulfiram (Antabuse)

- Tricyclics
- Anticonvulsants
- Cimetidine
- Benzodiazepines
- Amphetamines and related drugs
- Antiarrhythmics
- Narcotics
- Barbiturates
- Methyldopa
- Nonsteroidal anti-inflammatory drugs
- Anticancer agents
- Recreational drugs

17. **How should my physical examination be tailored for a psychotic patient?**
Always note the vital signs and pulse oximetry readings. Defer any examinations that require undressing. Start with the head, neck, and neurologic examination. In most cases, emergency physicians will have built sufficient rapport with patients in time for the cooperation necessary for a more intimate examination. Tell the patient exactly what you are doing and what you are going to do during the examination. This helps to provide structure for the psychotic patient and avoids confusion or misunderstanding. Touching the patient with a stethoscope first often is less threatening than direct physical contact.

18. **Is laboratory screening necessary in an appropriate work-up of an acute psychotic patient?**
Most laboratory investigations provide little help during the acute evaluation of a psychotic episode. The following tests are recommended if an organic cause is considered or an admission is anticipated: complete blood count, electrolytes, toxicology screens, urinalysis, thyroid function tests.

19. **Summarize the key points to consider in the differentiation of organic from functional psychosis.**
See Table 99-1.

20. **Name the life-threatening causes of acute psychosis.**
WHHHIMP mnemonic:
- **W** = **W**ernicke's encephalopathy
- **H** = **H**ypoxia or hypoperfusion of the central nervous system
- **H** = **H**ypoglycemia
- **H** = **H**ypertensive encephalopathy
- **I** = **I**ntracerebral hemorrhage
- **M** = **M**eningitis/encephalitis
- **P** = **P**oisonings

21. **Are there any other clinical "rules of thumb" in the work-up of the acute psychotic patient?**
- Fever and psychosis = meningitis
- Acute psychosis and alcoholism = Wernicke's encephalopathy
- Headache and psychosis = tumor or intracranial hemorrhage
- Abdominal pain and psychosis = porphyria
- Sweating and psychosis = hypoglycemia or delirium tremens
- Autonomic signs and psychosis = toxic or metabolic encephalopathy

TABLE 99-1. MADFOCS MNEMONIC		
	Organic	Functional
M = Memory deficit	Recent impaired	Remote impaired
A = Activity	Hyperactivity and hypoactivity	Repetitive activity
	Tremor	Posturing
	Ataxia	Rocking
D = Distortions	Visual hallucinations	Auditory hallucinations
F = Feelings	Emotional lability	Flat affect
O = Orientation	Disoriented	Oriented
C = Cognition	Some lucid thoughts	No lucid thoughts
	Perceives occasionally	Unfiltered perceptions
	Attends occasionally	Unable to attend
	Focuses occasionally	Unable to focus
S = Some other findings	Age >40	Age <40
	Sudden onset	Gradual onset
	Physical exam often abnormal	Physical exam normal
	Vital signs may be abnormal	Vital signs usually normal
	Social immodesty	Social modesty
	Aphasia	Intelligible speech
	Consciousness impaired	Alert, awake
	Confabulation	Ambivalence

22. **Summarize the potentially reversible causes of psychosis.**
    DEMENTIA mnemonic:
    - **D** = **D**rug toxicity
    - **E** = **E**motional disorders
    - **M** = **M**etabolic disorders
    - **E** = **E**ndocrine disorders
    - **N** = **N**utritional disorders
    - **T** = **T**umors and trauma
    - **I** = **I**nfection
    - **A** = **A**rteriosclerotic complications

23. **What are the three basic questions to answer regarding the disposition of the psychotic patient?**
    - Is there risk of suicide or homicide?
    - Is there realistic social support or supervision?
    - What is the patient's initial response to medication?

24. **When should hospitalization be recommended?**
    - If this is the patient's first psychotic episode
    - If the patient is a danger to self or others
    - If the patient is unable to care for self appropriately
    - If the patient has no social support system
    - If the functional psychotic patient is not sufficiently clear after initial ED tranquilization
    - If an acute organic psychosis does not clear while the patient is in the ED

WEBSITE

Massachusetts College of Emergency Physicians, Massachusetts Psychiatric Society: Consensus guidelines on the medical clearance exam for the evaluation and management of the psychiatric patient in the emergency department. 1999. www.macep.org/ practice_information/medical_clearance.htm, January 2003.

BIBLIOGRAPHY

1. American College of Emergency Physicians: Clinical policy for the initial approach to patients presenting with altered mental status. Ann Emerg Med 33:251–281, 1999.
2. Battaglia J, Moss S, Rush J, et al: Haloperidol, lorazepam, or both for psychotic agitation? A multicenter, prospective, double-blind, emergency department study. Am J Emerg Med 15:335, 1997.
3. Broderick KB, Lerner EB, McCourt JD, et al: Emergency physician practices and requirements regarding the medical screening examination of psychiatric patients. Acad Emerg Med 9:88–92, 2002.
4. Frame DS, Kercher EE: Acute psychosis: Functional vs. organic. Emerg Med Clin North Am 9:123–136, 1991.
5. Hillard JF: Emergency treatment of acute psychosis. J Clin Psychiatry 59:57, 1998.
6. Hockberger RS, Richards J: Thought disorders. In Marx JA, et al (eds): Rosen's Emergency Medicine: Concepts Clinical Practice, 5th ed. Mosby, St. Louis, 2002, pp 1541–1548.
7. Kercher EE: Acute psychosis. In Rund DA, Barkin RM, Rosen P, Sternbach GL (eds): Essentials of Emergency Medicine, 2nd ed. Mosby, St. Louis, 1996, pp 647–655.
8. Yildiz A, Sachs GS, Turgay A: Pharmacological management of agitation in emergency settings. Emerg Med J 20:339–346, 2003.
9. Zun LS, Leikin JB, Stotland NL, et al: A tool for the emergency medicine evaluation of psychiatric patients. Am J Emerg Med 14:329–333, 1996.

CHAPTER 100

DEPRESSION AND SUICIDE

Douglas A. Rund, MD, and Richard A. Nockowitz, MD

DEPRESSION

1. **What are the symptoms of depression?**

   The cardinal symptoms of depression are a **dysphoric or sad mood, and a loss of interests or enjoyment.** To diagnose depression, one of these must be present at least half of the time over a 2-week period. There must also be at least four of the following symptoms during this same period: sleep disturbance, feelings of guilt or worthlessness, lack of energy, decreased concentration or ability to make decisions, appetite disturbance (usually diminished), psychomotor changes (agitated or slowed), and suicidal thinking. The mnemonic **SIG E CAPS** can be remembered by thinking of what you want to do for depressed patients (figuratively): "prescribe energy capsules."

   Four of the following are necessary for the diagnosis of depression, one of which must be the "I"—loss of interests or depressed mood:

S = **S**leep disturbance	**C** = **C**oncentration
I = **I**nterests/mood	**A** = **A**ppetite disturbance
G = **G**uilt	**P** = **P**sychomotor changes
E = **E**nergy	**S** = **S**uicidal thinking

2. **Why is depression considered a mood disorder?**

   Mood refers to a person's internal state, as subjectively experienced and reported by that person. *Affect* is a person's outward appearance, as objectively experienced by another. The term *mood disorder* has essentially replaced *affective disorder* in much of the psychiatric literature and communications. The main mood disorders are major depression (or unipolar disorder), which is exclusively depression, and manic-depression (or bipolar disorder), which is depression with a history of at least one manic episode.

3. **What is the difference between primary and secondary depression?**

   Major depression is classified as **primary** if the symptom complex appears before or is causally unrelated to any other significant medical or psychiatric illness. It is considered **secondary** when it follows and is causally related to other medical or psychiatric illness.

4. **List medical conditions that might cause secondary depression.**

   Endocrine disorders
   - Hypothyroidism
   - Diabetes mellitus
   - Cushing's syndrome

   Neurologic disorders
   - Cerebrovascular accidents
   - Subdural hematoma
   - Multiple sclerosis
   - Brain neoplasm
   - Parkinson's disease
   - Seizure disorder
   - Dementia

Connective tissue diseases
- Systemic lupus erythematosus
Neoplasms
- Pancreatic cancer

5. **List medications that might cause secondary depression.**
- Antihypertensives (beta blockers)
- Hypnotics and sedatives (benzodiazepines and barbiturates)
- Corticosteroids
- Cimetidine
- Ranitidine

6. **Why should the clinician always inquire about alcohol use when evaluating depression?**
Alcohol use and abuse is an extremely common comorbid condition with depression and should always be queried for several reasons. First, alcohol use can be disinhibiting with regard to behavior, putting a depressed and suicidal person at increased risk of impulsively acting on suicidal tendencies. Second, depression cannot be treated effectively if there is ongoing alcohol abuse. Third, alcohol is a depressant and is a common cause for depression, a problem known as **alcohol-induced mood disorder.** It may be that the patient's depression is secondary to alcohol use and is treated best by abstaining from alcohol, rather than by administering an antidepressant. This situation is suggested when the onset of the mood disturbance occurs during an extended period of regular (usually daily) alcohol use, rather than before it.

7. **When should I suspect depression when a patient presents with what seems to be a medical complaint?**
Screen for depression when patients present with nonspecific complaints, such as "sick all over," "weak and dizzy," or "just feeling bad." Using the SIG E CAPS mnemonic (*see* question 1) aids in diagnosis. Often depression is expressed in physical rather than emotional terms. Nonspecific physical complaints, such as fatigue, exhaustion, headache, gastrointestinal complaints, muscle aches, and nonspecific pain, are common. Anxiety is seen commonly with depression and can manifest as shortness of breath, nervousness, irritability, and difficulty swallowing, among other symptoms. Panic attacks, a severe form of anxiety that often occurs in the context of depression, are a common cause of emergency department (ED) presentations of atypical chest pain.

8. **Are psychotic features ever a manifestation of depression?**
Sometimes. If psychotic symptoms accompany depression, it signifies a more severe and dangerous form of depression. When this is the case, psychiatric consultation and often psychiatric hospitalization are indicated. Patients with **psychotic depression** are at higher risk for suicide, especially when they have hallucinations commanding them to harm themselves. Other common psychotic symptoms are hearing guilt-provoking or self-critical voices, called *auditory hallucinations*; and fixed, false beliefs that can be persecutory or paranoid in nature, referred to as *delusions*.

9. **Name therapies available for treatment of depression.**
Antidepressant medications, psychotherapy, and electroconvulsive therapy.

10. **What antidepressant medications are used to treat depression?**
Tricyclic antidepressants (TCAs) and monoamine oxidase inhibitors (MAOIs) are the two original classes of antidepressants, both of which have fallen into relative disuse because of their side effects and dietary restrictions (in the case of MAOIs). Serotonin reuptake inhibitors are still the most commonly prescribed class of antidepressants, mainly because of comparable efficacy,

greater ease of use, and fewer adverse effects. These are fluoxetine (Prozac), paroxetine (Paxil), sertraline (Zoloft), citalopram (Celexa), fluvoxamine (Luvox), and S-citalopram (Lexapro). However, newer and perhaps better medications that act on multiple neurotransmitter systems are now available, and also have better side-effect profiles than the older TCAs or MAOIs. These include venlafaxine (Effexor), bupropion (Wellbutrin), mirtazapine (Remeron), and duloxetine (Cymbalta). Lithium, psychostimulants, and thyroid hormone are common adjunctive treatments.

Stahl SM: Essential Psychopharmacology: The Prescribers Guide. Cambridge University Press, Cambridge, 2005.

11. What are some psychotropic-related emergencies or precautions?
MAOIs in combination with sympathomimetic agents can cause hyperadrenergic crisis, and their combination with meperidine (Demerol) or dextromethorphan can cause cardiovascular instability and central nervous system excitability. Neuroleptics can cause dystonias, including laryngeal spasm and neuroleptic malignant syndrome (delirium, rigidity, fever, and autonomic abnormalities), both medical emergencies. Anticholinergic toxicity may occur because many psychotropics have anticholinergic properties and often are used in combination; these include benztropine mesylate (Cogentin), trihexyphenidyl (Artane), diphenhydramine (Benadryl), TCAs, and low-potency and mid-potency neuroleptics. Many other commonly used agents have dose-related toxic side effects, particularly the *mood stabilizers,* which include lithium and the anticonvulsants valproic acid and carbamazepine.

12. When should the emergency physician prescribe antidepressant therapy?
Because antidepressants generally take weeks to begin working and often require monitoring of side effects and dose titration, prescribing them in the ED should be avoided whenever possible. Exceptions include a patient who is already on treatment and needs a refill or a patient who is initiating new treatment after an emergent consultative evaluation by a psychiatrist. Ideally, in both of these cases, a 2- to 4-day supply of medication can be prescribed, and the patient should follow up with outpatient psychiatric care.

13. What is the most serious complication of depression?
Suicide. Major depression accounts for an estimated 50% of all suicides.

14. Which patients should be hospitalized for depression?
Depressed patients who express suicidal intent or have a plan for suicide and psychotic depressed patients should be admitted. Also, patients who have just made a violent suicide attempt, have tried to avoid rescue, or are refusing help should be admitted for further observation. Do not forget to institute suicidal precautions while these patients are in the ED.

SUICIDE

15. What is the proper approach to a patient who has attempted suicide?
Medical management of any life-threatening condition precedes psychiatric evaluation. It is important, however, that as the treatment proceeds, the ED team maintain a nonjudgmental approach. Punishment or ridicule is neither therapeutic nor proper conduct for medical professionals. Nearly all patients who attempt suicide are at least ambivalent about the wish to live or die. Demeaning or harsh treatment of such patients, especially by health professionals who are symbols of medical authority, worsens the already low self-esteem and may make subsequent psychiatric care more difficult.

16. Describe suicide precautions.
Because some patients have been known to repeat a suicide attempt while in the ED, suicide precautions are necessary. Such precautions include searching the patient and recovering

weapons, pills, or other potential means of self-injury; keeping the patient under close observation; recovering any potential dangerous items from the immediate care area (e.g., needles, scalpels, glass, razors); and not allowing the patient to go anywhere (e.g., bathroom) unaccompanied. When constant staff observation is not possible, physical restraints may be necessary to protect the severely suicidal patient from further self-harm.

17. Are "accidents" ever suicide attempts?

It is important to remember that victims of trauma may have actually attempted suicide. Single-victim accidents, such as a car driven at high speed into a concrete structure, a pedestrian hit by a high-speed vehicle, or a fall, are classic examples of suicide attempts presenting as trauma. Medical management should be followed by an assessment of suicide intent, including a discussion with family members and perhaps psychiatric consultation.

18. What psychiatric disorders are associated with attempted suicide?

Major depression, alcohol and drug dependence, schizophrenia and other thought disorders, personality disorders, panic disorder, adjustment disorders, and organic brain syndromes.

19. How do I evaluate the risk of a subsequent suicide in a suicide attempter?

The following elements are part of an emergency assessment of suicide risks: age, gender, marital status, social supports, physical illness, previous attempts, family history of suicide, risk of the attempts versus likelihood of rescue, secondary gain, nature of any psychiatric illness, alcohol or drug abuse, attitude, affect, and future plans of the suicide attempter. If, after reviewing these factors, the emergency physician is still unsure of the patient's risk, psychiatric consultation is often helpful.

20. How does age relate to suicide risk?

Older patients (especially >45 years) are statistically more likely to complete suicide than younger patients. Such patients may experience loss of spouse, loneliness, physical illness, or economic hardship in addition to depression. A worrisome increase in suicide among younger persons has emerged, however. Suicide is now the third leading cause of death in children older than 5, youth, and young adults (19–24 years of age).

American Association of Suicidology: www.aso.org

21. What role does gender play?

The rates of completed suicide in men are higher than those for women, whereas the rates of attempted suicide are higher for women than for men. This difference has to do with the lethality of the means. Men attempt suicide more often by violent means, such as shooting, stabbing, hanging, or jumping from a height, whereas women typically use less violent and less effective methods, such as drug overdose.

22. What is the relationship of marital status to risk of successful suicide?

Never having been married carries the highest risk, followed in decreasing magnitude of risk by being widowed, separated, divorced, and married.

23. What about other social support?

Unemployment, loneliness, loss of home, and relative isolation increase the risks of suicide. Church, family, or community support helps to mitigate suicide risk.

24. Is there a relationship between physical illness and suicide risk?

Yes. Patients with a medical illness, especially a painful, incurable one, may seek a "way out" through suicide. The most common nonpsychiatric diagnoses associated with suicide are chronic medical conditions, such as cancer, chronic obstructive pulmonary disease, and chronic pain. Renal dialysis patients have a suicide rate 400 times higher than the general population, and human immunodeficiency virus (HIV) patients may also have a higher than average rate.

25. Does a history of prior suicide attempts signify increased risk?
Yes, especially if each subsequent attempt escalates in severity. The risk of completed suicide is more than 100 times the average in the first year after an attempt—200 times greater for people older than 45 (National Mental Health Association: www.nmha.org). An exception may exist if the previous attempts all have been minor and considered to be manipulative acts.

26. What is the relationship of family history to suicide risk?
Patients with a family history of suicide, alcoholism, or depression have a higher suicide risk than patients without such a family history. A family history of suicide in first-order relatives (e.g., parent or sibling) should cause particular concern.

27. How does the risk of the suicide attempt and the likelihood of rescue affect a suicide evaluation?
In general, a more serious or risky attempt is considered a more likely predictor of subsequent attempts than a minor attempt. An attempt carried out in such a way that rescue is probable is associated with a lower risk of subsequent successful suicide. The patient's *belief* about the lethality of the attempt is at least as important as the physician's assessment of the seriousness of it.

KEY POINTS: SERIOUS SUICIDE ATTEMPTS

1. Patients thought what they did in their attempt to commit suicide was likely to kill them.

2. They did it in such a way as to have a low chance of being rescued.

3. They are not talking much about how they are feeling now.

4. They have little social support and are unwilling to reach out to others or accept help from available resources.

5. They still want to die.

28. What is secondary gain as it applies to suicide attempt?
Sometimes a suicide attempt seems to have a goal other than death. This goal, which is termed *secondary gain*, may be increased attention from parents, friends, or lovers. In attempts with no expected gain other than death, the potential for subsequent successful suicide is great. With the increase in successful suicides among the young, the physician must be careful in ascribing suicide attempts to the desire for attention or secondary gain until a reasonably thorough evaluation can be completed.

29. What is the value of assessing the suicidal patient's attitude and affect?
The patient who appears exhausted, helpless, hopeless, or lonely represents high risk. The patient who attempts suicide because of anger or in an effort to gain revenge has a much better prognosis than one who appears quiet, sad, fatigued, or apathetic.

30. **Why is it important to inquire about a specific plan?**
Never hesitate to ask the patient about any plans regarding suicide. The patient who continues to express suicidal ideation after one attempt is at risk for a subsequent attempt. The risk is highest if the plan is detailed, violent, or feasible.

31. **What is the SAD PERSONS Scale?**
In 1983, Patterson et al. used known high-risk characteristics to develop the mnemonic SAD PERSONS Scale. The scale was designed to be used by nonpsychiatrists to assess the need for hospitalization in suicidal patients. Hockberger and Rothstein modified the scale to facilitate use in the ED (see Table 100-1). A score of 5 or less indicates that a patient probably can be discharged safely. Scores of 6 or more require psychiatric consultation, and a score of 9 or more indicates the probable need for psychiatric hospitalization.

32. **In general, which suicidal patients should be hospitalized?**
   - **Absolute indications** for hospitalization after suicide attempts (involuntarily, if necessary) usually include the following: presence of psychosis; a violent, nearly lethal preplanned attempt; and continued suicidal ideation with definite plans for a repeated attempt.

TABLE 100-1. MODIFIED SAD PERSONS SCALE

Mnemonic		Characteristic	Score
S	Sex	Male	1
A	Age	<19 or >45 y	1
D	Depression or hopelessness	Admits to depression or decreased concentration, appetite, sleep, libido	2
P	Previous attempts or psychiatric care	Previous inpatient or outpatient psychiatric care	1
E	Excessive alcohol or drug use	Stigmata of chronic addiction or recent frequent use	1
R	Rational thinking loss	Organic brain syndrome or psychosis	2
S	Separated, widowed, or divorced		1
O	Organized or serious attempt	Well-thought-out plan or life-threatening presentation	2
N	No social supports	No close family, friends, job, or active religious affiliation	1
S	Stated future intent	Determined to repeat attempt or ambivalent	2

Scoring: A positive answer to the presence of depression or hopelessness, lack of rational thought processes, an organized plan or serious suicide attempt, and affirmative or ambivalent statement regarding future intent to commit suicide are each scored 2 points. Each other positive answer is scored 1 point.
From Hockberger RS, Rothstein RJ: Assessment of suicide potential by non-psychiatrists using the SAD PERSONS score. J Emerg Med 99:6, 1988, Hockberger RS, Smith M: Depression and suicide ideation In Wolfson A.B (ed): Clinical Practice of Emergency Medicine, 4th ed. Philadelphia, Lippincott Williams & Wilkins, 2005, pp 637–639.

- **Relative indications** include age older than 45; high risk-to-rescue ratio; serious mental illness; alcoholism; drug addiction; living alone with poor social support; and hopelessness, helplessness, or exhaustion.

KEY POINTS: INDICATIONS FOR SUICIDE PRECAUTIONS AND PSYCHIATRIC CONSULTATION

1. Violent, near-lethal, preplanned attempt

2. Psychotic patient

3. Elderly patient

4. Expression of continued wish to die by suicide

CHAPTER 101

MANAGEMENT OF THE VIOLENT PATIENT

Danielle Raeburn, MD, and Katherine M. Bakes, MD

1. **Is violence a problem in the emergency department (ED)?**

   Yes. Only a small percentage of ED patients are violent, disruptive, or abusive to staff; yet they require a disproportionate amount of staff attention and resources. About 4% of patients in the ED need restraints during their stay. The reasons for restraints vary according to a prospective observational study from an urban ED, violent and disruptive behavior being responsible 29.2% of the time, agitation another 25.2%, and alcohol or drug intoxication 7.4%. Restraints were less frequently used for confusion (6.4%) or dementia (1.7%), but note that 40% of the patients who were restrained had multiple reasons for restraints. Also notable is that approximately 30% of patients require a combination of physical and chemical restraint.

   > Lavoe FW: Consent, involuntary treatment and the use of force in an urban ED. Ann Emerg Med 21:25–32, 1992.
   >
   > Zun LS: A prospective study of the complication rate of use of patient restraint in the ED. J Emerg Med 24:119–124, 2003.

2. **What can hospitals do to decrease the risk of violence?**

   - Limit access to the hospital via a few entrances that are staffed and monitored by trained security personnel.
   - Metal detectors should be used to screen patients and visitors for weapons.
   - Continuous surveillance, closed-circuit television monitors should be used to help ensure safety in the parking areas and the immediate grounds of the hospital.
   - Multiple methods of summoning police or security must be available to the ED without having to go through the hospital operator.

3. **What can be done to preempt a violent episode?**

   - Be aware of early signs of impending violent behavior, such as agitation, abusive language, and challenges to authority.
   - Completely undress all patients and place in a gown. Remove any weapons on their person.
   - Do not leave instruments that can be used as weapons near a potentially violent patient.

4. **What is the initial approach a physician can take to control an agitated or violent patient?**

   The first approach should be verbal redirection. When interacting with the patient, the physician should appear calm and in control but empathetic. The physician should tell the patient that he or she is in a safe environment and that the ED staff is there to help. Keep hands in a neutral position, not crossed across your chest or behind your back. Make an attempt to make the patient more comfortable (perhaps with something to drink or a warm blanket). Be clear with the patient what will and will not be tolerated and that the ED must maintain control to prevent any harm to the patient or others. Active listening may go a long way toward calming the patient. Stationing security officers in the patient's presence may dissuade further inappropriate behavior. Most importantly, care providers must be aware of their own emotions when dealing with agitated patients. Do not take it personally! Yelling back at or exchanging threats with the patient only further escalates the situation.

KEY POINTS: DE-ESCALATING A VIOLENT PATIENT

1. Use verbal redirection.

2. Use nonconfrontational body language.

3. Reassure the patient's safety.

4. Use empathy.

5. Maintain and emphasize control over the ED.

6. Be honest and direct.

5. What if that doesn't work?

When aggressive behavior cannot be managed by verbal de-escalation and a patient becomes an increasing risk of violence or elopement, physical and/or chemical restraint can be used. For physical restraint, four-point (both wrists and both ankles) locking leather cuffs should be used. A team of five staff members should place the restraints, one care provider for each limb and one at the head of the patient to provide an ongoing explanation to the patient of what is happening and why. It is preferable that the physician not be involved in this action because it may further jeopardize his or her therapeutic relationship with the patient. Soft restraints or two-point restraints are usually best choices in the disoriented patient at risk of pulling lines and tubes. Going directly to four-point restraints in the violent patient is the safest option for both the patient and staff, and if chemical restraint must be added, it can be done so easily. When the patient becomes calm, he or she is often brought down to two-point restraints or out of restraints completely.

6. What do I need to remember when physically restraining a patient?

The restraints must be snug enough to hold him or her but not impede circulation. Always be sure there is enough room to allow one finger to move easily between the patient's skin and the cuff. Always place siderails in the up position. Never place the patient prone (suffocation risk). Patients at risk of aspiration should be positioned on their side. When restraints are in place, they must be monitored for their continued need. Subsequent reevaluations may reveal that restraining measures can be downgraded or discontinued. The patient's behavior, attempts at less restrictive measures, and monitoring of the patient's mental status and vital signs after restraints are placed all must be documented. The Joint Commission on Healthcare Accreditation (JCAHO) has specific guidelines for use of physical restraints. There are hospital protocols regarding restraints, and the physician should be familiar with these guidelines.

7. Am I legally allowed to restrain someone?

Yes. The courts have held both physicians and hospitals liable for injuries that have occurred when violent or otherwise incapacitated patients escape hospital grounds or are discharged. The ED staff must therefore prevent certain patients from leaving until they can be examined and thoroughly evaluated. If the patient somehow leaves the department and the manpower isn't available to keep the patient, avoid heroics and call the local authorities. Regarding a patient's right to refuse antipsychotic medication, this does not apply to patients who exhibit violent or psychotic behavior acutely in the ED. You may administer medication "in an emergency situation in which to do so [refuse medication] . . .would result in a substantial likelihood of physical harm to the patient, other patients, or to staff members at the institution."

Hill S, Petit J: Psychiatric emergencies. Emerg Med Clin North Am 18:201–315, 2000.
American Psychiatric Association: Seclusion and Restraint, Task Force Report No.22. Washington, DC, American Psychiatric Association, 1984.

8. **What are the indications for chemical restraint?**
   - If verbal de-escalation is unsuccessful and the patient remains violent despite physical restraints
   - For patient and staff safety if very difficult or impossible to place physical restraints

9. **What medications are recommended for chemical restraint?**
   Two classes of drugs generally are used for chemical restraint: (1) butyrophenones, such as haloperidol and droperidol and (2) benzodiazepines, such as lorazepam and diazepam.

   Butyrophenones: The antipsychotic effects of these medications take days to work, but their usefulness in the acute setting with any patient (with or without psychosis) is due to their sedating properties. Droperidol has been used extensively and quite successfully for many years but is presently not recommended because of a 2001 Food and Drug Administration "black box" warning. The concern is for the potential for this class of medications (including haloperidol) to prolong the QT interval and possibly lead to torsades de pointes, a potentially fatal dysrhythmia. A large retrospective review of droperidol being used for agitation in an urban setting showed no cardiovascular events. At this time, **haloperidol,** 5–10 mg intramuscular (IM) or intravenous (IV), is the preferred agent for chemical restraint.

   Benzodiazepines: These are useful in agitation, mania, psychosis, alcohol withdrawal, benzodiazepine withdrawal, and sympathomimetic toxidromes like cocaine or amphetamine toxicity. Initial doses of 1–4 mg IM or IV of *lorazepam* may be given. Except in cases of liver disease, diazepam generally is preferred over lorazepam because it is cheaper and not as long acting. This allows for more frequent reassessment of the patient. *Diazepam* may be given as follows: 5–10 mg IV, IM, or per rectum (PR) for an initial dose and repeated doses of 2–10 mg every 20–30 minutes as needed.

   Another choice is *midazolam* **alone or in combination with haloperidol.** Midazolam, 5 mg IM, has been shown to be more rapid in sedation onset than lorazepam or haloperidol and also has the benefit of having a shorter time to arousal. No randomized study has yet compared midazolam to the shorter acting diazepam, but they are probably comparable in efficacy, and diazepam has the added benefit of being cheaper.

   In summary, if you want expeditious sedation and patient control, use diazepam/haloperidol or lorazepam/haloperidol in combination. Midazolam alone or with haloperidol is a safe alternative. If you are concerned about length of sedation, the shortest half-life is with midazolam or diazepam alone.

   Chase PB, Biros MH: A retrospective review of the use and safety of droperidol in a large, high-risk, inner-city ED patient population. Acad Emerg Med 9:1402–1410, 2002.
   Nobay F, Simon DC, Levitt MA, et al: A prospective, double-blind, randomized trial of midazolam versus haloperidol versus lorazepam in the chemical restraint of violent and severely agitated patients. Acad Emerg Med 11:744–749, 2004.
   Sorrentino A: Chemical restraints for the agitated, violent, or psychotic pediatric patient in the ED: Controversies and recommendations. Curr Opin Pediatr 16:201–205, 2004.

10. **What if two doses of haloperidol have not sedated the patient?**
    Don't give a third dose. What is very helpful is to supplement the haloperidol with a benzodiazepine; the two together are more effective than each alone. If you used haloperidol 5 mg IM and repeated this once, try adding lorazepam 2 mg IM or IV or diazepam 5 mg IM or IV. You can then add increasing doses of benzodiazepines, but you probably will not need it.

    Battaglia SA, Ownby RL, Penalver A, Domingueq RA: Haloperidol, lorazepam, or both for psychotic agitation? A multicenter, prospective, double-blind, ED study. Am J Emerg Med 15:335–340, 1997.

11. **How do you use chemical restraint for sedation in a pediatric patient?**

Only half of the psychotropic medications used for restraint in adults have been approved for use in children. The most frequently used medication for rapid sedation in children is *lorazepam*. The benefits, again, are rapid onset, short half-life, and multiple routes of administration. The dose in children is 0.05–0.1 mg/kg/dose either IV, IM, or orally (PO). As far as neuroleptics go, *haloperidol* is safe and effective. Haloperidol 0.025–0.075 mg/kg/dose (max 2.5 mg) can be given IM or PO, and even though not yet approved by the Food and Drug Administration (FDA) for IV use, it is effective IV. If you decide to administer haloperidol and lorazepam together, this can be done in the same syringe in one IM dose. This is also safe and effective in the pediatric population but may lead to prolonged sedation.

Kao LW, Moore GP, Jackimczyk KC, et al: The combative patient: chemical restraints. In Marx (ed): Rosen's Emergency Medicine: Concepts and Clinical Practice, 5th ed. Mosby, 2002, pp 2595–2599.

Sorrentino A: Chemical restraints for the agitated, violent, or psychotic pediatric patient in the ED: Controversies and recommendations. Curr Opin Pediatr 16:201–205, 2004.

KEY POINTS: PREFERRED DRUGS FOR CHEMICAL RESTRAINT

1. Haloperidol alone, given IM

2. Haloperidol in combination with lorazepam, both given IM

---

12. **Summarize the main side effects to watch for with these drugs.**

All benzodiazepines can cause hypotension and respiratory depression. The butyrophenones may cause hypotension and extrapyramidal or other dystonic reactions. Hypotension is rare, but dystonic reactions occur in approximately 1% of patients. The most common extrapyramidal symptoms are oculogyric crisis, torticollis, and opisthotonos, which are irregular movements of the eyes, neck, and back, respectively. Neuroleptic malignant syndrome (NMS) is characterized by rigidity, hypertension, hyperthermia, and altered mental status and can been seen after administration of an antipsychotic medication. Treatment for NMS involves supportive care and dantrolene.

Some clinicians recommend prophylaxis with diphenhydramine or benztropine mesylate (Cogentin) with haloperidol administration and for 2–3 days after treatment. Alternatively, dystonic and extrapyramidal symptoms are easily controlled by these medications when they occur.

Sorrentino A: Chemical restraints for the agitated, violent, or psychotic pediatric patient in the ED: Controversies and recommendations. Curr Opin Pediatr 16:201–205, 2004.

KEY POINTS: MAJOR SIDE EFFECTS OF HALOPERIDOL

1. Akathisias

2. Dystonic reactions

3. Neuroleptic malignant syndrome (rare)

4. Anticholinergic effects

5. Hypotension

6. Lowered seizure threshold

13. **Why did the patient become violent in the first place?**
    - Acute intoxication
    - Acute withdrawal
    - Metabolic disorder
    - Trauma
    - Infectious disease
    - Environmental injury
    - Cardiovascular disorder
    - Psychiatric disorders
    - Intracranial disorder
    - Hypoxia
    - Overdose

    Note that the rate of violence is the same between patients with mental illness and those without mental illness. A better predictor of violence is personality disorder and/or substance abuse.

    Buckley PF, Noffsinger SG, Smith DA, et al: Treatment of the psychotic patient who is violent. Psychiatr Clin North Am 26:231–272, 2003.

KEY POINTS: COMMON MEDICAL CONDITIONS THAT MANIFEST AS VIOLENT BEHAVIOR

1. Hypoxia

2. Hypoglycemia

3. Acute intoxication or withdrawal

4. Meningoencephalitis

5. Intracranial injury or bleed

6. Hyponatremia/hypernatremia

7. Drug side effects

---

14. **Give a quick reference on dosing/administration.**
    See Table 101-1.

15. **Does the ED staff need any treatment?**
    The effect of major unpredictable violence and mayhem on ED employees can be devastating. Physical and psychological trauma is only part of the long-lasting effects. Such episodes may affect future job performance. A comprehensive program patterned after the critical incident stress debriefing model should be established to provide immediate and long-term psychological support, and staff should be encouraged to avail themselves of this support when the need arises.

16. **How should these patients be monitored?**
    In any patient who has received chemical restraint that alone (i.e., benzodiazepines) or in combination with a central nervous system (CNS) depressant such as ethanol (EtOH) has the potential to suppress respirations, strong consideration should be given to continuous pulse oximetry monitoring.

TABLE 101-1. QUICK REFERENCE FOR DOSING AND ADMINISTRATION

Medication	Adult Dose	Pediatric Dose	Route	Onset of Action	Duration of Action	"Time to Arousal"	Side Effects
Lorazepam	0.5–4 mg	0.05–0.1 mg/kg/dose	IV/IM/PO	5–10 min IV/IM 20–30 min PO	4–8 h IV	2 mg (alone) = 217 min	Respiratory depression Paradoxical reactions
Diazepam	2–10 mg			1–5 min IV	30–60 min IV		Respiratory depression Paradoxical reactions
Midazolam	1–2.5 mg	0.1 mg/kg/dose (1 mg max)	IV/IM/PO	1–5 min IV 15 min IM		5 mg (alone) = 81 min	Respiratory depression
Haloperidol	2–5 mg	0.025–0.075 mg/kg/dose max 2.5 mg	IM/PO/IV	20–30 min IM 45–60 min PO	4–8 h	5 mg (alone) = 126 min	EPS (dystonia, akathisia) Hypotension QTc prolongation Lower seizure threshold Anticholinergic effects NMS
Droperidol*	2.5–10 mg	0.03–0.07 mg/kg/dose max 2.5 mg	IV/IM	5–10 min			Same as haloperidol

Continued

TABLE 101-1. QUICK REFERENCE FOR DOSING AND ADMINISTRATION—CONT'D

Medication	Adult Dose	Pediatric Dose	Route	Onset of Action	Duration of Action	"Time to Arousal"	Side Effects
For EPS							
Benztropine (Cogentin)	1–4 mg	0.02–0.05 mg/kg/dose	IV/IM/PO				
Diphenhydramine	25–50 mg	1.25 mg/kg/dose	IV/IM/PO				

*Black box warning.
EPS = extrapyramidal symptoms. IM = intramuscular, IV = intravenous, NMS = neuroleptic malignant syndrome, PO = orally.
Wigner N: emedicine "restraints" 2002; available at www.emedicine.com; Hill S, Petit J: Psychiatric emergencies. Emerg Med Clin North Am 18:201–315, 2000; Sorrentino A: Chemical restraints for the agitated, violent, or psychotic pediatric patient in the ED: Controversies and recommendations. Curr Opin Pediatr 16:201–205, 2004; Nobay F, Simon DC, Levitt MA, et al: A prospective, double-blind, randomized trial of midazolam versus haloperidol versus lorazepam in the chemical restraint of violent and severely agitated patients. Acad Emerg Med 11:744–749, 2004.

CHAPTER 102

DOMESTIC VIOLENCE

Debra Houry, MD, MPH, and Kim M. Feldhaus, MD

1. **Isn't domestic violence more of a law enforcement issue than it is a health issue?**

   No. Research shows that 50% of all women presenting to emergency departments (EDs) for care have experienced abuse from an intimate partner or ex-partner at some point in their lives and that 30% of women have experienced domestic violence within the past year. Injuries and illnesses caused by abuse affect their lives more frequently than diseases such as hypertension, cancer, or diabetes. Interpersonal violence has tremendous health implications in the United States.

   Abbott J, Johnson R, Koziol-McLain J, et al: Domestic violence against women: Incidence and prevalence in an emergency department population. JAMA 273:1763–1767, 1995.

2. **Define domestic violence.**

   Domestic violence, in a broad sense, refers to all violence occurring within a family unit. By this definition, partner abuse, child abuse, and elder abuse are subsets of domestic violence. *Domestic violence* is the term most commonly used to refer to the victimization of one partner by his or her intimate partner or partners. *Intimate partner violence* (IPV) is a more specific term, and it is used in this chapter. IPV includes physical acts, such as battering and sexual assault, and nonphysical acts, such as emotional abuse, economic abuse, threats to harm children and property, and prevention of access to health care or prenatal care. Most battered women state that the nonphysical abuse is more humiliating and distressing to them than physical beatings.

3. **What are the risk factors for IPV?**

   IPV occurs in all socioeconomic classes and in all races. Women at greatest risk include those with male partners who abuse alcohol or use drugs; are unemployed; have less than a high school education; or are the former husband, estranged husband, or former boyfriend of the woman. Women who are younger than 30 years; who are single, divorced, or separated; or who abuse drugs or alcohol classically have been viewed as at increased risk for IPV. It is unclear, however, if some of these risk factors lead to the partner abuse or are a result of living in an abusive situation.

4. **Are men *ever* victims of partner abuse?**

   Yes, but 95% of IPV victims are women, and women almost exclusively endure the pattern of recurrent nonphysical and physical abuse. In any conflict that has escalated to the point of violence, the persons involved become mutual combatants. The woman is 13 times more likely to be injured than the man, however, and 30% more likely to be killed.

5. **If IPV is so common, why have none of my patients experienced it?**

   Many of your patients may be experiencing partner abuse. Often, physicians do not know because they do not ask about it.

6. **What is the result of a missed diagnosis of IPV?**

   Failure to diagnose IPV may return the woman to a dangerous situation and increase her risk of future injury. It also furthers the victim's sense of entrapment and helplessness. Inappropriate medications may be prescribed (tranquilizers and antidepressants) without a search for the underlying causes of these symptoms. Patients may be labeled as being hysterical, paranoid, and irrational.

7. **State some of the reasons why physicians choose not to inquire about IPV.**
   The most commonly cited reason is **lack of time.** Health care providers believe that this issue is too time consuming to deal with, especially in a busy ED. Other reasons include the belief that it is none of the physician's business, the belief that women would "tell" if they wanted to, the belief that there is nothing that can be done, the belief that the woman deserved the abuse, and the belief that a woman could just leave the situation if she wanted to.

8. **State some of the reasons why victims of partner abuse might not disclose the abuse to health care providers, even if asked.**
   Women may be embarrassed and humiliated that it is happening to them. There may be cultural or religious beliefs that lead her to believe that this is normal or to be expected. She may have been told that she deserved the abuse. Her abuser might have threatened to harm her, her children, or other loved ones if she discloses to others; or she may believe that no one can help her.

9. **What are some of the structural and system barriers that might prevent a woman from disclosing abuse?**
   Lack of privacy is a real concern in the ED. Women should be interviewed alone, without children or partners present. If necessary, hospital security may be recruited to ensure their safety. Also, family members or children should not be used as translators when inquiring about abuse.

10. **How many women who present to an ED for care are there because of injuries or illness caused by IPV?**
    Studies indicate that approximately 10–14% of women who present to an ED are there because of illness or injuries related to partner abuse. Approximately 2–3% of all women seen in an ED have an acute injury caused by domestic assault.

11. **What clues to IPV might be evident in a patient's history?**
    Most importantly, a history that is inconsistent with the physical examination findings should raise physician suspicion for IPV. You should also consider partner abuse in patients with threatened miscarriages (because of abdominal trauma), patients with suicidal intentions or attempts (frequently occur after a "fight" with a partner), patients who are depressed, patients who have evidence of drug and alcohol abuse, patients with frequent visits for chronic pain complaints, and patients who report no prenatal care (their partners may prevent them from accessing care).

12. **What clues may be present on physical examination in a victim of IPV?**
    Common injury patterns include injuries to the face, neck, and throat (especially signs or symptoms of strangulation), chest, breasts, abdomen, and genitals. Any injury that does not "fit" with the history obtained should create suspicion of abuse. Other physical examination findings of concern include evidence of sexual assault or frequent, recurrent sexually transmitted diseases.

Muelleman RL, Lenaghan PA, Pakieser RA: Battered women: Injury locations and types. Ann Emerg Med 28:486–492, 1996.

KEY POINTS: PHYSICAL EXAM FINDINGS IN IPV

1. Injuries to face, neck, throat, chest, abdomen ("central" pattern)

2. Injuries to chest and abdomen

3. ANY injury that does not "fit" with the history

4. Evidence of sexual assault or frequent, recurrent sexually transmitted diseases

5. Injuries in multiple stages of healing

---

13. **How can I increase my recognition of partner abuse?**
    First, ask about IPV. Any woman who presents with an injury should be specifically asked who injured her. Second, raise your level of suspicion in women without injuries. Remember the clues that might be present in the history or physical examination. If you are considering partner abuse, ask about it.

14. **What questions about partner violence can I ask a woman without injuries?**
    1. Have you ever been hurt or injured by a partner or ex-partner?
    2. Are there situations in your relationship where you have felt afraid?
    3. Has your partner ever abused you or your children?
    4. Do you feel safe in your current relationship?
    5. Is there a partner from a past relationship who is making you feel unsafe now?

15. **What about screening all women for IPV?**
    Good idea! Because of the prevalence of this problem, many organizations have advocated screening all women for the presence of IPV. One screening tool that has been tested clinically is the Partner Violence Screen. This consists of these three questions: (1) Have you been hurt or injured in the past year by anyone? If so, by whom? (2) Do you feel safe in your current relationship? (3) Is there a partner from a previous relationship who is making you feel unsafe now? This tool is 71% sensitive for detecting IPV. Women who screen positive for IPV are 11 times more likely to experience physical violence in the next 4 months than women who screen negative for IPV.

    Feldhaus KM, Koziol-McLain J, Amsbury HL, et al: Accuracy of 3 brief screening questions for detecting partner violence in the emergency department. JAMA 277:1357–1361, 1997.

16. **What comments or questions would be inappropriate when discussing IPV with women?**
    - "What did you do to him?"
    - "What did you do that made him so mad?"
    - "This has happened before, and you are still married to him?"
    - "Why didn't you tell anyone?"
    - "You let him do that to you?"
    - "I wouldn't let anyone do that to me."
    - "Why don't you just leave?"

17. **What do I do if my patient has an injury caused by her partner?**
    1. Treat her injuries.
    2. Document her history and her injuries carefully in the medical records.

3. Provide support and empathy; women should be informed that IPV is a common problem, that no one deserves this abuse, and that help is available. Helping victims access community resources should be a primary goal of ED treatment.
4. Inquire about the woman's safety and that of her children. Not all women want or require shelter placement. Women who are experiencing increasingly severe physical injuries or whose batterers have access to firearms are at risk for severe or lethal injuries. Some of these interventions may be by a social worker or by a domestic violence advocate, depending on the clinical setting.

18. **Summarize some important points to remember when documenting IPV.**
Document what happened in the patient's own words, and document the relationship to her batterer. Record all areas of bruising or tenderness; a body map may be helpful. Photographs may be used, but care should be taken to follow local legal guidelines for photographing injuries. Be *sure* to obtain the patient's permission. Any treatment and intervention should be documented. In cases in which abuse is highly suspected and the patient is denying abuse, document the reason that you suspect abuse (e.g., the history does not match the physical examination findings). A well-documented medical record can mean the difference between convicting an abuser and allowing him to go free.

19. **Don't I have any legal responsibilities?**
You might. Forty-five states have a law that mandates reporting intentionally inflicted injuries; however, these laws vary greatly as to what injuries must be reported. See Table 102-1 for your state's mandatory reporting requirements.

Houry D, Sachs CJ, Feldhaus KM, et al: Violence-inflicted injuries: Reporting laws in the fifty states. Ann Emerg Med 39:56–60, 2002.

20. **I am practicing in a state that has mandated reporting of IPV, and my patient is begging me not to report her to the police. She says he will kill her if she tells anyone about what happened. What do I do?**
By law, you are required to call the police; however, forcing an intervention on a patient without her consent violates her autonomy and furthers her sense of entrapment. Women need to be informed that the law requires that this be done, and some women are relieved that this decision has been taken out of their hands. The patient is not required to talk to the police when they arrive. States with mandated reporting should have a law enforcement response that provides for patient safety (e.g., strict restraining order policies, mandated arrest of the perpetrator, fast tracks to process domestic violence cases quickly, and adequate shelters to provide safe homes for victims). Knowledge of the typical law enforcement response to partner abuse calls helps you to reassure the victim when she does not want the police involved. Explain to the patient why you are involving the police; remind her that this is a crime; involve your social services agencies if possible, and ensure that she is going to a safe place. Use your best judgment with the goal of preventing further battering. There is a difference between doing something to a patient ("I am going to report you to the police"), and doing something *with* a patient ("We are going to make a police report together about this crime").

Rodriquez MA, McLoughlin E, Nah G, et al: Mandatory reporting of domestic violence to the police: What do emergency department patients think? JAMA 286:580–583, 2001.

21. **My patient just told me about an episode of battering that occurred several months ago. What do I do now?**
If there is no recent assault, a police report is not required. You should let the patient know that this is a common problem, that help is available, and that she does not deserve the abuse. An inquiry into her safety is warranted. Women who are experiencing increasingly severe physical injuries or whose batterers have access to guns are considered to be at extreme risk for significant injuries and death.

TABLE 102-1. LEGAL REQUIREMENTS FOR REPORTING INJURIES BY STATE

State (Statute)	Injuries from Weapons	Injuries from Crimes	Injuries from Domestic Violence
Alabama	No	No	No
Alaska (Statute 08.64.369)	Yes	Yes	No
Arizona (Rev Stat 13-3806)	Yes	Yes	No
Arkansas (Code Ann 12-12-602)	Yes	No	No
California (Pen Code 11172 AB74x19)	Yes	Yes	Yes
Colorado (Rev Stat 12-36-135)	Yes	Yes	Yes
Connecticut (Acts 269)	Yes	No	No
Delaware (Code Ann 24-17-1762)	Yes	No	No
District of Columbia (Ann 2-1361)	Yes	No	No
Florida (Stat Ann 790.24)	Yes	Yes	No
Georgia (Code Ann 31-7-9)	No	Yes	No
Hawaii (Rev Stat 453-14)	Yes	Yes	No
Idaho (Code 39-1390)	Yes	Yes	No
Illinois (Code Ann 20-2630-3)	Yes	Yes	No
Indiana (Code Ann 35-47-1)	Yes	No	No
Iowa (Code Ann 147.111)	Yes	Yes	No
Kansas (Stat 21-4213)	Yes	No	No
Kentucky (Stat Ann 209.020)	No	Yes	Yes
Louisiana (Rev Stat 403.5)	Yes	No	No
Maine (Rev Stat 17A Ch 21.512)	Yes	No	No
Maryland (Ann Code 336, art 27)	Yes	No	No
Massachusetts (Gen Laws 112-12)	Yes	No	No
Michigan (Comp Laws 750.411)	Yes	Yes	No
Minnesota (Stat Ann 626.52)	Yes	No	No
Mississippi (Code Ann 45-9-31; 93-21-1)	Yes	No	Yes
Missouri (Rev Stat 578-350.1)	Yes	Yes	No
Montana (Code Ann 37-2-302)	Yes	No	No
Nebraska (Rev Stat 28-902)	No	Yes	No
Nevada (Rev Stat Ann 629.041)	Yes	No	No
New Hampshire (Rev Stat Ann 631.6)	Yes	Yes	No
New Jersey (Stat Ann 2C: 58–8)	Yes	No	No
New Mexico	No	No	No
New York (Penal Code 265.25)	Yes	No	No
North Carolina (Gen Stat 90-21.20)	Yes	Yes	No
North Dakota (Cent Code 43-17-41)	Yes	Yes	No
Ohio (ORC 2921; 2151)	Yes	Yes	Yes
Oklahoma (Stat 2105-846.1)	No	Yes	No
Oregon (Rev Stat 146.750)	Yes	No	No

Continued

TABLE 102-1. LEGAL REQUIREMENTS FOR REPORTING INJURIES BY STATE—CONT'D

State (Statute)	Injuries from Weapons	Injuries from Crimes	Injuries from Domestic Violence
Pennsylvania (Cons Stat Anns 18-5106)	Yes	Yes	No
Rhode Island (Gen Laws 12-29-9; 11-47-48)	Yes	No	Yes
South Carolina	No	No	No
South Dakota (Codified Laws 23-13-10)	Yes	No	No
Tennessee (Stat 36-3-621; 38-1-101)	Yes	Yes	Voluntary
Texas (Fam Code 91.003, 161.041)	Yes	No	Yes
Utah (Code Ann 26-23a)	Yes	Yes	No
Vermont (Stat Ann 13-4012)	Yes	No	No
Virginia (Code Ann 54.1-2967)	Yes	No	No
Washington	No	No	No
West Virginia (Code Ann 61-2-27)	Yes	No	No
Wisconsin (Stat Ann 146.995)	Yes	Yes	No
Wyoming	No	No	No
Total (including DC) "yes"	42	23	7

*Verified as of March 2001.
From Houry D, Sachs CJ, Feldhaus KM, et al: Violence-inflicted injuries: reporting laws in the fifty states. Ann Emerg Med 39:56–60, 2002.

KEY POINTS: WHAT TO DO WITH AN IPV VICTIM

1. Treat her injuries.
2. Document her history and her injuries carefully. (Consider drawing a picture or taking a photo.)
3. Provide support and empathy.
4. Inquire about the woman's safety and that of her children.
5. Refer to community resources or social worker.
6. Notify law enforcement if required by your state.

22. **Why is she going home to her batterer? Why doesn't she just leave him?**
Why a woman does not leave her batterer is the wrong question to ask. It implies that the woman is to blame and that if she would just leave everything would be okay. Battered women are most likely to be killed during the act of leaving or after they have left their abuser. There are

many other valid reasons why women stay in an abusive situation. She may have no money or job skills; she may have nowhere else to go, or she may feel she must stay to protect her children.

23. What can we do about IPV?

A more appropriate response to IPV is to ask ourselves why society tolerates this behavior and how we, as health care providers, might change those attitudes.

BIBLIOGRAPHY

1. Abbott J: Assault-related injuries: What do we know, and what should we do about it?. Ann Emerg Med 32:363–366, 1998.

2. Haywood YC, Haile-Mariam T: Violence against women. Emerg Med Clin North Am 17:603–615, 1999.

3. Houry D, Feldhaus K, Peery B, et al: A positive domestic violence screen predicts future domestic violence. J Interpers Violence 19:955–966, 2004.

4. Houry D, Parramore C, Fayard G, et al: Characteristics of household addresses that repeatedly contact 911 to report intimate partner violence. Acad Emerg Med 11:662–667, 2004.

5. Kyriacou DN, Anglin D, Taliaferro E, et al: Risk factors for injury to women from domestic violence against women. N Engl J Med 341:1892–1898, 1999.

COST CONTAINMENT AND RISK MANAGEMENT IN EMERGENCY MEDICINE

Stephen V. Cantrill, MD

CHAPTER 103

COST CONTAINMENT

1. What is cost containment in emergency medicine?

An approach to limit medical care expenses without compromising quality of care.

2. Why is cost containment so important?

Medical care currently consumes nearly 15% of the gross domestic product (GDP), and health care costs traditionally have increased at a rate far above inflation. Because the federal government directly or indirectly pays for at least 42% of health care, they are quite concerned about this ongoing increase. One study concluded that one third of medical care may be unnecessary. If medicine continues to fail to deal with these issues, the federal government may step in and "help" us deal with them. The proliferation of health-maintenance organizations (HMOs) and capitated-care contracts has placed additional pressure on physicians to curtail unnecessary health care costs, often with the health care provider sharing in the financial risk of providing patient care. Also, many practice environments are developing physician practice profiling systems to identify practitioners who order excessive numbers of tests and procedures.

Winslow CM, Solomon DH, Chassin MR, et al: The appropriateness of carotid endarterectomy. N Engl J Med 318:721–727, 1988.

3. In what area do emergency physicians have the most control in terms of containing costs?

Ancillary tests (clinical laboratory and radiology) constitute 44% of patient emergency department (ED) charges—the largest component. These tests are done at the request of the emergency physician and represent an area directly under our control.

4. List some reasons for excessive test ordering in emergency medicine.

- Peer pressure (e.g., wanting to please a consultant)
- Out-of-date hospital policies
- Intellectual curiosity
- Ignorance of the costs of tests
- Patient expectations
- Defensive medicine
- Reflex ordering/old habits

None of these reasons is adequate justification for ordering tests that are not medically indicated based on the patient's presentation.

5. Can just knowing the cost of the tests have an effect?

Yes. This has been demonstrated by several studies, including one in which just having the patient charges for tests on the order slip reduced overall patient test charges by 27%.

Hampers LC, Cha S, Gutglass DJ, et al: The effect of price information on test-ordering behavior and patient outcomes in a pediatric emergency department. Pediatrics 103:877–882, 1999.

6. **What is the "golden question" to ask before ordering any test?**
The question is "How useful will this test be in establishing a diagnosis, assisting in treatment, or making the appropriate disposition?" If the answer is "it won't," serious thought should be given regarding the necessity of ordering the test.

7. **List some additional strategies to reduce inappropriate test ordering.**
   - Avoid ordering reflexively. Carefully consider the benefits before ordering a test.
   - Do not order a test because "it would be nice to know," unless you are willing to pay for the test yourself.
   - Learn how much routine laboratory tests and radiographs cost. Prepare yourself for a shock.
   - Establish guidelines for the use of new technologies. Medicine is notorious for developing and using new tests without discontinuing tests that are old or outdated.
   - Avoid ordering studies for medicolegal reasons. Good medicine is good law. Order only studies that are medically indicated.
   - Use patient education to reshape patient expectations when possible.
   - Cancel studies that were ordered but later found to be unnecessary.

8. **Shouldn't we order tests to "cover" ourselves?**
No. Again, good medicine is good law. The criteria for ordering studies should be strictly medical, not based on the physician's notion of what would be helpful to have in a court of law. Laboratory or radiographic studies should not be used as a substitute for a proper history and physical examination.

Cantrill SV, Karas S (eds): Cost-Effective Diagnostic Testing in Emergency Medicine: Guidelines for Appropriate Utilization of Clinical Laboratory Radiology Studies, 2nd ed. Dallas, American College of Emergency Physicians, 2000 pp 25–26.

9. **Name some commonly over-ordered tests.**
   - Extremity radiographs
   - Urine culture and sensitivity
   - Chest radiographs
   - Throat culture (excluding streptococcal screen)
   - Abdominal radiographs
   - Blood type and crossmatch
   - Rib radiographs
   - Blood ethanol level
   - Electrolyte panel
   - Arterial blood gases
   - Complete blood count

10. **How much can be saved with no compromise in patient care?**
In a multicenter study of 20 hospital EDs, both teaching and nonteaching, a cost-containment educational program was used. Seventeen tests or groups of tests or studies (including those listed earlier) were targeted. A 12.5% decrease in targeted test charges was shown. No decrease in the perceived quality of care could be shown. Careful implementation of clinical decision rules, such as the Ottawa ankle rule, can save up to 35% in ordering x-rays, with no decrease in sensitivity. Implementation of specific cost-effective guidelines has been shown to decrease the hospital ED charge by 28%, with the laboratory charge decreased by 46%. This clearly demonstrates that the costs of medical testing in the ED can be contained by careful, thoughtful ordering without compromising patient care.

Cantrill SV, Karas S (eds): Cost-Effective Diagnostic Testing in Emergency Medicine: Guidelines for Appropriate Utilization of Clinical Laboratory Radiology Studies, 2nd ed. Dallas, American College of Emergency Physicians, 2000 pp 2–5.

Guterman SJ, VanRooyan MJ: Cost-effective medicine: The financial impact that practice guidelines have on outpatient hospital charges in the emergency department. J Emerg Med 16:215–219, 1998.

Leddy JJ, Kesari A, Smolinski RJ: Implementation of the Ottawa ankle rule in a university sports medicine center. Med Sci Sports Exerc 34:57–62, 2002.

11. Can good medication-prescribing habits impact the cost of patient care?
Without question! Common, costly, unnecessary practices in prescribing practices include prescribing antibiotics when no true medical indication exists (e.g., for a viral urinary tract infection [URI]), prescribing the latest and greatest antibiotic that gives unnecessarily broad coverage, and prescribing by brand name when a generic has demonstrated adequate bioequivalence. Avoiding these practices will not only help control costs but will also improve the quality of your care.

12. How is the center for medicare and medicaid services (CMS) concerned about appropriateness of testing?
CMS now requires that documentation be supplied to support that the diagnostic testing ordered was reasonable and medically necessary. Often, routine "screening" tests are disallowed, even if the ordering physician thought them to be appropriate. Retrospective audits have been performed, with some institutions having to return tens of millions of dollars to the federal government for not being able to demonstrate the medical necessity of many diagnostic studies.

Center for Medicare and Medicaid Services: http://www.cms.hhs.gov

KEY POINTS: COST CONTAINMENT

1. Only diagnostic studies should be ordered in the emergency department that directly impact the diagnosis and/or treatment of the patient's presenting problem.

2. The Centers for Medicare and Medicaid Services will not reimburse a hospital for diagnostic testing if the documentation does not support that the tests were reasonable and necessary.

RISK MANAGEMENT

13. What is risk management?
Efforts to identify (and, when possible, improve or rectify) situations that place a service provider in jeopardy. Good risk management not only deals with situations as they arise (e.g., dealing appropriately with a patient's complaint about care) but also anticipates health-delivery problems before they occur (e.g., establishing in advance the procedures for dealing with a patient who wishes to leave against medical advice).

14. Why are emergency physicians at high risk for malpractice lawsuits?
The primary reason is the lack of an established physician-patient relationship. The patient often feels little rapport with a physician unknown to the patient before the visit to the ED. The visit is usually not at the patient's wish, occurring at an unscheduled time and in a situation in which the

patient is under stress and sometimes pain. All of these factors may contribute to feelings of anger and hostility, laying the groundwork for feelings of dissatisfaction about the provided care. A second major reason is that in emergency medicine, the decisions are often irrevocable. If a mistake or misjudgment is made on a patient who is admitted to the hospital, a second chance to correct the error usually exists because the patient is still accessible. In patients wrongly discharged from the ED, sometimes no such second chance exists.

15. **What must be proved in a malpractice case?**
    1. Duty to treat. Was there an obligation for the physician in question to treat the patient? In emergency medicine, this answer is almost always yes. By working in an ED, an emergency physician automatically assumes the duty to treat any patient presenting to the ED and requesting care.
    2. Actual negligence. Was the care provided actually negligent? This often involves showing (to the jury's satisfaction) that the care provided fell below what is to be considered the standard of care. This point is the one most often contested by the opposing sides in a malpractice suit. Negligence may result from acts of commission or omission.
    3. Damages. Did the patient suffer actual damages? This can include the nebulous pain and suffering.
    4. Proximate cause. Did the negligence cause the damages? It must be shown to the jury's satisfaction that the alleged damages were truly the result of the alleged negligent care.

16. **Give some examples of high-risk patients.**
    - The hostile or belligerent patient. These patients are difficult to deal with and sometimes get less than complete, careful evaluation. Intoxicated patients represent a significant subgroup of this class of patients. Demanding patients also fall into this class. When confronted with patients in this category, remember that "you don't have to love them to give them proper care."
    - The patient with a problem that may be a potential life threat. With these patients, the challenge is to discover and address the life threat (see Chapter 1). Inappropriately discharging these patients often results in a risk-management problem.
    - The returning patient. The patient who returns unscheduled to the ED should raise a red flag. What problem is being missed? These patients deserve extra care in reevaluation. The threshold for admitting an unscheduled returning patient should be low.
    - The "private" patient. Patients may be sent to the ED by a private physician for diagnostic studies or treatment but not to be seen and evaluated by the emergency physician. In general, any patient in the ED becomes the responsibility of the emergency physician. If something goes wrong with the care of these patients, the emergency physician also may be held liable. It is advisable to have very clear established policies concerning "private" patients in the emergency department. These patients should be seen by the emergency physician on duty if the patient so requests, if there is a delay in the arrival of the private physician, or if their triage category so warrants.

KEY POINTS: RISK MANAGEMENT

1. Treat every patient as you would want your mother treated.

2. If possible, avoid writing admission orders.

3. Always address the potential life threats, based on the patient's presentation.

17. **What clinical problems tend to get emergency physicians into malpractice difficulty?**
   There is regional variation in clinical problems that tend to cause malpractice problems for emergency physicians, but the following entities are generally major causes: (1) acute coronary syndromes, (2) meningitis/sepsis (especially in young children), (3) missed fractures (including spine and pelvis), (4) appendicitis, (5) ectopic pregnancy, (6) retained foreign bodies, (7) aortic aneurysms, (8) tendon/nerve injuries associated with wounds, (9) intracranial hemorrhage (subdural, epidural, and subarachnoid hemorrhages), and (10) wound infections.

18. **What is the most common error emergency physicians make with regard to their malpractice insurance policy?**
   Failure to read carefully and understand the conditions of the policy (i.e., what is covered, what is not covered, what is required for a malpractice occurrence to be covered, what are the settlement options, and what are the "tail" requirements to provide coverage for past patient encounters when the current policy is no longer in force).

19. **What common deficiencies in the medical record exacerbate malpractice problems for emergency physicians?**
   In a malpractice case, your record of a patient's visit can be your greatest friend or your worst foe. The following problems will place the record on the side of the opposing team:
   - An illegible record. Think about how the record will look when it is enlarged to 4 feet by 4 feet by the plaintiff's attorney to show to the jury. Dictated or typed records avoid this problem.
   - Not addressing the chief complaint or nurses' and paramedics' notes. Make sure your evaluation addresses why the patient came to the ED and what others observed and documented about the patient.
   - Not addressing abnormal vital signs. As a rule, patients must not be discharged from the ED with abnormal vital signs. Whenever this is done, the record must contain a discussion of why the physician is taking this action.
   - An incomplete recorded history. As with all other parts of the medical record, an attempt will be made to convince the jury that "not recorded equals not done." The history must include information concerning all potential serious problems consistent with the patient's presentation. Significant negatives should be recorded as well.
   - Labeling the patient with a diagnosis that cannot be substantiated by the rest of the record. This not only may cause difficulty if the physician's "guess" is wrong but also leads to premature closure on the part of the next physician to treat the patient, removing the slim chance of correcting the diagnostic error if the patient returns to the ED because of no improvement.
   - Inadequate documentation of the patient's course in the ED with inadequate attention to the patient's condition at discharge. Often the patient's condition may improve dramatically while in the ED, justifying discharge, but this fact is not reflected in the record. If this case becomes a malpractice problem, it appears that the patient was discharged in the original (unimproved) condition.
   - Inadequate discharge (follow-up, aftercare) instructions. The greatest risk in dealing with patients is being wrong in our judgment. The best insurance is careful and complete patient discharge instructions that include when and where to follow up and under what conditions to return to the ED. It is striking how little effort is put into this component of the record. After completing your evaluation and treatment of a patient, ask yourself, "What if I am wrong, and what is the worst possible complication that can occur?" Address these possibilities completely in your discharge instructions, and document them carefully in the record.

20. **What "systems problems" often lead to lawsuits?**
   Systems problems are not under the emergency physician's control, but still can cause difficulty. Such problems include inadequate follow-up on radiology rereads of radiographs,

inadequate follow-up of cardiology rereads of electrocardiograms (ECGs), inadequate follow-up of delayed clinical laboratory results (e.g., cultures), poor availability of previous medical records, inadequate handling of patient complaints (your chance possibly to head off a malpractice suit), and inadequate physician and ED staffing patterns (leading to prolonged patient waits and subsequent patient hostility).

21. **When a patient refuses care, what are the two criteria that must be present?**
If a patient desires to leave the ED against medical advice, the patient must (1) be competent to refuse care and (2) understand the possible untoward sequelae that could result from refusal of care. All patients have the right to refuse care if these two criteria are met. Common sense (and most risk managers) would tell you to err on the side of treating the patient if there is any doubt as to competence.

22. **What clinical problem-solving approach is most helpful in avoiding lawsuits?**
When dealing with any patient, make sure you address the life threats: major problems that could exist, given this presentation for this patient. The safe approach is to assume the presence of these life threats, then set about to disprove them (see Chapter 1).

23. **What physician behaviors may help avoid lawsuits?**
1. Be courteous and kind to the patient and to the patient's family.
2. Take time to communicate with the patient. It takes only seconds to tell the patient what is going on, what the results of diagnostic studies are, and what you are thinking concerning his or her case. Make sure all patient questions and concerns are addressed.
3. Dress neatly.
4. Explain and apologize for inordinate delays in patient care.
5. Make sure the medical record accurately reflects the care provided and the thought processes behind the care.
   This approach can be summarized in a simple statement: "Treat every patient as you would want your mother treated." This, of course, assumes you love your mother.

24. **How can writing admission orders for admitted patients cause problems for the emergency physician?**
In many situations, writing admission orders for patients has made the emergency physician liable for untoward events occurring to the patient in the hospital before he or she is seen by the private physician. There is often significant peer pressure for the emergency physician to write such orders. This practice is potentially dangerous and must be discouraged.

Henry GL, Sullivan DJ: Emergency Medicine Risk Management: A Comprehensive Review. 2nd ed. Dallas, American College of Emergency Physicians, 1997.

25. **What are the criteria for reporting a physician to the national practitioner data bank (NPDB)?**
The NPDB was established by the federal government in 1989 to track potential problem physicians. The criteria for reporting a physician to the NPDB are (1) any payment made for a claim or judgment against a physician, (2) any action taken by a state medical licensing board against a physician, and (3) any disciplinary action lasting more than 30 days taken against a physician by a group or institution. A hospital must query the NPDB about any physician applying for staff privileges and at the time of reappointment of a physician to the medical staff.

26. **How can clinical policies (standards of care) *decrease* malpractice risk for the emergency physician?**
Many groups and organizations are developing standards of care—clinical policies, clinical guidelines, protocols, or standards. If it can be shown that a physician's care was consistent

with an accepted standard, it may help to show the appropriateness of the care and the lack of negligence.

27. How can clinical policies potentially *increase* malpractice risk for emergency physicians?

Malpractice risk can be increased by applicable clinical policies or other standards of care if the emergency physician is not aware of those standards that apply to his or her practice or if he or she chooses not to follow a standard without carefully documenting the reasons for not doing so.

28. Does emergency medicine residency training decrease my malpractice risk?

One study revealed emergency medicine residency-trained physicians had significantly less malpractice indemnity than non-emergency medicine residency-trained physicians. This difference was not due to differences in the average indemnity but was due to significantly fewer closed claims against emergency medicine residency-trained physicians with indemnity paid. This resulted in a cost per physician-year of malpractice coverage for non-emergency medicine residency-trained physicians that was more than twice that of emergency medicine residency-trained physicians ($4905 versus $2212).

Branney SW, Pons PT, Markovchick VJ, et al: Malpractice occurrence in emergency medicine: Does residency training make a difference? J Emerg Med 19:99–105, 2000.

CHAPTER 104

EMTALA, JCAHO, AND HIPAA

Andrew L. Knaut, MD, PhD, and Carolyn S. Knaut, JD

1. **What is EMTALA?**

   Emergency Medical Treatment and Labor Act; not, as some would assert, Easy Method to Attract unwanted Legal Action. In 1986, Congress enacted EMTALA as part of the Consolidated Omnibus Reconciliation Act (COBRA). Its intended purpose is to prevent the "dumping" of patients; that is, the inappropriate transfer or discharge of uninsured patients in an unstable condition solely for the economic benefit of the treating hospital. Put simply, EMTALA requires any hospital that participates in Medicare to do a medical screening exam (MSE) on each patient requesting medical evaluation at any portion of their facility that functions as a "dedicated emergency department (ED)" to determine if an emergency medical condition exists without regard to the patient's ability to pay for services rendered. If such a condition is found to exist, the hospital and the treating physician must use all of the resources normally available to them in stabilizing the emergency medical condition before that patient can be discharged or transferred to another facility. Because more than 98% of hospitals in the United States participate in Medicare, the influence of EMTALA on emergency medical care is far reaching. Failure to comply with its provisions can mean criminal sanctions, stiff financial penalties, and exclusion from participating in governmental programs such as Medicare and Medicaid.

   Examination and treatment for emergency medical conditions and women in labor. 42 USC § 1395dd.

2. **Define emergency medical condition.**

   Any condition that without immediate medical attention might result in the patient's loss of life; a serious impairment of bodily function; severe pain; or, in the case of a woman in active labor, the death or disability of the unborn child.

3. **Why does such a statute even exist?**

   Access to medical care in the United States has never been defined as a fundamental right. For much of the 20th century, private hospitals were under no obligation to offer emergency care to the uninsured. Consequently, indigent or "undesirable" patients were often denied such care and forced either to seek care elsewhere or go without any assistance whatsoever. By the mid-20th century, a two-tiered emergency health care system existed in which the properly insured received better care than the poor. To mitigate the situation, Congress enacted the Hill Burton Act in 1946 requiring any hospital receiving federal funds for construction or other expenses to open its doors to all persons residing within its territorial area. The statute lacked any real means of enforcement, however, and compliance was poor. Over the course of the 1960s and 1970s, the number of civil legal actions taken against hospitals that denied emergent medical treatment to indigent patients grew dramatically. As a result, important legal theories emerged as to how and why hospitals could be held liable for withholding medical care. Essentially, these theories held that any hospital presenting itself as a place offering emergency care must provide that service competently and in a timely fashion to anyone in the public who relied on such advertisement in seeking emergent treatment during a time of need. Paralleling this development was the evolving concept that any hospital receiving public moneys through such programs as Medicare and Medicaid reimbursement in turn held a duty to serve all sectors of the public equally. Ultimately, these concepts culminated in the 1986 enactment of EMTALA. Many amendments over the years have sharpened the focus and increased both the scope and the enforcement powers of the statute.

4. **As a physician, can I personally be penalized for an EMTALA violation?**
Yes. The hospital, the individual physician who provided care, or both can be penalized for an infraction of EMTALA. Formal sanctions include a $50,000 fine for each violation and termination of the Medicare provider agreement that is in essence key to allowing both hospitals and individual physicians to deliver medical care in this country. Moreover, the statute allows patients involved in an EMTALA violation to take private cause of action against the offending institution.

5. **How is this any different than being sued for malpractice?**
The most immediate difference to any physician implicated in an EMTALA violation is the fact that malpractice insurers generally do not cover monetary sanctions imposed for an infraction of the statute. As a result, the penalties amount to a major out-of-pocket expense for the practitioner. Another important difference is that EMTALA is not intended to police standards of medical care per se, but rather to ensure that every patient is treated equally without regard to ability to pay. The patient does not have to suffer a poor outcome, nor does a practitioner have to commit negligence for a physician or a hospital to be cited for an EMTALA violation. If a patient suffers a poor outcome from treatment and alleges malpractice in the state courts, EMTALA is invoked only if it can be proven that the care was substantially different from what the hospital would provide uniformly to any other patient presenting with similar complaints and circumstances.

Gerber v. Northwest Hosp. Center Inc., 943 F. Supp. 571 (D. Md. 1996).
Summers v. Baptist Medical Center Arkadelphia, 91 F.3d 1132 (8th Cir. 1996).

6. **Does EMTALA apply when a patient in need presents to any part of a hospital's campus, even if it is not an ED?**
Not exactly. In the past, EMTALA stated only that the statute applied to any patient presenting on hospital property with a perceived emergent medical condition. This generated considerable confusion because the courts defined "hospital property" broadly to include any physical area within a 250-yard radius of the hospital itself. This meant that EMTALA applied the moment a patient entered a parking lot, pharmacy, outpatient clinic, or other physical component of a hospital's campus. Under the old interpretation, a hospital was even obligated to fulfill EMTALA requirements if a patient presented to an ambulance owned and operated by that hospital, regardless of the location.

Recently, the Center for Medicare and Medicaid Services (CMS) clarified this issue. In what it has termed the final version of EMTALA, enacted on November 10, 2003, CMS has stated that a hospital's EMTALA obligation is only triggered when a patient presents to a "dedicated ED" operated by the hospital. If a patient presents to any other area within a 250-yard radius of the hospital campus declaring or exhibiting what a prudent layperson would define as a medical emergency, that patient must be moved to a dedicated ED within the hospital to receive an appropriate medical screening examination.

Barker TR, Urbanowicz P, Joy L: Health lawyers teleconference: EMTALA update. J Health Law 37:7–40, 2004.
McDonnell WM: Will EMTALA changes leave emergency patients dying on the hospital doorstep? J Health Law 38:77–93, 2005.

7. **What is a dedicated ED?**
A hospital location is defined as a dedicated ED if it meets any one of three criteria: (1) it is licensed by the state to function as an ED, (2) it holds itself out to the public as a place providing care for emergent medical conditions on an urgent basis without requiring a previously scheduled appointment, or (3) if a representative sample of its patient population seen over the

previous year demonstrated that at least one third of all outpatient visits were for urgent patient complaints that did not require a previously scheduled appointment.

Kamoie B: EMTALA: Dedicating an ED near you. J Health Law 37:41–79, 2004.

8. **Is a hospital still obligated under EMTALA to medically screen and stabilize any patient presenting to an ambulance it owns and operates?**
No. Hospital-run ambulance services are now exempt from EMTALA if they operate under community-wide EMS protocols or EMS protocols mandated by state law that direct the ambulance to transport patients to the closest appropriate facility.

Peth HA: The Emergency Medical Treatment and Active Labor Act (EMTALA): Guidelines for compliance. Emerg Med Clin North Am 22:225–240, 2004.

9. **How does EMTALA define a proper MSE?**
The simple answer: the adequate screening of a patient for an emergency medical condition using the resources normally available to the hospital's ED. The complex reality is that those resources are stated to include any laboratory studies; radiologic examinations such as computed tomography (CT), magnetic resonance imaging (MRI), or angiography; and the services of any on-call consultant normally available to the dedicated ED. Consequently, an adequate MSE can range from a quick history and physical to confirm the presence of an upper respiratory tract infection to a complex work-up involving multiple tests, diagnostic procedures, consultations from specialists, and hospital admission for further evaluation and treatment.

10. **Who can perform the MSE?**
EMTALA states simply that "qualified medical personnel" must perform the MSE. The statute does not specify whether that means a physician, a nurse, or some other provider such as a physician's assistant or a nurse-practitioner. Instead, EMTALA allows each hospital's governing body or the director of its ED to determine who is qualified to perform screenings for the hospital. One person who clearly *cannot* perform an MSE is a triage nurse. The courts have held consistently that triage by a nurse is not adequate medical screening. Many hospitals have been cited for EMTALA violations because their triage nurses evaluated patients and then referred them to an outside clinic or a private physician's office without a formal evaluation in the ED.

Frew SA: Triage errors continue to plague California with EMTALA citations. Transfer News 7:1–2, 2003.

11. **When has the MSE been satisfactorily completed under EMTALA?**
When a physician or medical care provider designated by the hospital to provide an MSE can document in good faith that no emergency medical condition exists, the patient has been "stabilized," and EMTALA no longer applies. If a dedicated ED initiates a MSE, stabilizes a patient to the best of its ability, and then appropriately transfers that patient to another facility in the manner described later, the EMTALA obligation is fulfilled. Lastly, according to the 2003 final version, EMTALA ceases to apply once a patient has been admitted to the hospital. Importantly, that cessation applies to patients formally admitted to the hospital but who may be housed in an ED awaiting an inpatient bed.

Barker TR, Urbanowicz P, Joy L: Health lawyers teleconference: EMTALA update. J Health Law 37:7–40, 2004.

12. **Is it an EMTALA violation if the patient decides to leave against medical advice before the MSE is complete?**
That depends on when during the triage and evaluation process the patient decides to refuse care and on his or her competency to do so. If, during the course of the MSE, a patient refuses further evaluation and treatment after discussion of the potential risks of such a decision, the patient is considered to have withdrawn the initial request for evaluation, and EMTALA no longer applies. The burden of proof falls on the hospital and the treating physician, however, to show

that no coercion was used to dissuade the patient from consenting to further treatment with suggestions or statements that the continued care could be prohibitively expensive. Proper charting and documentation in such situations are essential. A more difficult situation arises when a patient is triaged to the waiting room and then decides to leave before being formally evaluated in the ED. On the surface, this situation can be interpreted as the patient withdrawing the initial request for medical evaluation. EMTALA and the courts have focused considerable attention on the potential for inequity in triage practices, with the uninsured or undesirable patient being subjected to long waiting times in the hopes that he or she will simply leave. In such situations, the hospital must be able to prove that no different standard of triage was used and that a reasonable effort was made to call the patient back to the ED to address the initial complaint.

Correa v. Hospital San Francisco, 69 F.3d 1184 (1st) Cir. 1995), *cert. denied*, 116 S. Ct. 1423, 517 U.S. 1136, 134 L.Ed. 2d 547.

13. **What is meant by "transfer" under EMTALA?**
EMTALA does not simply deal with patient transfers and the transferring facilities. EMTALA defines *transfer* as the movement of a patient away from the hospital, not simply as the act of transporting a patient to another hospital. By this definition, even a patient sent home from the ED is considered to have been transferred under the statute. If such a patient is subsequently found to have been discharged in unstable condition, claim of an EMTALA violation could be made.

14. **When does EMTALA say it's OK to transfer a patient?**
EMTALA applies only to the transfer of unstable patients. If a patient is deemed stable (i.e., an emergency medical condition is no longer present, and no significant medical deterioration is likely during or after the transfer), a transfer can proceed without the statute being applicable. Unstable patients can be transferred under one of three conditions.
1. The patient requests the transfer. In that case, an informed request for the transfer must be signed by the patient, and it is important for the hospital and the treating physician to document that a discussion of cost did not enter into the patient's decision to ask for a transfer.
2. An unstable patient needs to be moved because the initial facility lacks the capability or the resources to treat the emergent condition adequately. This might occur when a multitrauma patient presents to a small rural ED and requires transfer to a Level I trauma center to receive proper care. Similarly, a patient with a complicated hand injury who presents to an ED with no hand specialist on call may need to be transferred to a facility capable of providing that service.
3. During a declared national emergency. The 2003 final version specifies that EMTALA penalties do not apply to an inappropriate transfer by a dedicated ED operating in a declared national disaster area.

Examination and treatment for emergency medical conditions and women in labor. 42 USC § 1395dd.
Peth HA: The Emergency Medical Treatment and Active Labor Act (EMTALA): Guidelines for compliance. Emerg Med Clin North Am 22:225–240, 2004.

15. **List the requirements for transferring an unstable patient.**
1. A physician must certify that the benefits of the transfer outweigh the risks and that when possible this has been discussed with the patient or responsible party.
2. Every effort shall be made to minimize the risk involved in the transfer in terms of proper treatment before the patient's departure.
3. The receiving facility has accepted the patient and has the capability to treat the emergency medical condition.
4. The receiving facility has been provided with all pertinent records of the patient's care to the point of transfer.
5. The transfer is conducted with proper equipment and personnel.

KEY POINTS: CONDITIONS THAT ALLOW TRANSFER OF AN UNSTABLE PATIENT UNDER EMTALA

1. The patient requests transfer.

2. The transferring facility lacks the resources to stabilize the patient adequately.

3. The transfer occurs during a declared national emergency.

16. **Can an on-call consultant refuse to see an unstable patient?**

    No. If an on-call physician fails or refuses to respond or come to the hospital in a timely fashion (i.e., within a reasonable time under the circumstances or within the time frame established by the hospital's medical staff bylaws), the hospital and the on-call physician may be in violation of EMTALA. The emergency physician must decide what time frame is reasonable under the circumstances. In that situation, the emergency physician may transfer the unstable patient to a facility with the capability of treating the emergent medical condition without personally violating EMTALA, but the emergency physician must document the name and address of the consultant who failed to treat the patient on the transfer form.

    McHugh FM: The new EMTALA regulations and the on-call physician shortage: In defense of the regulations. J Health Law 37:61–84, 2004.

17. **How is the hospital's on-call list determined?**

    The 2003 final version of EMTALA allows hospitals considerable discretion in determining their on-call lists "in a manner that best meets the needs of the hospital's patients" and in accordance with the hospital's capability and the availability of on-call physicians. The policies and procedures must be determined in advance and must be well documented.

18. **Can a hospital refuse to accept a transfer under EMTALA?**

    A receiving hospital cannot refuse an appropriate transfer if they have the capability to treat the patient.

19. **If I receive an inappropriate transfer at my hospital, do I have an obligation to report an EMTALA violation?**

    EMTALA states that any hospital that receives an inappropriate transfer must report the suspected EMTALA violation within 72 hours or face penalties. This is, however, an obligation of the hospital, not of an individual physician.

20. **What is JCAHO?**

    The Joint Commission on Accreditation of Healthcare Organizations. Its origins date to 1917, when the American College of Surgeons (ACS) published its *Minimum Standards for Hospitals* in an effort to establish basic national standards to be met by every hospital operating in the United States. Over the ensuing decades, the ACS assumed responsibility for conducting site visits at hospitals throughout the country to enforce those minimum standards. In 1951, the Joint Commission on Accreditation of Hospitals (JCAH) arose as a nonprofit, nongovernmental institution dedicated to further defining a set of standards recommended as essential to the safe and effective delivery of health care by hospitals throughout the nation. In 1952, the ACS transferred its Hospital Standardization Program to JCAH. In 1965, Congress empowered JCAH substantially by linking each hospital's eligibility to participate in the newly created Medicare program with accreditation by JCAH. As the scope of JCAH expanded to include accreditation of such nonhospital entities as clinical laboratories, home health care networks, and managed care organizations, the organization changed its title in 1987 to the Joint Commission on Accreditation of Healthcare Organizations (JCAHO). Currently, JCAHO accredits and certifies more than 15,000 health care organizations and programs.

A journey through the history of the Joint Commission: http://www.jcaho.org/about+us/history.htm

21. What sort of standards does JCAHO set?

JCAHO maintains its *Accreditation Manual for Hospitals* with the declared aim of promoting appropriate medical care, protecting patient safety, and fostering performance improvement within health care organizations. The manual itself is divided into 11 chapters detailing minimum acceptable standards in such areas as patient care, infection control and prevention, information management, human resources management, and patient/family education. In 2002, JCAHO announced its *Shared Visions: New Pathways* initiative designed to replace simple compliance with published standards with a more dynamic emphasis on identifying and disseminating new ways to enhance patient safety and prevent adverse patient outcomes. Examples of this new focus include improving accuracy in identifying patients prior to the performance of procedures or the administration of medications, enhancing the safety and effectiveness of medical equipment such as infusion pumps and monitor alarms, minimizing health care workers' risk of acquiring infections, and identifying high-risk medications that require special education and training on the part of administering health care personnel. The Sentinel Event Policy mandates that institutions report adverse patient events and document corrective measures initiated to prevent their recurrence.

Facts about Shared Visions: New Pathways: www.jcaho.org/accredited+organizations/svnp/svnp+facts. htm

22. How are JCAHO standards enforced?

Every Medicare-participating organization must pass an on-site JCAHO survey every 3 years to maintain its accreditation. Beginning in 2006, these surveys will be random and unannounced for all organizations. JCAHO surveyors review documentation of each organization's compliance with accreditation standards and utilize a "tracer methodology" that tracks and evaluates the care provided to selected patients over the course of their encounter with the organization. Chart audits, as well as interviews with randomly selected staff members, are central features of this component of the site survey.

23. How do JCAHO requirements influence the practice of emergency medicine?

Many of the hospital-wide standards set by JCAHO apply to patient care and administration within the ED. JCAHO requires detailed documentation of such ED activities as the application and monitoring of patient restraints; medication and laboratory test ordering; conscious sedation administration and monitoring; and staff training with regard to patient safety, best-practice identification, and bioterrorism preparedness. In January 2005, JCAHO enacted a new Leadership Standard titled "Managing Patient Flow." This new standard is intended to spark initiatives within hospitals to alleviate ED overcrowding and mitigate the unsafe practice of housing admitted patients in the ED as they wait long hours for the assignment of an inpatient bed. The standard requires hospital administrators to document their efforts to study and alleviate patient flow problems within their institution. Its impact on ED overcrowding remains to be seen.

JCR publishes solutions to hospital overcrowding. JCR News Releases: www.jcaho.org/new+room/ jcr+news+releases/jcr_011005.htm

KEY POINTS: JCAHO POINTS OF INTEREST ESPECIALLY PERTINENT IN THE ED

1. Monitoring patient restraints

2. Conscious sedation administration and monitoring

3. Ordering of medications and diagnostic studies

4. Staff training in safety, best practices, and bioterrorism preparedness

5. ED overcrowding

24. **What is HIPAA?**

The **H**ealth **I**nsurance **P**ortability and **A**ccountability **A**ct. Enacted by Congress in 1996, HIPAA was designed to protect individuals from the unauthorized or inappropriate use of their personal health information. The act's privacy regulations went into full force on April 14, 2004. HIPAA applies to any health care entity (HCE), public or private, that creates, stores, or transmits health information pertaining to specific individuals. This includes information in oral, written, or electronic form. HIPAA not only details when and how personal health data may be accessed and shared but also delineates standard transaction formats and data code sets that must be used in transferring such information.

Public Law 104-191. August 21, 1996. Health Insurance Portability and Accountability Act.

25. **What prompted the enactment of such a statute?**

Patient privacy and the confidentiality of the physician–patient relationship have been recognized as fundamental ethical and moral obligations in medicine since the time of Hippocrates. With the rise of informatics and the evolution of medical care, individual patient information is now often shared among numerous practitioners, quality assurance auditors, billing coders, and third-party payers. As a result, the potential for unauthorized or inappropriate access to patients' personal information has escalated exponentially. HIPAA is intended to delineate the manner in which personal health data can be accessed, by whom, and for what reason.

Martinez JA: Regulatory issues. In Harwood-Nuss A (ed): The Clinical Practice of Emergency Medicine, 4th ed. Philadelphia, Lippincott Williams & Wilkins, 2005, pp 1818–1822.

26. **What is protected health information (PHI)?**

PHI is all information pertaining to an individual's medical or psychiatric status, treatment, or payment for health-related services. PHI is linked to specific patients by individually identifiable health information, which HIPAA defines as the person's name; specific contact information; place of residence by geographic subdivision smaller than the state; social security, medical record, or specific account numbers; photographs; biometric identifiers such as finger prints or voice recognition; or any other unique identifier characteristic or code.

27. **What is the difference between the use and the disclosure of PHI?**

HIPAA defines use of PHI as the sharing, employment, application, utilization, examination, or analysis of PHI within the HCE that maintains the PHI. In general, use of PHI within the HCE for treatment, payment, and normal health care operations without the individual's consent is permissible under HIPAA. The sharing of PHI among physicians, nurses, or other health care providers involved in the direct care of a patient is considered use and is not restricted under HIPAA. Disclosure is the release of PHI to entities outside of the HCE, such as the press, law enforcement, or marketers. PHI disclosure is much more restricted under HIPAA.

28. According to HIPAA, when is it okay to disclose PHI?

PHI may be disclosed under the following circumstances: with the individual's written consent; for certain judicial, law enforcement, or public health purposes such as the reporting of a communicable disease; for workers' compensation claims; and in matters of national defense and security.

29. How is the statute enforced, and what are the penalties for a HIPAA violation?

The Office of Civil Rights oversees enforcement of HIPAA privacy standards. Individuals may lodge HIPAA grievances with the HCE or the federal government. Penalties for an established violation include potential monetary fines and jail sentences for the offender(s). Inadvertent violations carry a $100 fine, not to exceed $25,000 per year. If the violation occurred with the knowledge of the offender, punishment can include fines up to $50,000 and up to 1 year in prison. If the violation was committed knowingly and with false pretenses, potential penalties include fines up to $100,000 and a maximum of 5 years in prison. Violation with the intent to sell or profit from PHI disclosure carries a fine of up to $250,000 and up to 10 years in prison.

30. What steps should be taken to prevent disclosure of PHI in the ED?

Maintaining patient privacy is problematic in a busy, crowded ED. Patients and visitors often overhear discussions pertaining to individuals unknown to them in the normal operation of the department. Such inadvertent disclosures are permissible under HIPAA, provided that the department has taken steps in good faith to minimize the likelihood of their occurrence. Examples of such measures include conducting patient interviews and examinations in individual examining rooms when possible; posting signs reminding staff members of the importance of maintaining patient privacy; removing easily identifiable patient information on chalk boards, computer screens, and x-ray view boxes from open view; and documenting staff training with regard to HIPAA issues.

KEY POINTS: BASIC HIPAA COMPLIANCE IN THE ED

1. Perform interviews and examinations in private areas whenever possible.

2. Remove patient identifiers from highly visible areas.

3. Document staff training with regard to HIPAA requirements.

MEDICAL OVERSIGHT AND DISASTER MANAGEMENT

Daniel W. Spaite, MD, and Elizabeth A. Criss, RN, MEd, CEN

1. **What is medical oversight?**

   This is the means by which physicians give direction and authority to nonphysicians to provide emergency medical care outside of the hospital and without a physician being present. Medical oversight can be provided either via the radio/phone or through written protocols or guidelines. Before organized emergency medical services (EMS), ill and injured patients were cared for and transported by personnel who had little more than basic first-aid training. There was essentially no physician input regarding training, scope of practice, or quality of care provided by prehospital personnel. The first standardized EMS curriculum, in 1976, required increased physician involvement in education, skill acquisition, and a requirement to provide medical oversight of prehospital personnel.

2. **Why is medical oversight of prehospital personnel and care important?**

   The importance of medical oversight lies in the concept that nonphysicians with appropriate education and training can provide advanced-level medical care safely and effectively. However, the safety and efficiency are a direct reflection of the quality of medical oversight and the relationship between providers and medical director.

3. **How is medical oversight provided?**

   It can be provided through radio or telephone communications with a physician or designee during patient contact, typically called direct medical oversight. It can also be provided through the use of physician-developed treatment protocols or standing orders (indirect medical oversight). The percentage of EMS calls that use direct, on-line medical oversight varies widely among EMS systems. Some rely heavily on standing orders and require little direct contact during patient encounters, whereas others require direct contact during each patient encounter.

KEY POINTS: COMPONENTS OF MEDICAL OVERSIGHT ✓

1. Includes components of both direct and indirect medical oversight

2. Direct involvement by the medical director in initial education, continuing education, research, and protocol development

3. Development of a quality improvement program with participation by all agencies and provider levels

4. **How important is physician involvement in education and training for prehospital personnel?**

   Physician involvement in the development of educational programs and the delivery of training provides an opportunity to interact with and provide guidance to the personnel who may be operating under his or her license. Having personal knowledge of the skill level of the prehospital providers develops a level of trust in their ability to assess and respond appropriately to most situations they encounter.

5. **Define the term *disaster*.**
A disaster is best described as an imbalance between needs and resources. It is not defined by the size of the event but rather by the community's ability to respond. It might be easy to see how a bleacher section collapse with 200 people injured is a disaster in any community; even the best resources will be quickly overwhelmed by the need. But consider the impact a one-vehicle roll over with five critical patients might have on the limited resources of a rural community. The area may have only one ambulance, a very small number of prehospital personnel with advanced skills, and no local hospital, which will necessitate that the ambulance and EMS personnel leave their area for a transport, stripping the community of all of the EMS resources. The similarity between these two is the extent to which the incident outstripped the available resources in the area.

6. **Why is there a need for disaster planning?**
The quality of medical care in general is tied directly to the experience of the practitioner. Proficiency of a given medical intervention depends on the frequent performance of that intervention. In a disaster, people are trying to do quickly what they do not ordinarily do, often in an unfamiliar environment, therefore it makes sense to plan and exercise the contingencies regularly. No matter how experienced someone is, the level of care, resources, and framework for resource management undergo major alterations during a disaster.

7. **Define the all-hazards approach to disaster planning.**
To have the right contingencies in place, it is essential to know what the potential hazards are in the area and the threat they pose. In an all-hazards approach, a review is done, usually yearly, on the natural, man-made, and technologic events that could happen in the area. Each event is ranked by likelihood and then by the extent of the impact it would have on the ability to provide patient care. Based on ranking an agency, hospital, or community can begin to develop emergency plans to deal with the most likely events, while also being aware of the potential for other events.

8. **What is an incident command system (ICS)?**
An ICS is a standardized structure that provides command and control of personnel and resources at a disaster or multiagency scene. An ICS begins with an incident commander and then, depending on the size of the incident, can be easily expanded to involve additional positions for logistics, planning, medical care, and finance. Using an ICS improves the ability of multiple agencies to work together because they are using common terminology and position descriptions. The National Incident Management System (NIMS) standardizes the ICS structure to be used by EMS agencies, fire departments, law enforcement, and hospitals in an effort to enhance response coordination at all levels and for all types of incidents (Fig. 105-1).

KEY POINTS: ROLE OF INCIDENT COMMAND SYSTEM

1. It provides a standardized structure that improves communications between organizations working a disaster, or the disaster site and a hospital.

2. An ICS is very flexible, allowing the incident commander to expand or contract the positions in the structure to meet the needs of the disaster.

3. The system helps the incident commander and other chief officers by limiting the span of control (number of subordinates) to no more than seven before more positions must be established.

4. The standardized naming and color-coding of each position assist arriving personnel with identification.

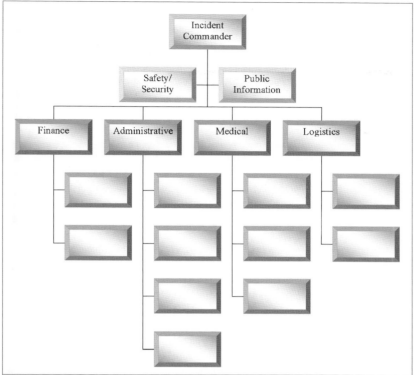

Figure 105-1. Typical incident command structure showing incident commander and components of the command section, the four main section chiefs, and potential further subdivisions.

9. **Is an ICS a requirement?**

Yes and no. For incidents involving a single agency, there is no mandate to utilize an ICS; however, it does provide structure in the face of chaos. For incidents involving multiple local agencies or any federal resources, an ICS is mandated. The NIMS mandates when the ICS structure is to be used. It also standardizes the position descriptions that will be used by EMS agencies, fire departments, law enforcement agencies, and hospitals. NIMS is a direct result of some of the communication and coordination issues that arose from September 11, 2001.

10. **How does triage occur at a scene?**

Triage means "to sort." Napoleon's surgeon is thought to be the first physician to use triage on a battlefield to sort out soldiers who could be treated in a near by hospital and returned to duty. Although several systems exist for triaging victims of multicasualty incidents, the basic concept generally identifies four groups of patients: (1) minor illness or injury (walking wounded), (2) serious but not immediately life-threatening illness or injury (e.g., an intra-abdominal injury or fractured femur not in shock), (3) critical or immediately life-threatening illness or injury (tension pneumothorax, hypovolemic shock), and (4) dead or resource-intensive victims. The most common triage system currently in use is Simple Triage and Rapid Transport (START). As with any triage system, colors help rescuers identify the order in which patients will receive care: red is immediate or life threatening; yellow is delayed or serious but not yet life threatening; green is for walking wounded, and black for resource-intensive victims or the dead.

11. **What makes START so unique?**

START, developed by the Newport Beach, California Fire Department and Hoag Hospital in 1983 and revised in 1994, is designed to triage a patient in 30 seconds. The triage officer evaluates respiratory rate, presence or absence of a radial pulse, and mental status. Depending on these findings, the patient is categorized as dead/dying, immediate, delayed, or minor (Table 105-1). For patients with a pulse but absent breathing, the triage officer provides basic airway maneuver and inserts an oropharyngeal airway (OPA); if the patient initiates spontaneous breathing, his or her status is upgraded to immediate. This sort of rapid assessment allows for maximum use of the limited resources that are usually available at a disaster scene.

TABLE 105-1. START TRIAGE		
Dead/Dying BLACK	Respirations: absent Perform headtilt and inset OPA; if unable to maintain airway even with help of OPA, then they meet this criterion	These patients must be re-evaluated as soon as possible to detect anyone who might be salvageable.
Immediate RED	Respirations: >30 *or* Perfusion: radial pulse not present *or* Mental status: unable to follow simple commands	One or more of these indicators present on initial assessment
Delayed YELLOW	Respirations: < 30 *or* Perfusion: radial pulse present *or* Mental status: able to follow simple commands Unable to ambulate without assistance	Must be relatively stable as defined by specific criteria
Minor GREEN	All three parameters within normal limits; able to ambulate to a designated location without assistance	Infants are included as minor if they respond appropriately for age.

OPA = oropharyngeal airway.

WEBSITE

For more information about the National Incident Management System, including educational opportunities: http://www.fema.gov/nims

BIBLIOGRAPHY

1. Alonso-Serra H, Blanton D, O'Connor RE: Physician Medical Direction in EMS. National Association of EMS Physicians Position Paper. Prehosp Emerg Care 2:153–157, 1998.

2. Auf der Heide E (ed): Community Medical Disaster Planning and Evaluation Guide. American College of Emergency Physicians, Dallas, 1995.

3. Augustine JJ: Medical direction and EMS. Emerg Med Serv 30(5):65–69, 2001.

4. Kuehl AK (ed): Prehospital Systems and Medical Oversight, 3rd ed. National Association of EMS Physicians: Kendall Hunt Publishing, Dubuque, IA, 2002.

5. Brennan JA, Krohmer JR (eds): Principles of EMS Systems, ed 3. Jones and Bartlett Publishers, Sudbury, MA, 2006.

6. Sobo EK, Andriese S, Stroup C, et al: Developing indicators for emergency medical services (EMS) system evaluation and quality improvement: A statewide demonstration project. Jt Comm J Qual Improve 27(3):138–154, 2001.

7. Stewart RD: Prehospital care: Education, evaluation, and medical control. Top Emerg Med 2:67–82, 1980.

8. Stone RM, Seaman KG, Bissell RA: A statewide study of EMS oversight: Medical director characteristics and involvement compared with national guidelines. Prehosp Emerg Care 4:345–351, 2000.

9. Storer DL, Dickinson ET, ACEP, et al: Physician Medical Direction of EMS Education Programs: Policy Resource and Education Paper. Prehosp Emerg Care 2:158–159, 1998.

CHAPTER 106

MEDICAL CARE AT MASS GATHERINGS

Peter T. Pons, MD

1. What constitutes a mass gathering?

Any event or occurrence that draws large numbers of spectators or participants.

2. Why is on-site medical care needed at mass gatherings?

Any time a large number of people is gathered together in one place, it is likely that there will be some medical emergencies. One can expect the full gamut of potential problems, from minor injuries to life-threatening emergencies such as cardiac arrest. A mass gathering essentially creates a small community or city, all in one location for a short period of time, needing its own emergency medical services (EMS) system to handle medical emergencies while the event is occurring. If no on-site medical care is provided, any medical emergency has to be handled by the local EMS system. Responding to calls for medical assistance at a special event or mass gathering can overburden the local EMS system and interfere with its handling of the normal daily EMS response.

3. What factors affect how much medical care needs to be provided at a mass gathering?

Many factors must be analyzed to determine the level of care to be provided, the type and number of medical personnel, and the amount of equipment and supplies: the type of event, the nature of the event venue, the location of the venue, and the number and characteristics of the attendees. Each of these factors influences the likelihood of and the potential for medical emergencies.

Arbon P, Bridgewate FH, Smith C: Mass gathering medicine: A predictive model for patient presentation and transport rates. Prehosp Disaster Med 16:150–158, 2001.

Milsten AM, Maguire BJ, Bissell RA, Seaman KG: Mass-gathering medical care: A review of the literature. Prehosp Disaster Med 17:151–162, 2002.

KEY POINTS: FACTORS THAT INCREASE STAFFING NEEDS AT MASS GATHERINGS

1. Outdoor event

2. Heat and humidity

3. Alcohol and drugs

4. Type of event: concert, sporting event

4. How does the type of event affect medical staffing?

Let's start by using a concert as an example. A classical music concert would attract a different audience than an event featuring a heavy-metal hard-rock group. There is a much greater potential for one or more medical emergencies to occur at the latter compared with the former.

This is true for many types of events. At sporting events, a fan might be struck by a ball at a baseball game, possibly injured by an out-of-control vehicle at an automobile race, or potentially involved in a major riot at a soccer game.

Milsten AM, Seaman KG, Liu P, et al: Variables influencing medical usage rates, injury patterns, and levels of care for mass gatherings. Prehosp Disaster Med 18:334–346, 2003.

5. **Does the event venue have any impact on planning for medical staffing?**
   Indoor events usually are seated events occurring in a climate-controlled environment. **Outdoor events** often expose participants to temperature extremes, and some events such as fairs involve walking about over various types of terrain. There are usually more medical problems at an outdoor event than at an indoor event. Heat exposure is a particularly significant risk factor to bear in mind when planning medical coverage at an outdoor event. More persons require medical attention if the ambient temperature is increased.
   Location is an important consideration. If the event is located at a site that is far from hospital facilities, planners might choose to provide for a more definitive and higher level of care, such as suturing and advanced life support, because prolonged transport and delayed care are likely. The event planner might add physicians and appropriate supplies and equipment to meet anticipated needs. Conversely, if the event is located in close proximity to a hospital, event planners may choose not to offer physician-level services but instead may rely on transport to a nearby medical facility.

Grange JT, Baumann GW, Vaezazizi R: On-site physicians reduce ambulance transports at mass gatherings. Prehosp Emerg Care 7:322–326, 2003.

Lukins JL, Feldman MJ, Summers JA, Verbeek PR: A paramedic-staffed medical rehydration unit at a mass gathering. Prehosp Emerg Care 8:411–416, 2004.

6. **Are there any other factors that affect the planned medical staffing?**
   It is important to ascertain whether alcoholic beverages will be served at the event or if there is a strong likelihood of drug or alcohol use by the event participants. Alcohol and drug use significantly increases the medical contact rate at an event.

7. **After analyzing these factors, are there any guidelines or suggested staffing levels?**
   A good place to start is anticipated attendance. For every 25,000 attendees, two paramedics should be assigned. If physician staffing is included, one physician per 25,000 attendees should suffice. If the event is something like an outdoor, all-day rock music festival in August and drug or alcohol use is anticipated, the number of medical personnel is increased from this starting point. If the event is a classical music performance in a concert hall, the number of medical staffers may be decreased. Other issues that affect medical staffing include the number and location of medical aid stations and the need for on-site medical response capability. Medical aid stations should be centrally located and always should be staffed by medical providers during event hours. Provision of on-site EMS response personnel also has an impact on staffing and equipment requirements. Bicycles or stretcher-equipped golf carts can be used in many venues and for many events. Ambulance vehicles may be needed for events involving large geographic areas, such as marathons. The mix of personnel needed to staff a mass gathering can often reflect routine EMS-emergency medical technicians (EMTs) and paramedics for on-site EMS, nurses to staff aid stations, and physicians to provide on-site definitive care and medical control.

Feldman MJ, Lukins JL, Verbeek RP, et al: Half-a-million strong: The emergency medical services response to a single-day, mass-gathering event. Prehosp Disaster Med 19:287–296, 2004.

8. **What should be done about on-site communications and medical system activation?**
   Because the planning effort should be creating a mini EMS system, communication is an integral component. A command post or communications center should be created with a

representative from all appropriate venue services, such as police or security, fire control, and EMS. All on-site employees or ushers should be educated in how to access or request medical assistance. Each on-site service should have a communications or radio system that is dedicated for that purpose and does not accommodate multiple purposes on the same frequency. The medical service should ensure a mechanism to obtain medical control and direction as warranted.

9. **How is patient transport, when necessary, accomplished?**
Ideally, there would be an ambulance and crew stationed at the venue with the primary purpose being patient transport. This increases the cost of providing on-site medical care. In some cases, the local EMS system is used to perform the transport after the on-site medical personnel have evaluated the patient and determined the need for transport to a hospital. If long-distance transport is involved because the event venue is located some distance from a hospital, consideration for helicopter use is appropriate.

10. **Okay, so who pays for all the medical services?**
There is no one answer. In some cases, the cost of on-site medical care is built into a venue contract and is considered an event expense by the promoter. In some cases, medical care is part of the annual venue budget. Sometimes, the cost is borne by the medical personnel provider, who then bills patients for medical services; and in some situations, the cost is covered entirely by the provider.

11. **Are there any other important considerations?**
One must also take into account security arrangements and the potential for a terrorist attack. Part of the overall analysis of an event is to determine the risk of the event being a terrorist target. A junior high school football game is likely not a target; however, a high-profile event with television coverage and participants from around the world might be an inviting target. In this case, additional contingency plans should be in place to ensure an appropriate medical and disaster response if a terrorist act involving large numbers of people should occur.

INDEX

Page numbers in **boldface type** indicate complete chapters.